Current Endourology

Senol Tonyali • Evangelos N. Liatsikos
İlker Seckiner • Ates Kadioglu
Editors

Current Endourology

Springer

Editors
Senol Tonyali
Department of Urology
Istanbul University Istanbul School of Medicine
Istanbul, Türkiye

Evangelos N. Liatsikos
Department of Urology
General University Hospital of Patras
Patras, Greece

İlker Seckiner
Department of Urology
Gaziantep University School of Medicine
Gaziantep, Türkiye

Ates Kadioglu
Division of Andrology, Department of Urology
Istanbul University Istanbul School of Medicine
Istanbul, Türkiye

ISBN 978-3-032-00009-5 ISBN 978-3-032-00010-1 (eBook)
https://doi.org/10.1007/978-3-032-00010-1

This Springer imprint is published by the registered company Springer Nature Switzerland AG
The registered company address is: Gewerbestrasse 11, 6330 Cham, Switzerland

Contents

Chapter 1
Techniques of Percutaneous Renal Access

Yusuf Ozlulerden and İlker Seckiner

Percutaneous Nephrolithotomy (PNL) is the preferred treatment method for kidney stones larger than 2 cm, multiple kidney stones, and staghorn kidney stones, as well as for kidney stones smaller than 2 cm where Extracorporeal Shock Wave Lithotripsy (ESWL) and retrograde intrarenal surgery are not suitable or successful [1]. In the 1950s, after percutaneous needle aspiration treatment experiences and antegrade pyelography applications in hydronephrosis kidneys were presented, percutaneous kidney interventions began to become widespread [2]. PNL in the treatment of kidney stones was first described by Fernström and Johansson in 1976 [3]. The first series consisting of five patients was published and the first description of PNL in the prone position was made.

The standard patient position in PNL is the prone position. However, prone-flexed, supine, supine-oblique, and modified lateral positions with legs apart have been described [4–7]. The prone position provides an advantage both during entry into the kidney and during operation after entering the kidney, by providing a wide area. Despite these advantages, the prone position also has disadvantages. It can cause respiratory problems, possible eye, spinal and peripheral nerve problems and circulatory problems. In addition, in the first stage of PNL, a ureteral catheter with two open ends is placed on the patient in the supine position, and then the anesthetized patient is turned into the prone position. This not only wastes time but also requires excessive effort. In order to eliminate all these disadvantages and at the same time to perform retrograde interventions via the ureteral route, PNL in the supine position has become widespread in the last 10 years. Despite its advantages, PNL in the supine position causes a more lateral access and provides a narrower

Y. Ozlulerden
Pamukkale University Faculty of Medicine, Department of Urology, Denizli, Turkey

İ. Seckiner (✉)
Department of Urology, Gaziantep University School of Medicine, Gaziantep, Türkiye

S. Tonyali et al. (eds.), *Current Endourology*,
https://doi.org/10.1007/978-3-032-00010-1_1

working area. European urology guidelines report that although both positions have advantages, complication and success rates are similar.

One of the first and most important steps of PNL surgery after positioning is to perform the entry procedure from the right place and in an appropriate manner. The most appropriate calyx should be selected to reach the stone. When making this choice, it is important to have a calyx that will allow access to the stone in the shortest distance and allow all stones to be cleaned. In pre-procedural patient planning, calyx selection can be planned by observing both the surrounding organ structures and kidney anatomy with radiological imaging methods, preferably CT scan. It can also be re-evaluated with retrograde pyelography before entry during the procedure. If possible, choosing the posterior and lower calyces reduces the risk of vascular injury. In addition, access through dilated calyces increases the success rate.

Percutaneous Nephrolithotomy Preoperative Patient Preparation

Routine laboratory tests should be performed, including complete blood count, kidney and liver function tests, electrolytes, complete urinalysis, and coagulation profile. If there is any bleeding diathesis, it should be corrected before surgery. It should be noted that one of the absolute contraindications for PNL is an uncorrected coagulopathy. Antiplatelet or anticoagulant drugs should be discontinued before elective PNL, and treatment of risky patients should be arranged in consultation with cardiology, hematology and anesthesia.

Another contraindication is the presence of active urinary tract infection. Patients with urinary tract infection or suspected urinary tract infection should be treated with specific antibiotics according to urine culture results. PNL should be planned after a negative post-treatment urine culture is obtained.

Preoperative imaging such as Intravenous Pyelography (IVP) and Computed tomography (CT) are used to reveal the anatomical details of the kidney, which are necessary to determine the number and location of stones and also to plan the percutaneous approach. Today, the most frequently preferred imaging method is non-contrast CT. Especially with recent technological advances and the ability to obtain quality images at lower radiation doses, CT has come to the forefront. Another advantage of CT is that it better shows the relationship with neighboring organs. In clinics where the prone position is applied, performing CT scans in the prone position helps evaluate the surrounding structures and access suitability. If necessary, the use of contrast-enhanced CT is also advantageous, especially in kidneys with anomalies. If functional evaluation is required, DMSA, DTPA or MAG-3 renal scintigraphic examinations can be used in special cases.

Anesthetic Technique for Percutaneous Nephrolithotomy

Prone PNL is usually performed under general anesthesia. However, recently PNL surgeries performed under epidural, iv sedation and local anesthesia have been described [8, 9]. Care should be taken in terms of intraoperative pain palliation, especially in patients scheduled for spinal/epidural anesthesia, and it should be considered that it may be inadequate in long-term procedures. If there is no medical problem that needs to be considered for PNL, there is no problem in performing the operation in the prone position. It should not be forgotten that in obese patients, there may be cardio-respiratory problems in the prone position, as intra-abdominal pressure will increase in the prone position [6]. Furthermore, the prone position may lead to potential increases in intraocular pressure and pose risks of spinal and peripheral nerve issues, as well as circulatory difficulties. These problems are especially prominent in obese patients with respiratory and circulatory problems. In addition, in the first stage of PNL, the ureteral catheter is placed on the patient in the supine position, and then the anesthetized patient is turned into the prone position. At this time, care must be taken as it may cause intubation tube malrotation and patient injury.

Instruments and Equipment Required for Percutaneous Nephrolithotomy:

1. Entry needle (preferably 18G)
2. Guidewire (Hydrophilic-tipped, superstiff)
3. Open-ended ureteral catheter (5-6F)
4. Dilation set (Balloon, Amplatz, metal dilator, etc.)
5. Nephroscope
6. Nephrostomy tube (Reentry, Nelaton catheter, etc.)
7. C-arm fluoroscopy device, Ultrasound (USG)
8. Stone retrieval forceps
9. Stone crushers (pneumatic, ultrasonic, laser)
10. Monitor and endovision system
11. Irrigation system

The entry into the kidney can be achieved through various methods. Although conventional methods remain the most commonly used, recent technological advancements have led to a rapid increase in developments related to navigational systems. In suitable cases, PNL can be applied with the assistance of CT and magnetic resonance (MR). However, recently, ultrasound or endoscopic methods have also been employed with the aim of minimizing radiation exposure [10]. Each technique has its own specific advantages and disadvantages.

Conventional Access Techniques

Fluoroscopy Guided Access

Within conventional methods, single-plane (monoplanar) entry, two-plane (biplanar) entry, and triangulation technique are the most commonly used fluoroscopy-guided access methods. While biplanar entry is considered safer, monoplanar entry technique is widely and successfully applied in many clinics [11]. Radiological imaging methods are required during the creation of a percutaneous tract. Typically, fluoroscopy is used for this purpose.

Monoplanar Access

Single-plane entry is generally preferred by experienced endourologists. When the patient is in the prone position, the C-arm X-ray device is in a straight position (at a 90° angle). The surgeon identifies the calyx to enter. If a direct stone image is not targeted, contrast material is given through the ureteral catheter, and the calyces are identified. The needle is advanced towards the targeted calyx, creating a 30° angle with the patient from an appropriate skin area. The entering the kidney is felt, and from the movement of the needle with the fluoroscopy, it can be understood that it is inside the kidney (Fig. 1.1a). The inner sheath of the needle is removed, and it is checked whether urine comes out, or sterile fluid (physiological saline) is given through the ureteral catheter to check if it comes out of the needle. After confirming

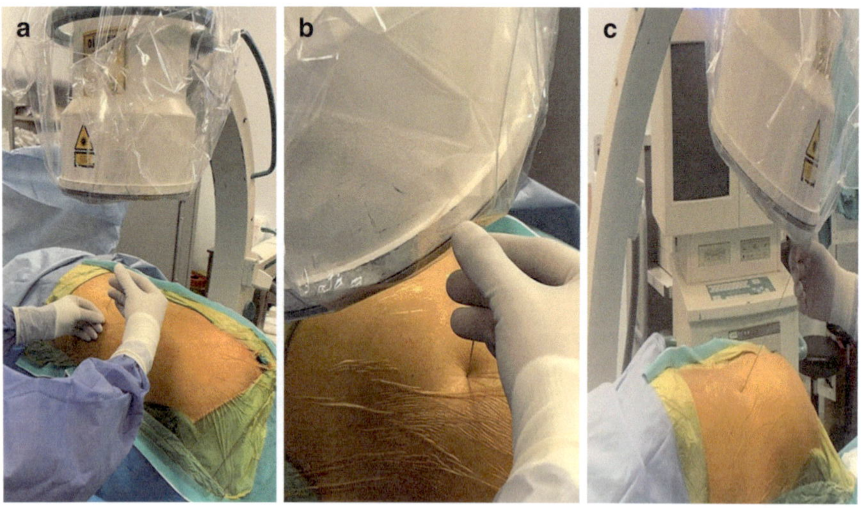

Fig. 1.1 Fluoroscopy guided access. (**a**) Monoplanar Access C-arm X-ray device is at a 90° angle. (**b**) Biplanar Access C-arm X-ray device is at a 30° angle. (**c**) Triangulation Technique C-arm X-ray device is at a 30° angle laterally and 30° angle vertically inferior

that we are inside the renal collecting system, the guidewire is advanced and placed inside the kidney. Ideally, the guidewire should be placed in the ureter, but this is not always possible.

Biplanar Access

In the two-plane entry technique, approximately 30° rotation is applied to the C-arm towards the operating surgeon. This ensures that the axis of the C-arm aligns with the same plane as the kidney, providing a direct perpendicular view of the posterior calyces. Once the calyx is identified, the skin area is marked with the aid of a clamp. After targeting the calyx to be entered, the needle is aligned with the same plane as the 30° fluoroscopy, allowing the needle to be seen as a point. This appearance on the fluoroscopy screen is referred to as the "bull's eye sign" (Fig. 1.1b). The needle is advanced in this position, and then the fluoroscopy is adjusted to 90° to determine the distance of the needle from the kidney. The needle is then appropriately placed into the kidney. After confirming that we are inside the renal collecting system, the guidewire is advanced and placed inside the kidney.

Triangulation Technique

In cases where entry into the upper calyx or intercostal entry is not preferred, one of the most commonly used techniques is triangulation. The C-arm is positioned at a perpendicular angle (90°) above the patient. While the C-arm is in this position, a clamp is used to mark the desired calyx entry point on the skin. This plane determines the medial distance of the needle entry to the desired calyx. The C-arm is then tilted 30° towards the surgeon to provide an upright view of the posterior calyx group. When the C-arm is at 30°, the skin area above the calyx is marked, more lateral to the first area. Using this point on the skin surface, the surgeon advances to 1–2 cm below the 12th rib and the third Point is marked. This third point is used for needle entry. The needle is advanced from this point to the 30° junction with the vertical plane. Thus, access to the kidney is achieved at the junction of the 3 axes (Fig. 1.1c). After it is confirmed that we are in the kidney collecting system, the guide wire is advanced and placed into the kidney.

With digital technological developments, three-dimensional fluoroscopic systems have emerged. The biggest advantage of these systems is to be able to see all dimensions of the kidney, including its depth, and thus to clearly reveal the anatomy of the calyceal system for which access is planned. In studies conducted on pigs, access to the kidney calyces with a three-dimensional fluoroscopic system was attempted and 100% success was achieved [12]. More animal studies and clinical studies are needed for the results of this technique on humans.

Needle Kiss Technique

C Arm is placed at a right angle (90°) position on the patient. While the C-arm is in this position, the calyx where entry is desired is marked. The 20G needle is advanced vertically until it enters the calyx. This plane determines the desired depth of needle entry into the calyx. Then, the C-arm is bent 30° towards the surgeon and the needle is aimed inside the calyx group and entry is made with another 18G needle. When it is observed that both needles meet at the same target, the inside of the needle is removed and when fluid is seen coming out, it is determined that it is in the right place [13] (Fig. 1.2). Afterwards, standard application continues.

Ultrasound Guided Access

The entry into the kidney under the guidance of ultrasonography (USG) can be highly successful when performed by experienced urologists (Fig. 1.3). Success rates are reported between 88% and 99%, while complication rates are reported between 4% and 8% [13, 14]. The most significant advantages of the technique of entering the kidney under USG guidance include the absence of radiation, clear understanding of the structure of tissues between the skin and kidney, and the precise location of organs around the kidney. Additionally, there is no need for contrast

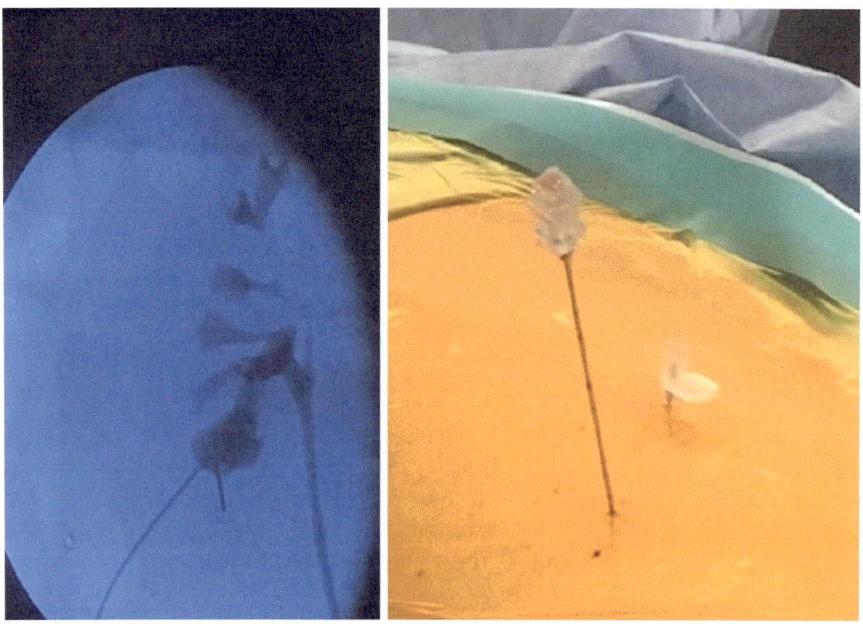

Fig. 1.2 Needle kiss technique

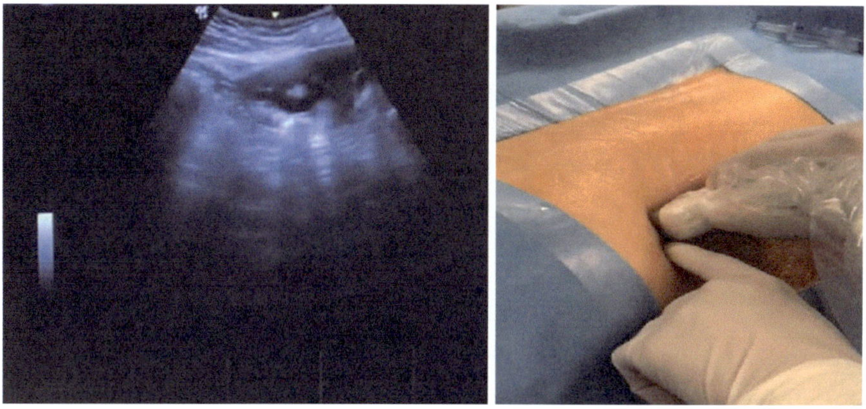

Fig. 1.3 Ultrasound guided access

material, and the use of color Doppler USG helps avoid intrarenal vascular damage. This technique can also be applied in the supine position and can provide a safe entry into the kidney, especially in pediatric patients. However, the operator's experience is crucial in determining whether the needle is inside the kidney. In addition, the ability to sonographically identify the guidewire during its placement after entering the kidney with the needle can be a challenge. At this stage, especially limited experience surgeons, may prefer for a combined approach with the assistance of fluoroscopy. This results in a significant reduction in the total radiation dose exposure.

Endoscopy Assisted Access

The origin of the process of reaching the kidney endoscopically, through the ureter, and entering the kidney by going out of the kidney with a perforating wire through the antegrade route and dilating over this wire, actually dates back to ancient times. In parallel with today's technological developments, it is easier to perform this process through flexible URS. Kawahara et al. reached the calyx to be entered in an antegrade way through flexible URS, and from there they performed PNL surgery by going out of the skin through a piercing wire and dilating retrogradely [15]. The advantages of this method are reported as less radiation exposure, less bleeding and less operation time. The most important advantage is that PNL surgery can be performed by easily entering non-dilated systems.

CT and MRI Guided Access

Another access alternative, especially for complex cases, is CT-guided access. This method can be preferred especially in those who are morbidly obese, in cases such as splenomegaly and hepatomegaly, in those with skeletal anomalies such as scoliosis and kyphosis, individuals with a history of major abdominal surgery, and those with minimal or no hydronephrosis [16]. Access with MRI is used on a very limited extent. In particular, the difficulty of seeing guidewires on MRI is a significant obstacle.

Laparoscopy Assisted Access

Laparoscopy-assisted access may be preferred in selected cases. It can be preferred especially in complex patients (retrorenal colon), location anomalies such as horseshoe kidney, ectopic kidney, and in cases accompanied by other diseases that require laparoscopy [17]. After laparoscopy, the kidney is released, the needle is advanced from a suitable point through the skin under camera vision to provide access to the kidney under direct vision, a guide wire is placed, and then the patient is placed back in the standard position and the procedure continues.

Navigation Assisted Access Techniques

Various technologies and techniques are being developed to overcome the disadvantages of ultrasound and fluoroscopy-based techniques for access to the renal collecting system. These include electromagnetic guided entry [18], iPad-assisted entry [19], real-time ultrasound guided entry and 3D CT-guided laser-assisted entry methods [16, 20]. These techniques are designed with the aim of reducing the use of fluoroscopy and minimizing major complications such as adjacent organ and large vessel injuries. However, besides the advantages of each method, it also has disadvantages such as cost and increased radiation exposure compared to conventional methods.

Robot Assisted Percutaneous Access

Robotics platforms have been experimented with for entry in PNL for a long time. Among the systems developed in this field, LARS, PAKY, and AcuBOT can be mentioned. These systems are developed to enable shorter and less trial-and-error entries compared to manual entry. However, due to the complex structures and high costs of robotic systems, they are not widely preferred.

Tips and Tricks

1. The use of 3D CT should be more prioritized in preoperative planning.
2. Supracostal access should be avoided if possible because of the high risk of thoracic complications (especially above 11th rib). Therefore, it would be useful to use triangulation technique for upper pol stones.
3. Fluoroscopy-guided percutaneous renal access is essential for successful percutaneous renal surgery. To minimize radiation exposure, entry with short shots should be preferred instead of continuous radiation.
4. The use of ultrasound is recommended to reduce radiation exposure and improve access success.
5. Endoscopy-assisted access techniques should be preferred especially in cases with complex stone burden.
6. If necessary, 2 or more entries can be safely performed. However, in cases with a high risk of bleeding, single access and combined treatment (ECIRS), use of a flexible nephroscope or staged treatment should be considered.

References

1. Ramakumar S, Segura JW. Renal calculi. Percutaneous management. Urol Clin North Am. 2000;27:617–22.
2. Casey WC, Goodwin WE. Percutaneous antegrade pyelography and hydronephrosis; direct, intrapelvic injection of urographic contrast material to secure a pyeloureterogram after percutaneous needle puncture and aspiration of hydronephrosis. J Urol. 1955;74(1):164–73.
3. Fernstrom I, Johansson B. Percutaneous pyelolithotomy. A new extraction technique. Scand J Urol Nephrol. 1976;10:257–9.
4. Honey RJ, Wiesenthal JD, Ghiculete D, Pace S, Ray AA, Pace KT. Comparison of supracostal versus infracostal percutaneous nephrolithotomy using the novel proneflexed patients position. J Endourol. 2011;25:947–54.
5. Valdivia JG, Valle J, Lopez JA, et al. Technique and complications of percutaneous nephroscopy: experience with 557 patients in the supine position. J Urol. 1998;160:1975–8.
6. Moraitis K, Philippou P, El-Husseiny T, Wazait H, Masood J, Buchholz N. Simultaneous antegrade/retrograde upper urinary tract access: Bart's modified lateral position for complex upper tract endourologic pathologic features. Urology. 2012;79:287–92.
7. Lezrek M, Ammani A, Bazine K, et al. The split-leg modified lateral position for percutaneous renal surgery and optimal retrograde access to the upper urinary tract. Urology. 2011;78:217–20.
8. Kanaroglou A, Razvi H. Percutaneous nephrolithotomy under conscious sedation in morbidly obese patients. Can J Urol. 2006;13:3153–5.
9. Cicek T, Gonulalan U, Dogan R, Kosan M, Istanbulluoglu O, Gonen M, et al. Spinal anesthesia is an efficient and safe anesthetic method for percutaneous nephrolithotomy. Urology. 2014;83:50–5.
10. Ko R, Soucy F, Denstedt JD, Razvi H. Percutaneous nephrolithotomy made easier: a practical guide, tips and tricks. BJU Int. 2008;101:535–9.
11. Hatipoglu NK, Bodakci MN, Penbegül N, et al. Monoplanar access technique for percutaneous nephrolithotomy. Urolithiasis. 2013;41(3):257–63.

12. Soria F, Delgado MI, Sanchez FM, Allona A, Jimenez Cruz JF, Morell E, et al. Effectiveness of three-dimensional fluoroscopy in percutaneous nephrostomy: an animal model study. Urology. 2009;73:649–52.
13. Perez D, Neeman BB, Dotan D, Raisin G, Chertin B, Kafka I. Ultrasound-guided percutaneous nephrolithotomy (PCNL) success rates in patients with elevated body mass index: a comparative study. Urolithiasis. 2023;51(1):111.
14. Corrales M, Doizi S, Barghouthy Y, Kamkoum H, Somani B, Traxer O. Ultrasound or fluoroscopy for percutaneous nephrolithotomy access, is there really a difference? A review of literature. J Endourol. 2021;35(3):241–8.
15. Kawahara T, Ito H, Terao H, Yoshida M, Ogawa T, Uemura H, et al. Ureteroscopy assisted retrograde nephrostomy: a new technique for percutaneous nephrolithotomy (PCNL). BJU Int. 2012;110:588–90.
16. Grüne B, Burger R, Bauer D, Schäfer A, Rothfuss A, Stallkamp J, Rassweiler J, Kriegmair MC, Rassweiler-Seyfried MC. Robotic-assisted versus manual Uro Dyna-CT-guided puncture in an *ex-vivo* kidney phantom. Minim Invasive Ther Allied Technol. 2023;4:1–7.
17. Sharma G, Jangid DK, Yadav SS, Mathur R, Tomar V. Retro-renal colon: role in percutaneous access. Urolithiasis. 2015;43:171–5.
18. Lima E, Rodrigues PL, Mota P, Carvalho N, Dias E, Correia-Pinto J, Autorino R, Vilaça JL. Ureteroscopy-assisted percutaneous kidney access made easy: first clinical experience with a novel navigation system using electromagnetic guidance (IDEAL stage 1). Eur Urol. 2017;72(4):610–6.
19. Rassweiler-Seyfried MC, Rassweiler JJ, Weiss C, Müller M, Meinzer HP, Maier-Hein L, Klein JT. iPad-assisted percutaneous nephrolithotomy (PCNL): a matched pair analysis compared to standard PCNL. World J Urol. 2020;38(2):447–53.
20. Ritter M, Rassweiler MC, Michel MS. The uro dyna-CT enables three-dimensional planned laser-guided complex punctures. Eur Urol. 2015;68(5):880–4.

Chapter 2
Transurethral Resection of Prostate

Taylan Oksay and Sefa Alperen Ozturk

Benign prostatic hyperplasia (BPH) is the most common benign neoplasm in aging men, with an incidence of 8% in the fourth decade and 90% in the ninth decade [47]. The clinical reflection of BPH, a pathological term, is that adenoma tissue enlarges and causes lower urinary tract symptoms (LUTS) after obstruction. LUTS seriously affects the quality of life in men. Treatment can be classified according to the severity of symptoms as mainly monitoring, lifestyle modifications, pharmacological agents, and surgery [22].

Transurethral resection of prostate (TUR-P) has been used for nearly a century and is a cornerstone of urological surgery. TUR-P was developed to prevent the complications associated with open prostatectomy and can be considered the first minimally invasive endoscopic surgery in the history of urology. TUR-P, which has become the gold standard treatment method in BPH surgery by technological progress in the instruments over time, still maintains its place as a reference method among other treatment options (EAU Guidelines 2023).

Over the last 30 years, the increased use of alpha-blockers, 5-alpha reductase inhibitors, phosphodiesterase type-5 inhibitors, phytotherapy, and combined treatments have shifted the first-line treatment option from TUR-P to oral medication [22, 38].

Significant decreases were observed in the number of TUR-P operations after other minimally invasive procedures were used alone or combined with oral pharmacotherapy. Wilson et al. detected a 31.6% decrease in the number of TUR-Ps performed over a ten years period [73]. A similar study compared TUR-P and prescribed oral treatments in Sweden between 1987 and 1994. While the number of operations performed decreased significantly, the authors observed that pharmacotherapy increased 15-fold [10]. According to a study conducted in the USA between the same periods, the decrease of 43% (253,000 vs. 145,000) in TUR-P operations

T. Oksay (✉) · S. A. Ozturk
Department of Urology, Suleyman Demirel University, Faculty of Medicine, Isparta, Türkiye

S. Tonyali et al. (eds.), *Current Endourology*,
https://doi.org/10.1007/978-3-032-00010-1_2

reveals that alternative treatments are being accepted worldwide. Another reason for this decrease is that minimally invasive techniques are more cost-effective than conventional TUR-P [17, 26, 30, 42, 46, 72].

Monopolar TUR-P (mTUR-P)

Comparing the first devices invented in the 1930s, modern TUR instruments have become more ergonomic with technological developments. Next-generation resectoscopes, innovations in optics and imaging instruments, diversity in the armamentarium, and significant advances in energy sources have enabled TUR to be performed more effectively and safely.

In the book published in 1634, Ambroise Pare, who thought that the voiding symptoms in men were due to bladder outlet stenosis, illustrated the blind incision method and the hardened bougie-like catheters he used in this procedure [39]. After notification that the lateral lobes of the prostate and especially the middle lobe also cause bladder outlet obstruction, various operation methods were being tried for resection in the eighteenth century. However, severe bleeding during the procedure could not be prevented. Enrico Bottini prevented bleeding during incision of the prostate and bladder neck with using a direct electric current instrument he developed. The operation was being performed blindly, which meant that the surgeon had not known which tissues were burned exactly [9]. In 1913, Hugh Hampton Young published the first cold punch resection of the prostate [75]. In this technique, after the prostate tissue was compressed into a hole at the tip of the resectoscope, a blade slid through the working canal was cut the prostate without using energy, similar to today's internal urethrotomy. Nevertheless, as with other techniques, bleeding was the biggest problem. In the following years, W.F. Braasch modified Young's technique by adding direct optical vision. However, bleeding was not prevented until the coagulation electrode was added to the resectoscope, which Thompson developed in 1935 [11]. Fenwick was cutting the prostate tissue using electrical energy in a different technique called 'galvanic écraseur '. Prostate tissue resected with the help of a wire ring coming out of the tip of the resectoscope, like tonsillectomy [25]. The disadvantages were difficulties manipulating the wire during surgery, wire carbonization caused by the energy used, and wire adhesion to the tissue. In 1926, Stern used the system produced with the diathermy technology developed by Wappler, which can be accepted as the ancestor of the loops used today [69]. In the late 1930s, this system was updated by McCarthy with a curved optical lens to provide a better vision. In the 1950s, the invention of wide-angle rod-shaped optics by Hopkins and Storz, the discovery of flexible light cables, and the improvements in working elements led to the completion of the prototypes of the systems used in TUR.

The resectoscope and its covers were made of bakelite, which can be easily broken in the past. Today they are made of steel and have insulated ceramic or plastic parts at the tips. The systems allow continuous irrigation, keep intravesical pressure constant, and improve vision during bleeding.

The resectoscopes used in the first years of TUR-P had small light bulbs at the tip to provide vision. These bulbs did not produce sufficient light and had to be replaced frequently. Then, hot light sources were invented, but they were overheated during the procedure, was putting both the surgeon and the patient in danger. Rod optics and cold light sources that Hopkins and Storz developed ushered TUR operations into a new era. While the wider angle and enlarged view increased the surgeon's ergonomics in operation, the cold light sources and cables significantly lowered costs. Residents' training was facilitated via the adaptation of modern cameras and imaging systems to optics and resectoscopes. The surgeon's neck pain caused by long-timed monocular operations and exposure to patient-contaminated irrigation fluid was prevented.

Another point that should be emphasized is the electro cauterization sources used in mTUR-P. An energy source that generates a high-frequency current is used in mTUR-P. Devices generally operate between 500–900 Ω and 100–200 W, producing nearly 400 °C temperatures on the tissues [6, 65]. The grounding cable coming from the energy source is pasted to the medial of the patient's thigh with a plate. The other line connected to the end of the cutting loop through the resectoscope. Thus, the circuit required for the electric current is completed. In other words, the patient becomes a part of the electrical circuit. Electric current flows through the patient, and the temperature increase is provided in the targeted tissue with the help of the loop. If the degree of heat reaches a sufficient level, the intracellular fluid evaporates in the tissues adjacent to the loop. The cells explode as a result of the vapor pressure formed. Thus, the loop can be moved easily within the tissue for cutting. The frequency and magnitude of the energy required for the coagulation process are less [6]. The energy source produces a continuous current for cutting and an intermittent current for coagulation [5]. One of the most critical points to be considered and kept in mind is the possibility of urethral stricture that may develop after the tissue heating due to the current flow in the part of the resectoscope inside the urethra. Stricture formation can be prevented by using lubricant gels with low electrical current conductivity before entering the urethra [6]. mTUR-P operation is a risky surgery in patients using a pacemaker. They should be carefully evaluated before operation. High-frequency current from the energy source can stop and reprogram the pacemaker, cause ventricular fibrillation, or damage the myocardium. A cardiology consultation should be requested before the procedure, and recommendations must be followed. During the procedure, the energy source should be placed as far from the pacemaker as possible and ensured that the plate was sticked to the patient. Otherwise, current may pass through the pacemaker. The patient's heart rhythm should be closely monitored [9]. In bipolar TUR era, it's not recommended to use mTUR in this patient group.

An irrigation solution is needed to provide a clear vision, wash the clot and cut tissues during the surgery. An ideal irrigation solution should be non-conductive and not affect diathermy. Solutions should be iso-osmolar to serum and have minimal side effects due to elimination upon absorption. Moreover, it should be cheap and not harm surgical instruments [14, 51]. Distilled water, glycine, mannitol, or sorbitol solutions are generally preferred for mTUR-P. Different concentrations of these solutions have been used, either hypoosmolar or iso-osmolar with serum. At first, distilled water was primarily used. However, hemolysis after absorption of distilled water from the bladder that results in acute renal failure due to hemoglobinuria caused a search for a different fluid [16].

Nesbit and Glickman recommended using 1.1% glycine solution in mTUR-P after their study in 1948 [50]. Glycine is a neutral amino acid. After absorption and metabolism of large amounts of glycine solution, hyperammonemia, nausea-vomiting, cortical edema, visual impairment, and blurred consciousness may occur during the procedure [14]. Acute renal failure and anuria may emerge due to the oxalate and hyperoxaluria produced during the glycine metabolism [19]. Excessive isoosmotic glycine solution absorption may result in hemodilution and a drop in serum sodium, hemoglobin, and albumin levels [51]. Mannitol is eliminated from the body via the kidneys. In healthy people, the half-life is 150 minutes. Although it is not harmful, excessive absorption increases extracellular volume and results in diuresis. This can lead to TUR syndrome, discussed further in the 'complications' section [51]. Sorbitol is metabolized in the liver. Excessive absorption of fructose may cause lactic acidosis in those with congenital disorders [18]. In the endoscopic treatment of symptomatic BPH, mTUR-P has become the gold standard treatment with the help of technological advancements in the process that started with Bottini [9, 22]. Although several minimally invasive techniques were used to avoid complications and undesirable side effects, mTUR-P remained on the throne. For many years, complications such as bleeding, bladder neck, and urethral strictures, restrictions in patients with pacemakers, the risk of skin burn, and the limited operation time could not be overcome.

Bipolar TUR-P (bTUR-P)

The first bipolar system used in urology practice is the plasmakinetic system produced by Gyrus (Gyrus Plasmakinetic (PK) system, Gyrus Medical Ltd., Cardiff, Wales) [67]. During the same period, various bipolar systems were developed by different manufacturers (ACMI, Olympus, Storz, Wolf) [56]. Although the working principle of these devices is the same, the bipolar current formation is different. The loop used in the Olympus device acts as an active electrode, while the resectoscope sheath forms the neutral electrode. The neutral electrode is located on the proximal portion of the ACMI device, whereas the active electrode is placed on the distal portion. In the co-axial resection system of Gyrus's plasmakinetic device, the loop is the active electrode while the passive part is at the distal end of the loop. In Storz, from two loops placed opposite each other, the upper part is the passive electrode, and the lower is the active electrode [56]. Unlike the mTUR-P, the current flows from the active electrode to the neutral electrode without traveling through the patient's body to complete the circuit.

A high voltage current is established between the electrodes when the energy source is activated by pressing the pedal. If the loop is not in contact closely with the tissue, this current is dispersed in the irrigation fluid. When the loop is brought close enough to the tissue, the current formed between the active and neutral ends transforms the NaCl solution into a vapor layer (plasma) of highly charged sodium particles. When the voltage exceeds 200 V, this plasma current can be seen as an orange color. After the loop is contacted with the tissue, fragmentation occurs due to molecular dissociation in the tissue. Carbon-carbon and carbon-nitrogen bonds are broken down in the tissue by the plasma energy, while water molecules are divided into H and OH molecules. As a result, the cell membranes in the tissue are fragmented, and a visible resection process takes place. On the other hand, much lower voltage energy (80–100 V) is required in the coagulation process than mTUR-P. NaCl, which is gasified with bipolar energy, penetrates the tissues better and provides coagulation. The temperature formed in the tissue is 40–70 °C in bTUR-P and 300–400 °C in mTURP [65]. Thus, thermal injury to surrounding tissue is minimized, and the chips remain fresher for pathological examination [56].

Indications

In most patients, a mixture of symptoms is present. In order to have a better insight about which symptoms are affecting quality of life, a thorough evaluation should be done. It is strongly recommended to use anamnesis, physical examination, and questioning forms to evaluate patients presenting to the outpatient clinic with LUTS. Urine analysis should not be skipped during the evaluation of the patient. PSA may be requested to establish a baseline value for laboratory tests if prostate cancer is suspected or believed to affect treatment choice [22]. Uroflowmetry and, if necessary, urodynamics should be performed to assess the voiding pattern. Suprapubic or transrectal USG should be performed to evaluate the prostate size and bladder capacity before surgery to plan the technique.

Surgery is required in patients who has; renal failure secondary to BPH, refractory urinary retention, recurrent urinary tract infection, bladder stones, and gross hematuria who do not respond to medical treatment and/or who prefer surgery instead of medical treatment [62]. According to the European Association of Urology (EAU) guidelines, TUR-P should be the first choice for prostates between 30 and 80 ml in volume; open prostatectomy, HoLEP, or bipolar enucleation should be the first choice for prostates larger than 80 ml [22]. Besides a tailored BPH surgical treatment should not only take into account the prostate volume, but also many other factors including possible adverse events and the patient's expectations.

Patient Preparation and Anesthesia

Oral medications should examined carefully, especially anticoagulant (AC) / anti-platelet (AP) use should be questioned in patients scheduled to undergo TUR-P. It is critical in terms of bleeding before and after surgery and the risk of developing hematomas during spinal/epidural anesthesia. The increased prevalence of cardiovascular diseases associated with aging contributes to the increased use of AC/AP. There is still no consensus regarding the timing of drug discontinuation in patients using AC/AP who needs surgery for BPH. Some surgeons prefer to discontinue AC/APs altogether, others to continue, and some prefer to switch to low molecular weight heparin (LMWH) before the procedure. The EAU guidelines recommend discontinuing the drugs five days before the procedure without any alternative AP and starting again when the risk of bleeding disappears (average of four days) in eligible patients. Postponing the surgery is recommended (1) in very high-risk patients who have had a drug-eluting stent placed in the last six months or (2) a metal stent has been placed within six weeks, and who have had a transient ischemic attack or (3) stroke in the last six months. If it cannot be postponed, performing the procedure under treatment is recommended. Delaying surgery for at least one month, if possible three months, in patients with recent thromboembolic history; and also recommends switching to LMWH before surgery in high-risk patients using warfarin [23].

According to a new meta-analysis of 13 studies involving 3767 patients, bleeding and blood transfusion rates were significantly greater in patients who received AC/AP in the perioperative period than those who did not [41]. The efficacy of bTUR-P was evaluated in patients who are/are not receiving AC/AP medication in a study from Switzerland. While acetylsalicylic acid (ASA) group results were similar to the control group, complications related to bleeding were observed more common in the clopidogrel arm. In the phenprocoumon arm, a coumadin-like drug, the findings were similar to clopidogrel. As a result of the study, it was emphasized that while acetylsalicylic acid did not affect the outcome of bTUR-P, the other two drugs increased bleeding, blood transfusion rates, and hospitalization time. However, bTUR-P could still be performed safely in these patients [61]. LMWH may prolong catheter extraction time due to hematuria [21].

In high-risk patients, discontinuation of AP/AC treatment should be discussed with the consultants. Nonsteroidal anti-inflammatory drug use should be discontinued ten days before the surgery, as it predisposes to bleeding [9].

Antibiotic prophylaxis lowers infection-related complications in patients undergoing TUR-P [59]. Trimethoprim, trimethoprim-sulfamethoxazole, second or third generation cephalosporins, and beta-lactamase inhibitor aminopenicillins are recommended for prophylaxis before TUR-P [24].

TUR-P can be performed under spinal, epidural, caudal, sacral, or general anesthesia. Usually, spinal anesthesia is preferred. Since the patient is awake under spinal anesthesia, the patient's early signs of TUR syndrome; blurred vision, temporary blindness and flashes of light, abdominal or shoulder pain developing after bladder perforation can be reported to the physician [9, 44].

The patient is placed in the dorsal lithotomy position on the operating table. Soft pads should be used to support the contact points. Metals (rings, necklaces, etc.) should be removed before performing mTUR-P. The surgical field is sterilized before the patient is covered sterile. The camera, cautery, and light cables are all sterilely linked to the resectoscope. After configuring the vision, the operation can begin.

Surgical Techniques

It is critical to apply the lubricant gel before entry from the external meatus to avoid urethral stricture formation and to ease the advancement of the obturator sheath. Patients with fossa navicularis or external meatal stenosis may require a bougie or Otis dilatation. Entry from the urethra can be done blindly with an obturator sheath or visually with a resectoscope. When using visual entry it is important to avoid urethral damage with the resectoscope sheath. The surgeon should examine the bladder and the prostatic space detailed for possible formations such as tumors, stones, diverticulums, and foreign bodies. Verumontanum, the urethral sphincter, lobes of the prostate, bladder neck, and ureteral orifices should be identified to ensure adequate orientation before resection. The appearance of the circular fibers in the bladder neck gives an opinion about the depth of resection. Simultaneously, the emergence of prostate stones and decreased vascularity indicate that the prostate capsule is close. In our experience, monopolar resection perforates the prostate capsule more easily than bipolar resection, because of the energy scattering even in coagulation. Capsule perforation exhibits a filthy yellow spongy appearance. The loop is brought closer to the tissue during resection and pulled far to near, like rowing. The loop is pulled distally at the same level as the tissue insertion depth and becomes even more superficial at the end of the pull. Contact between the hot loop and the optic or resectoscope may cause damage to the equipment.

To date, numerous TURP techniques have been defined. Various advantages and disadvantages of the techniques have been revealed. The most widely accepted techniques used in practice can be summarized as follows;

Barnes Technique

Roger W. Barnes first described this technique in 1951. The middle lobe, if present, is resected first. Starting from the protruding part of the middle lobe, short resections are made to reach the lateral margins. The resection is then deepened until the circular fibers of the bladder are visible. After the middle lobe resection, the vessels in the bladder neck are coagulated to control the bleeding. Then, the side lobe is resected, preferably started with the larger one. The resection begins at 6 o'clock and ascends to 12 o'clock. It is then deepened and descended from 12 to 6 o'clock. This procedure is repeated until the bladder neck fibers are visible. When protruded parts have finished, the resectoscope towards the verumontanum. Then, the adenoma in the prostatic lodge is resected as described above. After completely removing one of the lateral lobes up to the capsule, the opposite lobe is passed. Apical resection is resected in the last part of the operation [7].

According to Barnes, starting the resection at the 6 o'clock position improves the orientation to anatomical landmarks such as the trigon, orifices, and verumontanum. Coagulation of vessels in the bladder neck facilitates hemostasis. However, recutting the coagulated vessels from bottom to top and from top to bottom during resection seems to be a disadvantage.

Nesbit Technique

Nesbit's technique is based on the principle of ascended to descended resection. This method is similar to the finger enucleation technique used in open prostatectomy. The first resection in the bladder neck is made at 12 o'clock. Then, resection is continued until circular fibers are seen in the bladder neck towards the 3 o'clock position. Afterward, a canal is opened from the bladder neck to the apical part of the prostate with a resection going down to the capsule from 12 o'clock to 3 o'clock. The same maneuvers are performed between 12 o'clock and 9 o'clock. The prostate adenoma tissue between the two canals is removed up to the capsule. Then the middle lobe, if any, is resected up to the capsule. By assisting digital rectal examination, remaining tissues in the prostatic lodge can be resected in this technique. The apical tissue is resected last.

A decrease in the flow of irrigation fluid during apical resection may distort the image. Furthermore, the thinner prostate tissue in the anterior zone necessitates extra caution for capsule perforation. Bleeding is decreased as a result of the resection between opened canals before. However, bleeding cannot be controlled entirely until the resection is descended to the 5–7 o'clock position.

Alcock and Flocks Technique

Middle lobe resection is performed in the beginning of the operation. The resection is continued until it reaches the border of the lateral lobes. Meanwhile, the vessels feeding the prostate are coagulated at the 5–7 o'clock position. Then, a canal is opened in the left lateral lobe at 3 o'clock position go down to the capsule. The adenoma is resected between the bladder neck and the verumontanum from the 3 to the 6 o'clock position. The same procedure is applied to the other lobe. After the upper parts of the lateral lobes are resected, the apical resection is completed [2].

The technique described by Alcock and Flocks appears to be more useful in patients with larger lateral lobes. Additionally, it is not recommended for large middle lobes due to the difficulty in opening the canal. As bleeding control is established early at the 5 and 7 o'clock positions, the bleeding rates are reduced [34]. Nesbit's method is not very suitable in cases where only the middle lobe is present, or the lateral lobes are not large enough. The Barnes method is more suitable for small adenomas due to excessive bleeding caused by cutting the same vessels multiple times during resection [8].

After the resection procedure is complete and adequate bleeding control is achieved, the bladder is irrigated to remove residual clots and resected prostate chips. Then, the 3-way 18–20 F urethral Foley catheter is inserted with the help of lubricant gel, and the catheter balloon is inflated between 30–50 cc, depending on the size of the resected prostate tissue. The catheter's balloon reduces bleedings such as leakage in the prostate lodge. If necessary a penile traction to the catheter is made avoiding the compression to the penile glans. While one of the drainage holes of a 3-way catheter is connected to the urine bag, the other hole is attached to a 0.9% NaCl solution to avoid clot formation and provide continuous bladder irrigation. The speed of the irrigation fluid is adjusted according to the color of the urine.

The catheter may become clogged during the patient's follow-up due to a clot, prostate chip, or filled urine bag. This will cause a 'globe vesical' and suprapubic pain. First the irrigation fluid should be stopped then the clogged catheter is attempted to be cleared with the help of an injector; if not, it should be changed with a new one. Unless the catheter does not work after these maneuvers, cystoscopy should be performed to remove any hematoma or prostate chips in the bladder. If a bleeding vessel is observed during cystoscopy, it should be coagulated under anesthesia. When the bleeding stops and after achieving a satisfactory urine color, bladder irrigation is discontinued then the patient's urethral catheter is removed within two or three days. We generally prefer early hours of the day instead of evening hours for catheter removal, because if a 'globe vesical' or bleeding occurs, it should be easy to handle it in the daytime. The patient, whose catheter is removed, is discharged after urinating comfortably twice by observing the urine color.

Efficacy

mTUR-P is prostate surgery with longest lasting results and it has the only durability data of BPH surgery nearly 20 years [57]. A systematic review and meta-analysis of 69 RCTs with a maximum follow-up of five years m-TURP showed significant improvements in all parameters of efficacy, with a mean Qmax improvement (+162%), a reduction in IPSS (−70%), QoL score (−69%), and PVR (−77%). Also this paper revealed no significant change in the improvement of IPSS, QoL score, PVR at 12 months between bTUR-P and mTUR-P. However, Qmax was higher in the bTUR-P arm [15]. Madersbacher S et al. analysed 29 RCTs and found a retreatment rate of 2.6% after a mean follow-up of sixteen months. Repeating TUR-P has been reported at a constant annual rate of approximately 1–2% [43]. Another study reported similar results for IPSS and Qmax at one-year follow-up. However, in longer follow up (>1 year), IPSS and Qmax results are found better in the mTUR-P arm [12]. Omar et al. concluded their meta-analysis with these words 'there is no overall difference between mTUR-P and bTUR-P in terms of clinical effectiveness.' bTUR-P is associated with fewer adverse events, including TUR syndrome, clot retention and need for blood transfusion [52].

Six prospective randomized trials comparing bTUR-P with mTUR-P on functional outcomes (IPSS, Qmax, PVR, and QoL score) reported no significant differences. The follow-up periods of these studies changed between 24–60 months [4, 13, 27, 29, 40, 74]. The shorter urethral catheter withdrawal and hospitalization time seem to favor bTUR-P [55].

Complications

Complications related to TUR-P can be classified into three parts; perioperative, early postoperative, and late postoperative.

Perioperative Complications

(a) **Bleeding:**

Arterial bleeding is common in patients with pre-operative urinary tract infections or edema in the prostate tissue based on chronic urinary retention. Venous bleeding usually occurs due to capsule perforation or cut off the sinusoidal veins [55]. Arterial bleedings at the bladder neck and apex are usually seen at the 12 o'clock position. If severe arterial bleeding limits the vision, the clear vision will be regained by applying pressure to the bleeding point with a resectoscope and squeezing the irrigation fluid. Circular movements should be used to coagulate the bleeding artery. Capsule perforation may lead venous sinus bleeding, in this case it is important not to use an excessive force applied during coagulation that may widen the capsule perforation and increase bleeding. Venous leakages can be stopped by inserting continuous three-way irrigation Foley catheter, inflating the balloon 40–50 cc and traction of the urethral catheter. Blood pressure levels must be normal at the termination of the procedure to ensure that significant bleeding points are not masked by hypotension. After urethral catheter is inserted, care should be given to the urine color for a while to figure out if there is a need for a bleeding control.

According to Chen et al., bTUR-P has significantly lower blood transfusion rates than mTUR-P. He underlined that bipolar TUR systems enable the coagulation of small vessels during resection and that high-powered coagulation can safely seal large veins [13]. In a recent systematic review Cornu et al. emphasized that bTUR-P is superior to mTUR-P in terms of bleeding complications, as blood transfusion need and hemoglobin drop rates are less [15]. However, a prospective randomized trial focusing on bleeding complications stated no difference in blood transfusion between the two techniques [68]. In a multicentric trial comparing the safety and efficacy of bTUR-P vs. mTUR-P in large prostates >100 ml, the authors found no significant changes in hemoglobin levels pre-and postoperatively [66].

(b) **Capsule Perforation and Extravasation of Irrigation Fluid:**

Symptomatic perforation of bladder neck and prostate capsule should occur rarely and it is mainly seen in the early stages of TUR-P training. Extravasation occurs following capsular perforation or when the bladder neck is separated from the prostatic urethra in case of excessive resection below the bladder neck. The irrigation fluid often leaks from the perforation area to the extraperitoneal or, rarely, intraperitoneal area. The patient with spinal anesthesia may experience abdominal pain, shoulder pain, nausea-vomiting, and dyspnea. General anesthesia often delays the diagnosis. Low oxygen saturation, tachycardia, and hypotension may arise during general anesthesia. Abdominal distension and a decrease in the amount of irrigation fluid that drains outside should alert the surgeon. In case of perforation, bleeding should be controlled immediately, and the operation should be terminated. A conservative approach of holding the urethral catheter longer than usual is sufficient in asymptomatic patients with extraperitoneal fluid. A percutaneous catheter can be used to drain a massive amount of irrigation fluid from the intraperitoneal area. Laparotomy should be considered in patients with severe symptoms. During open surgery, the bowel loops near the perforation area should be checked against possible bowel injury. Skolarikos et al. found no difference in capsular perforation rates between mTUR-P and bTUR-P (15% and 26% respectively). However, two patients in the mTUR-P arm experienced severe perforation [66]. Despite that Chen et al. reported higher rates with mTUR-P (40% versus 20%) [13].

Rectal perforation is an infrequent complication. Neal has reported the incidence as 0.25% [49]. Intraoperative general surgery consultation should be requested if rectal perforation is suspected. Colostomy and concurrent suprapubic cystostomy should be performed to separate intestinal content and the urine [9].

(c) **TUR Syndrome:**

TUR syndrome is characterized by blurred consciousness, visual disturbances, nausea-vomiting, hypertension, and bradycardia [31]. Apart from these findings, seizure, coma, restlessness, and headache symptoms can also be observed [33]. When general anesthesia has been employed, the only manifestations of delusional hyponatremia in such patients may be increasing hypertension and increasing pulse or venous pressure.

A prospective multicenter evaluation of 10,654 patients have shown an incidence of 1.2% in prostate volume < 30 ml, 1.4% between 30–60 ml and 3% >60 ml [58]. When non-conductive hypoosmolar irrigation medium (glycine, mannitol, sorbitol) is excessively absorbed into the systemic circulation through the prostatic venous sinuses and the peri-prostatic tissues during mTUR-P, it causes hypervolemia and dilutional hyponatremia (Na <125 mEq/L). It is associated with longer resection times and larger prostates. To prevent this complication attention must be given to the coagulation while making resection, time of the operation should not exceed 1 hour and the height of the irrigation fluid should not exceed 60 cm from the patient during the operation.

If perforation occurs of if venous sinuses open during resection and if the operation get longer, a loop diuretic (furosemide, 40 to 120 mg) should be administered. In addition, IV fluids should be changed to normal saline. If the sodium level is below 125 mEq/L, a hypertonic saline (3%) sodium solution should be administered intravenously within 3–6 hours, and blood sodium levels should be closely monitored [32]. Of the other traditionally used solutions, sorbitol can cause hyperglycemia, care must be given in patients with diabetes, and glycine should not be used in patients with hepatic dysfunction because of concerns about hyperammonemia.

The incidence of TUR syndrome has decreased significantly during the last few decades from 3% to <1% [55]. The role of bipolar systems in the prevention of TUR syndrome cannot be ignored. Its hemostatic advantages and the use of saline rather than other solutions (glycine, mannitol and sorbitol) for resection are the main factors preventing TUR syndrome. Most of the RCT's and prospective studies comparing these two techniques indicates that TUR syndrome rates are lower in bTUR-P [12, 13, 15, 27, 29, 36, 40, 48, 52, 63, 71, 74].

Early Postoperative Complications

(a) **Bleeding and Clot Retention:**

Bleeding might emerge during the early or late periods of TUR-P. The approach to bleeding and the evaluation of the two techniques are described in the perioperative complications section.

Several studies in literature emphasized that clot retention rates are higher in mTUR-P [27, 40]. These findings support the simultaneous seal effect of the bipolar system during resection that Chen et al. stated in his study [13]. As a result, bTUR-P has more advantages over hospitalization and catheterization time [40].

(b) **Urinary Tract Infections (UTI)**:

UTI is one of the most common complications in the early postoperative period [1]. The rate of UTI is more than two fold as high in patients who have a catheter placement for urinary retention before surgery. It is mandatory to eradicate preoperative UTI before TUR-P. There was no correlation between the size of the resected prostate and the presence of UTI [58]. A study stated that the risk of UTI increased in operations lasting longer than 70 minutes [55]. If high fever occurs in the postoperative period, the risk of epididymitis, orchitis, or urethritis should be considered. Urine culture should be taken from the patient with suspected UTI. According to the antibiogram result, current prophylactic antibiotic therapy should be revised. During the healing phase, the presence of pyuri is expected. It is not necessary to treat it with antibiotics, even it is not approved with a positive urine culture.

(c) **Urine retention and incontinence:**

Palmisano et al. reported the rate of re-operation in acute urinary retention as 3.1% in the first month after TUR-P [54]. In a meta-analysis, this rate varies between 0–13.3% [1]. Contrary to common belief, acute urinary retention following TUR-P is mostly related to detrusor muscle insufficiency rather than inadequate resection [20]. Patients with prolonged voiding symptoms caused by obstruction should be evaluated carefully. Poorly controlled diabetes mellitus, patients with a potential neurogenic cause of urinary retention and patients with chronic urinary retention have an increased risk of having weak streams or inability to void postoperatively.

Acute urinary retention after inadequate resection is typically caused by residual prostate tissue in the apical region or incompletely removed prostatic tissue, usually anterior part that fall into the prostatic fossa after resection of lateral lobes, closing the urethra like a flap. In patients who are unable to void after TUR-P, a urethral catheter should be placed for drainage. Anti-inflammatory and alpha-blocker drugs can be started for treatment. After one week, the catheter is withdrawn, and the patient should be observed for voiding. Cystoscopy should be performed for residual tissue in those who do not benefit from this treatment. If there is no obstruction in the prostatic fossa and urethra, urodynamic should be performed for bladder functions. Most patients with poor bladder tonus who void inadequately have to be managed with intermittent self-catheterization.

The most feared complication of prostate surgery is incontinence and patients must be forewarned of about 0.5% possibility of this complication. The most common type of incontinence in the early period after TUR-P is urge incontinence, secondary to irritation from resected prostatic fossa or detrusor instability. Appropriate anticholinergic and anti-inflammatory drugs can be used in the treatment. If incontinence persists for more than six months, urethrography and cystourethroscopy should be performed for detailed examination. Additional intervention is required if there is urethral stricture, bladder neck sclerosis, or residual prostate tissue. Cystoscopy should be performed to assess the sphincter's integrity. If necessary, video-urodynamics should be used to determine sphincteric deficiency. The initial approach in treating incontinence associated with sphincter injury is conservative treatment and medication (duloxetine). Unless the patient does not benefit from first step treatment, the injection, a male sling, adjustable balloon devices, or an artificial sphincter can be used [64]. Urinary incontinence rates were found similar for mTUR-P and bTUR-P, both in short-term and long-term follow-ups [27].

Late Postoperative Complications

(a) **Urethral Stricture and Bladder Neck Stenosis:**

Urethral strictures can occur in any part of the urethra (Fig. 2.1a). The most common cause of external meatus stricture is forcing the urethra with an inappropriate diameter resectoscope. Strictures in other parts of the urethra can arise due to the trauma from resectoscope. It's important to make proper preliminary urethral dilatation and instrument lubrication to avoid this. Using the thinnest available instruments and limiting the resection time to 1.5 hours, the incidence of stricture can be decreased. Lubricant gel should be applied before entry, and if the procedure takes longer than expected, gel should be applied periodically to the urethra and resectoscope. Assessment of the entire urethra by panendoscopy before inserting the resectoscope blindly lessens the incidence of false passage formation and permits more accurate assessment of the urethral channel.

Incidence of bladder neck stenosis for mTUR-P and bTUR-P is 2% (0–21) versus 0.5% (0–4) (Fig. 2.1b). Usually seem to occur more commonly in patients with small, fibrotic prostates [55]. Although the cause is unknown, indiscriminate fulguration and excessive catheter traction of the bladder neck have been implicated. Bladder neck incision is used in the treatment. If this does not allow the bladder neck to open, a "Mercedes Benz–type" incision or a four-quadrant, cross-like incision of the bladder neck should be performed. Open surgical repair with a Y-V plasty is the treatment option in repeating bladder neck contractures.

Data given from the previous studies were contradictory. Most of the studies with long-term follow-up indicate that the rate of urethral stricture and bladder neck stenosis are comparable for mTUR-P and bTUR-P [4, 13, 27, 45, 74]. However, other research implies that the rate of urethral stricture is higher in bTUR-P. Prolonged resection times in large prostate volumes, high ablative

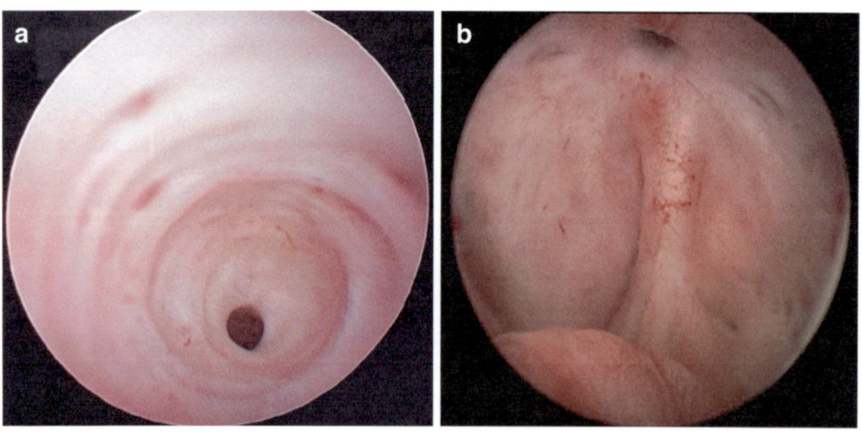

Fig. 2.1 (**a**) Urethral stricture (**b**) Bladder neck sclerosis

Table 2.1 Comparison of safety and efficacy between mTUR-P and bTUR-P

	Number of Patients	Follow-up time (months)	Efficacy	Safety
Seckiner et al.	48	12	Non-significant	More hyponatremia in mTUR-P
Autorine et al.	70	48	Non-significant	Non-significant
Xie et al.	220	60	Non-significant	More hyponatremia and hemoglobin decrease in mTUR-P
Giulianelli et al.	160	36	Non-significant	More hemoglobin decrease in mTUR-P
Otaola-Arca et al.	84	12	Non-significant	Non-significant

energy levels, larger resectoscope diameters, and any flow leakage through the sheath, particularly in the semi-bipolar system, have all been associated with increased urethral stricture formation [37, 40, 70].

(b) **Retrograde ejeculation:**

The incidence of retrograde ejaculation after TUR-P is 53.4–77.5% [48]. Patients should be made aware that this condition will occur in the postoperative period. Previously, disruption of the integrity of the bladder neck was believed to be the primary cause; but recent studies have shown that a newly described technique protects up to 90% from retrograde ejaculation [3, 60]. This novel approach advises not to resect the paracollicular and localized tissue located 1 cm proximal to the verumontanum because musculus ejaculators and verumontanum is important structures mainly related to the ejaculation [28, 35].

(c) **Erectile Dysfunction:**

The incidence of erectile function is 6.5% [43]. Injury of the neurovascular bundle close to the prostate capsule during resection is the leading cause. Additionally, the effect of retrograde ejaculation on erectile dysfunction should not be ignored.

Overall the summary of some RCT's that compared the efficacy and safety of mTUR-P and bTUR-P is shown in Table 2.1.

Conclusion

TUR-P remains the gold standard for the treatment of men with BPH between 30–80 ml prostates. When done correctly and methodically, TUR-P not only is an effective and durable therapy for BPH but also can be performed safely with minimal complications. Although bipolar systems improvements in surgical technologies seem to diminish perioperative morbidity by eliminating transurethral resection syndrome and minimizes bleeding risk, both monopolar and bipolar technologies have very good and comparative results in terms of efficacy. Especially at the beginning of their learning curve, bTUR-P allows surgeons the opportunity to perform their operations more safely and comfortably. Endoscopic enucleation surgeries (bipolar or laser enucleation) are getting popular nowadays because of more anatomical resection can be possible, TUR-P remains a priority as the surgery with the longest follow-up, but we will see how prostate surgery will shape up in time. TUR-P doesn't have a long learning curve, but it can be mastered only with time and practice. Success and the incidence of complications of transurethral surgery is proportional to the experience of the surgeon.

Tips and Tricks

- bTUR-P (and/or bipolar enucleation) is the treatment of choice for prostates between 30–100 gr in our practice. The main point in choosing surgery type should be the experience in technic, operation room technical facilities and patient expectations.
- If present, we always start from the protruding part of the middle lobe, and care should be given to the ureteral orifices. After resecting the upper part of the middle lobe, you shouldn't continue to resect the bladder neck itself to reach the parts of the lobe in the bladder. Instead of this, you should hook and lift the resting part with the resectoscope loop and resect it high over the bladder neck.
- Undermining the bladder trigone by over-resection of the proximal prostatic urethra is problematic for various reasons. Catheter placement both postoperatively and in the case of a failed voiding trial may be difficult. Foley catheter should be placed using a guidewire passed from the resectoscope to the bladder. The surgeon should consider delayed catheter removal if the patient is high risk of voiding trial.
- We are ordering furosemide 20 mg every one hour while the operation prolonged, or a venous sinus opened during the operation.
- Especially in patients with big volume prostates, prostatic lobes should be resected one by one. If any problems occur that we need to terminate the operation, one lobe resection might be enough in most cases for urination problems.

References

1. Ahyai SA, Gilling P, Kaplan SA, Kuntz RM, Madersbacher S, Montorsi F, Speakman MJ, Stief CG. Meta-analysis of functional outcomes and complications following transurethral procedures for lower urinary tract symptoms resulting from benign prostatic enlargement. Eur Urol. 2010;58(3):384–97. https://doi.org/10.1016/j.eururo.2010.06.005.
2. Alcock NG. Ten months experience with transurethral prostatic resection1. J Urol. 1932;28(5):545–59. https://doi.org/10.1016/S0022-5347(17)72684-5.

3. Alloussi SH, Lang C, Eichel R, Alloussi S. Ejaculation-preserving transurethral resection of prostate and bladder neck: short- and long-term results of a new innovative resection technique. J Endourol. 2014;28(1):84–9. https://doi.org/10.1089/end.2013.0093.
4. Autorino R, Damiano R, Di Lorenzo G, Quarto G, Perdonà S, D'Armiento M, De Sio M. Four-year outcome of a prospective randomised trial comparing bipolar plasmakinetic and monopolar transurethral resection of the prostate. Eur Urol. 2009;55(4):922–9. https://doi.org/10.1016/j.eururo.2009.01.028.
5. Babayan RK. Development of transurethral resection of the prostate (TURP). In: The history of technologic advancements in urology. 1st ed. Cham: Springer; 2018. p. 49–57.
6. Barba M, Fastenmeier K, Hartung R. Electrocautery: principles and practice. J Endourol. 2003;17(8):541–55. https://doi.org/10.1089/089277903322518545.
7. Barnes RW. Method and rhythm in transurethral prostatic resection. J Urol. 1951;65(4):603–7. https://doi.org/10.1016/s0022-5347(17)68527-6.
8. Baş O, Yıkılmaz TN. Transurethral prostate resection techniques. In: Şener NC, Zengin K, editors. Indications and resection methods of prostate. Ankara: Derman Tıbbi Yayıncılık; 2015.
9. Blandy JP, Reynard JM, Notley R. Transurethral resection. CRC Press; 2004.
10. Blomqvist P, Ekbom A, Carlsson P, Ahlstrand C, Johansson J-E. Benign prostatic hyperplasia in Sweden 1987 to 1994: changing patterns of treatment, changing patterns of costs. Urology. 1997;50(2):214–20. https://doi.org/10.1016/S0090-4295(97)00241-0.
11. Braasch WF. Median Bar Excisor. JAMA J Am Med Assoc. 1918;70(11):758–9. https://doi.org/10.1001/jama.1918.02600110016005.
12. Burke N, Whelan JP, Goeree L, Hopkins RB, Campbell K, Goeree R, Tarride J-E. Systematic review and meta-analysis of transurethral resection of the prostate versus minimally invasive procedures for the treatment of benign prostatic obstruction. Urology. 2010;75(5):1015–22. https://doi.org/10.1016/j.urology.2009.08.015.
13. Chen Q, Zhang L, Fan Q-L, Zhou J, Peng Y-B, Wang Z. Bipolar transurethral resection in saline vs traditional monopolar resection of the prostate: results of a randomized trial with a 2-year follow-up. BJU Int. 2010;106(9):1339–43. https://doi.org/10.1111/j.1464-410X.2010.09401.x.
14. Collins JW, MacDermott S, Bradbrook RA, Keeley FX, Timoney AG. A comparison of the effect of 1.5% glycine and 5% glucose irrigants on plasma serum physiology and the incidence of transurethral resection syndrome during prostate resection. BJU Int. 2005;96(3):368–72. https://doi.org/10.1111/j.1464-410X.2005.05633.x.
15. Cornu J-N, Ahyai S, Bachmann A, de la Rosette J, Gilling P, Gratzke C, McVary K, Novara G, Woo H, Madersbacher S. A systematic review and meta-analysis of functional outcomes and complications following transurethral procedures for lower urinary tract symptoms resulting from benign prostatic obstruction: an update. Eur Urol. 2015;67(6):1066–96. https://doi.org/10.1016/j.eururo.2014.06.017.
16. Creevy CD. Hemolytic reactions during transurethral prostatic resection. J Urol. 1947;58(2):125–31. https://doi.org/10.1016/s0022-5347(17)69530-2.
17. Das AK, Leong JY, Roehrborn CG. Office-based therapies for benign prostatic hyperplasia: a review and update. Can J Urol. 2019;26(4 Suppl 1):2–7.
18. Dimberg M, Allgén LG, Norlén H. Absence of lactate accumulation on transurethral resection of the prostate using 2.5% sorbitol solution as an irrigating fluid. Scand J Urol Nephrol. 1988;22(2):119–24. https://doi.org/10.1080/00365599.1988.11690396.
19. Dimberg M, Norlén H, Allgén LG, Allgén T, Wallin M. A comparison between two hypotonic irrigating solutions used in transurethral resections of the prostate: sorbitol (2%)-mannitol (1%) and 1.5% glycine solutions. Scand J Urol Nephrol. 1992;26(3):241–7. https://doi.org/10.3109/00365599209180876.
20. Djavan B, Madersbacher S, Klingler C, Marberger M. Urodynamic assessment of patients with acute urinary retention: is treatment failure after prostatectomy predictable? J Urol. 1997;158(5):1829–33. https://doi.org/10.1016/s0022-5347(01)64139-9.

21. Dotan ZA, Mor Y, Leibovitch I, Varon D, Golomb J, Duvdevani M, Ramon J. The efficacy and safety of perioperative low molecular weight heparin substitution in patients on chronic oral anticoagulant therapy undergoing transurethral prostatectomy for bladder outlet obstruction. J Urol. 2002;168(2):610–3; discussion 614.
22. EAU Guidelines on the Management of Non-neurogenic Male LUTS - DISEASE MANAGEMENT - Uroweb. In: Uroweb - Eur. Assoc. Urol. https://uroweb.org/guidelines/management-of-non-neurogenic-male-luts/chapter/disease-management. Accessed 10 Feb 2024.
23. EAU Guidelines on the Thromboprophylaxis. THE GUIDELINE- Uroweb. In: Uroweb- Eur. Assoc. Urol. https://uroweb.org/guidelines/thromboprophylaxis/chapter/guideline. Accessed 10 Feb 2024.
24. EAU Guidelines on Urological Infections. THE GUIDELINE - Uroweb. In: Uroweb - Eur Assoc Urol. https://uroweb.org/guidelines/urological-infections/chapter/the-guideline. Accessed 10 Feb 2024.
25. Fenwick EH. In: urinary surgery. Bristol: Wright; 1985. p. 151–3.
26. Fitzpatrick J. Which BPH treatment is the most clinically efficacious and cost-effective? Nat Clin Pract Urol. 2007;4(7):358–9. https://doi.org/10.1038/ncpuro0806.
27. Geavlete B, Georgescu D, Multescu R, Stanescu F, Jecu M, Geavlete P. Bipolar plasma vaporization vs monopolar and bipolar TURP-A prospective, randomized, long-term comparison. Urology. 2011;78(4):930–5. https://doi.org/10.1016/j.urology.2011.03.072.
28. Gil-Vernet JM, Alvarez-Vijande R, Gil-Vernet A, Gil-Vernet JM. Ejaculation in men: a dynamic endorectal ultrasonographical study. Br J Urol. 1994;73(4):442–8. https://doi.org/10.1111/j.1464-410x.1994.tb07612.x.
29. Giulianelli R, Albanesi L, Attisani F, Gentile BC, Vincenti G, Pisanti F, Shestani T, Mavilla L, Granata D, Schettini M. Comparative randomized study on the efficaciousness of endoscopic bipolar prostate resection versus monopolar resection technique. 3 year follow-up. Arch Ital Urol Androl Organo. 2013;85(2):86–91. https://doi.org/10.4081/aiua.2013.2.86.
30. Green Z, Westwood J, Somani BK. What's new in Rezum: a transurethral water vapour therapy for BPH. Curr Urol Rep. 2019;20(7):39. https://doi.org/10.1007/s11934-019-0903-7.
31. Gupta K, Rastogi B, Jain M, Gupta PK, Sharma D. Electrolyte changes: an indirect method to assess irrigation fluid absorption complications during transurethral resection of prostate: a prospective study. Saudi J Anaesth. 2010;4(3):142–6. https://doi.org/10.4103/1658-354X.71505.
32. Hahn RG. The transurethral resection syndrome. Acta Anaesthesiol Scand. 1991;35(7):557–67. https://doi.org/10.1111/j.1399-6576.1991.tb03348.x.
33. Hahn RG. Fluid absorption in endoscopic surgery. Br J Anaesth. 2006;96(1):8–20. https://doi.org/10.1093/bja/aei279.
34. Hawtrey CE, Williams RD. Historical evolution of transurethral resection at the University of I owa: Alcock and Flocks. J Urol. 2008;180(1):55–61. https://doi.org/10.1016/j.juro.2008.03.018.
35. Hermabessiere J, Guy L, Boiteux JP. Human ejaculation: physiology, surgical conservation of ejaculation. Progres En Urol. 1999;9(2):305–9.
36. Ho HSS, Cheng CWS. Bipolar transurethral resection of prostate: a new reference standard? Curr Opin Urol. 2008;18(1):50–5. https://doi.org/10.1097/MOU.0b013e3282f194db.
37. Ho HSS, Yip SKH, Lim KB, Fook S, Foo KT, Cheng CWS. A prospective randomized study comparing monopolar and bipolar transurethral resection of prostate using transurethral resection in saline (TURIS) system. Eur Urol. 2007;52(2):517–22. https://doi.org/10.1016/j.eururo.2007.03.038.
38. Izard J, Nickel JC. Impact of medical therapy on transurethral resection of the prostate: two decades of change. BJU Int. 2011;108(1):89–93. https://doi.org/10.1111/j.1464-410X.2010.09737.x.
39. Johnson T. The works of that famous Chirurgien Ambrose pare. Translated by T. Johnson. London; 1634. p. 665.

40. Komura K, Inamoto T, Takai T, Uchimoto T, Saito K, Tanda N, Minami K, Oide R, Uehara H, Takahara K, Hirano H, Nomi H, Kiyama S, Watsuji T, Azuma H. Incidence of urethral stricture after bipolar transurethral resection of the prostate using TURis: results from a randomised trial. BJU Int. 2015;115(4):644–52. https://doi.org/10.1111/bju.12831.
41. Liang X, Wu W, Huang Y, Zhang S, Huang J, Zeng T, Zhong F, Yong L, Duan X, Chao C, Gurioli A, Deng T, Wu W. Safety of surgery in benign prostatic hyperplasia patients on antiplatelet or anticoagulant therapy: a systematic review and meta-analysis. Urol J. 2020;18(2):151–9. https://doi.org/10.22037/uj.v16i7.5974.
42. Lokeshwar SD, Harper BT, Webb E, Jordan A, Dykes TA, Neal DE, Terris MK, Klaassen Z. Epidemiology and treatment modalities for the management of benign prostatic hyperplasia. Transl Androl Urol. 2019;8(5):529–39. https://doi.org/10.21037/tau.2019.10.01.
43. Madersbacher S, Marberger M. Is transurethral resection of the prostate still justified? BJU Int. 1999;83(3):227–37. https://doi.org/10.1046/j.1464-410x.1999.00908.x.
44. Malhotra V. Transurethral resection of the prostate. Anesthesiol Clin N Am. 2000;18(4):883–97., x. https://doi.org/10.1016/s0889-8537(05)70200-5.
45. Mamoulakis C, Schulze M, Skolarikos A, Alivizatos G, Scarpa RM, Rassweiler JJ, de la Rosette JJMCH, Scoffone CM. Midterm results from an international multicentre randomised controlled trial comparing bipolar with monopolar transurethral resection of the prostate. Eur Urol. 2013;63(4):667–76. https://doi.org/10.1016/j.eururo.2012.10.003.
46. Manyak MJ, Ackerman SJ, Blute ML, Rein AL, Buesterien K, Sullivan EM, Tanio CP, Strauss MJ. Cost effectiveness of treatment for benign prostatic hyperplasia: an economic model for comparison of medical, minimally invasive, and surgical therapy. J Endourol. 2002;16(1):51–6. https://doi.org/10.1089/089277902753483736.
47. McVary KT. BPH: epidemiology and comorbidities. Am J Manag Care. 2006;12(5 Suppl):S122–8.
48. Michielsen DPJ, Debacker T, De Boe V, Van Lersberghe C, Kaufman L, Braeckman JG, Amy J-J, Keuppens FI. Bipolar transurethral resection in saline—an alternative surgical treatment for bladder outlet obstruction? J Urol. 2007;178(5):2035–9.; discussion 2039. https://doi.org/10.1016/j.juro.2007.07.038.
49. Neal DE. The National Prostatectomy Audit. Br J Urol. 1997;79(Suppl 2):69–75. https://doi.org/10.1111/j.1464-410x.1997.tb16924.x.
50. Nesbit RM, Glickman SI. The use of glycine solution as an irrigating medium during transurethral resection. J Urol. 1948;59(6):1212–6. https://doi.org/10.1016/s0022-5347(17)69504-1.
51. Norlén H, Allgén LG, Vinnars E, Bedrelidou-Classon G. Glycine solution as an irrigating agent during transurethral prostatic resection. Glycine concentrations in blood plasma. Scand J Urol Nephrol. 1986;20(1):19–26. https://doi.org/10.3109/00365598609024475.
52. Omar MI, Lam TB, Alexander CE, Graham J, Mamoulakis C, Imamura M, Maclennan S, Stewart F, N'dow J. Systematic review and meta-analysis of the clinical effectiveness of bipolar compared with monopolar transurethral resection of the prostate (TURP). BJU Int. 2014;113(1):24–35. https://doi.org/10.1111/bju.12281.
53. Otaola-Arca H, Álvarez-Ardura M, Molina-Escudero R, Fernández MI, Páez-Borda Á. A prospective randomized study comparing bipolar plasmakinetic transurethral resection of the prostate and monopolar transurethral resection of the prostate for the treatment of Benign Prostatic Hyperplasia: efficacy, sexual function, quality of life, and complications. Int Braz J Urol. 2021;47(1):131–44. https://doi.org/10.1590/S1677-5538.IBJU.2019.0766.
54. Palmisano F, Boeri L, Fontana M, Gallioli A, De Lorenzis E, Zanetti SP, Sampogna G, Spinelli MG, Albo G, Longo F, Gadda F, Dell'Orto PG, Montanari E. Incidence and predictors of readmission within 30 days of transurethral resection of the prostate: a single center European experience. Sci Rep. 2018;8(1):6575. https://doi.org/10.1038/s41598-018-25069-5.
55. Rassweiler J, Teber D, Kuntz R, Hofmann R (2006) Complications of transurethral resection of the prostate (TURP)—incidence, management, and prevention. Eur Urol. 50(5):969–79; discussion 980. https://doi.org/10.1016/j.eururo.2005.12.042.

56. Rassweiler J, Schulze M, Stock C, Teber D, De La Rosette J. Bipolar transurethral resection of the prostate--technical modifications and early clinical experience. Minim Invasive Ther Allied Technol. 2007;16(1):11–21. https://doi.org/10.1080/13645700601159410.
57. Reich O, Gratzke C, Stief CG (2006) Techniques and long-term results of surgical procedures for BPH. Eur Urol. 49(6):970–978; discussion 978. https://doi.org/10.1016/j.eururo.2005.12.072.
58. Reich O, Gratzke C, Bachmann A, Seitz M, Schlenker B, Hermanek P, Lack N, Stief CG, Urology Section of the Bavarian Working Group for Quality Assurance. Morbidity, mortality and early outcome of transurethral resection of the prostate: a prospective multicenter evaluation of 10,654 patients. J Urol. 2008;180(1):246–9. https://doi.org/10.1016/j.juro.2008.03.058.
59. Roderick C, Violette P. Antibiotic prophylaxis in urological surgery. In: Evidence-based urology, 2. UK: Wiley-Blackwell; 2018. p. 67–87.
60. Ronzoni G, De Vecchis M. Preservation of anterograde ejaculation after transurethral resection of both the prostate and bladder neck. Br J Urol. 1998;81(6):830–3. https://doi.org/10.1046/j.1464-410x.1998.00658.x.
61. Rühle A, Blarer J, Oehme F, Marini L, Mattei A, Stucki P, Danuser H. Safety and effectiveness of bipolar transurethral resection of the prostate in patients under ongoing Oral anticoagulation with Coumarins or antiplatelet drug therapy compared to patients without anticoagulation/antiplatelet therapy. J Endourol. 2019;33(6):455–62. https://doi.org/10.1089/end.2018.0879.
62. Sandhu JS, Bixler BR, Dahm P, Goueli R, Kirkby E, Stoffel JT, Wilt TJ. Management of lower urinary tract symptoms attributed to benign prostatic hyperplasia (BPH): AUA guideline amendment 2023. J Urol. 2024;211(1):11–9. https://doi.org/10.1097/JU.0000000000003698.
63. Seckiner I, Yesilli C, Akduman B, Altan K, Mungan NA. A prospective randomized study for comparing bipolar plasmakinetic resection of the prostate with standard TURP. Urol Int. 2006;76(2):139–43. https://doi.org/10.1159/000090877.
64. Silva LA, Andriolo RB, Atallah ÁN, da Silva EM. Surgery for stress urinary incontinence due to presumed sphincter deficiency after prostate surgery. Cochrane Database Syst Rev. 2014;2014(9) https://doi.org/10.1002/14651858.CD008306.pub3.
65. Singh H, Desai MR, Shrivastav P, Vani K. Bipolar versus monopolar transurethral resection of prostate: randomized controlled study. J Endourol. 2005;19(3):333–8. https://doi.org/10.1089/end.2005.19.333.
66. Skolarikos A, Rassweiler J, de la Rosette JJ, Alivizatos G, Scoffone C, Scarpa RM, Schulze M, Mamoulakis C. Safety and efficacy of bipolar versus monopolar transurethral resection of the prostate in patients with large prostates or severe lower urinary tract symptoms: post hoc analysis of a European multicenter randomized controlled trial. J Urol. 2016;195(3):677–84. https://doi.org/10.1016/j.juro.2015.08.083.
67. Smith D, Khoubehi B, Patel A. Bipolar electrosurgery for benign prostatic hyperplasia: transurethral electrovaporization and resection of the prostate. Curr Opin Urol. 2005;15(2):95–100. https://doi.org/10.1097/01.mou.0000160623.13366.e8.
68. Stucki P, Marini L, Mattei A, Xafis K, Boldini M, Danuser H. Bipolar versus monopolar transurethral resection of the prostate: a prospective randomized trial focusing on bleeding c omplications. J Urol. 2015;193(4):1371–5. https://doi.org/10.1016/j.juro.2014.08.137.
69. Stwen M. Resection of obstructions at the vesical orifice: new instruments and a new method. JAMA J Am Med Assoc. 1926;87(21):1726–30. https://doi.org/10.1001/jama.1926.02680210032010.
70. Tefekli A, Muslumanoglu AY, Baykal M, Binbay M, Tas A, Altunrende F. A hybrid technique using bipolar energy in transurethral prostate surgery: a prospective, randomized comparison. J Urol. 2005;174(4 Pt 1):1339–43. https://doi.org/10.1097/01.ju.0000173075.62504.73.
71. Treharne C, Crowe L, Booth D, Ihara Z. Economic value of the transurethral resection in saline system for treatment of benign prostatic hyperplasia in England and Wales: systematic review, meta-analysis, and cost-consequence model. Eur Urol Focus. 2018;4(2):270–9. https://doi.org/10.1016/j.euf.2016.03.002.

72. Ulchaker JC, Martinson MS. Cost-effectiveness analysis of six therapies for the treatment of lower urinary tract symptoms due to benign prostatic hyperplasia. Clin Outcomes Res CEOR. 2018;10:29–43. https://doi.org/10.2147/CEOR.S148195.
73. Wilson JR, Urwin GH, Stower MJ. The changing practice of transurethral prostatectomy: a comparison of cases performed in 1990 and 2000. Ann R Coll Surg Engl. 2004;86(6):428–31. https://doi.org/10.1308/147870804731.
74. Xie C-Y, Zhu G-B, Wang X-H, Liu X-B. Five-year follow-up results of a randomized controlled trial comparing bipolar plasmakinetic and monopolar transurethral resection of the prostate. Yonsei Med J. 2012;53(4):734–41. https://doi.org/10.3349/ymj.2012.53.4.734.
75. Young HH. A new procedure (punch operation) for small prostatic bars and contracture of the prostatic orifice. JAMA J Am Med Assoc. 1913;60(4):253–7. https://doi.org/10.1001/jama.1913.04340040001001.

Chapter 3
Holmium/Thulium Laser Enucleation of the Prostate

Onur Acikgoz, Mehmet Yilmaz, and Engin Kaya

Preparing for Laser Enucleation of the Prostate Surgery: The Operation Room

Preoperative Equipment Control

Before the patient enters the operating room, all preparations are made and device controls are completed (Fig. 3.1).

The basic endoscopic and surgical instruments used in transurethral resection of the prostate (TUR P) are also used in laser enucleation of the prostate. Different sizes of endoscopic instrument can be used for enucleation. As a resectoscope, 26 fr outer sheet (24 fr inner sheet) and 22 fr outer sheet (19 fr inner sheet) can be used during enucleation. Cystoscopes of various sizes, internal urethrotome, urethral dilators should be kept ready as they may be needed in each case (Fig. 3.2).

O. Acikgoz
Kadikoy Florence Nightingale Hospital, Department of Urology, Istanbul, Turkey

M. Yilmaz (✉)
Mediclin Kraichgau-Klinik, Urology, Bad Rappenau, Germany

E. Kaya
Istanbul Health and Technology University, Department of Urology, Istanbul, Turkey

S. Tonyali et al. (eds.), *Current Endourology*,
https://doi.org/10.1007/978-3-032-00010-1_3

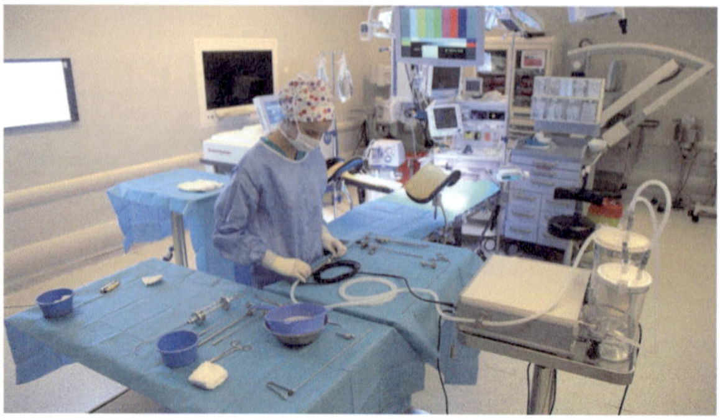

Fig. 3.1 General view of the operating room preparation

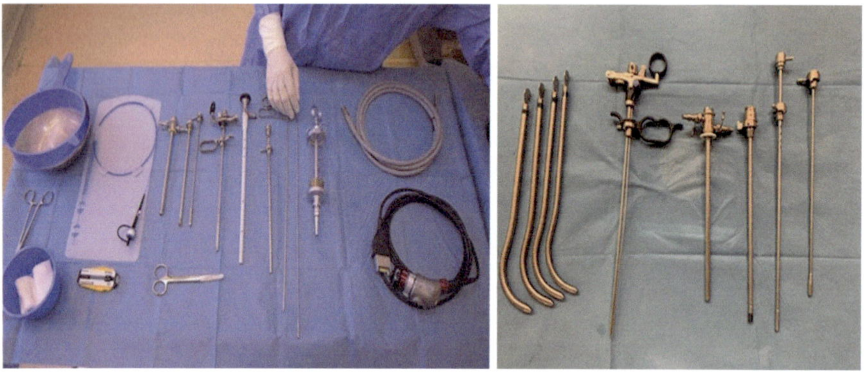

Fig. 3.2 Endoscopic instruments used in laser enucleation surgery

Preoperative Laser Generator Control

Holmium: YAG

Laser generator control should be routinely performed by a technician before all cases. The most important point for the protection of the laser fiber is the control of the structure called the **blast shield**, which protects the laser. Blast shield has a very important role in transferring the laser beams to the laser fiber. To effectively transmit laser beams to the fiber, the lens must be clean. Micro-fractures in the laser fiber can cause the laser beams to diverge and contaminate the blast shield (Fig. 3.3). If this contamination is not checked and cleaned, the blast shield may not function and may cause a malfunction in the laser device. Unlike normal power lines, all Holmium:YAG generators require a high-energy line. Another point is to pay attention to the power transformer switches of these devices. These switches are important for fast closing in case of emergency (Fig. 3.4). When using Holmium:YAG generators, the room temperature should be kept below 19 °C to assist the cooling system of the laser generator.

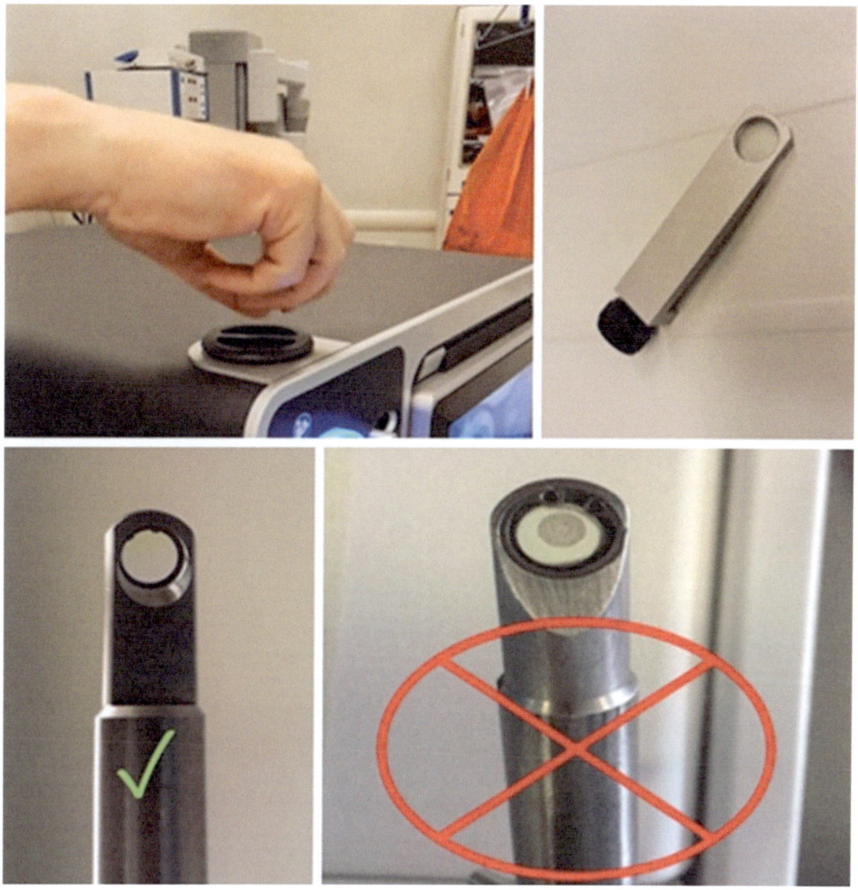

Fig. 3.3 Blast shield and control

Thulium: YAG

Thulium: YAG device has some differences compared to Holmium: YAG. First of all, this device does not have a blast shield. Secondly, normal electric current is used. Finally, it is not necessary to lower the room temperature when using this generator (Fig. 3.5a).

Thulium Fiber Laser (TFL)

TFL has significant advantages over other laser generators. It has high performance with less energy consumption. It does not require a special electrical outlet in the operating room, it is compatible with standard electrical outlets. With its simple

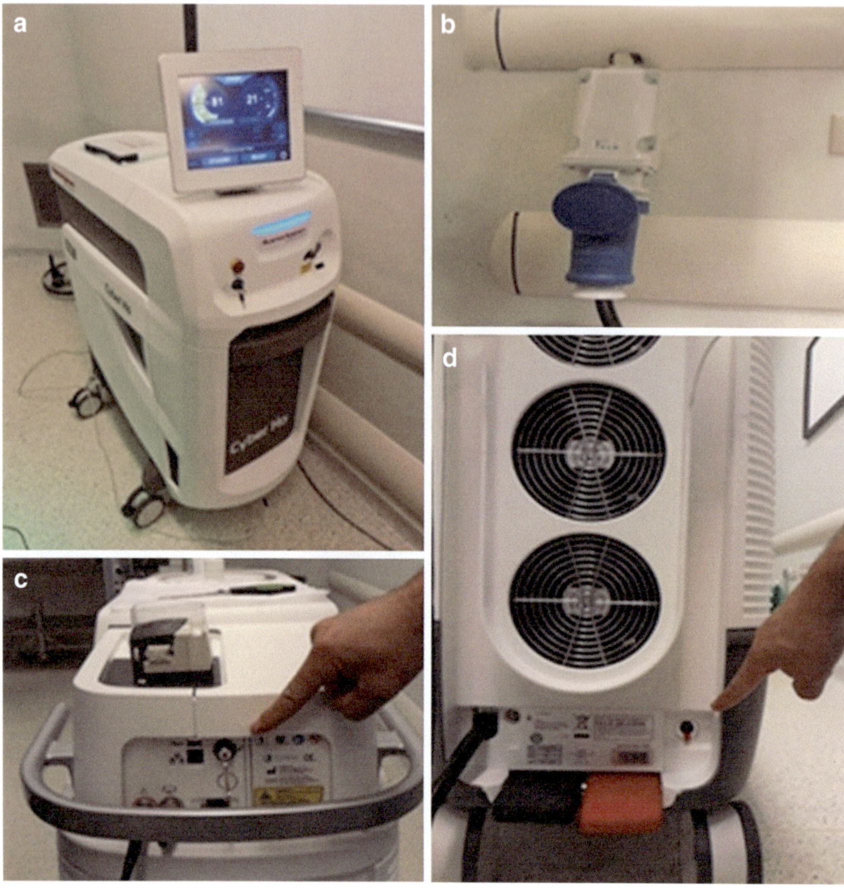

Fig. 3.4 (**a**) Holmium: YAG laser device. (**b**) The high-energy power line used for Holmium: YAG. (**c**, **d**) power transformer switches of laser generator

device design, it occupies little space and can easily change place in the operating room (Fig. 3.5b).

Position

The screen should be just in front of the surgeon and care should be taken not to hold the screen higher than the surgeon's height. Other screen or screens are used by the nurse, assistant or even the patient to monitor the operation. On the surgeon's right side, the assistant monitors the surgery and controls the equipment. In all cases, an experienced nurse is right behind the surgeon. All equipment is under her/his control during the process (Fig. 3.6).

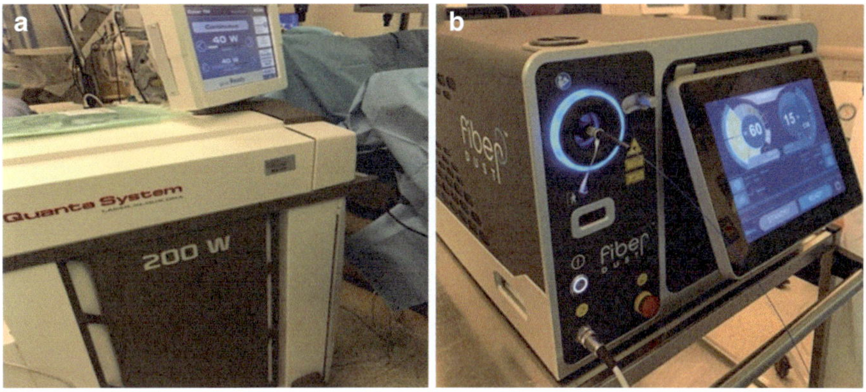

Fig. 3.5 (**a**) Thulium:YAG laser generator. (**b**) Thulium Fiber laser generator

Tissue Morcellator

After enucleation of the prostate, the adenoma pushed into the bladder is morcellated with a morcellator device and removed (Fig. 3.7). For morcellation, a 26-Fr nephroscope is used through which morcellator blade will pass. The footswitch that initiates the morcellation can preferably be located to the right or left of the surgeon. It is recommended to have foreign body forceps ready to remove small pieces of adenoma that may remain in the bladder after morcellation.

Laser Enucleation of the Prostate Techniques

In the last 25 years after Gilling described HoLEP and his own technique, various laser enucleation techniques and modifications have been defined in order to shorten the laser enucleation learning curve and minimize postoperative urinary incontinence [40]. In this section, Gilling's classical technique and its modifications, two lobe and en-bloc enucleation techniques and their modifications will be summarized.

Classic 3-Lobe Enucleation of the Prostate Technique

The classic technique was described by Gilling in 1998 and is known as Gilling's 3-lobe technique, which involves enucleation of the median lobe of the prostate and two lateral lobes separately in retrograde fashion [18, 53]. The classic technique begins with bilateral incisions in the bladder neck at the 5 and 7 o'clock positions. These incisions are extended vertically into the verumontanum and deepened until the surgical capsule. These incisions are joined transversely for median lobe

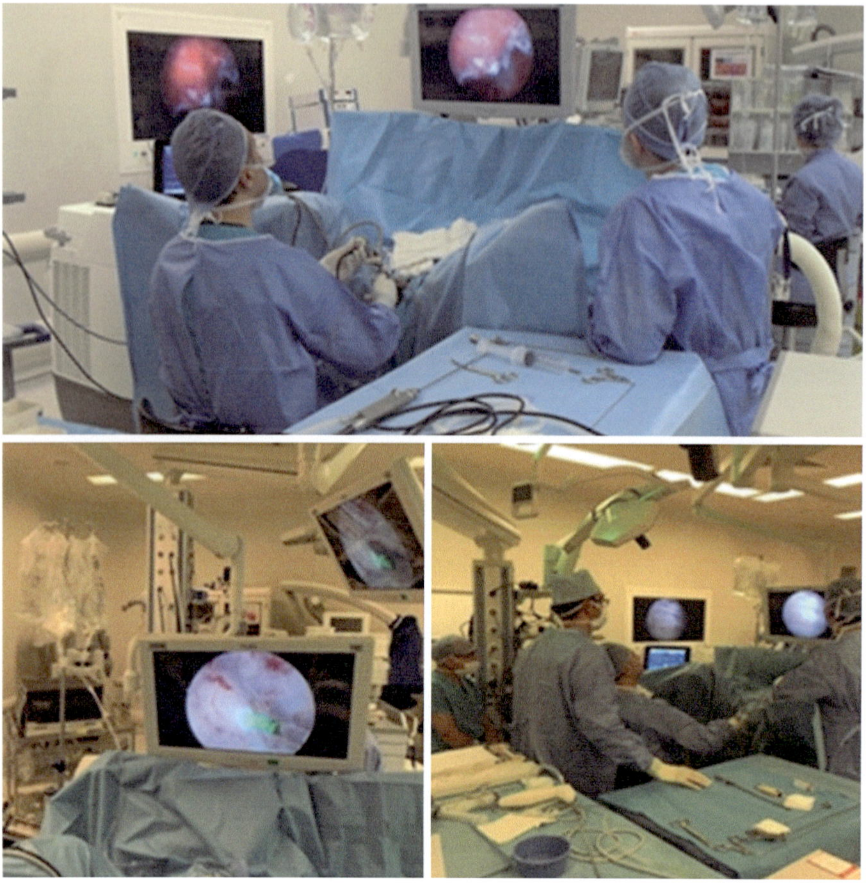

Fig. 3.6 Positions of surgeon, assistant, nurse and screens during the procedure

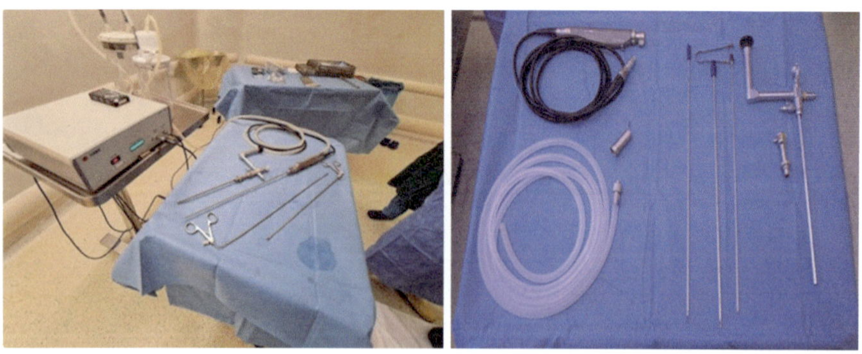

Fig. 3.7 Tissue morcellator and endoscopic instruments used during morcellation: Morcellator interconnections, tubing system and 26-Fr nephroscope through which the morcellator blade will pass

enucleation above the verumontanum. With blunt dissections, the median lobe is dissected from the surgical capsule. Next, both lateral lobes are enucleated. The medial edges of both lateral lobes, created by the incisions in the previous step to remove the median lobe, are extended towards the apex to more clearly define the apical anatomy. The lateral lobes are enucleated on both sides by lengthening the initial bladder neck incisions laterally and circumferentially at the apex, working toward the 2 and 10 o'clock positions. The depth created by the initial bladder neck incisions guides the surgical plan and subsequent dissections. Enucleation of the left lateral lobe is performed by circumferentially blunt dissections until the 2 o'clock position is reached. At the 12 o'clock position of the bladder neck, an elongated longitudinal incision is made distally and this incision is deepened to the level of the surgical capsule. The space between the adenoma and the surgical capsule is enlarged laterally and circumferentially by blunt dissection and "sweeping" maneuvers. The enucleation grooves from the upper and lower parts are joined at the 2 o'clock position of the apex and the left lateral lobe is fully enucleated and pushed into the bladder for morcellation. Then the same process is repeated for the right lateral lobe. Enucleation of the right lateral lobe is performed by circumferentially blunt dissections until the 10 o'clock position is reached, and the enucleated right lobe is also pushed into the bladder. After pushing the lateral lobes into the bladder, hemostasis is performed using laser. It should be noted that prolonging the incision at the 12 o'clock position will increase the risk of external urethral sphincter (EUS) injury.

Modifications of the 3-Lobe Technique

Kim et al. modified the 3-lobe technique to better protect the EUS around the prostate apex at the 12 o'clock position [27, 40]. In this modified technique, a small longitudinal incision is first made on either side of the verumontanum to define the prostatic capsule. Enucleation of the median lobe is initiated by deep and longitudinal incisions at 5 and 7 o'clock, from the bladder neck to the first incisions made on either side of the verumontanum. These incisions on both sides are then joined transversely proximal to the verumontanum for enucleation of the median lobe. Median lobe enucleation is completed by laser and blunt dissections. A small vertical incision is then made at the 12 o'clock position of the bladder neck and this incision is extended downward on both sides. In enucleation of both lateral lobes, the lateral lobes are lifted upwards with bottom-up dissections from 7 to 9 o'clock on the right side and from 5 to 3 o'clock on the left side (mucosal wing formation). Inverted V-shaped apical mucosal incisions are then made involving both lateral lobes. To separate the adenoma from the capsule without leaving any tissue, the left prostate adenoma part between 12 and 2 o'clock positions is approached from both sides, from bottom to top and from top to bottom, and the left side of the reverse V incision and the first apical incision made at 12 o'clock are joined anteriorly (anterior conjoining). At 1 or 2 o'clock position, the enucleation plane for the left lateral lobe is determined, enucleation of the left lateral lobe is performed, and the lobe is pushed into the bladder. The right prostate adenoma is circumferentially swept from bottom to top to enucleate the right lateral lobe. Enucleation is easily advanced from 7 o'clock position to the 10 o'clock position as the previous inverted V-shaped mucosal incision separates the mucosal layer.

Tunc et al. developed the "Omega Sign" technique with the aim of preserving the EUS structure by leaving a mucosal flap at the apex of the prostate between 2–10 o'clock and thus minimizing postoperative urinary incontinence [56]. In this technique, the first mucosal incisions begin at the 5 and 7 o'clock positions by aligning the ureteral orifices proximally at the bladder neck. These incisions are deepened until the fibers of the surgical capsule are visible. Additional mucosal incisions of 2–3 cm are made bilaterally from the proximal border of the verumontanum to the mucosal folds of the lateral lobes at the level of the prostatic apex. Posteriorly, the lateral lobes are dissected in the proximal and lateral directions, revealing the surgical plan. The proximal ends of the mucosal incisions at the level of the verumontanum are joined with the distal ends of the first incisions made at 5 and 7 o'clock positions starting from the bladder neck. As a result, two grooves form on either side of the median lobe. The grooves at 5 and 7 o'clock positions are joined with the incision proximal to the verumontanum. The median lobe is completely enucleated and pushed into the bladder by sweeping movements and blunt dissections. Then, the resectoscope is rotated at the level of the verumontanum and the distal end of the incision to be made at the 12 o'clock position is marked, then the incisions are extended approximately 1 cm laterally on both sides from this end. On both sides, these incisions are deepened until the fiber of the capsule is visible between 2 and 10 o'clock. The 5 and 7 o'clock incisions at the level of the prostatic apex are combined at the lateral end of 12 o'clock incision and at 2 and 10 o'clock positions in both lateral lobes. Enucleation of the lateral lobes is then performed. Enucleation of the lateral lobes at the beginning of surgery is extended retrogradely to the 10 o'clock position in the right lobe and 2 o'clock in the left lobe. Enucleation of the lateral lobes is completed at 2 and 10 o'clock position using blunt dissections and laser if necessary. The lobes are pushed into the bladder. Thus, the "Omega Sign", which is formed together with the preserved mucosal tissue in the anterior, becomes visible in the surgical site. The appearance of the "Omega Sign" confirms that all steps have been performed properly and EUS coaptation can also be observed. It has been suggested that incisions made between 2 and 10 o'clock positions in both lobes and leaving a mucosal flap between 2–10 o'clock contribute to the preservation of the EUS structure. The most important step forming the mucosal flap is the mucosal incisions, where the proximal part of the Omega-shaped EUS and the apex of the prostate are separated just before enucleation.

Endo et al. added the definition of anteroposterior dissection to the classical three-lobe technique, claiming that it would prevent sphincter damage [13]. In this modified technique, the enucleation of the median lobe is the same as the classical technique, but the enucleation of the lateral lobes differs. The lower edge of the lateral lobe is dissected from the surgical capsule between the apex and the bladder neck. This dissection is not extended upwards, only an edge that is stripped from the capsule is created. The urethral mucosa at 12 o'clock just above the verumontanum is then vaporized up to the surgical capsule. This vaporized area is extended towards the bladder neck. The lateral lobe is dissected from the surgical capsule in the middle of the adenoma. The lateral lobe is dissected from the area formed and separated in the first step towards the bladder neck. This maneuver mobilizes the adenoma. Then, this separated portion is extended anteroposteriorly and downwards towards 6 o'clock apical adenoma. This step of the technique is called "anteroposterior dissection". After this dissection, the apical urethral mucosa between 12 and 5 o'clock positions is naturally separated from the prostate capsule without damaging the EUS. The remaining apical arch-shaped urethral mucosa is completely separated from the adenoma and can then be cut without sphincteric damage. After removal of the left lateral adenoma, the intact ring structure formed by EUS is observed. It has been noted that dissecting the lateral lobe anteroposteriorly and vertically from 12 to 6 o'clock is the same as simulating finger movements during open prostatectomy. It has been suggested that this dissection provides both complete dissection of the apical adenoma and excision of the urethra without a mucosal incision.

Another modified version of the three-lobed technique was described by Gong et al. [21]. Enucleation begins at the apex. A short horizontal incision is made along the demarcation line between the left lateral lobe and the urethra near the proximal verumontanum, without exceeding the verumontanum, and this incision is extended circumferentially to the 3 o'clock position in the left lateral lobe. The same procedure is applied for the right lateral lobe; The first horizontal incision made proximal to the verumontanum is continued towards the right lateral lobe and the dissection is extended to the 9 o'clock position in the right lateral lobe. The median lobe is dissected towards the bladder neck. After dilation of the bladder neck, the posterior half-surface of the prostate (between 3, 6, and 9 o'clock positions) is released inferolaterally from the capsular base. The left lateral lobe separates from the median lobe at the 5 o'clock position. The incision in the left lateral lobe is then extended from 3 to 11 o'clock. Between 12 and 1 o'clock the urethral mucosal band is dissected, thus freeing the left lateral lobe from the anterior capsule. Enucleation of the right lateral lobe is performed similarly to the left lateral lobe. Since the right apical incision is made circumferentially from 9 o'clock to 11 o'clock, a urethral mucosal strip is formed between the 11 and 12 o'clock positions. The right lateral lobe is easily separated from the surgical capsule when the mucosal strip is dissected .

Two-Lobe Enucleation Techniques

Enucleation can be performed with the 2-lobe technique [11, 14]. According to Enikeev et al., surgery begins with a 6 o'clock incision in the bladder neck and is deepened until the circular capsular fibers are visible [14]. At the level of the seminal crest, the incision is continued counterclockwise, laterally to 5 o'clock position, towards the bladder neck. An incision is then made from the bladder neck to the verumontanum at 12 o'clock position. These incisions are then joined and the enucleated left lobe is pushed into the bladder. The same process is repeated for the right lobe enucleation.

Recently, Liu et al. described the "seven-step two lobe''HoLEP technique [35]. The first incision is made retrogradely from the side of the verumontanum at 5 o'clock position to the cleavage between the median and left lobe. The same process is repeated for the right side. A transverse incision is made at the anterior to the verumontanum and the bilateral surgical planes are thus combined. The median lobe, which joins the bilateral lobes, is slightly elevated to form a dihedral angle between the adenoma and the capsular plane. The posterior capsular plane is then dissected and the plane is expanded from apical 4–8 o'clock to approximately 5–7 o'clock proximal to the fan-shaped bladder neck. From the end of 5 o'clock incision in step 1, a retrograde incision is made across the left cleavage into the bladder neck. A retrograde dissection is then performed to create a cleavage between the lobes. It is deepened with laser incision and blunt separation movements until reaching the posterior space created in step 3. The same process is repeated on the opposite side and the median lobe is thus isolated. The isolated median lobe is released by dissections and pushed into the bladder. Strips holding the sphincter mucosa are observed at 4 and 8 o'clock positions. An upward circular incision is made from the left strip margin at the level of the distal verumontanum and joined with a contralateral circular incision at 12 o'clock position distal to the anterior commissure. The incisions are then deepened to completely separate the mucosa. Separation of the lateral lobes begins at 4 o'clock position. The endoscope is rotated to 12 o'clock along the surgical plane to create lateral and medial spaces. The surgical plane is extended along the midline above the anterior commissure to conform to the contralateral plane created from 8 o'clock. When the bilateral planes converge, the apical adenoma separates from the EUS and then circularly dissects towards the bladder neck until the two lobes are fully mobilized and pushed into the bladder.

En Bloc Enucleation Techniques

En bloc enucleation is a laser enucleation technique of the prostate that has been used since 2010. Scoffone and Cracco developed the 'en-bloc no touch' technique [48]. First, it is started with a small incision on the left lateral side of the verumontanum and the surgical plan is expanded retrogradely. The left lateral lobe is dissected longitudinally and retrogradely at 5 o'clock position from the apex to the bladder neck, enucleated laterally and moved from 5 o'clock position to 3 o'clock position. The enucleation is then advanced from 3 o'clock position to 12 o'clock position, then the dissections are continued in the right lateral lobe towards 9 o'clock position by passing the anterior commissure at 12 o'clock position. The first incision is then made in the left lateral aspect of the verumontanum. Through this incision, the apex of the right lateral lobe is reached with a horizontal incision over the verumontanum. The median lobe and right lateral lobe are then enucleated in a single block from 5 to 9 o'clock position. For the fan-shaped anterior mucosal tissue between 10 and 2 o'clock, two oblique incisions are made in the mucosa of the lateral lobes, at least 1 cm from the sphincter, in the adenoma, starting at 10 and 2 o'clock and converging at 12 o'clock, leaving a residual mucosal flap. A final horizontal incision is made at 12 o'clock by gently stretching the mucosa away from the sphincter, toward the bladder neck as proximally as possible. The enucleated adenoma is pushed into the bladder.

Ito et al. described the 'complete en-bloc' enucleation technique [24]. In this technique, the mucosa is incised from the side of the verumontanum to establish the correct surgical plan for enucleation in the right lobe apex. The plane between the adenoma and the surgical capsule is advanced retrogradely towards the bladder neck. Then, the fibers of the anterior fibromuscular stroma are cut at 10 o'clock position to expose the bladder lumen. After reaching the bladder lumen, enucleation is performed antegradely under the right and middle lobes. The left lobe is dissected antegradely and en-bloc enucleation of the entire adenoma is completed. When the adenoma completely separates from the capsule, a sphincteric mucosal band forms in the apical urethra. The apical mucosal band is cut without damaging the EUS. The enucleated adenoma is pushed into the bladder lumen. After the entire adenoma is removed, a solid ring structure is observed, in which the sphincter is formed. The advantage of this surgical technique is that the surgical plan can be preserved throughout the procedure.

Minagawa et al. described another en bloc enucleation technique [37]. The mucosa is cut bilaterally from the side of the verumontanum to expose the surgical capsule. The urethral mucosa at 12 o'clock position just above the verumontanum is incised into the surgical capsule. To separate the area between the right and left adenoma, the incision is made until the anterior fibromuscular stroma is visible at its apex. Enucleation extends proximal and from the bladder neck anteroposteriorly and inferiorly; this is followed by enucleation of the adenoma towards the prostate apex at 6 o'clock position. Since the adenoma is enucleated in the upper region from the urethral sphincter, the urethral mucosa of the apex is naturally pushed aside to form an arch-shaped mucosal band at 3 o'clock position in the left lateral lobe and at 9 o'clock position in the right lateral lobe. It is observed that the apical urethral mucosa collapses naturally into an arch without damaging the ring formed by the sphincter muscle. The lateral adenoma apex behind this mucosal arch is completely separated from the surgical capsule and urethral mucosa. The incisions are joined just proximal to the verumontanum and the tissue layers are joined left and right at 6 o'clock. The remaining connection between the adenoma and the surgical capsule leaves the bladder neck inferiorly to the verumontanum. The en-bloc adenoma is then pushed into the bladder. After the en-bloc adenoma is removed, it is observed that the intact ring structure formed by the sphincter is preserved. It has been suggested that this en bloc procedure preserves the surgical plane between the prostate adenoma and the capsule and leaves no residual prostate adenoma.

Miernik and Schoeb developed the '3 horse shoe-like incision HoLEP' technique, which is the en block HoLEP method in which a three-horse shoe incisions are made [36]. The first incision is made around the seminal colliculus in an inverted U shape (first horse shoe incision) and the median lobe is dissected for enucleation.

Apical prostate adenomas on both sides are enucleated until a mucosal band forms in both lateral lobes. The mucosal band between the external sphincter and both lateral lobes is cut with a single incision and another inverted U incision is made from 10 to 2 o'clock position (second horse shoe incision). This ensures complete mobilization of the apical part of the prostate. The resectoscope shaft is then placed between the anterior commissure and the surgical capsule at 12 o'clock position. Then, dissection is continued towards the bladder neck with laser and blunt dissection. Thus, a canal is formed between the surgical capsule and the anterior commissure of the bladder neck at 11–1 o'clock. Here, a third inverted U incision is made into the bladder neck to partially separate the adenoma from the bladder neck (third horse shoe incision); both lateral lobes are now circumferentially enucleated. Then, the lateral sides of both lateral lobes are circularly mobilized until the lateral part of the median lobe on both sides is reached. The median lobe is then mobilized retrogradely to the level of the bladder neck. The attachment on the bladder neck between 4 and 8 o'clock is cut with laser. Unlike other en bloc methods, this technique does not make longitudinal incisions in the prostatic urethra. It has been suggested that complications arising from longitudinal incisions that do not follow anatomical landmarks can be potentially prevented by this technique, and enucleation can be performed without leaving any residual tissue with this technique.

Another en-bloc enucleation technique, 'En Bloc with early apical release' was defined by Saitta et al. [46]. The mucosal incision is initiated by the proximal edge of the external sphincter at the apex of the prostate, where an incision is made from 11 to 1 o'clock. The incision is then made parallel to the verumontanum up to the margin of the sphincter and joined with the anterior incision made earlier. The same process is performed on the opposite side. This step results in complete separation of the apex from the sphincter. Dissection of the apex is performed by deepening the para-sphincteric tissue from 6 to 12 o'clock with laser and mild blunt dissections until the entire right apex is freed from the sphincter. The same steps are performed on the opposite side, apex anteriorly, at 12 o'clock until it is completely free from the sphincter. Next, the crista urethralis is cut over the verumontanum to separate the apex from the sphincter. The enucleation plan is followed circumferentially and the bladder neck is approached. The bladder neck is then cut circumferentially, observing the ureteral orifices. Enucleation is completed. This method of early release of the sphincter from the prostatic capsule is suggested to be a crucial step in sphincter preservation as it prevents sphincter stretching.

Kim et al. described the 'all-in-one' prostate enucleation technique with Thulium laser in 2015 [28]. In this technique, enucleation begins at the apex. An incision is made around the inverted U-shaped verumontanum. The incision is continued until the surgical capsule is identified. A marking incision is made at the apex at 12 o'clock to prevent the urethral sphincter. Then, the upper incision line at 12 o'clock and the end of the inverted U-shaped incision line at 5 and 7 o'clock are circumferentially connected. A deep incision is then made along the lateral circumferential line until the surgical capsule is visible from 5 or 7 o'clock to 12 o'clock. The enucleation process continues until the bladder neck. Near the bladder neck, the release of the enucleated adenoma proceeds latero-inferiorly from 12 o'clock. The region between 5 and 7 o'clock, which belongs to the median lobe, is released last.

Sancha et al. developed the en-block enucleation technique with lithium triborate (LBO) (Greenlight) laser [20]. Bilateral incisions are made on both sides of the verumontanum, the surgical plane is created between the capsule and the adenoma, and the planes are combined medially, proximal to the verumontanum (capsular localization maneuver). A careful mechanical dissection is made towards the bladder neck at 6 o'clock and a 6 o'clock incision is made upwards from the bottom of the adenoma to vaporize the adenomatous tissue. Incisions are made at 5 and 7 o'clock without trying to reach the surgical capsule. The capsular localization maneuver is performed, and instead of cutting the plane at 6 o'clock, the dissection follows the direction of the previous incisions at 5 o'clock and 7 o'clock. The remaining adenomatous tissue is vaporized and two channels are created at 5 and 7 o'clock that reach the surgical capsule. The median lobe is then mechanically dissected and pushed into the bladder. A circumferential incision is made to mark the boundary between the apex of the adenoma and the EUS. Crista urethralis is not cut. Capsular localization maneuver is performed on the right side and enucleation is performed. The apex is cut and freed from the sphincter. The dissection is directed ventrally and the bladder is entered spontaneously at 11 o'clock, following the anatomical plan between the capsule and the adenoma. Then the bladder neck is cut towards 12 and 7 o'clock. When the right side is completely separated from the capsule, the same steps are performed on the other side. While all lateral and anterior aspects of the adenoma are free, the crista urethralis is cut at 6 o'clock and its posterior surface is released. To push the adenoma "en bloc" into the bladder, the attachment is cut at the bladder neck at 6 o'clock.

Different techniques are used in laser enucleation of the prostate. In this context, the question comes to the fore: "Which enucleation technique is the best and which technique should we use?" It would be logical for the surgeon to choose the technique on which the surgeon has the most experience and completes the learning curve, best performed by the surgeon and minimizes residual adenoma tissue, and has low rates of postoperative urinary incontinence.

Laser Enucleation of the Prostate: Tips in the Learning Curve

Although laser enucleation of the prostate is the most popular benign prostate hyperplasia (BPH) surgery in recent years, it has not been as widespread as other transurethral methods due to its long learning curve. The reasons for the long learning curve can be summarized with a few items: Since the endoscopic enucleation of the prostate (EEP) procedure is performed in 3D prostate surgery on a 2D screen, it is difficult to understand and manipulate the entire surgical anatomy of the prostate. In addition, unlike other conventional transurethral prostate surgeries, EEP is performed retrograde fashion rather than antegrade. In addition, making the first mucosal incision at the correct depth and at the appropriate point, finding and maintaining the correct surgical plan between the surgical capsule and the adenoma, using the laser appropriately during enucleation, and performing blunt dissections with the correct angle and force are some of the difficulties faced by surgeons who are newly starting the EEP procedure [52]. These difficulties are the reasons of the obstacles (except for the equipment cost) to the widespread use of EEP surgery.

Studies in the literature report that the learning curve of HoLEP is 40–50 cases [6, 42, 43]. Du et al. showed that postoperative transient stress urinary incontinence (SUI) in the first 50 cases of HoLEP surgery was more common than in patients after 50 cases [8]. In a very recent systematic review, it has been shown that 30–40 cases for HoLEP, at least 20–30 cases for Greenlight laser, Although heterogeneous data, 30 cases for ThuLEP, 40–50 cases for bipolar prostate enucleation are necessary to reach a plateau in the learning curve [15]. Therefore, it can be concluded that 30–50 cases are necessary for the plateau for EEP.

This section will focus on the parameters that are important in the learning curve of EEP surgery.

The Role of the Mentor in the Learning Curve

Mentor-based education is effective for learning EEP and shortening the learning curve [16, 39, 52, 54]. Enikeev et al. stated in a randomized study that 30 cases performed with a mentor are required for a safe and effective EEP [14]. In 2010, a mentoring program structured by Holmium User Group was initiated for urologists who intended to perform HoLEP [1]. Urologists participating in this program have 2.5 operating days and under the supervision of mentors, they make selected cases, starting with small prostates and in the continuation large prostates. Shin et al. suggested that the HoLEP learning curve can be shortened with the mentor-based "hand-grab navigated technique' '[52]. In this technique, the mentor actively guides the urologist's hand holding the camera and demonstrates the necessary maneuvers.

In a multicenter, prospective study, it was shown that one-third of urologists without mentors abandon EEP surgery because of the increased risk of complications [45]. For urologists who want to learn EEP, starting with a mentor is a logical choice.

The Role of Prostate Size in the Learning Curve

It is important to choose the appropriate prostate size during the EEP learning curve. Shah et al. showed that the surgeon adapted to the procedure after an average of 20 cases in small prostates [51]. Haraguchi et al. reported HoLEP learning curve for medium-sized prostate more reproducible throughout that small or large according to prostate and medium-sized always start to learn with prostate [22]. Although the possibility of bleeding is less in small prostates, it is difficult to distinguish the surgical plane between a surgical capsule and an adenoma. On the other hand, while the surgical capsule can be distinguished better in large prostates, loss of orientation is more likely in these prostates since it is more difficult to maintain the surgical plane. Teoh et al. recommended that a size range of 50–80 g would be an appropriate choice for the ideal prostate size at the beginning of the learning curve [54].

The Role of Endoscopic Surgery Experience in the Learning Curve

Brunkhorst et al. stated that surgeons with >500 TURP experience had a learning curve of 40–60 cases for HoLEP [6]. Al-Hakim et al. suggested that transurethral surgery experience is necessary for successful HoLEP surgery [9]. Gazel et al. investigated the association of laparoscopic surgery experience with the HoLEP learning curve with a questionnaire study, since they have common aspects such as blunt dissections and separation of tissues from each other, tissue resistance felt tactilely, and working in a 3-dimensional surgical field with 2D screen images [19]. In the study, it was stated that surgeons with high laparoscopic experience had a short HoLEP learning curve.

Simulation, Training Programs and Operation Videos

Simulations and training programs have an important place in surgical training because inexperienced surgeons get used to the operations, the learning curve accelerates and there is no possibility of harming a real patient. Therefore, if possible, it is beneficial to include simulator and training models in surgical training programs [54]. In 2015, Kuronen-Stewart et al. presented the UroSim HoLEP simulator, a virtual reality simulator [30]. The authors stated that the simulator is useful to the users. However, this simulator does not give users a real laser application and irrigation fluid experience. Another HoLEP simulator, which includes a prostate model consisting of two layers, inner and outer layer, has also been validated and evaluated as usable for surgical training by experienced and inexperienced urologists [3]. The European Urology Association Section of Urotechnology (ESUT) AEEP (anatomic endoscopic enucleation of the prostate) Working Group demonstrated for the first time the usability of a fresh frozen cadaver training model in AEEP training [55]. Although realistic anatomy and tissue similarity are among the most important advantages of this model, the inability to simulate bleeding and the expensiveness of obtaining cadavers are among the limitations of the model. Apart from training programs, many operation videos available on the internet can be used to become familiar with the procedures and better understand the surgical steps, and can increase the basic knowledge level before practicing [54].

Intraoperative Highlights

One of the most important challenges in the EEP learning curve is to determine the depth of the laser incision in the prostate mucosa, thus finding the correct surgical plan between the surgical capsule and prostate adenoma and maintaining this plan throughout the enucleation procedure. To identify the prostatic capsule, the mucosa must begin to be incised from the bladder neck or near the verumontanum [41]. Ureteral orifices and verumontanum can be designated as a guide for checkpoints and incisions for the enucleation procedure [19]. For example, when starting with a bladder neck incision, the 5 and 7 o'clock points are aligned with the ureteral orifices and the end point of the incision is determined as the verumontanum [57]. A mentor who is present during the operation can guide inexperienced surgical incision depth and length, introduce the correct surgical plan, and continue the operation if orientation is lost. In addition, it may be useful to watch a large number of operations from live or video recordings before starting the surgical application, in order to distinguish the surgical capsule structure from adenoma.

The most common concern of EEP surgery is postoperative stress urinary incontinence. Inexperienced surgeons may damage the external sphincter by overstretching the 12 o'clock position during apical dissection or by the thermal effect of the laser [25]. While enucleating anterior prostatic tissue, it is important to leave a mucosal flap at the apex of the prostate at the 12 o'clock position, to protect the urethral sphincter and to maintain continence [41, 57]. However, since the anatomical borders of the urethral sphincter at the 12 o'clock position are not precise, difficulties may be encountered in preserving this region. Scoffone and Cracco have pointed out several important points to protect the urethral sphincter at 12 o'clock [48]. According to the authors, the incision should be made at least 1 cm from the sphincter and gently flex the adenoma towards the bladder neck as the prostate apex cuts through the mucosa. Thus, the incision is made as far from the sphincter as possible. Saidta et al. suggested that early separation of the external sphincter from the apex of the prostate at the 12 o'clock allows better visualization of the surgical plan and reduces the postoperative incontinence rate [47].

It is known that a plateau is reached more quickly in tissue morcellation compared to prostate enucleation in the learning curve [25]. The most important complication to be encountered during morcellation is bladder injury. Morcellators in use in the market are safe and effective devices [17]. However, there are some important points to consider from the learning curve during morcellation: The bladder must be kept sufficiently full to avoid possible bladder injuries. For continuous control of safe morcellation, adequate hemostasis should be performed to ensure a clear endoscopic view, and the irrigation fluid flow should be sufficient.

Incontinence and Ejaculation Disorders, and Complications After Laser Enucleation of the Prostate

Incontinence and Ejaculation

Incontinence after 'Laser Enucleation of Prostate' (LEP) was observed at high rates, especially in the period when the technique was first described. Thanks to enucleation techniques suitable for the anatomical structure of the external urethral sphincter (EUS), which were developed to maintain continence, acceptable and largely temporary incontinence rates began to be seen. Stress-type (SUI) or urge-type (UUI) incontinence can be seen after LEP. Observing similar incontinence rates in all laser types used for LEP, especially Holmium-YAG (HoLEP) and Thulium-YAG (ThuLEP), suggests that the problem of incontinence after LEP is related to the enucleation technique rather than the energy source used [26, 59].

Urgency and UUI after LEP are usually described by patients as mild [31]. The main reason is thought to be the high amount of energy applied to the prostate capsule during enucleation [50]. UUI rates vary between 1–16% in the literature. In a study with small series conducted in the years when the technique was first applied, Fraundorfer et al. reported that the incidence of UUI was 16% in the early period following urethral catheter removal after HoLEP, and this rate regressed to 5% in the first month [18]. In more recent and high-series another study, the rates of UUI after HoLEP were reported as 4% immediately after catheter removal and 1% at postoperative 1 month [57]. In many studies, UUI rates are reported as 1–2% in short-term follow-ups, and it is a rare complaint especially in controls longer than 6 months. Conservative approaches that will contribute to the storage function of the bladder and, if necessary, the use of antimuscarinic agents can be considered in the relief of symptoms.

SUI seen after LEP is reported in the literature in the range of 4.9–12.5%. These rates are higher than those seen in 'Transurethral Resection of Prostate-TURP' (2%) and 'Open Prostatektomi-OP' (3–9%), the most frequently compared surgeries [40]. However, it should be noted that these rates are not permanent and decrease gradually in the postoperative period. Shah et al., in their study which they shared their first HoLEP experiences, found the rates of early SUI as 10.7%, but reported the rates of permanent incontinence as 0.7% [50, 51]. Similarly, Elzayat et al. reported their rates of SUI after HoLEP as 4.2% and indicated that this rate decreased to 0.5% in the follow-ups [12]. More recent studies continue to emphasize the transient character of incontinence after LEP.

Another point that should be mentioned about SUI after LEP is that much less SUI rates are reported today, thanks to some techniques developed especially considering the structure of EUS. It can be said that the common aspects of these techniques are that they provide enucleation in accordance with EUS structure and/or they cut the connection between prostatic adenoma and EUS before enucleation starts. In this way, the EUS is prevented from being exposed to traction during the retrograde enucleation and loss of function in the postoperative period. In this regard, Tunc et al. reported the rates of SUI in the 1st month as 1% after the HoLEP performed with the technique they described, and as 0.2% in the ongoing SUI in the 6th month follow-up [57]. Similarly, Gong et al. reported 1.58% of SUI in their study, in which they published the results of their modified techniques, and stated that this problem resolved within 3 months postoperatively [21].

In order to prevent or at least reduce the incontinence seen after LEP to reasonable rates, the first thing to consider is that the prostatic adenoma is released from EUS before enucleation begins. In addition, it is important that the incision to be made to separate both lateral lobes from each other at the 12 o'clock position is not extended to the verumontanum and kept at the appropriate length-depth. Reducing the laser power used during apical dissection/enucleation as much as possible will decrease the possibility of damage to the sphincter. Last but not least, doing blunt dissection as much as possible during enucleation and avoidance of laser application to the prostate capsule unless necessary are points to be considered in terms of reducing UUI rates.

Ejaculation disorders are among the most common problems after prostate enucleation, regardless of whether the technique is open or endoscopic. In the literature, approximately 75% retrograde ejaculation (RE) frequency is reported after LEP [5, 58]. In the results of HoLEP performed by leaving some prostate tissue adjacent to the verumontanum to protect ejaculation, Kim et al. Reported their overall ejaculation preservation success as 46.2% [58]. However, it should be emphasized that even with the ejaculation-preserving technique, the rate of patients with the same ejaculate olüme as in the preoperative period is as low as 15.4%. Studies evaluating sexual functions do not reveal significant differences in terms of ED and orgasmic functions (except for RE) [5, 10, 33].

Complications

The percentage of complications seen after LEP is comparable to or better than other modalities used in the surgical treatment of BPH. In meta-analyses compared to monopolar TURP, LEP seems more advantageous in terms of hemoglobin decrease and blood transfusion rates [61]. Furthermore, in studies comparing LEP with Bipolar TURP, no statistically significant difference was found in terms of complication rates in addition to functional results, however, postoperative irrigation time was found to be shorter in the LEP arm [7, 44]. Additionaly, in two meta-analyses comparing LEP and AP, similar to other surgical method comparisons, less blood loss and the need for blood transfusion were found in the LEP arm; however, there was no statistically significant difference in the incidence of other complications such as urinary tract infection, need for re-intervention for clot or bleeding control, pneumonia and ischemic diseases, bladder neck contracture and urethral stricture [32, 34].

In the light of this comparative data, considering the frequency of non-specific complications after LEP; the rate of blood transfusion is 1.7–2.2%, urethral stricture

2.4–7%, urinary tract infection 3.2–6.8%, bladder neck contracture 0–3.9%, and the need for postoperative early cystoscopic intervention 2.2% [2, 4, 29, 49, 50].

Complications which specific to endoscopic enucleation techniques after LEP include perforations that may occur in the prostate capsule or under the bladder neck during enucleation, and mucosal or ureteral orifice injuries that may occur in the bladder during morcellation.

Prostatic capsule perforation is seen at a rate of 1.5–9.6% in the literatüre [29, 50]. It usually develops as a result of forcing the prostatic capsule with the resectoscope during enucleation. In particular, the presence of fibrotic and resistant fibers between the prostatic adenoma and the capsule, which makes blunt enucleation difficult, may increase the possibility of perforation. Another condition that may predispose to capsule perforation is related to the shape of the prostate. It is known that the long transverse diameter of the prostate makes especially lateral lobe enucleation difficult [60]. In such prostates, having to use the resectoscope at a compelling angle during lateral lobe enucleation may cause inability to move the instruments as desired and this may facilitate the development of complications.

In order to prevent prostatic capsule perforation, it is important to perform dissection and enucleation in a way that lifts the adenoma from the capsule without advancing the surgical instrument forward. In addition, resistant fibrotic fibers that make enucleation difficult should be separated by laser without insisting on blunt dissection. Capsule perforation noticed during surgery is managed according to the depth and size of the perforation. While the procedure may be continued in small perforations that do not cause intense fluid leakage out of the surgical site, in large perforations and/or perforations with intra-abdominal findings, the procedure should be terminated and the patient should be followed up with a urethral catheter.

False passage formation under the bladder neck is a rare (<1%) complication that almost always occurs during median lobe enucleation [29]. In particular, the presence of a large or asymmetrical median lobe increases the risk. To avoid this complication, during median lobe enucleation, the resectoscope should be withdrawn occasionally to view the surgical site from a wider angle and the distance of the enucleation margin to the bladder neck should be checked. The approach to perforations under the bladder neck is the same as for prostatic capsule perforations.

The frequency of intravesical mucosal injury that may occur during morcellation has a wide range of 1.3–18.2% [23, 29, 38, 50]. However, in current studies, rates less than 4% are generally reported. Ureteral orifice injury, which is another complication that may develop due to morcellator use, can also be seen during the use of laser on the bladder neck. Especially in prostates with median lobe that is large or indented into the bladder, care should be taken to protect the ureteral orifices when using lasers during separation of the median lobe from the bladder neck. Apart from this, in order to prevent intra-bladder injuries due to the morcellator, it is important to control bleeding before morcellation for a good optical image, to ensure proper filling of the bladder, and to keep the blade of the morcellator away from the bladder wall. Mucosal injuries in the bladder are usually superficial and do not require additional treatment or can be treated by prolonging the urethral catheterization time. However, in the presence of more serious injury, appropriate surgical repair is also among the options.

References

1. Aho T, Herrmann TR. Description of a modular mentorship programme for holmium laser enucleation of the prostate. World J Urol. 2015;33:497–502.
2. Ahyai SA, Gilling P, Kaplan SA, Kuntz RM, Madersbacher S, Montorsi F, Speakman MJ, Stief CG. Meta-analysis of functional outcomes and complications following transurethral procedures for lower urinary tract symptoms resulting from benign prostatic enlargement. Eur Urol. 2010;58:384–97.
3. Aydin A, Ahmed K, Brewin J, Khan MS, Dasgupta P, Aho T. Face and content validation of the prostatic hyperplasia model and holmium laser surgery simulator. J Surg Educ. 2014;71:339–44.
4. Bach T, Netsch C, Haecker A, Michel MS, Herrmann TR, Gross AJ. Thulium:YAG laser enucleation (VapoEnucleation) of the prostate: safety and durability during intermediate-term follow-up. World J Urol. 2010;28:39–43.
5. Briganti A, Naspro R, Gallina A, Salonia A, Vavassori I, Hurle R, Scattoni E, Rigatti P, Montorsi F. Impact on sexual function of holmium laser enucleation versus transurethral resection of the prostate: results of a prospective, 2-center, randomized trial. J Urol. 2006;175:1817–21.
6. Brunckhorst O, Ahmed K, Nehikhare O, Marra G, Challacombe B, Popert R. Evaluation of the learning curve for holmium laser enucleation of the prostate using multiple outcome measures. Urology. 2015;86:824–9.
7. Chen YB, Chen Q, Wang Z, Peng YB, Ma LM, Zheng DC, Cai ZK, Li WJ, Ma LH. A prospective, randomized clinical trial comparing plasmakinetic resection of the prostate with holmium laser enucleation of the prostate based on a 2-year followup. J Urol. 2013;189:217–22.
8. Du C, Jin X, Bai F, Qiu Y. Holmium laser enucleation of the prostate: the safety, efficacy, and learning experience in China. J Endourol. 2008;22:1031–6.
9. El-Hakim A, Elhilali MM. Holmium laser enucleation of the prostate can be taught: the first learning experience. BJU Int. 2002;90:863–9.
10. Elshal AM, El-Assmy A, Mekkawy R, Taha DE, El-Nahas AR, Laymon M, El-Kappany H, Ibrahiem EH. Prospective controlled assessment of men's sexual function changes following holmium laser enucleation of the prostate for treatment of benign prostate hyperplasia. Int Urol Nephrol. 2017;49:1741–9.
11. Elshal AM, El-Nahas AR, Ghazy M, Nabeeh H, Laymon M, Soltan M, Ghobrial FK, El-Kappany HA. Low-power vs high-power holmium laser enucleation of the prostate: critical assessment through randomized trial. Urology. 2018;121:58–65.
12. Elzayat EA, Habib EI, Elhilali MM. Holmium laser enucleation of the prostate: a size-independent new "gold standard". Urology. 2005;66:108–13.
13. Endo F, Shiga Y, Minagawa S, Iwabuchi T, Fujisaki A, Yashi M, Hattori K, Muraishi O. Anteroposterior dissection HoLEP: a modification to prevent transient stress urinary incontinence. Urology. 2010;76:1451–5.
14. Enikeev D, Glybochko P, Rapoport L, Gahan J, Gazimiev M, Spivak L, Enikeev M, Taratkin M. A randomized trial comparing the learning curve of 3 endoscopic enucleation techniques (HoLEP, ThuFLEP, and MEP) for BPH using mentoring approach-initial results. Urology. 2018;121:51–7.
15. Enikeev D, Morozov A, Taratkin M, Misrai V, Rijo E, Podoinitsin A, Gabdullina S, Herrmann TRW. Systematic review of the endoscopic enucleation of the prostate learning curve. World J Urol. 2021;39:2427–38.
16. Feng L, Song J, Zhang D, Tian Y. Evaluation of the learning curve for transurethral Plasmakinetic enucleation and resection of prostate using a mentor-based approach. Int Braz J Urol. 2017;43:245–55.
17. Franz J, Suarez-Ibarrola R, Putz P, Sigle A, Lusuardi L, Netsch C, Lehrich K, Herrmann TRW, Gratzke C, Miernik A. Morcellation after endoscopic enucleation of the prostate: efficiency and safety of currently available devices, vol. 8. Eur Urol Focus; 2021. p. 532–44.

18. Fraundorfer MR, Gilling PJ. Holmium:YAG laser enucleation of the prostate combined with mechanical morcellation: preliminary results. Eur Urol. 1998;33:69–72.
19. Gazel E, Kaya E, Yalcin S, Tokas T, Yilmaz S, Aybal HC, Aydogan TB, Tunc L. The role of laparoscopic experience on the learning curve of HoLEP surgery: a questionnaire-based study. Turk J Urol. 2020;46:129–33.
20. Gomez Sancha F, Rivera VC, Georgiev G, Botsevski A, Kotsev J, Herrmann T. Common trend: move to enucleation-is there a case for GreenLight enucleation? Development and description of the technique. World J Urol. 2015;33:539–47.
21. Gong YG, He DL, Wang MZ, Li XD, Zhu GD, Zheng ZH, Du YF, Chang LS, Nan XY. Holmium laser enucleation of the prostate: a modified enucleation technique and initial results. J Urol. 2012;187:1336–40.
22. Haraguchi T, Takenaka A, Yamazaki T, Nakano Y, Miyake H, Tanaka K, Kuwayama M, Takechi Y, Fujisawa M. The relationship between the reproducibility of holmium laser enucleation of the prostate and prostate size over the learning curve. Prostate Cancer Prostatic Dis. 2009;12:281–4.
23. Iacono F, Prezioso D, Di Lauro G, Romeo G, Ruffo A, Illiano E, Amato B. Efficacy and safety profile of a novel technique, ThuLEP (Thulium laser enucleation of the prostate) for the treatment of benign prostate hypertrophy. Our experience on 148 patients. BMC Surg. 2012;12 Suppl 1:S21.
24. Ito T, Tamura K, Otsuka A, Shinbo H, Takada S, Kurita Y, Miyake H. Development of a complete En-Bloc technique with direct bladder neck incision: a newly modified approach for holmium laser enucleation of the prostate. J Endourol. 2019;33:835–40.
25. Kampantais S, Dimopoulos P, Tasleem A, Acher P, Gordon K, Young A. Assessing the learning curve of holmium laser enucleation of prostate (HoLEP). A systematic review. Urology. 2018;120:9–22.
26. Kaya E, Yılmaz S, Açıkgöz O, Aybal HC, Yılmaz M, Gazel E, Yalcın S, Suarez-Ibarrola R, Tunc L. Laser enucleation for prostates larger than 100 mL: comparison of HoLEP and ThuLEP. Andrologia. 2021;53:e14125.
27. Kim M, Lee HE, Oh SJ. Technical aspects of holmium laser enucleation of the prostate for benign prostatic hyperplasia. Korean J Urol. 2013;54:570–9.
28. Kim YJ, Lee YH, Kwon JB, Cho SR, Kim JS. A novel one lobe technique of thulium laser enucleation of the prostate: 'All-in-One' technique. Korean J Urol. 2015;56:769–74.
29. Kuo RL, Paterson RF, Siqueira TM Jr, Watkins SL, Simmons GR, Steele RE, Lingeman JE. Holmium laser enucleation of the prostate: morbidity in a series of 206 patients. Urology. 2003;62:59–63.
30. Kuronen-Stewart C, Ahmed K, Aydin A, Cynk M, Miller P, Challacombe B, Khan MS, Dasgupta P, Aho TF, Popert R. Holmium laser enucleation of the prostate: simulation-based training curriculum and validation. Urology. 2015;86:639–46.
31. Larner TR, Agarwal D, Costello AJ. Day-case holmium laser enucleation of the prostate for gland volumes of < 60 mL: early experience. BJU Int. 2003;91:61–4.
32. Li M, Qiu J, Hou Q, Wang D, Huang W, Hu C, Li K, Gao X. Endoscopic enucleation versus open prostatectomy for treating large benign prostatic hyperplasia: a meta-analysis of randomized controlled trials. PLoS One. 2015;10:e0121265.
33. Li Z, Chen P, Wang J, Mao Q, Xiang H, Wang X, Wang X, Zhang X. The impact of surgical treatments for lower urinary tract symptoms/benign prostatic hyperplasia on male erectile function: a systematic review and network meta-analysis. Medicine (Baltimore). 2016;95:e3862.
34. Lin Y, Wu X, Xu A, Ren R, Zhou X, Wen Y, Zou Y, Gong M, Liu C, Su Z, Herrmann TR. Transurethral enucleation of the prostate versus transvesical open prostatectomy for large benign prostatic hyperplasia: a systematic review and meta-analysis of randomized controlled trials. World J Urol. 2016;34:1207–19.
35. Liu K, Xiao C, Hao Y, Ma L. 'Seven-step two-lobe' HoLEP: a modification to gain efficiency of the enucleation applying relatively low-power holmium laser devices. World J Urol. 2021;39:2627–33.

36. Miernik A, Schoeb DS. "Three horse shoe-like incision" holmium laser enucleation of the prostate: first experience with a novel en bloc technique for anatomic transurethral prostatectomy. World J Urol. 2019;37:523–8.
37. Minagawa S, Okada S, Sakamoto H, Toyofuku K, Morikawa H. En-bloc technique with anteroposterior dissection holmium laser enucleation of the prostate allows a short operative time and acceptable outcomes. Urology. 2015;86:628–33.
38. Montorsi F, Naspro R, Salonia A, Suardi N, Briganti A, Zanoni M, Valenti S, Vavassori I, Rigatti P. Holmium laser enucleation versus transurethral resection of the prostate: results from a 2-center, prospective, randomized trial in patients with obstructive benign prostatic hyperplasia. J Urol. 2004;172:1926–9.
39. Netsch C, Bach T, Herrmann TR, Neubauer O, Gross AJ. Evaluation of the learning curve for thulium VapoEnucleation of the prostate (ThuVEP) using a mentor-based approach. World J Urol. 2013;31:1231–8.
40. Oh SJ. Current surgical techniques of enucleation in holmium laser enucleation of the prostate. Investig Clin Urol. 2019;60:333–42.
41. Oh SJ, Shitara T. Enucleation of the prostate: an anatomical perspective. Andrologia. 2020;52:e13744.
42. Peyronnet B, Robert G, Comat V, Roupret M, Gomez-Sancha F, Cornu JN, Misrai V. Learning curves and perioperative outcomes after endoscopic enucleation of the prostate: a comparison between GreenLight 532-nm and holmium lasers. World J Urol. 2017;35:973–83.
43. Placer J, Gelabert-Mas A, Vallmanya F, Manresa JM, Menéndez V, Cortadellas R, Arango O. Holmium laser enucleation of prostate: outcome and complications of self-taught learning curve. Urology. 2009;73:1042–8.
44. Qian X, Liu H, Xu D, Xu L, Huang F, He W, Qi J, Zhu Y, Xu D. Functional outcomes and complications following B-TURP versus HoLEP for the treatment of benign prostatic hyperplasia: a review of the literature and meta-analysis. Aging Male. 2017;20:184–91.
45. Robert G, Cornu JN, Fourmarier M, Saussine C, Descazeaud A, Azzouzi AR, Vicaut E, Lukacs B. Multicentre prospective evaluation of the learning curve of holmium laser enucleation of the prostate (HoLEP). BJU Int. 2016;117:495–9.
46. Saitta G, Becerra JEA, Del Alamo JF, Gonzalez LL, Elbers JR, Suardi N, Gomez-Sancha F. 'En Bloc' HoLEP with early apical release in men with benign prostatic hyperplasia. World J Urol. 2019a;37:2451–8.
47. Saitta G, Becerra JEA, Del Álamo JF, González LL, Elbers JR, Suardi N, Gómez-Sancha F. 'En bloc' HoLEP with early apical release in men with benign prostatic hyperplasia. World J Urol. 2019b;37:2451–8.
48. Scoffone CM, Cracco CM. The en-bloc no-touch holmium laser enucleation of the prostate (HoLEP) technique. World J Urol. 2016;34:1175–81.
49. Seki N, Mochida O, Kinukawa N, Sagiyama K, Naito S. Holmium laser enucleation for prostatic adenoma: analysis of learning curve over the course of 70 consecutive cases. J Urol. 2003;170:1847–50.
50. Shah HN, Mahajan AP, Hegde SS, Bansal MB. Peri-operative complications of holmium laser enucleation of the prostate: experience in the first 280 patients, and a review of literature. BJU Int. 2007a;100:94–101.
51. Shah HN, Mahajan AP, Sodha HS, Hegde S, Mohile PD, Bansal MB. Prospective evaluation of the learning curve for holmium laser enucleation of the prostate. J Urol. 2007b;177:1468–74.
52. Shin DG, Kim HW, Park SW, Park CS, Choi S, Oh TH, Lee DH, Lee CY, Kim JM, Lee JZ. New surgical instruction method for Homium laser enucleation of the prostate, "hand-grab navigated technique," to shorten the learning curve: the results of multicenter analysis. Low Urin Tract Symptoms. 2018;10:247–52.
53. Tan AH, Gilling PJ. Holmium laser prostatectomy: current techniques. Urology. 2002;60:152–6.

54. Teoh JY, Cho CL, Wei Y, Isotani S, Tiong HY, Ong TA, Kijvikai K, Chu PS, Chan ES, Ng CF, T. Asian Urological Surgery, G. Education. Surgical training for anatomical endoscopic enucleation of the prostate. Andrologia. 2020;52:e13708.
55. Tunc L, Bozzini G, Scoffone CM, Guven S, Hermann T, Porreca A, Misrai V, Ahyai S, Zor M, Aksoy E, Gozen AS. Determination of face and content validity of cadaveric model for holmium anatomic endoscopic enucleation of the prostate training: an ESUT AEEP group study. Eur Urol Open Sci. 2021a;32:28–34.
56. Tunc L, Yalcin S, Kaya E, Gazel E, Yilmaz S, Aybal HC, Yilmaz M, Tokas T. The "omega sign": a novel HoLEP technique that improves continence outcomes after enucleation. World J Urol. 2021b;39:135–41.
57. Tunc L, Yalcin S, Kaya E, Gazel E, Yılmaz S, Aybal HC, Yılmaz M, Tokas T. The "omega sign": a novel HoLEP technique that improves continence outcomes after enucleation. World J Urol. 2021c;39:135–41.
58. Wilson LC, Gilling PJ, Williams A, Kennett KM, Frampton CM, Westenberg AM, Fraundorfer MR. A randomised trial comparing holmium laser enucleation versus transurethral resection in the treatment of prostates larger than 40 grams: results at 2 years. Eur Urol. 2006;50:569–73.
59. Xiao KW, Zhou L, He Q, Gao XS, Chen G, Ma YC, Li H, Wang KJ. Enucleation of the prostate for benign prostatic hyperplasia thulium laser versus holmium laser: a systematic review and meta-analysis. Lasers Med Sci. 2019;34:815–26.
60. Yalcin S, Gazel E, Somani BK, Yilmaz S, Tunc L. Prostate shape significantly affects the HoLEP procedure time and energy usage: a retrospective pilot study. Minim Invasive Ther Allied Technol. 2019;28:220–6.
61. Zhang Y, Yuan P, Ma D, Gao X, Wei C, Liu Z, Li R, Wang S, Liu J, Liu X. Efficacy and safety of enucleation vs. resection of prostate for treatment of benign prostatic hyperplasia: a meta-analysis of randomized controlled trials. Prostate Cancer Prostatic Dis. 2019;22:493–508.

Chapter 4
Robotic and Laparoscopic Prostate Adenomectomy

Mustafa Kirac

Introduction

Benign prostatic hyperplasia (BPH) is one of the most important health problems of the aging man. An estimated 1.1 to 1.2 billion people per year around the world have lower urinary tract complaints. In these patients, BPH is most of the lower urinary tract complaints. The quality of life of patients deteriorates due to the symptoms that occur as they get older. In advanced cases, complications such as urinary retention, bleeding, kidney dysfunction and bladder stones secondary to BPH occur, and patients sometimes require surgical operation. When the decision for surgical treatment is made, it is important which technique will be applied to which patient. As is known, open simple prostatectomy (OSP) is the standard surgical treatment for patients with enlarged prostate. Retropubic or suprapubic (transvesical) open prostatectomy is conventionally performed for prostate volumes greater than 80 g [1]. However, most surgeons and most clinics revise the 80 gram limit based on their own experience. Some experienced surgeons perform an endoscopic approach to prostates that are 80 grams or slightly larger. We know that endoscopic techniques such as monopolar or bipolar TUR-P (transurethral resection of the prostate), HoLEP (holmium laser enucleation of the prostate), ThuLEP (thulium laser enucleation of the prostate) are also applied in prostate volumes over 80 grams.

OSP, which is conventionally performed to large-volume prostates, has some disadvantages. Perioperative and postoperative complication rate of OSP can be up to 42% [2]. It has been demonstrated that OSP causes more complications such as prolonged hospitalization time, late return to work time, increased bleeding and transfusion rate, and prolonged catheterization time. The high morbidity and complication rate caused by OSP has led to the emergence of more minimally invasive

---

M. Kirac (✉)
Üsküdar University, Department of Urology, Istanbul, Türkiye

S. Tonyali et al. (eds.), *Current Endourology*,
https://doi.org/10.1007/978-3-032-00010-1_4

techniques for the treatment of expanding adenomas and new searches in this direction.

Terminology

As with every new technique, many different terminologies are used in robotic and laparoscopic prostate adenomectomy. As is known, this surgery is a laparoscopic method, not an endoscopic method. The abdomen is entered and the prostate is reached by the peritoneal or extraperitoneal route. The terms 'robotic/laparoscopic simple prostatectomy', 'robotic/laparoscopic transvesical prostatectomy', 'robotic/laparoscopic adenomectomy', 'robot-assisted' describe this technique. In fact, all of these terms express what is meant to be said. However, the European Association of Urology (EAU) has recently adopted the term 'minimally invasive simple prostatectomy (MISP)' for this. According to the EAU, this terminology is a general expression that covers both laparoscopic and robotic techniques at the same time. The term 'robotic simple prostatectomy (RSP)' can be used when using a robot, and the term 'laparoscopic simple prostatectomy (LSP)' can be used when a laparoscopic surgery is performed. It can be said that this is the most appropriate terminology for urologists to use a common language. However, different expressions will not pose a problem in terms of defining the technique.

Indications

As is known, OSP is a gold standard treatment modality for large-volume prostates if surgery is planned. Recently, alternative techniques to OSP have been developed thanks to technological advances. These techniques, called endoscopic enucleation, are holmium laser enucleation of the prostate (HoLEP) and thulium laser vapoenucleation of the prostate (ThuVEP) [3]. Laparoscopic or robotic simple prostatectomy techniques are enucleation methods and are therefore indicated for large-volume prostates. European and American urology associations express similar views on this issue. According to the guideline published by the American Urological Association, three methods (HoLEP, ThuVEP, RBP/LBP) for prostates over 80 grams are defined as surgical techniques to be selected according to the surgeon's experience [4]. On the other hand, the European urology guideline states that minimally invasive simple prostatectomy (MISP) is a suitable method for men with a prostate larger than 80 ml. The level of evidence for this expression is 1A [1].

In conclusion, if patients are eligible for surgery, simple prostatectomy via robotic or laparoscopic technique is an appropriate and feasible method in patients with prostate over 80 grams.

Surgical Technique

Mariano et al. performed the first laparoscopic simple prostatectomy in 2002, and this operation was replaced by robotic techniques mostly later on [5]. Sotelo et al. described the first robotic simple prostatectomy in 2008. Both techniques can be performed through transperitoneal or retroperitoneal approach [6]. In addition, prostate enucleation can be performed by the transvesical (Freyer) or transcapsular (Millin) approach in both techniques. Modified techniques have been described recently. Castillo et al. described a modified technique that included longitudinal capsular and vesical incision, plication of the prostatic capsule, and posterior-only urethro-vesical anastomosis [7]. Clavijo et al. described intrafascial RSP with principles similar to the intrafascial radical prostatectomy technique [8]. In this section, we will describe the robotic transperitoneal transvesical simple prostatectomy technique.

Patient Preparation

The urine of each patient with surgical indication should be sterilized. Preoperative urine culture should be done and if there is an infection, it must be treated. A consent form containing detailed information about the surgery should be given to the patients at least one day before the operation. The risk of bleeding, thromboembolic complications, vascular and organ injuries, and complications that may develop secondary to anesthesia should be explained to patients in detail. In the morning of the operation, patients are given an enema and they are put on knee embolism socks in order to reduce the risk of postoperative thromboembolism. Routine bowel cleansing is unnecessary.

The anesthesia preparation of patients is completed a few days before the operation. Pre-evaluation of the patient in terms of anesthesia is very important. For the evaluation of patients especially with co-morbidities and for preoperative medication, these patients should be hospitalized at least one day before the operation. The relevant departments should evaluate patients with chronic obstructive pulmonary disease or cardiac problems preoperatively and their eligibility for anesthesia should be determined. After the patients are taken to the operating room and it is understood that the robotic system works perfectly and there is no problem, they are delivered to the anesthesia team. Patients should be administered preoperative antibioprophylaxis with third generation cephalosporins or quinolones before anesthesia in the operating room.

Operating Room

The operating room should be a wide room where the robot can fit comfortably, away from noise, and where the auxiliary equipment and the robot can move easily. A surgical nurse, an assistant surgeon and a console surgeon may perform the operation with the attendance of allied health personnel. The following figure (Fig. 4.1) shows the robotic operation room layout.

Surgical Instruments

The surgical instruments and robotic system to be used should be checked prior to anesthesia. The surgical nurse should prepare a table with instruments that may be needed for open surgery when necessary. Instruments used for standard RSP are as follows:

Laparoscopic Instruments:

1. Hot water thermos
2. Veress needle
3. Gas hose
4. Laparoscopic aspirator with irrigation and aspiration features, 5 mm, 45 cm long
5. Trocar, 10–12 mm (2 pcs)
6. Endobag, 10 mm
7. Ligation clips

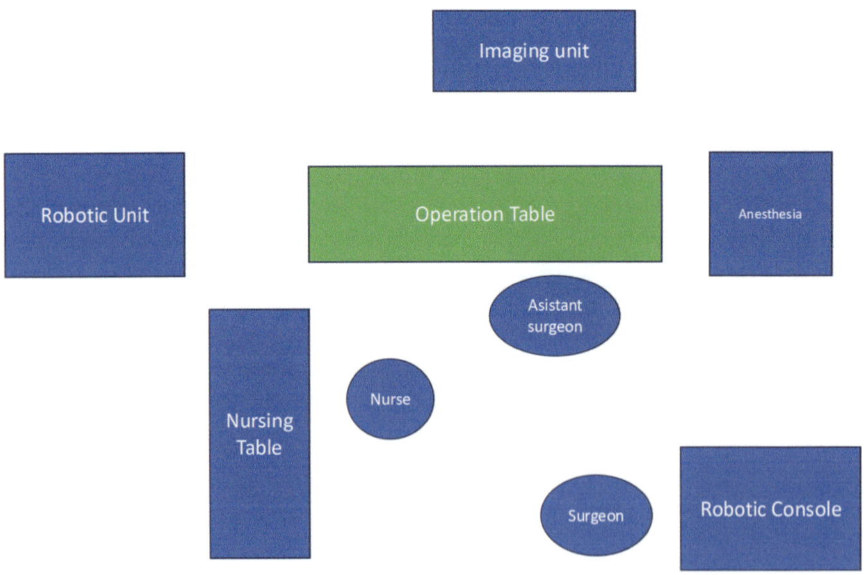

Fig. 4.1 The placement of operation room

Robotic tools and materials:

1. da Vinci-S Monopolar Curved Scissors, 8 mm (1 piece)
2. da Vinci-S Maryland Bipolar Forceps, 8 mm (1 piece)
3. da Vinci-S Prograsp Forceps, 8 mm (1 piece)
4. da Vinci-S Large Needle Driver, 8 mm (2 pcs)
5. Robotic trocar, 8 mm (3 pcs)
6. Robotic trocar seal, (3 pcs)
7. Tip cover (for monopolar curved scissors) (1 piece)
8. Camera arm adapter (1 piece)
9. Camera head adapter (1 piece)
10. Robotic monopolar and bipolar cautery cable (1 piece)
11. Robotic camera and camera arm cover
12. Covers for robotic arms
13. Robotic light cable (1 pcs)
14. Robotic endoscope, 0° and 30°

Starting the Robotic System

For the possibility of any technical problems, the robot should be started and checked first. If there is no problem, the patient should be administered general anesthesia. All cable connections between the surgical console, the system with robotic arms, the bedside unit and the display monitor must be made. After these checks, the operation should be started.

Operation

Anesthesia team performs necessary controls and medication after anesthesia. When everything is in order, the surgical team initiates the operation. The operation steps are as follows, respectively:

1. Position of the patient

   While the patient is on the operating table, his/her arms should be fixed and wrapped around the trunk in the adduction position. The legs and thighs are supported by placing silicone pads or surgical greens under them. In order to prevent the patient from slipping off the table, a shield is placed on the patient's shoulders and silicone pads are placed between the shield and the shoulder. Then, the operating table is given Trendelenburg position of 30 degrees. A metal shield is attached to the operating table at a distance of about one span from the patient's head and face. Shield draping is made to isolate the operation site. An 18 F urethral catheter is inserted after the patient's operation site has been sterilized and draped. Patient position is shown in Fig. 4.2.

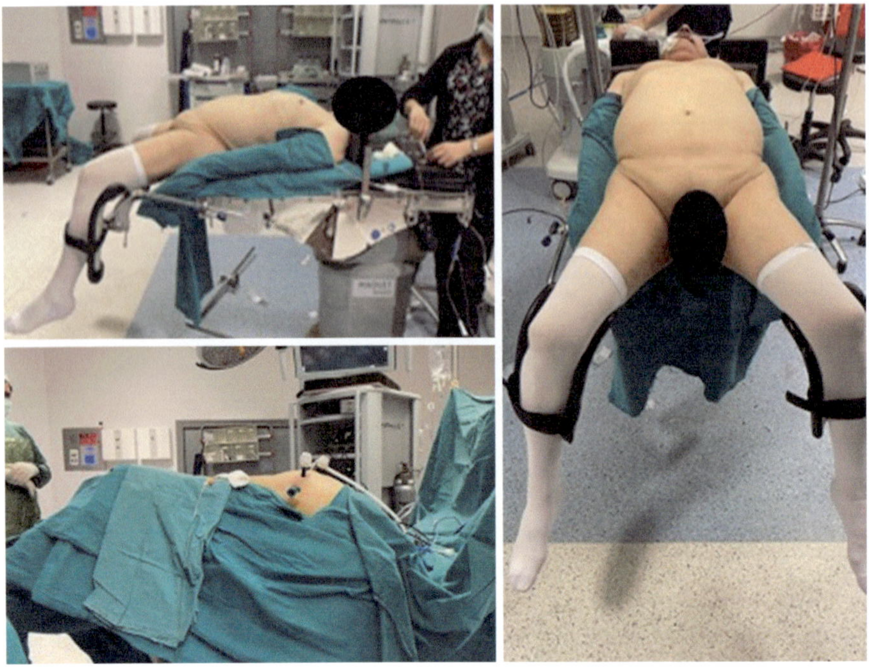

Fig. 4.2 Patient position

2. Placement of trocars

   A total of 5 trocars are used in robotic simple prostatectomy. Trocars including 3 pieces of 8 mm for the robotic arms, 1 piece of 12 mm for the camera port and 1 piece of 10–12 mm for the assistant port are used. İnsufflation is performed using a Veress needle through an incision 2 cm superior to the umbilicus. Next, when sufficient pressure is reached, a camera trocar of 12 mm is inserted. Next, other trocars are inserted, observing the epigastric vessels under direct vision and light. One robotic trocar of 8 mm is inserted in the center of a horizontal line drawn on the 4-finger right side of the umbilicus. The second robotic trocar of 8 mm is inserted at the point where the 4-finger lateral of the line drawn first intersects with 2–3 cm below the umbilicus. The third robotic trocar of 8 mm is inserted at the point where a horizontal line 10–12 cm from the left lateral of the umbilicus intersects with the transverse line 1–2 cm below the umbilicus. The 12 mm assistant port is inserted between the camera trocar and the third robotic trocar. This placement should be modified. Trocar localizations are shown in Fig. 4.3.

3. Intraperitoneal access

   After the trocars are inserted, the robot camera with a 0-degree optical lens is inserted. Urinary bladder is visualized. Intestinal segments spread over the rectovesical space and bladder dome, if any, are elevated. If there are intraperitoneal adhesions that prevent access to the bladder dome, these should be carefully released.

4. Opening the bladder and placement of suspension sutures

   At this stage, 300 cc of saline is injected into the bladder from the inserted Foley catheter and the intraperitoneal reflection of the bladder is observed. The bladder is vertically exposed as full layer. Suspension suturing should be made in the bladder after exposure. The bladder is suspended bilaterally on the abdominal upper wall using No. 0 vicryl fixated on a plane needle that can pass through the abdominal wall in full-thickness. If necessary, the lower corner of the bladder incision can be grasped and retracted using the robot's Prograsp forceps. Next, the camera is inserted into the bladder and localizations of bilateral orifices are primarily observed (Fig. 4.4)

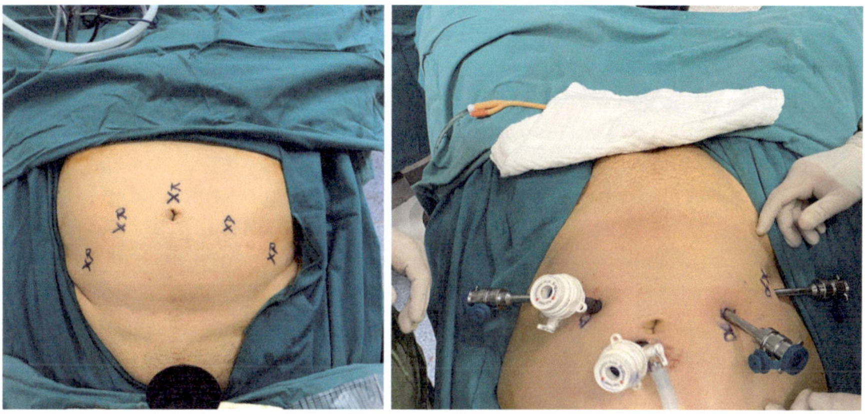

Fig. 4.3 Trocar placement

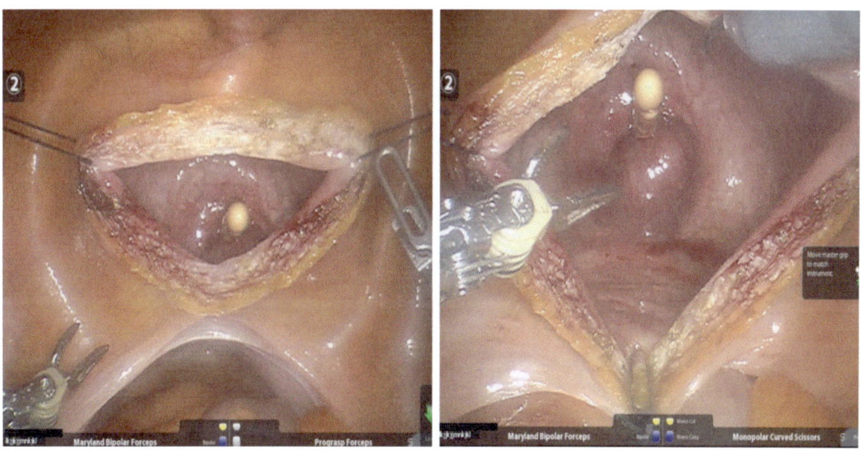

Fig. 4.4 Bladder ekartation with sutures placed on the abdominal wall

5. Marking the prostate from the bladder neck

   The prostate and bladder mucosa are evaluated at this stage and in the appropriate position, the mucosa is marked all around by means of a cautery. While marking, it should be checked again that it is away from the ureteral orifices. The enucleation phase will be easier if the mucosa is incised a little deeper while marking (Fig. 4.5).

6. Enucleation of the prostate

   The enucleation step is the most important phase of the surgery that must be performed carefully. It can be very easy with proper planning. However, undesirable results may occur in a wrong planning. The 6 o'clock radius should be chosen for enucleation. Next, the prostate is carefully dissected from the base to the lateral segments. In case of bleeding during enucleation, the vessels can be cauterized under direct vision. The most critical point at this time is enucleation of the apical tissues. During enucleation of the apex, the prostate shrinks anatomically and the apex begins to rotate from the pelvic floor. The catheter can be seen at this time and the urethra is cut. After enucleation, residual tissues in the locus can also be excised (Fig. 4.6).

7. Hemostatic control and suturing the bladder neck

   One of the main advantages of RSP is to ensure more comfortable hemostasis. Under direct vision, hemorrhagic areas can be controlled by means of a bipolar or monopolar cautery. Suturing the bladder neck is important to ensure more effective hemostasis. This step is optional. However, performing the procedure ensures effective hemostasis and helps anatomical recovery. Suturing of the bladder neck can be circumferential and continuous, or it can be made from 5 and 7 o'clock radii. We prefer circumferential and continuous suturing (Fig. 4.7).

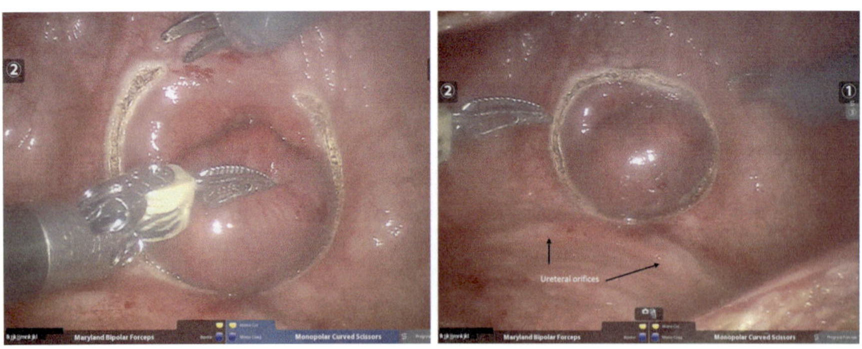

Fig. 4.5 Marking the bladder neck and for enucleation of the prostate, view of the ureteral orifices

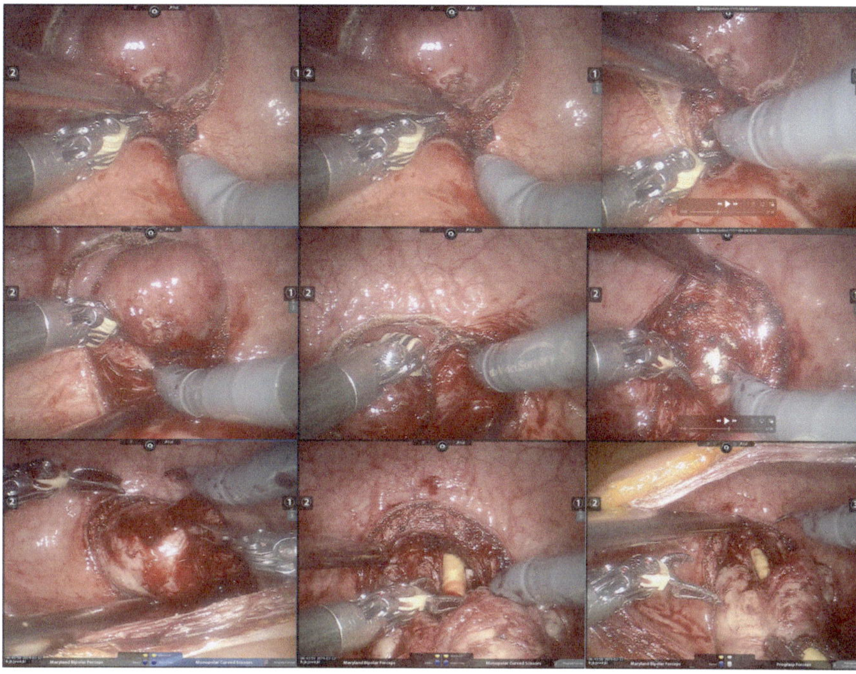

Fig. 4.6 Enucleation of the prostatic adenoma

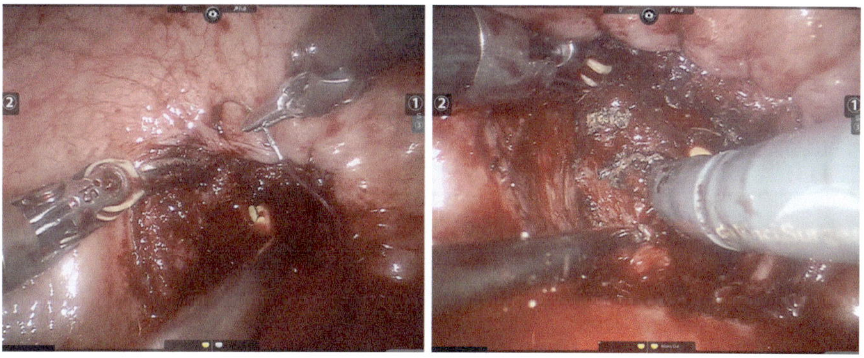

Fig. 4.7 Hemostatic control and suturing the bladder neck

8. Closure of the bladder and insertion of a drain

   After ensuring hemostasis, a 3-way Foley catheter is inserted into the bladder. Its balloon is inflated around 30–40 cc. Next, the bladder is closed. To do this, the mucosa, detrusor and peritoneum can be closed separately or all layers can be closed with a single suture (Fig. 4.8). After the bladder is closed, tightness must be strictly checked.

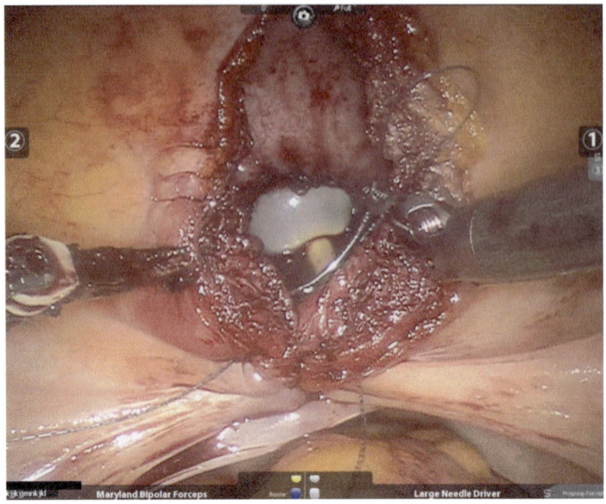

Fig. 4.8 Closing the bladder

Efficacy and Complication

Since 2002, when it was first performed, the use of minimally invasive simple prostatectomy has been gradually increased. Increasing robotic surgery centers and the presence of experienced surgeons in these centers have made this surgery more feasible. The efficacy of this technique has been evaluated and reported in many studies and case series. There is no prospective randomized study evaluating the efficacy of MISP in the literature. However, case series and comparative studies have shown that MISP is a safe and effective procedure in patients with prostates of 80 g and above [9]. In studies involving the RSP technique, a longer operation time has been reported compared to other methods (OSP, LSP, laser enucleation), however, no difference was found in terms of efficacy and complication rates.

Lucca et al. compared MISP and OSP in a study involving 764 patients and 27 meta-analyses [10]. Of the 27 operations in this study, 8 were operations performed with robotic technique. According to the results of this study, mean Q-max increase was 14.3 ml/s, mean IPSS improvement score was 17.2, mean operation time was 141 minutes, mean blood loss was 284 ml, mean hospital stay was 1.6 days, and complication rate was 13.6% [1, 10]. According to these results, mean blood loss, hospital stay and catheterization time were determined to be significantly shorter than OSP values. The improvement in IPSS and Q-max values was similar in both groups.

In a multicentric study by Autorino et al. [11] involving 1330 patients, 487 patients with RSP and 843 patients with LBP were evaluated. According to the results of this study, the mean operation time was 154 minutes, the mean blood loss was 200 ml, and the mean hospital stay was 2 days in 487 patients with robotic operations. According to the general results of this study, the mean prostate volume was 100 ml, blood transfusion was 3.5%, the rate of return to open surgery was 3.5%, and the complication rate was 10.6%. It was emphasized that there was no difference in efficacy in both methods and that the MISP technique could be performed effectively and safely.

In another study [12] in which robotic and open techniques were compared and included 59 patients, the groups were compared and the results were reported. The hospital stay was significantly shorter (1.5 & 2.6 days), less blood loss (339 & 587 ml) was found in patients with robotic surgery, and the rates of Q-max, IPSS, improvement in quality of life, and reduction in PVR and PSA values were similar in both groups. Results of a study from Turkey in which Kirac et al. performed robotic simple prostatectomy on 42 patients were published [13]. According to the results of this study, the mean prostate volume was 128 cc, the mean operation time was 112 minutes, the mean blood loss was 210 ml, and the mean hospital stay was 1.6 days. Based on these results, the authors demonstrated that RSP surgery can be performed safely and effectively.

On the other hand, when Umari et al. compared 81 patients with RBP and 45 patients with HoLEP, they found no difference in terms of operation time and complications [14]. When Zhang and et al. compared the results of 32 patients with RBP and 600 patients with HoLEP, they found that the operation time was lower in the HoLEP group [15].

Besides the effectiveness of RSP surgery, another factor to be evaluated is cost. This is actually a complex problem and varies according to countries and systems used. Data on this subject are variable. While there are studies reporting that the robotic method is more expensive than the open technique [16], there are also authors who state that it is less costly [17]. It is difficult to make a definite judgment since there is no cost analysis made under the conditions of our country. However, the cost of robotic surgery is considered to be higher in our country.

In conclusion, robotic and laparoscopic simple prostatectomy is a good method for patients with prostate over 80 g and requiring surgery. These open techniques can be applied especially in large prostates.

Tips and Tricks

The tricks of robotic simple prostatectomy surgery are as follows:

1. We definitely perform it for prostates over 80 grams.
2. Transperitoneal and transvesical (Freyer) procedures are ideal and easy.
3. We use exactly the same places as the robotic radical prostatectomy technique as trocar insertion sites.
4. The vertical opening of the bladder provides a more convenient field of view than the transverse opening.
5. Before enucleation, we always check the localizations of the ureteral orifices.
6. We initiate enucleation at 6 o'clock radius.
7. Post-enucleation hemostasis is very important. We cauterize the hemorrhagic areas using bipolar cautery. If the hemorrhage is large, we apply tamponade by inflating the balloon of the Foley catheter for 8 to 10 minutes in the prostatic locus.

8. After hemostasis is ensured, we suture the bladder neck all around with 3/0 vicryl. Thus, the bladder neck heals more anatomically.
9. There is no need to place a cystostomy in the bladder.
10. The bladder can be closed in a single layer.
11. We remove the urethral catheter on the postoperative day 6 or 7.

References

1. EAU guidelines 2021. Management non-neurogenic LUTS. https://uroweb.org/guideline/treatment-of-non-neurogenic-male-luts/
2. Elshal AM, El-Nahas AR, Barakat TS, Elsaadany MM, El-Hefnawy AS. Transvesical open prostatectomy for benign prostatic hyperplasia in the era of minimally invasive surgery: perioperative outcomes of a contemporary series. Arab J Urol. 2013;11:362–8.
3. Meyer D, Weprin S, Zukovski EB, Porpiglia F, Hampton LJ, Autorino R. Rationale for robotic-assisted simple prostatectomy for benign prostatic obstruction. Eur Urol Focus. 2018;4:643–7.
4. Foster HE, Barry MJ, Dahm P, Gandhi MC, Kaplan SA, Kohler TS, Lerner LB, Lightner DJ, Parsons JK, Roehrborn CG, et al. Surgical management of lower urinary tract symptoms attributed to benign prostatic hyperplasia: AUA guideline. J Urol. 2018;200:612–9.
5. Mariano MB, Graziottin TM, Tefilli MV. Laparoscopic prostatectomy with vascular control for benign prostatic hyperplasia. J Urol. 2002;167:2528–9.
6. Sotelo R, Clavijo R, Carmona O, Garcia A, Banda E, Miranda M, Fagin R. Robotic simple prostatectomy. J Urol. 2008;179:513–5.
7. Castillo O, Vidal-Mora I, Rodriguez-Carlin A, Silva A, Schatloff O, Borgna V. Modified urethrovesical anastomosis during robot-assisted simple prostatectomy: technique and results. Prostate Int. 2016;4:61–4.
8. Clavijo R, Carmona O, De Andrade R, Garza R, Fernandez G, Sotelo R. Robot-assisted intrafascial simple prostatectomy: novel technique. J Endourol. 2013;27:328–32.
9. Kordan Y, Canda AE, Köseoğlu E, Balbay D, Laguna MP, de la Rosette J. Robotic-assisted simple prostatectomy: a systematic review. J Clin Med. 2020;9(6):1798.
10. Lucca I, Shariat SF, Hofbauer SL, Klatte T. Outcomes of minimally invasive simple prostatectomy for benign prostatic hyperplasia: a systematic review and meta-analysis. World J Urol. 2015;33:563–70.
11. Autorino R, Zargar H, Mariano MB, Sanchez-Salas R, Sotelo RJ, Chlosta PL, et al. Perioperative outcomes of robotic and laparoscopic simple prostatectomy: a European-American multi-institutional analysis. Eur Urol. 2015;68(1):86–94. https://doi.org/10.1016/j.eururo.2014.11.044. Epub 2014 Dec 4.
12. Sorokin I, Sundaram V, Singla N, Walker J, Margulis V, Roehrborn C, Gahan JC. Robot-assisted versus open simple prostatectomy for benign prostatic hyperplasia in large glands: a propensity score-matched comparison of perioperative and short-term outcomes. J Endourol. 2017;31(11):1164–9.
13. Kirac M, Ergin G, Kibar Y, Köprü B, Biri H. Robotic simple prostatectomy is a safe and effective technique for benign prostatic hyperplasisa: Our single center initial short-term follow-u results for 42 patients. Turk J Urol. 2021;47(4):313–8.
14. Umari P, Fossati N, Gandaglia G, Pokorny M, De Groote R, Geurts N, Goossens M, Schatterman P, De Naeyer G, Mottrie A. Robotic assisted simple prostatectomy versus holmium laser enucleation of the prostate for lower urinary tract symptoms in patients with large volume prostate: a comparative analysis from a high volume center. J Urol. 2017;197:1108–14.

15. Zhang MW, El Tayeb MM, Borofsky MS, Dauw CA, Wagner KR, Lowry PS, Bird ET, Hudson TC, Lingeman JE. Comparison of perioperative outcomes between holmium laser enucleation of the prostate and robot-assisted simple prostatectomy. J Endourol. 2017;31:847–50.
16. Sutherland DE, Perez DS, Weeks DC. Robot-assisted simple prostatectomy for severe benign prostatic hyperplasia. J Endourol. 2011;25:641–4.
17. Matei DV, Brescia A, Mazzoleni F, Spinelli M, Musi G, Melegari S, Galasso G, Detti S, de Cobelli O. Robot-assisted simple prostatectomy (RASP): does it make sense? BJU Int. 2012;110:E972–9.

Chapter 5
Medical Management and Prevention of Urinary Stone Disease

Harun Ucmak, Mehmet Giray Sonmez, and Gokhan Gokce

Prevention

Nephrolithiasis is influenced by a number of genetic and environmental factors. Diet is a major environmental component. The developments in the surgical treatment of urinary system stones were not reflected in the medical treatment at the same rate, but with the understanding of the mechanisms in the formation of the stones, the studies on medical treatment have accelerated and the importance of the preventive approach has increased. Conservative treatment can be applied to all stone patients regardless of stone type or individual risk factors. Because stone recurrence was reported at high rates (50%) in five years of follow-up. The authors analyze the effect of diet on renal stone formation in an effort to demonstrate that better control of this environmental component may attenuate this disease [1–3].

Hydration

Many studies have shown that increasing fluid intake reduces the risk of stone formation. Stone recurrence is reduced by 60% with increasing fluid intake [4]. Increased fluid consumption results in excretion of a higher volume of urine which is less saturated and theoretically benefits all stone formers. It has been found that excessive fluid intake decreases urinary calcium phosphate, calcium oxalate and monosodium urate saturation and increases the calcium oxalate crystallization

H. Ucmak · M. G. Sonmez (✉)
Department of Urology, Meram Medical Faculty, Necmettin Erbakan University, Konya, Turkey

G. Gokce
Department of Urology, Sivas Medicana Hospital, Sivas, Turkey

S. Tonyali et al. (eds.), *Current Endourology*,
https://doi.org/10.1007/978-3-032-00010-1_5

threshold [5–7]. In addition, increased fluid intake may help prevent kidney stones by reducing contact time to potentially absorbent surfaces and increasing the passage of crystal products from nephrons [8]. In fact increasing fluid intake has been demonstrated to have a positive effect on two urinary inhibitors, citrate and Tamm-Horsfall protein. Hydration augments urinary citrate excretion, which is thought to result from an increased fluid flux in the proximal tubule resulting in the delivery of more bicarbonate to the cells of this portion of the nephron [9, 10]. The ensuing intracellular alkalosis blunts citrate reabsorption, leading to increased excretion of this inhibitor. Urinary dilution has been found to increase the inhibitory activity of Tamm-Horsfall protein on calcium oxalate monohydrate crystal aggregation in the urine of stone formers [11].

Current guidelines recommend drinking enough fluids to produce at least 2.5 liters of urine Daily [12]. Fluid intake should be spread throughout the day, especially within three hours of a meal, during strenuous physical activity, just before bedtime. In addition, those working in hot weather and hot environments should be more careful about fluid intake [13]. Almost all beverages, including coffee, tea, beer, and fruit juices, are acceptable. The fluids that should be avoided are tomato, grapefruit, and cranberry juice, because tomato juice is high in sodium whereas grapefruit and cranberry juices are rich in oxalate. The influences of water hardness on the formation of kidney stones have been debated for a number of years. Water hardness reflects the amount of dissolved calcium and magnesium. As a result of the studies, it was concluded that water hardness does not affect stone formation. Mineral water consumption may play a role in stone formation. One study found that among patients who initially drank at least 160 mL/d of soft drinks, those who quit had a higher 3-year freedom from recurrence than did those who continued to drink mineral water. However, this only held true for patients who drank phosphoric acid-containing mineral waters, which consist primary of the colas, and not in patients who drank citric acid-containing mineral waters, which include most clear soft drinks [14, 15].

Protein

In epidemiological studies, an increase in upper urinary tract stone formation was found in individuals consuming predominantly animal protein. In populations whose protein consumption is very high, kidney stone formation is 4 times higher [13]. A number of metabolic changes that are considered as a risk factor for stone formation is induced by increased protein consumption. These include increased calcium and uric-acid excretion, and decreased citrate excretion [16]. The magnitude of these changes can be significant. An extra 75 g of protein to the diet of normal subjects has been reported to raise urinary calcium excretion by approximately 100 mg/d [17]. Increased protein consumption also augments glomerular filtration, thus delivering more calcium to the nephron, which promotes its excretion [18]. Some investigators have suggested that stone formers are more sensitive to the calciuric action of protein. Animal protein has a high purine content, which explains the associated increase in uric-acid excretion. Hyperuricosuria is a risk factor for uric-acid stone occurrence and may play a role in calcium-stone formation. The associated acidosis results in a decrease in urinary pH that could potentiate uric-acid lithiasis. Because of these negative effects, all renal stone patients should be careful in the consumption of animal proteins [16].

Calcium

When discovered, approximately 50 to 60 years ago, hypercalciuria was observed frequently in individuals with calcium oxalate stone disease and that urinary calcium excretion could be decreased by lowering the intake of dietary calcium, a calcium-restricted diet became a mainstay in the treatment of stone patients [19]. Recent studies have shown that restriction of dietary calcium intake is unnecessary. However, calcium restriction should be applied in patients, if there is a connection between dietary calcium and stone formation. Calcium restriction reduces the amount of calcium to which oxalate will bind in the intestine and causes an increase in oxalate absorption. Calcium supplementation should not be administered except if patient suffers from enteric hyperoxaluria. In enteric hyperoxaluria, calcium supplementation should be made to bind intestinal oxalate and facilitate its excretion. It was found that especially milk-derived calcium increased stone recurrence, but non-milk-derived calcium (orange juice, soy milk, tofu) was found to be inversely proportional to stone formation. In addition, if too much calcium restriction is prescribed in the diet, the calcium balance must be maintained by the increase in bone resorption and this will eventually cause osteoporosis, especially in the elderly [20, 21].

Target calcium intake should be 1200 mg, which is the equivalent of four 8-oz glasses of milk. Dietary calcium is preferred to calcium supplementation because supplements may be associated with an increased risk of stone formation [22]. Patients should combine their calcium intake with a low-salt diet because sodium chloride leads to urinary calcium excretion. For every 2300 mg, or 1 teaspoon of salt intake, there is a 23 mg increase in urinary calcium excretion [23].

Sodium

Increased sodium intake may promote a variety of metabolic changes that may be detrimental to stone formers, including increases in urinary pH, calcium, and cystine excretion and a decrease in citrate excretion [24]. One of the conservative measures to take in kidney stone patients is the restriction of salt intake. Increased sodium consumption causes natriuresis. Therefore, natriuresis causes calciuresis, a decrease in the amount of citrate in the urine due to the loss of bicarbonate, and an increase in the risk of urate crystal formation [25]. With the addition of 250 mmol sodium chloride per day to the meals, there was a significant decrease in the amount of citrate in the urine and an increase in the urinary pH. It has also been found to cause calcium oxalate crystallization [23].

Oxalate

Dietary oxalate is absorbed all along the alimentary tract, with a time course that indicates that at least one half is absorbed in the small intestine. Higher oxalate intake has been shown to increase urinary oxalate levels [26]. Although the data are conflicting, the consensus is that higher urinary oxalate levels increase the risk of nephrolithiasis [27]. Even a slight increase in urinary excretion of oxalate causes calcium oxalate supersaturation. The oxalate diet is much more crucial, especially for patients with hyperoxaluria. Most oxalate-rich foods are considered "heart-healthy" foods (spinach, potatoes, and nuts). These foods account for 44% of the oxalate intake of the average American. The simplest way to minimize your oxalate intake is to monitor your consumption of these foods. Chocolate is a high source of dietary oxalate for young women and should be consumed with caution. In addition, a study conducted with female stone patients, it was shown that grapefruit increases the tendency to oxalate stones due to its high oxalate content [28].

Vitamins

The role of ascorbic acid in stone disease has been controversial. Due to the increase in urinary oxalate secretion, it is recommended not to take high amounts of vitamin C, especially in those with calcium oxalate stones. Vitamin C can be taken up to 4 g per day without increasing the risk of stone formation [29]. Vitamin B-6 (pyridoxine), on the other hand, may reduce urinary oxalate. Pyridoxine is a cofactor for alanine glyoxylate aminotransferase (AGT), which is the enzyme that catalyzes the conversion of glyoxylate to glycine. When there is a deficiency of AGT or low levels of pyridoxine, glyoxylate may be converted to oxalate. Studies have demonstrated an inverse association between vitamin B-6 intake and the risk of stone formation and have provided evidence that combining dietary therapy with pyridoxine supplementation is effective in hyperoxaluric stone-forming patients. The optimal dosage of supplemental vitamin B-6 has not been determined [30, 31]. It has been seen that calcium and vitamin D supplementation play an important role in the nucleation and growth of metabolic stones. In addition, excessive consumption of calcium supplements and vitamin D may result in the formation of urinary stones by causing excessive calcium excretion [32].

Medical Management

In addition to conservative approach suggestions, medical treatment is also quite important in urinary system stone disease. Stone analysis and specific medical treatment should also be applied in addition to conservative methods especially in the patient group with high recurrence risk. Before starting medical treatment, specific treatment should be constructed according to detailed metabolic examination and stone analysis results in addition to the basic patient evaluation.

Stone patients with high recurrence risk

- Presentation of stone disease in childhood or adolescence
- Familial stone disease
- Brushite-containing stones (calcium phosphate; CaHPO4.2H,0)
- Uric acid and urate containing stones
- Infection stones
- Solitary kidney
- Hyperparathyroidism
- Nephrocalcinosis
- Gastrointestinal diseases (jejuno-ileal bypass, intestinal resection, Crohn's disease, malabsorption, etc.)
- Sarcoidosis
- Cystinuria
- Primary hyperoxaluria
- Renal tubular acidosis
- Xanthinuria
- Lesh-Nyan syndrome
- Cystic fibrosis
- Drug-induced stone formation
- Anomalies causing stone formation (medullar sponge kidney, uretero-pelvic junction stenosis, calyceal diverticule and cyst, ureteral stricture, vesico-ureteral reflux, horseshoe kidney, ureterocele) [33–35].

Calcium Oxalate Stones

In addition to basic evaluation, specific assessment should also be performed in calcium oxalate stone patients, creatinine, basic electrolytes containing (sodium, potassium chlorine, ionized calcium), parathormone, uric acid values should be checked biochemically. Urine pH, density, 24-hour urine calcium, oxalate citrate and magnesium levels should be checked. Following the examinations, treatment modality should be determined based on etiology.

Drug treatment can be considered if the stones continue to recur despite conservative precautions, the patient has chronic kidney disease or metabolic bone disease or in certain patient groups (eg: flight staff) and patients with severe urinary

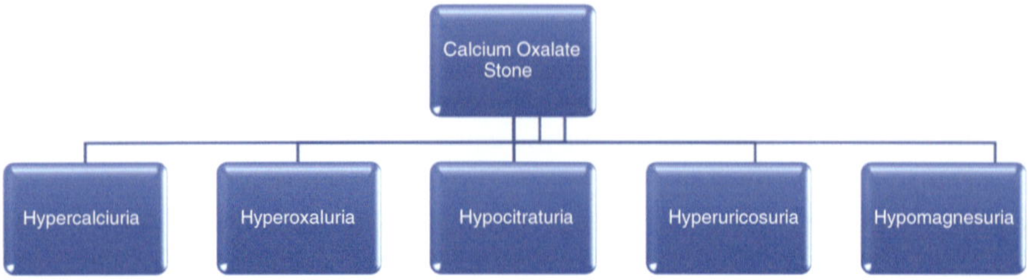

Fig. 5.1 Metabolic anomalies which may cause calcium oxalate stones [33] (EAU Guidelines)

metabolic anomalies [12, 33, 36]. Many metabolic anomalies may cause calcium oxalate stones (Fig. 5.1). Medical treatment should be planned according to the metabolic anomaly.

Hypercalciuria

Dietary calcium should not be restricted unless a strong relationship is established between stone formation and calcium taken through diet in hypercalciuria condition.

Potassium citrate can be given as 30–60 mEq/day in mild hypercalciuria (calcium release 5-8 mmol/day). Increasing citrate release through urine, potassium citrate causes calcium oxalate accumulation through binding calcium and citrate [37].

Thiazide and thiazide-like agents showing their effects through increasing calcium absorption in proximal and distal tubules in case of calcium release over 8 mmol should be added to treatment. Hydrochlorothiazide (25–50 mg/day), trichloromethyazide (4 mg/day), bendroflumethyazide (5 mg/day), chlortalidone (25–50 mg/day) and indapamid (1.25–2.5 mg/day) are some of the agents which can be used. But it should be considered that thiazide diuretics may have effects such as diabetes, gut hypocalciurea, erectile dysfunction and hyperuricemia. Potassium citrate should also be included in medical treatment for protection against the hypokalemic and hypocitraturic effects of thiazides. Therapeutic dose is 15–30 mEq twice a day. It is suitable for both CaOx and CaP stones when increased fluid intake and dietary precautions fail in preventing stone recurrence [37]. It was shown that allopurinol or febuxostat could be useful in patients with hyperuricosuric calcium stones [38]. Allopurinol was shown to be effective in lowering urinary uric acid and stone recurrence in hyperuricosuric calcium oxalate stone patients without any other metabolic anomaly. Despite the lack of any data supporting its use, hypouricosuric effect of feboxostat makes us consider that this drug could be effective in the treatment of stone patients intolerating allopurinol [39]. Medical treatment algorithm in hypercalciuria is shown in Fig. 5.2.

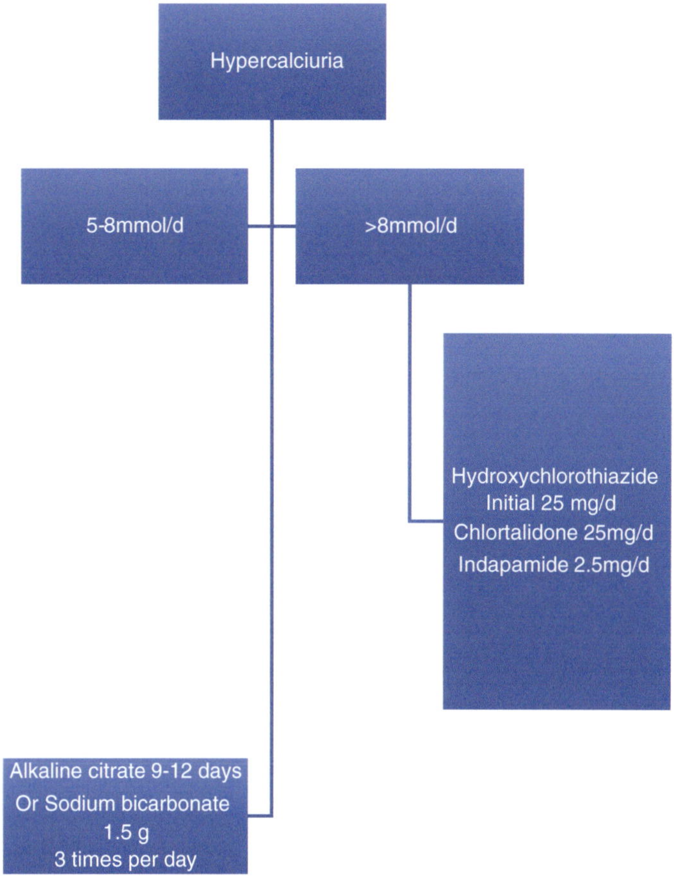

Fig. 5.2 Medical treatment algorithm in hypercalciuria [33] (EAU Guidelines)

Hypocitraturia

Low urinary citrate release (hypocitraturia) is among the most common and treatable causes of kidney stones. It was first reported by Boothby and Adams in 1934 and was then confirmed by Kissin and Locks in 1941. This information was highly ignored or attributed to bacterial citrate consumption. It was officially acknowledged when Hodgkinson suggested hypocitraturia as a unique urinary chemical disorder in nephrolithiasis patients in 1962 [40].

Hypocitraturia can be seen in 15–63% of stone patients. 10% of these stone patients have hypocitraturia as the isolated factor. Forming soluble salt through combining with calcium, citrate prevents the formation of calcium oxalate and calcium phosphate crystal.

Hypocitraturia is officially defined as daily urine citrate release below 320 mg but this amount has been questioned by many authors as it depends on the statistical

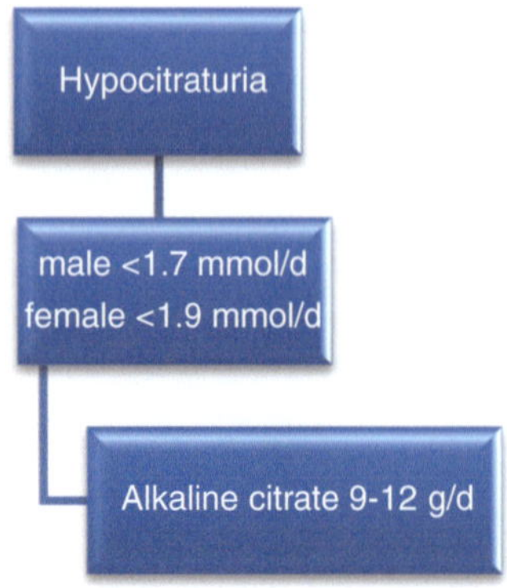

Fig. 5.3 Medical treatment algorithm in hypocitraturia [33] (EAU Guidelines)

analysis of 24-hour urine. Today, it is not possible to report optimal values of citrate even in standard laboratory results [40].

Potassium citrate is used for its treatment. Daily dose is 30–60 mEq. Tolerability of potassium citrate decreases in long-term use due to its side effects such as diarrhea, nausea-vomiting and dyspepsia. Intaking with food and dose decreasing can be solutions for this condition. Potassium citrate should not be used in peptic ulcer, active urinary system infection, renal failure (GFR < 0.7 mL/kg/min) and intestine passage disorders [34, 40]. Medical treatment algorithm in hypocitraturia is shown in Fig. 5.3.

Hyperoxaluria

Hyperoxaluria is an important pathogenic factor in the formation of calcium oxalate stones which constitute the most common type in humans. It can be caused by the genetic causes of hepatic over-production (primary hyperoxaluria) or gastrointestinal conditions causing fat malabsorption and increased oxalate absorption in gastrointestinal tract (enteric hyperoxaluria) [33, 40]. Normally, 10–15% of the oxalate in urine is taken through diet. But an increase takes place in calcium-binding bile salt and fatty acids in intestinal diseases causing malabsorption (inflammatory intestinal diseases, intestine resection, jejeno-ileal bypass, chronic diarrhoea, etc.). Calcium to be bonded to oxalate decreases in intestinal lumen and urinary oxalate release increases [41]. It may also occur in case of metabolic acidosis and hypokalemia-related hypocitraturia and decreased magnesium release through urine in malabsorption syndromes. Oxalate-rich food and fatty food should be restricted in enteric hyperoxaluria. Patients with diarrhoea may also have low urine pH, low urine volume and hypocitraturia. This is another underlying condition which should be fixed as it increases stone formation [41].

Oral calcium supplementation should also be provided in addition to diet [42]. Binding to the oxalate in the intestine, calcium decreases intestinal absorption. Even though calcium release through urine increases a little through calcium

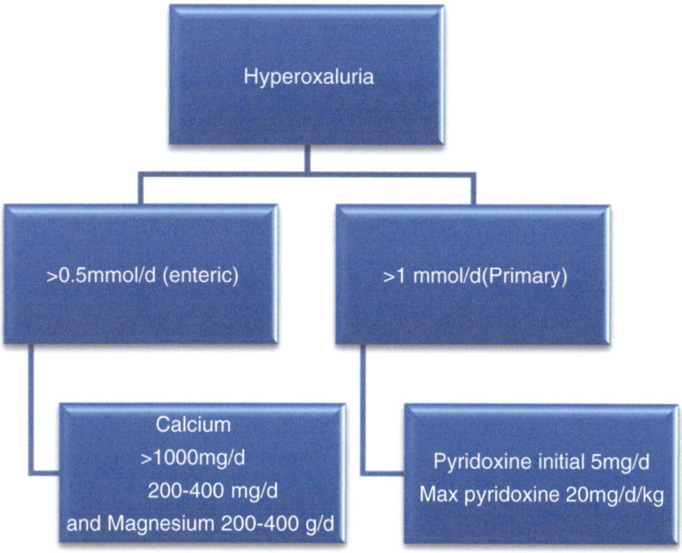

Fig. 5.4 Medical treatment algorithm in hyperoxaluria [33] (EAU Guidelines)

supplementation, it generally remains within normal limits. In addition to normal diet, a minimum of 500 mg calcium supplementation should be given daily to these patients with food. Just like calcium, oral magnesium can also be added to the diet in enteric hyperoxaluria. Binding with oxalate just like calcium, magnesium also decreases intestinal absorption and also lowers calcium oxalate saturation in the urine through binding with free oxalate in the urine. The suggested dose is 200–400 mg/day [42]. Oxalate amount can be over the normal value although some patients do not have an intestinal disease (idiopathic hyperoxaluria). Calcium should be limited in these patients and ascorbic acid (vitamin C) should be cut if it is taken [31]. If it continues despite these precautions, pyridoxine treatment can be applied. Oxalate levels are over 1 mmol/day as glioxalate metabolism in liver is corrupted in primary hyperoxaluria. Severe nephrocalcinosis is observed in these patients. High dose pyridoxine (600-800 mg/day) can be useful in these patients. Potassium citrate and magnesium supplementation can also be provided. Transplantation of kidney together with liver when considering the cure in these patients plays a significant role in kidney loss prevention stage to solve the underlying etiology [43]. Medical treatment algorithm in hyperoxaluria is shown in Fig. 5.4.

Hyperuricosuria

Hyperuricosuria may cause the formation of both uric acid stone and calcium oxalate stones through increasing oxalate crystallization. Low-purine diet can be enough in mild presentations but it may fail as problems occur most of the

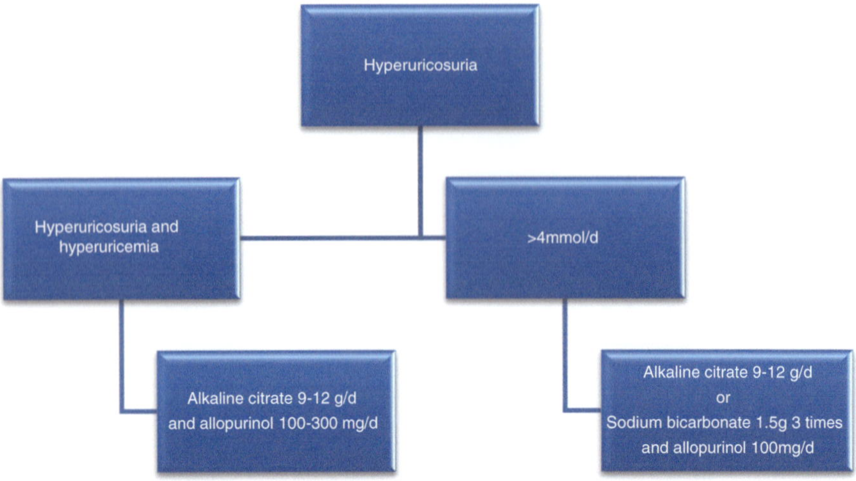

Fig. 5.5 Medical treatment algorithm in hyperuricosuria [33] (EAU Guidelines)

time in practice. In this condition, these patients can be given 30–60 mEq/day potassium citrate and 100–300 mg/day allopurine. Inhibiting xanthine oxidase, allopurinol inhibits uric acid formation from xanthine. It should be preferred especially in individuals with gut story [44]. Urinary urate level also decreases with decreasing serum uric acid level. There are also controversial views claiming that the treatment methods such as potassium citrate or sodium bicarbonate alkalinizing urine pH are satisfactory by themselves. Consensus has been reached on starting the treatment only with potassium citrate in cases without comorbid hyperuricaemia. Medical treatment algorithm in hyperuricosuria is shown in Fig. 5.5.

Hypomagnesuria

It is seen together with the other anomalies in 6–11% and in isolation in less than 1% of stone patients.

It forms a complex with magnesium, oxalate and calcium salts. Thus it is effective through preventing calcium oxalate and calcium phosphate crystallization. It is generally seen together with hypocitraturia. Mg was shown to increase urine pH and citrate levels and decrease free Ca saturation in vitro. Low Mg level in urine can be caused by low dietary intake or malabsorption disorders occurring with chronic diarrhea. It is generally related to thiazide diuretic use. Magnesium oxide or magnesium hydroxide replacement is generally provided in treatment. It should not be suggested in renal failure [44]. Medical treatment algorithm in hypomagnesuria is shown in Fig. 5.6.

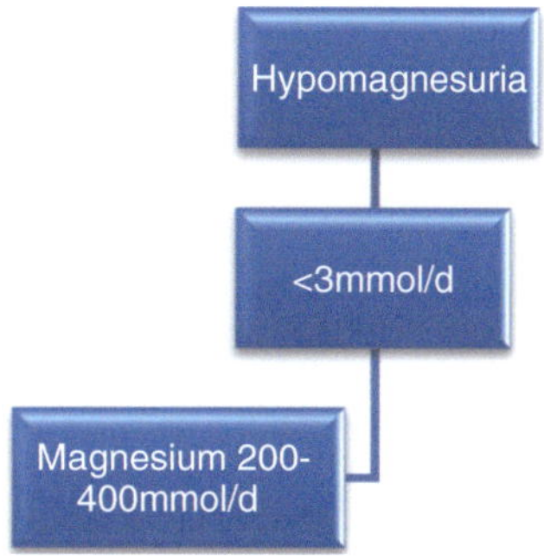

Fig. 5.6 Medical treatment algorithm in hypomagnesiuria [33]. (EAU Guidelines)

Low pH

Urinary pH constantly below 5.8 is generally seen in individuals with uric acid stone but it may also occur in calcium oxalate stones. Low urinary pH fastens calcium oxalate crystallization. This condition is generally seen in individuals consuming high amounts of animal-based food. 30–60 mEq/day potassium citrate can be used in treatment. Consumption of animal-based food should also be limited [12, 33, 34].

Calcium Phosphate Stones

Calcium phosphate is basically seen in two different minerals: carbonate apatite and brushite. Nearly 15–20% of all stone patients have calcium phosphate stone. Stones including calcium monohydrogen phosphate, brushite in other words, constitute 25% of these stones. Brushite stones are ESWL-resistant and symptomatic stones with a high volume. According to crystallization theory;

- Carbonate apatite crystallization forms in the presence of urinary pH over 6.8 and possible infection.
- Brushite crystallization forms when the urine reaches high calcium and phosphate saturation at a urine pH between 6.5 and 6.8. No relationship can be shown with infection.

Calcium phosphate stones generally accompany calcium oxalate stones. They are covered in active stone patients group when they are made up of calcium phosphate alone. Isolated calcium phosphate stones and renal tubular acidosis (RTA) generally occur together. The kidney cannot satisfactorily acidify the urine in RTA and dilavent and trivalent forms of phosphate increase at high pH values and this causes supersaturation of calcium phosphate. Two other possible causes of calcium phosphate stones are hyperparathyroidism and urinary system infections.

Distinction of this stone type from infection stones is very important. This is due to the fact that potassium citrate use is contraindicated in infection stones due to its

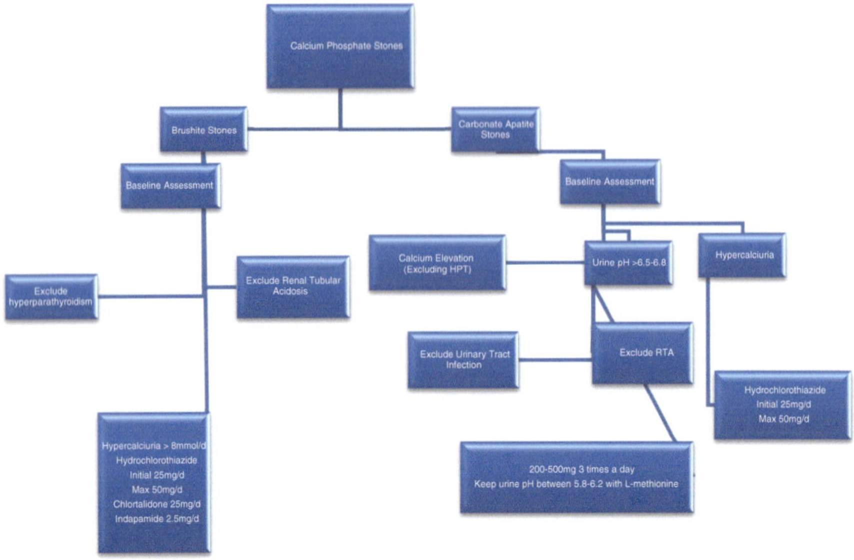

Fig. 5.7 Medical treatment algorithm in Calcium Phosphate stones [33] (EAU Guidelines)

urine alkalinization character. While surgery is generally necessary if the patient has hyperparathyroidism, RTA presence can be treated medically. Thiazide diuretics are quite effective to lower high urine calcium level of the patient. Although RTA is not present in hypercalciuria, urine acidification can be useful in case of urine pH constantly above 6.2 and 200–500 mg doses of L-methionine can be given three times a day for this [33–36]. Medical treatment algorithm in Calcium Phosphate stones is shown in Fig. 5.7.

Uric Acid Stones

Patients with uric acid stones constituting 5–10% of urinary system stones are under high recurrence risk. Creatinine and uric acid levels in blood biochemisty and uric acid levels, urine pH, density, 24-hour urine volume and uric acid level should be examined in metabolic examination. High fluid intake and its expansion throughout the day have high important especially in nocturnal diuresis. Purine-rich food should be avoided in diet.

Although hyperuricosuria can be a factor in the formation etiology of uric acid stones, the most important factor is low urine pH (constantly <6.0). Increasing of urine pH in the course of treatment constitutes the most important aspect of the treatment. A daily dose of 30–60 mEq potassium is suitable to achieve this [45].

Hyperuricosuria which is another metabolic problem in uric acid stones may occur due to conditions such as purine-rich diet, endogen over-production (enzyme

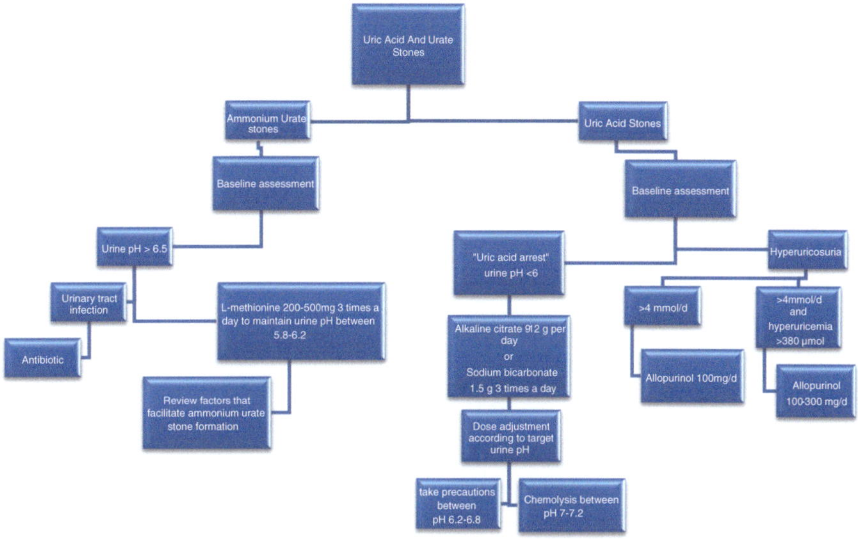

Fig. 5.8 Medical treatment algorithm in Uric Acid stones [33] (EAU Guidelines)

defects), tumour lysis syndrome, drugs and gut. 100–300 mg/day allopurinol is also suitable in addition to low purine diet in treatment [46]. 40–80 mg/day febuxostat can be used instead of allopurinol as an alternative [47]. Medical treatment algorithm in uric acid stones is shown in Fig. 5.8.

Infection Stones

Infection stones constitute 5–15% of all stones and may contain struvite (magnesium ammonium phosphate) or carbonate apatite or ammonium urate or their combination. These stones form in the presence of urease synthetizing bacteria and urine pH over 7.2 [48].

Proteus mirabilis forms more than half of urease positive urinary system infections. Proteus, klebsiella, pseudomonas and staphylococcus are some of other bacteria types causing infection stone formation. Together with calcium phosphate stones, these stones constitute the most important cause of staghorn stones. Infection stones are twice more common in women.

The most important stage in treatment should be the provision of urine acidification through antibiotherapy, ammonium chloride or L-methionine 3 × 200–500 mg/day to decrease urinary system infection recurrence after the complete cleaning of the stones through surgery or chemolysis. Acetohydroxamic acid can be used for urease inhibition in severe infections. Hemiacridine 10% solutions are agents applied through nephrostomy to dissolve infection stones but negative urine culture

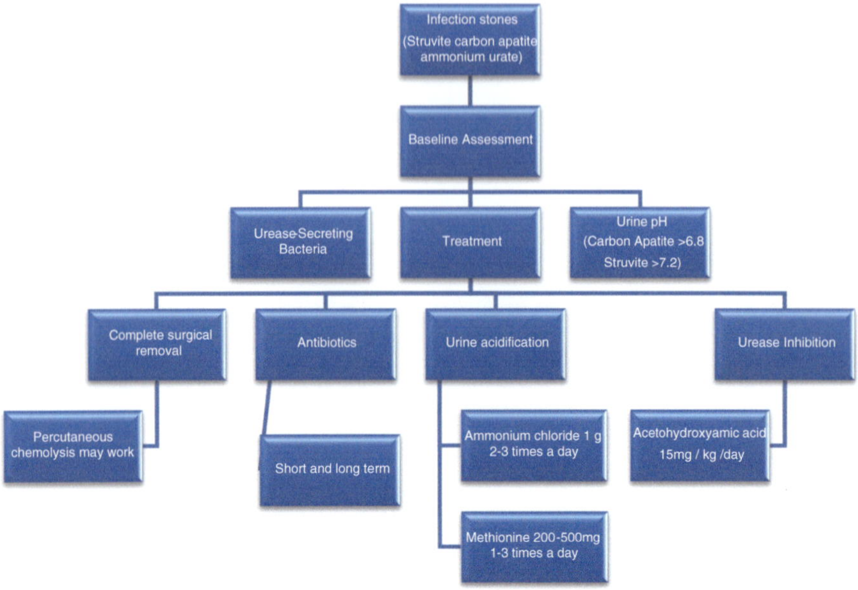

Fig. 5.9 Medical treatment algorithm in infection stones [33] (EAU Guidelines)

and exclusion of extravasation are important [33, 48]. Medical treatment algorithm in infection stones is shown in Fig. 5.9.

Cystine Stones

All cystine stone patients have high recurrence risk. Cystinuria is present in its etiology. Cystinuria is a condition forming with extreme release of 4 basic amino acid (cystine lysine ornithine arginine) through urine. Only cystine among these aminoacids is not included in water-soluble form in urine normal pH. 24 hour urine, density, creatinine and urine pH should be examined in these patients. Urine alkalinization, cystine binding agents and cystine levels should be examined in cystinuria patients [38, 49]. Limitation of salt and methionine-containing food such as meat, egg, wheat and nuts and daily urination over 3 litres are especially important in cystine stones. Urine alkalinization and cystine binding agents are used in medical treatment. Medical treatment algorithm in cystine stones is shown in Fig. 5.10.

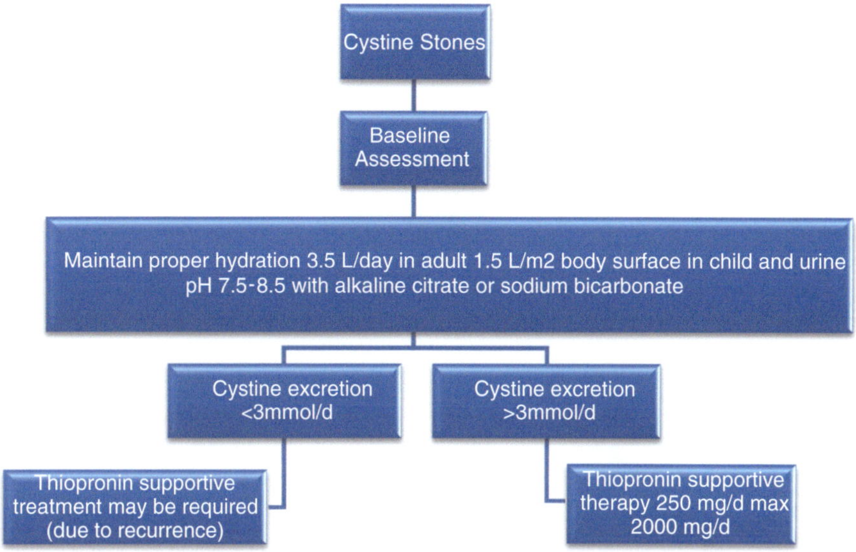

Fig. 5.10 Medical treatment algorithm in Cystine stones [33] (EAU Guidelines)

Ammonium Urate Stones

Ammonium urate stones have high recurrence risk although they form rarely. Although alkaline urine forms the basis of stone formation, it may be related to urinary track infections, malabsorption and malnutrition. Urine acidification can be provided through ammonium chloride or L-methionine [50]. (Shown on the uric acid stones table in the guide [33].

Dihydroxy Adenine Stones

Increased release of dihydroxiadenine through urine due to adenine phosphoribosyl transferase enzyme deficiency causes the formation of these stones. High dose allopurinol treatment can be given.

Xanthine Stones

Oxidase enzyme deficiency forms xanthine. Xanthine and hypoxanthine release increases in urine. Xanthine stones form due to the less soluble nature of xanthine. They may form in patients using allopurinol which is a xanthine oxidase inhibitor due to the presence of uric acid stone. No single drug is available for use in treatment. High fluid intake is the only treatment [51].

Drug-Induced Stones

Drugs can cause stone formation in two ways.

- Drugs causing stone formation through the crystallization of their ingredients (Cetriaxone, indinavir, sulphonamide, etc.). The drug should be cut in this condition and an alternative treatment should be applied.
- Drugs causing stone formation through damaging urine composition (acetazolamide, calcium, furosemide, etc.). The treatment should be planned accordingly following the detection of the formed metabolic anomaly [33–36].

Patients with Urinary Diversion

Patients with urinary diversion are under increased risk of stone formation in kidney collective system, ureters, conduit and continent reservoirs. Hypercalciuria, hypocitraturia, infections, mucus secretion and stasis are factors increasing stone formation and recurrence risk in these patients. Preventive approaches in these patients;

- Patients should be kept under control for metabolic anomalies and the formed anomalies should be fixed.
- Urinary infections should be treated accordingly.
- Continent reservoir should be irrigated intermittently [12, 33].

Chemolysis

Chemolysis of urinary system stones through oral or percutaneous irrigation can be the first treatment option. But this treatment is generally only used for the elimination of residual stones following endourological methods due to its long-term nature.

Percutaneous Chemolysis

Chemolysis can be present only in certain stones. Thus, the stone composition should be known.

Some points should be considered in percutaneous irrigation.

- Intrapelvic pressure should not exceed 20–25 cm H2O during irrigation. Hence, a minimum of two nephrostomy catheters should be present.

Table 5.1 Percutaneous chemolysis-applicable solutions based on stone composition

Stone composition	Solution
Uric acid	Trihydroxylmethyl aminomethane 0.3–0.6 mol/L
Cystine	Trihydroxylmethyl aminomethane 0.3–0.6 mol/L N-acetyl cysteine 200 mg/L
Calcium phosphate (brushite)	Hemiacidrin Solution G
Struvite carbonate apatite	Hemiacidrin Solution G

- There should be no extravasation.
- It should not be applied during active infection.
- Irrigation should be ended immediately in case of flank pain.
- Serum elecrolytes should be checked periodically [52].

Percutaneous chemolysis-applicable solutions based on stone composition are available in Table 5.1.

Oral Chemolysis

It is effective only for uric acid stones. Urine alkalinization can be provided through potassium citrate and sodium bicarbonate. High diuresis (2.5–3 L/day) should be provided together with alkalinization. Drug dose is adjusted according to Ph values [52].

Tips and Key-Points

All stone patients should be provided conservative medical treatment suggestions such as fluid intake, dietary and lifestyle changes. Specific medical treatment should also be applied in addition to these suggestions in patients with high recurrence risk. These patients should also be given suggestions based on stone analysis and detailed metabolic evaluation results in addition to the basic examination.

References

1. Grases F, Costa-Bauza A, Prieto RM. Renal lithiasis and nutrition. Nutr J. 2006;5:23.
2. Ljunghall S, Hedstrand H. Epidemiology of renal stones in a middle-aged male population. Acta Med Scand. 1975;197(6):439–45.
3. Khan SR, Pearle MS, Robertson WG, Gambaro G, Canales BK, Doizi S, Traxer O, Tiselius HG. Kidney stones. Nat Rev Dis Primers. 2016;25(2):16008.

4. Fink HA, Akornor JW, Garimella PS, MacDonald R, Cutting A, Rutks IR, Monga M, Wilt TJ. Diet, fluid, or supplements for secondary prevention of nephrolithiasis: a systematic review and meta-analysis of randomized trials. Eur Urol. 2009;56(1):72–80.
5. Pak CY, Galosy RA. Propensity for spontaneous nucleation of calcium oxalate. Quantitative assessment by urinary FPR-APR discriminant score. Am J Med. 1980;69(5):681–9.
6. Pak CY, Sakhaee K, Crowther C, Brinkley L. Evidence justifying a high fluid intake in treatment of nephrolithiasis. Ann Intern Med. 1980;93(1):36–9.
7. Sorensen MD, Eisner BH, Stone KL, Kahn AJ, Lui LY, Sadetsky N, Stoller ML. Impact of calcium intake and intestinal calcium absorption on kidney stones in older women: the study of osteoporotic fractures. J Urol. 2012;187(4):1287–92.
8. Finlayson B, Khan SR, Hackett RL. Mechanisms of stone formation--an overview. Scan Electron Microsc 1984;(Pt 3):1419-1425.
9. Hess B, Michel R, Takkinen R, Ackermann D, Jaeger P. Risk factors for low urinary citrate in calcium nephrolithiasis: low vegetable fibre intake and low urine volume to be added to the list. Nephrol Dial Transplant. 1994;9(6):642–9.
10. Simpson DP. Citrate excretion: a window on renal metabolism. Am J Phys. 1983;244(3):F223–34.
11. Jaeger P, Hess B, Takkinen R, Zipperle L. Nutritional determinants of nephrolithiasis. Adv Nephrol Necker Hosp. 1995;24:217–25.
12. Pearle MS, Goldfarb DS, Assimos DG, Curhan G, Denu-Ciocca CJ, Matlaga BR, Monga M, Penniston KL, Preminger GM, Turk TMT, White JR, American Urological Assocation. Medical management of kidney stones: AUA guideline. J Urol. 2014;192(2):316–24.
13. Ferrandino MN, Pietrow PK, Preminger GM. Evaluation and medical management of urinary lithiasis. In: Wein AJ, Kavoussi LR, Novick AC, Partin AW, Peters CA, editors. Campbell-Walsh urology. 10th ed. Philadelphia: Saunders Elsevier; 2012. p. p1287–323.
14. Shuster J, Jenkins A, Logan C, Barnett T, Riehle R, Zackson D, Wolfe H, Dale R, Daley M, Malik I, et al. Soft drink consumption and urinary stone recurrence: a randomized prevention trial. J Clin Epidemiol. 1992;45(8):911–6.
15. Shuster J, Finlayson B, Scheaffer R, Sierakowski R, Zoltek J, Dzegede S. Water hardness and urinary stone disease. J Urol. 1982;128(2):422–5.
16. Breslau NA, Brinkley L, Hill KD, Pak CY. Relationship of animal protein-rich diet to kidney stone formation and calcium metabolism. J Clin Endocrinol Metab. 1988;66(1):140–6.
17. Licata AA, Bou E, Bartter FC, Cox J. Effects of dietary protein on urinary calcium in normal subjects and in patients with nephrolithiasis. Metabolism. 1979;28(9):895–900.
18. Schuette SA, Zemel MB, Linkswiler HM. Studies on the mechanism of protein-induced hypercalciuria in older men and women. J Nutr. 1980;110(2):305–15.
19. Henneman PH, Benedict PH, Forbes AP, Dudley HR. Idiopathic hypercaicuria. N Engl J Med. 1958;259(17):802–7.
20. Curhan GC, Willett WC, Rimm EB, Stampfer MJ. A prospective study of dietary calcium and other nutrients and the risk of symptomatic kidney stones. N Engl J Med. 1993;328(12):833–8.
21. Curhan GC, Willett WC, Speizer FE, Spiegelman D, Stampfer MJ. Comparison of dietary calcium with supplemental calcium and other nutrients as factors affecting the risk for kidney stones in women. Ann Intern Med. 1997;126(7):497–504.
22. Borghi L, Schianchi T, Meschi T, Guerra A, Allegri F, Maggiore U, Novarini A. Comparison of two diets for the prevention of recurrent stones in idiopathic hypercalciuria. N Engl J Med. 2002;346(2):77–84.
23. Sakhaee K, Harvey JA, Padalino PK, Whitson P, Pak CY. The potential role of salt abuse on the risk for kidney stone formation. J Urol. 1993;150(2 Pt 1):310–2.
24. McCarron DA, Rankin LI, Bennett WM, Krutzik S, McClung MR, Luft FC. Urinary calcium excretion at extremes of sodium intake in normal man. Am J Nephrol. 1981;1(2):84–90.
25. Silver J, Rubinger D, Friedlaender MM, Popovtzer MM. Sodium-dependent idiopathic hypercalciuria in renal-stone formers. Lancet. 1983;2(8348):484–6.
26. Holmes RP, Goodman HO, Assimos DG. Dietary oxalate and its intestinal absorption. Scanning Microsc. 1995;9:1109–18. discussion 1118-20

27. Curhan GC, Taylor EN. 24-h uric acid excretion and the risk of kidney stones. Kidney Int. 2008;73(4):489–96.
28. Taylor EN, Curhan GC. Oxalate intake and the risk for nephrolithiasis. J Am Soc Nephrol. 2007;18(7):2198–204.
29. Wandzilak TR, D'Andre SD, Davis PA, Williams HE. Effect of high dose vitamin C on urinary oxalate levels. J Urol. 1994;151(4):834–7.
30. Curhan GC, Willett WC, Speizer FE, Stampfer MJ. Intake of vitamins B6 and C and the risk of kidney stones in women. J Am Soc Nephrol. 1999;10(4):840–5.
31. Ortiz-Alvarado O, Miyaoka R, Kriedberg C, Moeding A, Stessman M, Monga M. Pyridoxine and dietary counseling for the management of idiopathic hyperoxaluria in stone-forming patients. Urology. 2011;77(5):1054–8.
32. Taylor EN, Stampfer MJ, Curhan GC. Dietary factors and the risk of incident kidney stones in men: new insights after 14 years of follow-up. J Am Soc Nephrol. 2004;15(12):3225–32.
33. Türk C, Neisius A, Petrik A, Seitz C, Skolarikos A, Thomas K. EAU Guidelines on Urolithiasis. Arnhem. https://uroweb.org/guideline/urolithiasis: EAU Guidelines Office; 2020.
34. Clayman RV, Patel RM, Pearle M. "STONE TREES": metabolic evaluation and medical treatment of the Urolithiasis patient made easy. J Endourol. 2018;32(5):387–92.
35. Daudon M, Jungers P, Bazin D, Williams Jr JC. Recurrence rates of urinary calculi according to stone composition and morphology. Urolithiasis. 2018;46(5):459–70.
36. Daudon M, Letavernier E, Frochot V, Haymann J-P, Bazin D, Jungers P. Respective influence of calcium and oxalate urine concentration on the formation of calcium oxalate monohydrate or dihydrate crystals. C R Chim. 2016;19(11–12):1504–13.
37. Leslie SW, Sajjad H. Hypercalciuria. In: StatPearls [Internet]. Treasure Island: StatPearls Publishing; 2021 Jan; 2017. Available from: https://www.ncbi.nlm.nih.gov/books/NBK448183/.
38. Igor S, Pearle MS. Medical therapy for nephrolithiasis: state of the art. Asian journal of urology. 2018;5(4):243–55.
39. Goldfarb DS, Arowojolu O. Metabolic evaluation of first-time and recurrent stone formers. Urol Clin. 2013;40(1):13–20.
40. Hofbauer, J., Höbarth, K., Szabo, N. And Marberger, M. "Alkali citrate prophylaxis in idiopathic recurrent calcium oxalate urolithiasis—a prospective randomized study." Br J Urol 1994;73(4): 362–365.
41. Worcester EM. Stones from bowel disease. Endocrinol Metab Clin. 2002;31(4):979–99.
42. Caudarella R, Rizzoli E, Pironi L, Malavolta N, Martelli G, Poggioli G, et al. Renal stone formation in patients with inflammatory bowel disease. Scanning Microsc. 1993;7(1):371–9.
43. Shafiq A, Ansari TM, Shad MA. Prevalence of renal calculı. Type, Age And Gender Specıfıc In Southern Punjab, Pakıstan The Professional Medical Journal. 2016;23(4):389–95.
44. Spivacow FR, Negri AL, del Valle EE, Calvin˜o I, Zanchetta J´R. Clinical and metabolic risk factor evaluation in young adults with kidney stones. Int Urol Nephrol. 2010;42(2):471–5.
45. Cameron MA, Sakhaee K. Uric acid nephrolithiasis. Urol Clin N Am. 2007;34(3):335–46.
46. Shadman A, Bastani B. Evaluation and management of kidney calculi. Iran J Kidney Dis. 2017;11(6):395–407.
47. Goldfarb DS, MacDonald PA, Gunawardhana L, Chefo S, McLean L. Randomized controlled trial of febuxostat versus allopurinol or placebo in individuals with higher urinary uric acid excretion and calcium stones. Clin J Am Soc Nephrol. 2013;8(11):1960–7.
48. Espinosa-Ortiz EJ, Eisner BH, Lange D, Gerlach R. Current insights into the mechanisms and management of infection stones. Nat Rev Urol. 2019;16(1):35–53. https://doi.org/10.1038/s41585-018-0120-z.
49. Evan AP, Coe FL, Lingeman JE, et al. Renal crystal deposits and histopathology in patients with cystine stones. Kidney Int. 2006;69(12):2227–35.
50. Lomas DJ, Jaeger CD, Krambeck AE. Profile of the ammonium acid urate stone former based on a large contemporary cohort. Urology. 2017;102:43–7.
51. Pais VM, Lowe G, Lallas CD, Preminger GM, Assimos DG. Xanthine urolithiasis. Urology. 2006;67(5):1084–e9.
52. Bernardo NO, Smith AD. Chemolysis of urinary calculi. Urol Clin N Am. 2000;27(2):355–65.

Chapter 6
Supine Percutaneous Nephrolithotomy

Emrah Yuruk, Ahmet Semih Guleser, and Omer Levent Tuncay

Percutaneous nephrolithotomy (PCNL) was first described in 1976 by Fernström and Johansson and has become the gold standard method for removing large kidney stones in recent years, as minimally invasive approaches steadily gained in popularity. When compared to open surgery, PCNL has advantages such as reduced blood loss, shorter hospital stays, and lower morbidity. PCNL was originally performed when the patient was in the prone position. The lack of availability of computed tomography (CT) at the time when PCNL was introduced raised concerns that the risk of colon injury could be high in other positions. With the current widespread use of CT, more detailed information can be obtained before surgery about the perirenal anatomy of the patient. However, the prone position still remains the most commonly used method because of the extensive experience that urologists have with regard to PCNL.

In 1987, Valdivia Uria first described a PCNL procedure in which the patient was in the supine decubitus position. Complication rates and results were found to be similar to those of patients who were placed in the prone position and had had CT scans for preoperative evaluation. In addition, studies found that the incidence of retro-renal colon in the supine position was 1.9%, while it was found to be 10% in the prone position. With the widespread use of CT, surgeons have realized that concerns about the increased risk of colon perforation with the supine position are not valid. Nevertheless, the prone position remains the dominant position, while the supine position is preferred in only 20% of PCNL procedures worldwide.

E. Yuruk
Department of Urology, Medicana International Istanbul Hospital, İstanbul, Turkey

A. S. Guleser
Department of Urology, ASG Clinic, İstanbul, Turkey

O. L. Tuncay (✉)
Department of Urology, Pamukkale University, Denizli, Turkey

S. Tonyali et al. (eds.), *Current Endourology*,
https://doi.org/10.1007/978-3-032-00010-1_6

Surgical Technique

Patient Position

One of the important problems with supine PCNL is that the anatomical orientation of the surgeon may be lost after the patient is draped. Therefore, it is recommended that the inferior border of the 12th rib, the iliac crest, and the posterior axillary line on the patients be marked before surgery. Radiolucent carbon operating tables are used in some centers, and since there are no radio-opaque parts on the edges of these tables, patients can be pulled up to the edges. This helps to reduce the probability of a collision occurring with the C-arm scope device during the movement of the nephroscope. The increased maneuverability of the nephroscope also allows surgeons to work at wider angles. An ideal endourology table should be able to move in the caudal direction, so that the entire urinary system can be visualized. When a surgical table with these features is not available, standard surgical tables can be used by being reversed. However, for patient safety, the Mayo table should be placed at the foot of the patient.

For the original supine position that was used by Valdivia Uria for PCNL, a 3-liter saline bag is placed on the patient's flank to improve surgical field vision. Several variations have been described over time, such as the lateral, complete, and modified supine positions. The Galdakao-modified Valdivia position, in which the patient's legs are in the modified lithotomy position, has recently become the one that is most preferred, as it allows simultaneous ureteroscopic and retrograde urethral access. The Guisti position (Fig. 6.1) was devised to solve problems in reaching the upper pole stones and to address the limited maneuverability of the nephroscope. In the Guisti position, which is a modification of the Galdakoa-Valdivia position, the patient is placed at the edge of the operating table. With the help of a small support, the operating side is raised no more than 20 degrees. The ipsilateral arm is placed over the rib cage. While the ipsilateral leg is left in a straight position on the operating side, the contralateral leg is opened, allowing the second surgeon to perform simultaneous retrograde interventions.

Fig. 6.1 Guisti's position

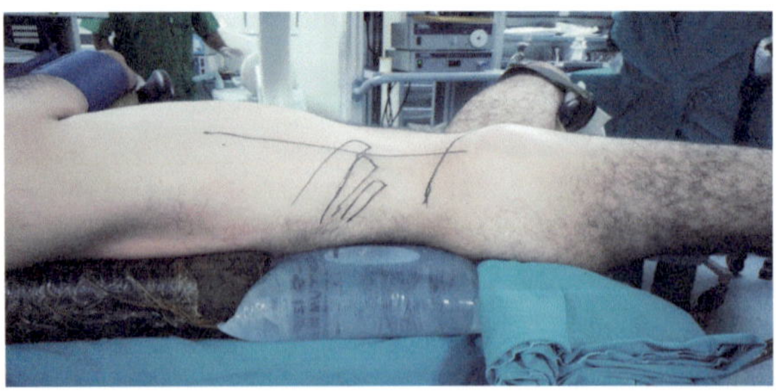

Percutaneous Puncture

Triangulation

The percutaneous puncture is initiated in the 0 degree neutral position. Needle orientation is almost parallel to the ground (Fig. 6.2). After the retrograde opaque material has been given, the needle is inserted under fluoroscopy. If the needle is in the correct trajectory, the targeted calyx appears depressed. This depression is easier to see when the patient is in the supine position, because the C-arm fluoroscopy is perpendicular to the needle. If the needle has entered the targeted calyx system on the fluoroscopic view but no urine is seen coming from the needle, the position of the access tract may need to be readjusted. To evaluate the puncture to be able to achieve the correct depth, the C- arm is rotated 30 degrees cephalad. If the needle is visible below the targeted calyx, the access trajectory should be placed more posteriorly. Conversely, if the needle is visible above the calyx, entry should be made anteriorly.

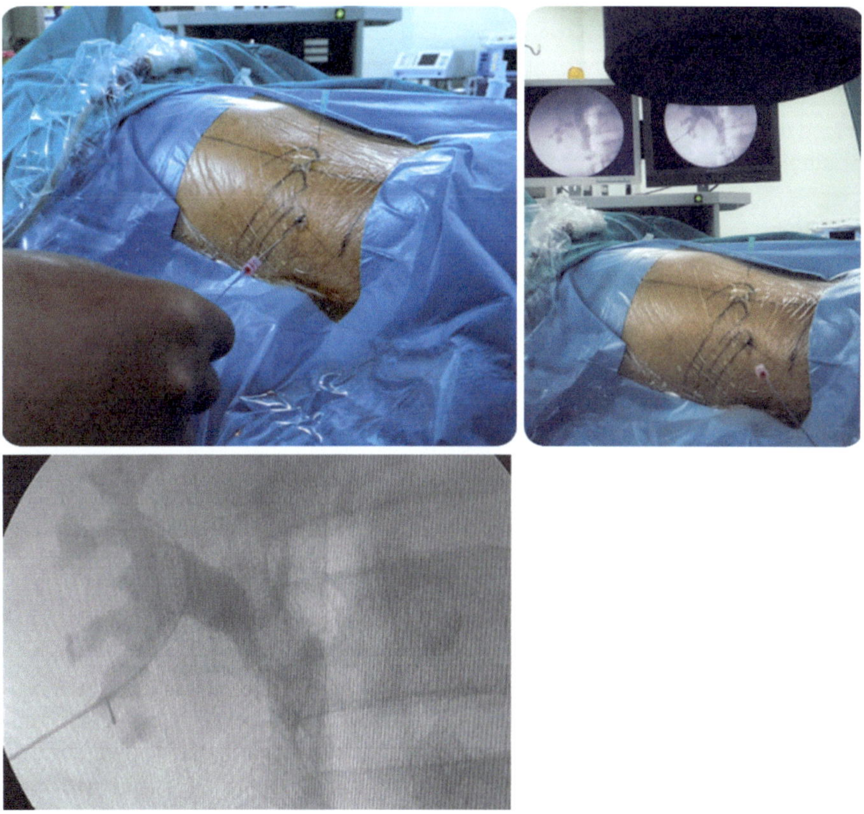

Fig. 6.2 Percutaneous renal puncture

Bullseye

Another approach to fluoroscopy-guided percutaneous renal access is a technique that was modified from the bullseye technique that is commonly used in PCNL procedures where the patients are in the prone position. First, the image is taken with the C-arm at 0 degrees. The C-arm is then imaged at an angle of 30 degrees, and the entry site for the targeted calyx is marked. In this way, the puncture point is determined exactly, and the needle is prevented from remaining either anterior or posterior. The C-arm is taken to 0 degrees again, and the needle is advanced toward the calyx from the marked point so that it is parallel to the ground. It can be seen through fluoroscopy that the targeted calyx is depressed to avoid any risk of progressing over the correct trajectory.

Ultrasound Guidance

Supine PCNL procedures can be ultrasound-assisted and completely ultrasound-guided, without the use of X-rays. However, experience is required to perform ultrasound punctures. Although some studies have reported that ultrasound-assisted and -guided PCNL can be used safely in the prone position, there is insufficient data with regard to supine PCNL. Since urologists are more familiar with fluoroscopy, the use of ultrasound is not as frequent, but it has the following advantages:

- It offers easier understanding of the needle depth.
- It allows the perirenal anatomy to be evaluated during the procedure, which can prevent lung, liver, and colon injuries.
- It results in reduced radiation exposure for patients and staff.

Supine PCNL Advantages

In the PCNL procedure, the supine position is superior to the traditional prone position in areas such as anesthesia management, operation time, intrarenal pressure, radiation exposure time, simultaneous intrarenal surgery, and access to upper pole stones. The advantages of the supine position are summarized in Table 6.1.

The supine position provides convenience to anesthesiologists in anesthesia management and makes cardiopulmonary system management more comfortable, especially in emergencies. In addition, in longer prone position surgeries, the possibility of nerve injuries, vascular damage, tracheal decompression, and ocular damage increases. Therefore, performing the PCNL procedure in the supine position reduces the incidence of these complications. Similarly, in the supine position, thromboembolic complications decrease as the pressure in the inferior vena cava is reduced. Due to the advantage of sheath placement in the supine position, intrarenal

Table 6.1 Advantages of supine PCNL

Anesthesia management is easier
Shorter surgical time
Collector system pressure is lower due to better fluid drainage
Avoiding complications due to position change during surgery
Simultaneous transureteral intervention easier
Since intra-abdominal pressure is low, it can be preferred in patients with obesity and lung disease
Access to the upper pole is easier in punctures made from the lower pole of the kidney

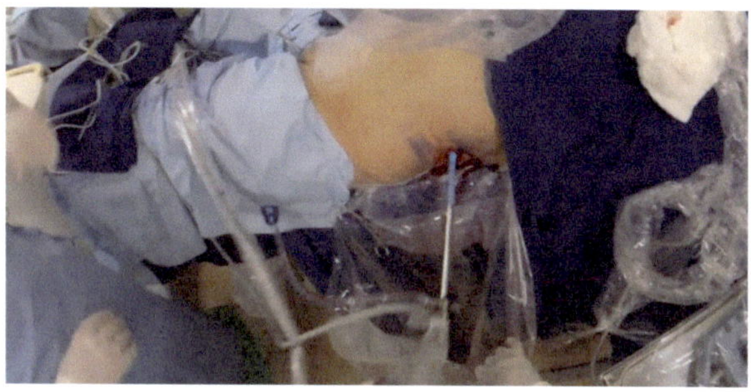

Fig. 6.3 Sheath position in supine PCNL

pressure and fluid absorption into the systemic circulation are less common. For this reason, it is thought that complications such as sepsis, which may develop due to infected stones, may occur less frequently. In addition, the fact that the patient's position does not need to be changed after retrograde catheter placement prevents problems such as dislocation of the intubation tube and single lung intubation. Also, not having to change the patient's position reduces the workload of the operating room staff in the operating room, and having to cover the patient only once shortens the operation time.

In supine PCNL, the position of the renal sheath is parallel to the ground or slightly angled towards the ground (Fig. 6.3). In this way, liquid drainage is increased, and a continuous vacuum effect is created. It becomes possible for the stone fragments to emerge from the kidney spontaneously, and better fluid drainage reduces the pressure in the renal pelvis. Working at lower pressure during surgery also theoretically reduces the risk of the patient developing sepsis.

In prone PCNL, the surgeon's hands are in the fluoroscopy field during entry into the renal calyces, which both impairs the fluoroscopy vision and increases the surgeon's radiation exposure. In supine PCNL, however, the fluoroscopic vision is not obstructed since the surgeon's hands are not directly exposed to the X-ray beam. Although it is thought that the radiation exposure is lower in supine PCNL, there are as yet insufficient studies to draw this conclusion. Another advantage of supine PCNL is that it allows renal access to be made more lateral to the skin. In this way, the C-arm can be moved more easily. Complications such as collision with the nephroscope and dislocation of the renal sheath during movement of the C-arm are less common. In addition, the comfort of the surgeon is higher during supine PCNL because the position of the renal sheath allows the surgeon to perform the procedure in a seated position.

In complex stone cases, the supine position allows simultaneous antegrade and retrograde transurethral manipulations. The use of the intrarenal surgical technique in PCNL reduces the rate of residual stones. Performing simultaneous transurethral manipulation in the prone position has some limitations and, for this reason, it is not common in traditional PCNL. The prevalence of the supine position has facilitated simultaneous manipulations during PCNL. In addition, simultaneous transurethral approaches allow the surgeon to check the correct position of the needle during renal access.

In a single session, bilateral PCNL can be performed safely and effectively in the supine position. Studies have shown that there is no difference in surgical time between the supine and prone positions in single-session bilateral PCNL. In addition, while the PCNL procedure is performed on one kidney in the supine position, intrarenal surgery on the contralateral kidney can be performed simultaneously by another surgeon. Thus, the operation and anesthesia time can be significantly reduced in selected patients with bilateral kidney stones.

In PCNL, the lower calyx is the most frequently punctured site because of easier access. It is not always possible to reach the stones in the upper pole from punctures made from the lower calyx. In the prone position, the upper pole can be reached in only 20% of renal units with lower pole entry. In this case, a second entry from the upper pole may be required to prevent residual stones, which may lead to thoracic complications. In supine PCNL, 80% of the upper pole can be reached from punctures made in the lower pole. Due to the thinner body wall and muscle and fat layers, the nephroscope can be manipulated at wider angles.

Supine PCNL Limitations

Although the supine position continues to gain popularity for PCNL, it is not as widely used as the prone position. Most surgeons avoid supine PCNL because they complete their learning curve using the prone position. There are several limitations to using the supine position (Table 6.2).

The mobility of the kidney in the supine position is usually greater than in the prone position. The pressure exerted by the abdominal wall in the prone position reduces renal mobility, but the absence of this pressure in the supine position causes renal mobility to increase. This makes renal access more difficult and causes the renal access tract to be longer. The mobile kidney complicates the procedure during renal access and dilatation, particularly in patients with a body mass index below 25 kg/m^2. Methods to reduce mobility include applying manual pressure on the abdominal wall during renal access, stretching the guide wire from both sides with a cystoscope after the bladder to be sent, using a smaller access sheath, and placing a retrograde urethral catheter.

Table 6.2 Disadvantages of supine PCNL

Renal puncture may be difficult due to renal mobility
The renal puncture tract is usually longer
Long or flexible nephroscope may be required
PCNL training is usually performed in the prone position

In the supine position, percutaneous access is made more laterally than in the prone position, which increases the length of the entry tract. As the length of the sheath inside the body increases, the maneuverability of the nephroscope decreases. This situation limits the use of a rigid nephroscope in the supine position, but a flexible nephroscope can be used to overcome this problem. The recently published American Urology Association guidelines recommend routine use of a flexible nephroscope in the PCNL procedure. A longer Amplatz sheath may be required in a supine PCNL due to the longer access tract.

Outcomes

The ideal result in patients undergoing stone surgery is the removal of all stone fragments in the collecting system. Factors such as the position and size of the stones in the kidney and the experience of the surgeon are directly related to stone-free rates. Though the prone position remains the most preferred position for the PCNL procedure, stone-free rates obtained with the supine PCNL technique are similar to those of the prone position (Falahatkar et al.). For each position, duration of hospital stay and stone-free rates were found to be similar in a randomized controlled trial. The operation time was found to be significantly reduced when using the supine position. In a meta-analysis by Liu et al., the stone-free rates were 83.4% and 81.6% in the prone and supine positions, respectively, and 84.5% and 83.5% in a meta-analysis by Wu et al. In another meta-analysis by Zhang et al., which included more studies, it was concluded that the stone-free rate was lower when the prone position was used (72.9% vs. 77.3%, $p < 0.001$). There is a general consensus that the supine position provides shorter surgical time and better respiratory results, and supine PCNL can be applied effectively and safely.

Complications

Although the most feared complications in PCNL are visceral organ injuries, they are rarely seen. It is thought that the risk of colon perforation should be higher in supine PCNL due to renal access from the anterior abdominal wall. In a study by Hopper et al. in which colon position was examined by CT, the retrorenal colon position was determined as 1.9% in the supine position and 10% in the prone position. Similarly, the retrorenal column position at the lower pole entrances was 15% in the prone and 6% in the supine. These findings suggest a potentially higher risk of colon injury in the prone position. Colonic perforation in the prone position was reported in 0.2–0.3% of patients, while colonic perforation in the supine position was not reported in the early series.

Although bleeding can occur at any stage of PCNL, injury to the main renal vessels is rare (<0.5%). Renal capsular or renal parenchymal hemorrhage may occur during percutaneous insertion or dilation. Although perinephritic hematoma is seen on CT scans in one out of every three patients, only 0.1% of patients require blood transfusion. Transfusion rates are reported similarly in supine PCNL; there is no significant difference in blood transfusion rates between the two techniques.

In supine PCNL, the sheath is positioned parallel to the ground. This orientation facilitates the drainage of the used fluid out of the collecting system and reduces the pyelovenous reflux. This is thought to reduce the development of postoperative fever and sepsis. However, there is no significant difference between the two techniques in terms of the development of fever and sepsis in the aforementioned studies.

References

1. Fernström I, Johansson B. Percutaneous pyelolithotomy: a new extraction technique. Scand J Urol Nephrol. 1976;10(3):257–9.
2. Hopper KD, Sherman JL, Luethke JM, Ghaed N. The retrorenal colon in the supine and prone patient. Radiology. 1987;162(2):443–6.
3. Valdivia Uría JG, Lachares Santamaría E, Villarroya Rodríguez S, Taberner Llop J, Abril Baquero G, Aranda Lassa JM. Percutaneous nephrolithectomy: simplified technic (preliminary report). Arch Esp Urol. 1987;40(3):177–80.
4. Valdivia JG, Scarpa RM, Duvdevani M, Gross AJ, Nadler RB, Nutahara K, et al. Supine versus prone position during percutaneous nephrolithotomy: a report from the Clinical Research Office of the Endourological Society Percutaneous Nephrolithotomy Global Study. J Endourol. 2011;25(10):1619–25.
5. Kerbl K, Clayman RV, Chandhoke PS, Urban DA, De Leo BC, Carbone JM. Percutaneous stone removal with the patient in a flank position. J Urol. 1994;151(3):686–8.
6. Falahatkar S, Moghaddam AA, Salehi M, Nikpour S, Esmaili F, Khaki N. Complete supine percutaneous nephrolithotripsy comparison with the prone standard technique. J Endourol. 2008;22(11):2513–8.
7. Ibarluzea G, Scoffone CM, Cracco CM, Poggio M, Porpiglia F, Terrone C, et al. Supine Valdivia and modified lithotomy position for simultaneous anterograde and retrograde endourological access. BJU Int. 2007;100(1):233–6.
8. Papatsoris AG, Zaman F, Panah A, Masood J, El-Husseiny T, Buchholz N. Simultaneous anterograde and retrograde endourologic access: "the Barts technique". J Endourol. 2008;22(12):2665–6.
9. Bach C, Goyal A, Kumar P, Kachrilas S, Papatsoris AG, Buchholz N, et al. The Barts "flank-free" modified supine position for percutaneous nephrolithotomy. Urol Int. 2012;89(3):365–8.
10. Hoznek A, Rode J, Ouzaid I, Faraj B, Kimuli M, de la Taille A, et al. Modified supine percutaneous nephrolithotomy for large kidney and ureteral stones: technique and results. Eur Urol. 2012;61(1):164–70.

11. Atkinson CJ, Turney BW, Noble JG, Reynard JM, Stoneham MD. Supine vs prone percutaneous nephrolithotomy: an anaesthetist's view: comments. BJU Int. 2011;108(3):306–8.
12. Cracco CM, Scoffone CM. ECIRS (endoscopic combined IntraRenal surgery) in the Galdakao-modified supine Valdivia position: a new life for percutaneous surgery? World J Urol. 2011;29(6):821–7.
13. Liu L, Zheng S, Xu Y, Wei Q. Systematic review and meta-analysis of percutaneous nephrolithotomy for patients in the supine versus prone position. J Endourol. 2010;24(12):1941–6.
14. Proietti S, Sortino G, Giannantoni A, Sofer M, Peschechera R, Luciani LG, et al. Single-session Supine Bilateral Percutaneous Nephrolithotomy. Urology. 2015;85(2):304–10.
15. Giusti G, Proietti S, Rodríguez-Socarrás ME, Eisner BH. Reply to Luca Boeri and Emanuele Montanari's Letter to the Editor re: Guido Giusti, Silvia Proietti, Moises E. Rodríguez-Socarrás, et al. Simultaneous Bilateral Endoscopic Surgery (SBES) for Patients with bilateral upper tract urolithiasis: technique and outcomes. Eur Urol. 2018;74:810–5. Eur Urol. 2019;75(6):e173–4.
16. Sofer M, Giusti G, Proietti S, Mintz I, Kabha M, Matzkin H, et al. Upper Calyx approachability through a lower Calyx access for prone versus supine percutaneous nephrolithotomy. J Urol. 2016;195(2):377–82.
17. Assimos D, Krambeck A, Miller NL, Monga M, Murad MH, Nelson CP, vd. Surgical management of stones: American Urological Association/endourological society guideline, Part II. J Urol. 2016;196(4):1161–9.
18. Usawachintachit M, Tzou DT, Hu W, Li J, Chi T. X-ray–free ultrasound-guided percutaneous nephrolithotomy: how to select the right patient? Urology. 2017;100:38–44.
19. Al-Dessoukey AA, Moussa AS, Abdelbary AM, Zayed A, Abdallah R, Elderwy AA, et al. Percutaneous Nephrolithotomy in the oblique supine lithotomy position and prone position: a comparative study. J Endourol. 2014;28(9):1058–63.
20. Karami H, Mohammadi R, Lotfi B. A study on comparative outcomes of percutaneous nephrolithotomy in prone, supine, and flank positions. World J Urol. 2013;31(5):1225–30.
21. Sofer M, Tavdi E, Levi O, Mintz I, Bar-Yosef Y, Sidi A, et al. Implementation of supine percutaneous nephrolithotomy: a novel position for an old operation. Cent Eur J Urol. 2017;70(1):60–5.
22. Patel RM, Okhunov Z, Clayman RV, Landman J. Prone versus supine percutaneous nephrolithotomy: what is your position? Curr Urol Rep. 2017;18(4):26.
23. Yuan D, Liu Y, Rao H, Cheng T, Sun Z, Wang Y, vd. Supine versus prone position in percutaneous nephrolithotomy for kidney calculi: a meta-analysis. J Endourol. 2016;30(7):754–63.
24. Wu P, Wang L, Wang K. Supine versus prone position in percutaneous nephrolithotomy for kidney calculi: a meta-analysis. Int Urol Nephrol. 2011;43(1):67–77.
25. Zhang X, Xia L, Xu T, Wang X, Zhong S, Shen Z. Is the supine position superior to the prone position for percutaneous nephrolithotomy (PCNL)? Urolithiasis. 2014;42(1):87–93.
26. Proietti S, Rodríguez-Socarrás ME, Eisner B, De Coninck V, Sofer M, Saitta G, et al. Supine percutaneous nephrolithotomy: tips and tricks. Transl Androl Urol. 2019;8(Suppl 4):S381–8.
27. Ghani KR, Andonian S, Bultitude M, Desai M, Giusti G, Okhunov Z, et al. Percutaneous nephrolithotomy: update, trends, and future directions. Eur Urol. 2016;70(2):382–96.
28. Zanetti SP, Boeri L, Catellani M, Gallioli A, Trinchieri A, Sarica K, et al. Retrograde intrarenal surgery (RIRS), regular and small sized percutaneous nephrolithotomy (PCNL) in daily practice: European Association of Urology Section of Urolithiasis (EULIS) survey. Arch Ital Urol Androl Organo Uff Soc Ital Ecogr Urol E Nefrol. 2016;88(3):212–6.

Chapter 7
Sacral Neuromodulation: Detailed Surgical Technique and Clinical Outcomes

Kadir Onem, Mehmet Cetinkaya, and Abdullah Acikgoz

Introduction

Sacral neuromodulation is a treatment method used in the treatment of pharmacotherapy-resistant overactive bladder, non-obstructive urinary retention and interstitial cystitis (bladder pain syndrome). In this article, the urological indications, mechanism of action, surgical technique of implantation, post-implantation patient management and clinical results of sacral neuromodulation will be discussed.

Parallel to the developing technology, body batteries, which can be made smaller by shrinking cardiac pacemakers, have also been used in sacral neuromodulation. Sacral neuromodulation (SNM) was first developed in the 1980s by Dr. Introduced by Tanagho and Schmidt [1]. In their study, they reported improvement in the detrusor and sphincter in neurogenic voiding disorders. Later, from London, Dr. Craggs and Dr. Fowler, University of Pittsburgh Dr. DeGroat and Dr. used by Chancellor to treat non-neurogenic overactive bladder [2–4]. After this use, the American Food And Drug Administration (FDA) approved the use of SNM for the treatment of urge incontinence in 1997. It subsequently approved its use in overactive bladder and non-obstructive urinary retention in 1999. To date, more than 25,000 patients with overactive bladder have been treated with sacral neuromodulation [5].

K. Onem (✉) · M. Cetinkaya · A. Acikgoz
Department of Urology, Medicalpark Samsun Hospital, Samsun, Turkey

S. Tonyali et al. (eds.), *Current Endourology*,
https://doi.org/10.1007/978-3-032-00010-1_7

Neuromodulation Mechanism Theories of Effect

Although the exact effect of neuromodulation on the voiding reflex is not yet clear, there are some theories and findings. One of these theories is the augmentation of inhibitory somatic afferent signals, which is claimed to be less in patients with overactive bladder [6]. These afferent fibers reach the pontine voiding center and regulate the voiding reflex with chronic stimulation [7]. In addition, chronic sacral neurostimulation has been shown to increase somotosensory cortical responses to evoked potentials in the posterior tibial nerve or pudandal nerve [8]. In this context, it is not surprising that posterior tibial nerve stimulations have similar effects to sacral neuromodulation.

In animal studies, chronic sacral neuromodulation has been shown to cause hypertrophy of the external urethral sphincter and increase in urethral closure pressure. However, it is not clear whether this effect is caused by direct stimulation of the Onuf nucleus or due to the neuromodulation effect [9].

Patient Selection and Indication

Overactive bladder clinic, which includes frequent urination, urgency and urge incontinence, is the patient group that urologists encounter quite often in daily practice. It is a fact that overactive bladder syndrome impairs quality of life and self-confidence [10]. In studies conducted with different methods the prevalence of overactive bladder has been reported between 8–43% [11–13]. In relation to these rates, stress and the prevalence of mixed urinary incontinence are also affected by age, pregnancy and birth [12]. According to American data, the financial loss of overactive bladder, including the diagnosis, treatment and labor process, is more than 9 billion dollars per year [14].

Conservative treatments are the first choice in the treatment of overactive bladder. At the beginning of these treatments are lifestyle changes, pelvic floor exercises and pharmacological treatment. However, despite these treatments, 40% of patients do not respond to conservative treatment [15]. In this group of patients who do not respond or who are resistant, many options can be offered, from intradetrusor botulinumtoxin injection to urinary diversion. These options include augmentation cystoplasty, detrusor myomectomy (autoaugmentation). Neuromodulation, which is less invasive and reversible, is a treatment method with a high success rate that can be used in patients with overactive bladder who are resistant to first-line treatment and who have been tried botulinumtoxin treatment in our country before deciding on more aggressive surgical treatment. When we look at the definition of refractory overactive bladder, it is defined as the American Urology Association and SUFU (Society of Urodynamics, Female Pelvic Medicine, Urogenital Reconstruction) guidelines in which a patient diagnosed with overactive bladder does not recover despite at least 4–8 weeks of behavioral therapy and/or pharmacotherapy (anticholinergic) application. is defined. Inability to tolerate pharmacotherapy can be considered a failure of anticholinergic therapy [16]. In this context, the AUA/SUFU guidelines recommend sacral neuromodulation as a third-line therapy in the treatment of treatment-resistant non-neurogenic overactive bladder, placing sacral neuromodulation in the same category as botulinumtoxin [16]. The European Association of Urology Incontinence Guidelines (EAU) recommends PTNS (percutaneous tibial nerve stimulation) in patients who do not benefit from anticholinergic therapy.

Neuromodulation can be done in several ways. These can be classified as selective pudendal nerve stimulation, external periurethral nerve stimulation, dorsal genital nerve stimulation, transcutaneous stimulation, direct bladder and spinal cord stimulation, and posterior tibial nerve stimulation. In this section, sacral neuromodulation will be discussed.

Sacral neuromodulation is mostly used in urology practice to stimulate the S3 (sometimes S4) root and reorganize the voiding reflex. In our country, the social security institution includes sacral neuromodulation for the treatment of overactive bladder, interstitial cystitis and non-obstructive urinary retention. After the ideal patient selection, there is a test period that can technically be done with either a temporary electrode (monopolar) or a permanent threaded (quadripolar) electrode. This test period usually ranges from 10 days to 15 days. If the patient's clinical response to the test period is greater than 50%, second-stage implantation is performed for a permanent stimulator or generator (IPG) is placed with the quadripolar electrode. Alternatively, instead of the temporary monopolar electrode placed in the office or outpatient clinic conditions, the electrode inserted in the second stage in the operating room can be inserted in the first stage (1st stage: first implantation of the quadripolar electrode). Then, likewise, if the patient has benefited more than 50% from the test period, stage 2 is passed (IPG implantation in addition to an existing threaded electrode). In the alternative method performed in this way, that is, in the method in which the quadripolar electrode is placed, only IPG is placed in the 2nd stage because the quadripolar electrode is placed in the 1st stage.

After the sacral implant 2nd stage is over, stimulation is continued in the program with the best response in the test period and the patient can control programmer

Implantation

Implantation is divided into two stages. The first stage is implantation for the test period and the second stage is the insertion of the IPG. In the first stage, either a temporary electrode or a quadripolar electrode is used. Positive response rate is higher when quadripolar electrode is used compared to using temporary electrode. This issue will be explored in the next paragraphs. Many urologists can perform temporary electrode placement in office-based outpatient settings. While using fluoroscopy in the monopolar electrode implantation (PNE) phase, it can also be performed using only anatomical landmarks and looking at motor and sensory response. Alternatively, if a quadripolar electrode is to be placed, it should be performed under fluoroscopy in operating room conditions.

Before the test period, all patients should have a 2–3 day voiding diary filled and symptom scoring should be done with a reliable evaluation form. The test period can be extended to an average of one week for the temporary electrode and up to 2 weeks for the permanent electrode. In this process, the electrodes are connected to an external stimulator that can be controlled by the patient. The patient should set the stimulator to an appropriate voltage that will not cause discomfort or pain. Then, the patient is asked to fill in the forms filled before the test period again and to fill out a voiding diary. Considering the patient's satisfaction and the improvement in the voiding diary, it is decided whether to proceed to the next stage (IPG implantation). In general, permanent IPG implantation is recommended if the patient's symptoms have improved by more than 50%.

Office Based Implantation

It is often called office-based implantation percutaneous nerve evaluation (PNE).

For temporary electrode placement, the patient is placed in the prone position. One or two pillows are placed under the patient's lower abdominal area. This is because the sacrum is better exposed. The sacrum is wiped with an antiseptic solution. The sacral notches (sacral notch) and the coccyx are palpated with fluoroscopy or on examination (Fig. 7.1). S3 generally stays in the projection of 1.2 cm lateral of the line intersection connecting this line and the midline (Fig. 7.2).

In addition, this point is approximately 9 cm above the end of the coccyx. After drawing horizontal and vertical lines in this area, local anesthesia was done by injecting local anesthetic under the skin from approximately s2 to s4.

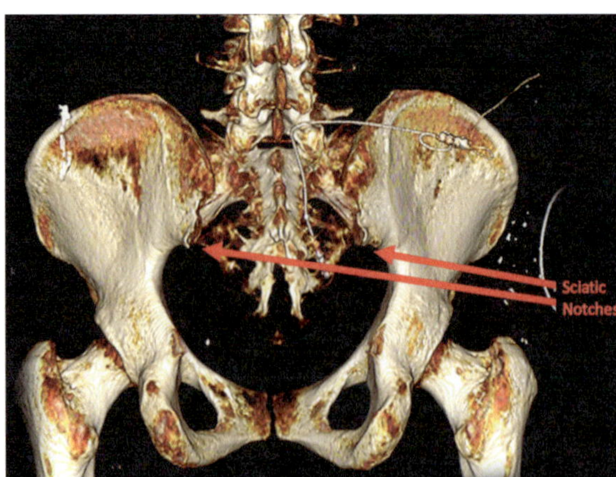

Fig. 7.1 Sciatic notches

Fig. 7.2 Detection of the line connecting the sciatic notches and the midline

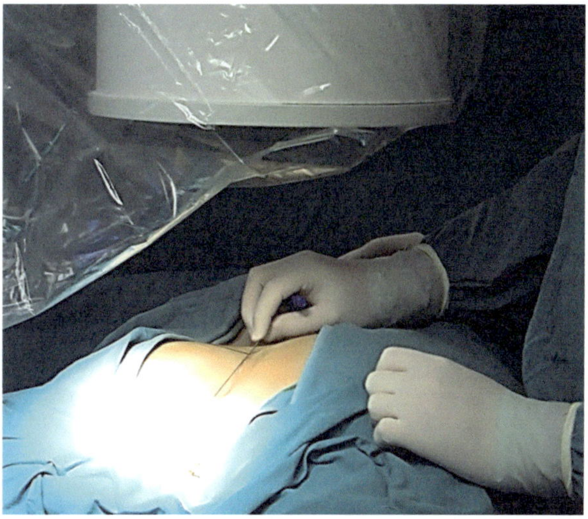

Fig. 7.3 Entry with the foramen needle

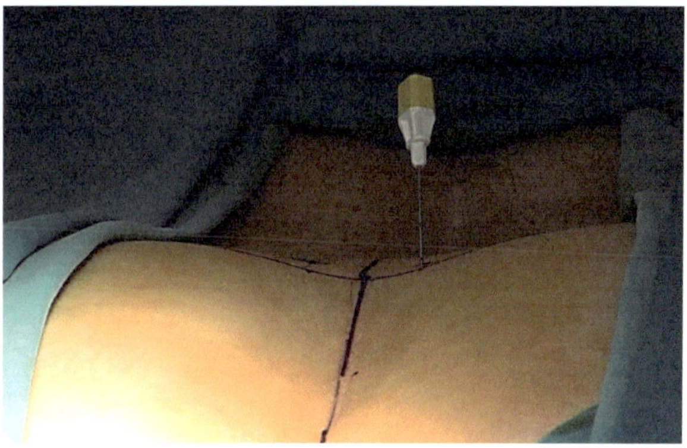

In the meantime, it is necessary not to enter the foramen for local anesthesia. With the foramen needle, it is entered towards the S3 foramen at an angle of 60 degrees from 1.5–2 cm lateral and superior to the intersection point of the lines (Fig. 7.3). Care should be taken to ensure that the direction of the needle is slightly medial to lateral (Fig. 7.4). If the foramen is not penetrated and the bone is felt, the needle should be withdrawn, changed in angle and pushed again, before it is completely removed from the skin, and the foramen should to be found in this way. Then stimulation should be given to see the motor and sensory response (Table 7.1, Fig. 7.5). Peroperative assistance is usually sought from the firm's technical staff to give warnings. There should be a grounding pad attached to the patient's body. This ground is connected to the external stimulator. He gives one side of the patient cable, which the doctor uses to stimulate the foramen needle, to the technical staff. Then the technical personnel perform the stimulation starting from low voltage.

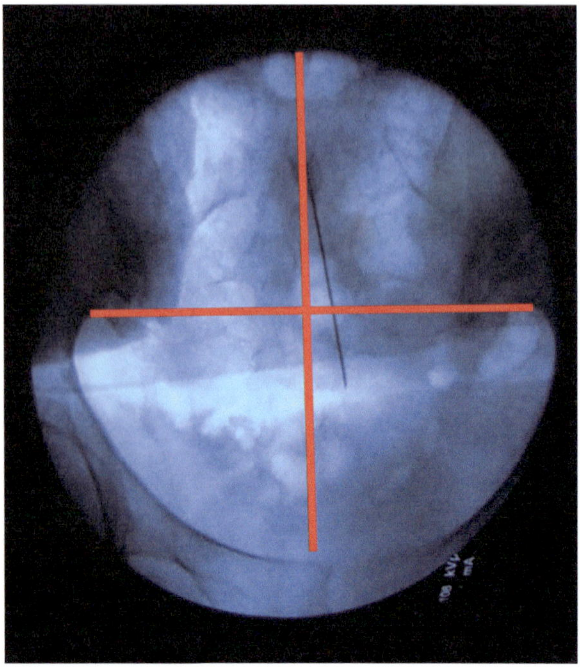

Fig. 7.4 Fluoroscopic view after foramen needle insertion. The direction of the needle should be slightly medial to lateral

Table 7.1 Motor and sensory responses with stimulation of sacral nerves

Sakral sinir	Motor	Duyusal
S2	Plantar flexion and especially lateral rotation of foot contraction of the anal sphincter or thight	Feeling in the leg and hip
S3	Plantar flexion of the big toe, anal contraction (below reflex) (Figs. 7.10, 7.11, 7.12 and 7.13)	Paresthesia or a pulling sensation in the rectum, scrotum, or vagina
S4	Anal contraction	A pulling sensation only in the rectum

If the desired response is not achieved, the needle should be pushed back and advanced and the test repeated (Fig. 7.6). In the meantime, if we suspect that we are not in the right foramen or if we cannot get a response by moving the needle back and forth, a lower or upper level foramen can be entered (Fig. 7.7).

It is useful to pay attention to the opening during this entry. It can be checked whether the second foramen needle enters the same foramen with the first foramen needle by placing the scope in the side position (Fig. 7.8). Because even though the entry levels from the skin are different, both foramen needles can enter the same foramen due to angulation. Preferably, bilateral testing can also be performed. For this purpose, the above-mentioned process is repeated by entering the opposite side with a second foramen needle (Figs. 7.6 and 7.9). If the correct answer is obtained, the stylet of the foramen needle is removed, a temporary monopolar electrode is

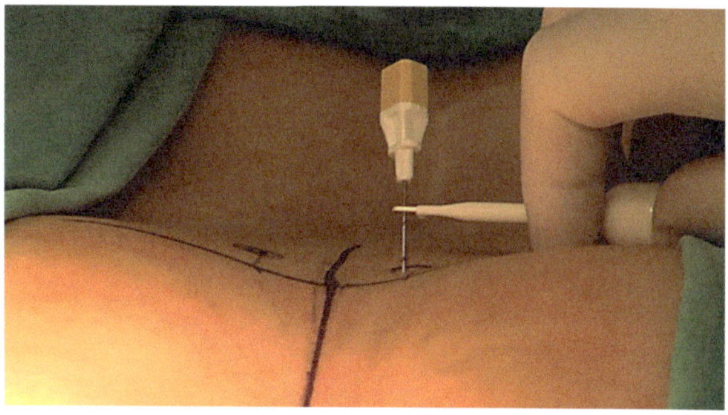

Fig. 7.5 Stimulation via foramen needle

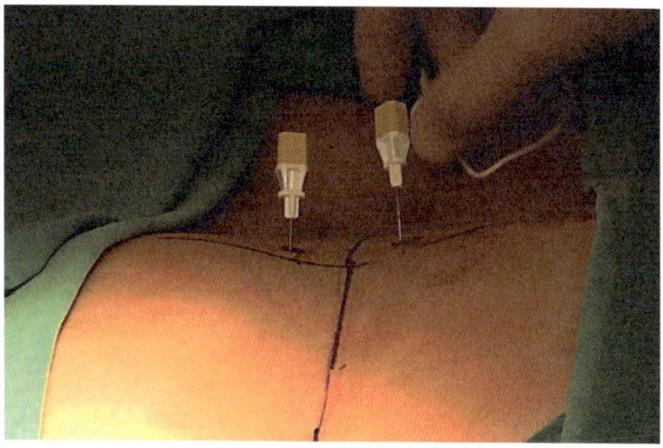

Fig. 7.6 Moving the foramen needles back and advanced

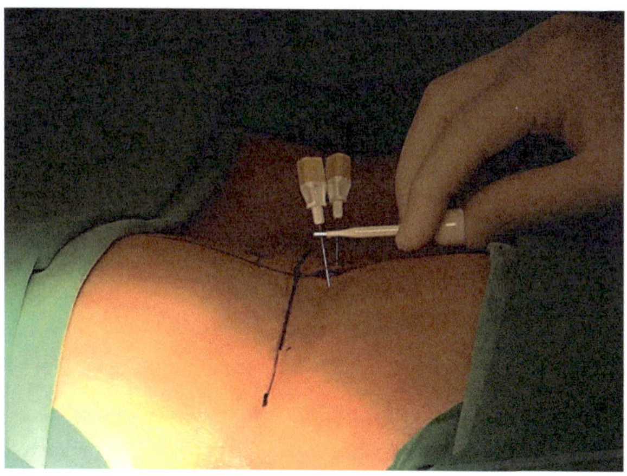

Fig. 7.7 Stimulation via second foramen needle

sent, and the procedure is terminated by retesting. Meanwhile, the outer part of the foramen needle is removed by carefully pulling back so that the monapolar electrode does not come out. It is connected to the external stimulator with a firm dressing. After the procedure, the patient is informed about the stimulation.

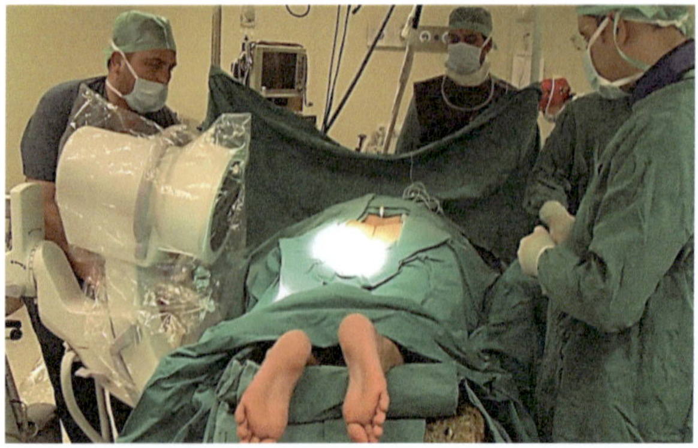

Fig. 7.8 Lateral (transverse or lateral) use of fluoroscopy

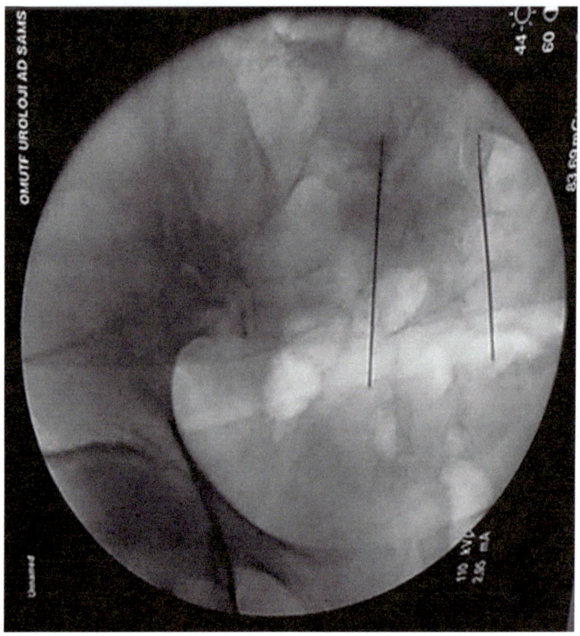

Fig. 7.9 Localization of foramen needles for bilateral testing

Motor and Sensory Response

Evaluation of intraoperative motor and sensory response gives us information about whether the electrodes are in the right place. The sensory response is usually felt as tingling, tugging and vibration in the vagina and rectum in women. In men, it is felt in the phallus, rectum, and scrotum. The motor response should be reflex contraction of the levator (below reflex) ani and plantar flexion of the big toe. Sometimes plantar flexion can be observed in all fingers instead of the big toe. In some patients, a more appropriate response may be obtained in S4.

There are studies showing that intraoperative motor response is more important than sensory response and is more predictive for subsequent success rate. In the study of Cohen et al., quadripolar electrode implantation was performed in 35 patients and response was observed in 21 of them. It is noteworthy that 95% of the patients who went to IPG implantation, that is, benefited from the test period, had a motor response, while this rate remained at only 21.4% in the patients who failed the test period [17]. In another study, patients were classified according to whether they received a sensory response or not. Of the 141 patients tested, 61% gave a sensory response, while 39% did not. It has been reported that there is no difference in demographic characteristics between the responding and non-responding groups. 90% of sensory responders and 87% of nonresponders went for IPG implantation. While the rates of removal of IPG at the end of 4 years were reported to be similar in both groups, IPG implantation provided significant improvement in all patients in terms of symptomatic improvement, but there was no significant difference between the groups [18].

In the test phase of sacral neurostimulation, although we wait for a motor response to find the right foramen, the stimulation is usually done below the voltage that generates this response. The patient can use this sensory sensation to see if neuromodulation is ongoing. The fact that the patient does not feel this sensation may be a sign that neurostimulation will no longer be effective.

Tined Lead Implantation

Fluoroscopy is needed for quadripolar electrode implantation. Preferably, the procedure should be performed in the operating room with light sedation or general anesthesia. It is important for us to see the motor response that the anesthesiologist does not use muscle relaxants. If a muscle relaxant is to be used, it should be reversed after the patient is asleep and positioned. Today, many doctors place stage I quadripolar electrodes instead of PNE. The reasons for this are mainly to prevent migration and related false negatives.

It is similar to the placement of the monopolar electrode and the pushing of the foramen needle up to the step of acquiring motor and sensory responses. After receiving a response with a foramen needle (Fig. 7.10). The stylet of the foramen needle is removed and the guiding guide is sent (Fig. 7.14). Then, in fluoroscopy, from the lateral position, how deep the guide goes is checked. The guide should not go too deep, it is sufficient that it has advanced around 1–1.5 cm after the sacral bone. In the next step, the guide is held while the foramen needle is withdrawn and only the guiding guide remains on the patient (Fig. 7.15). The point where the guide enters the skin is cut with a scalpel, making it easier for the dilator to pass through the skin (Fig. 7.16). Then, the dilator and dilator sheath are pushed together under the guidance of fluoroscopy so as to enclose the (Fig. 7.17). The radiopaque sign of the sheath, which is pushed under the guidance of fluoroscopy, should come up to half of the sacral bone in lateral view (Fig. 7.18).

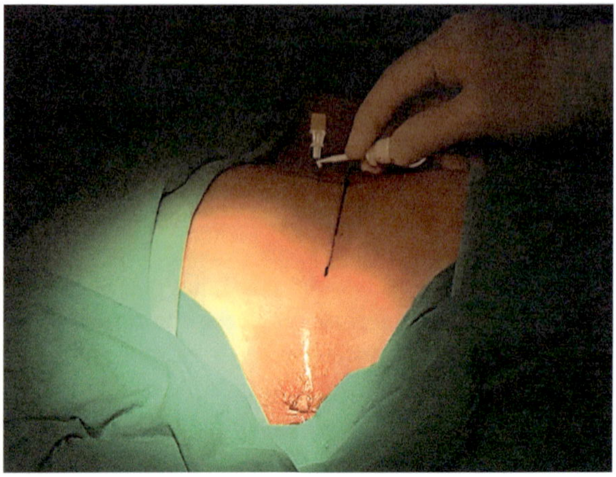

Fig. 7.10 Stimulation with a foramen needle and seeing the reflex in the anus

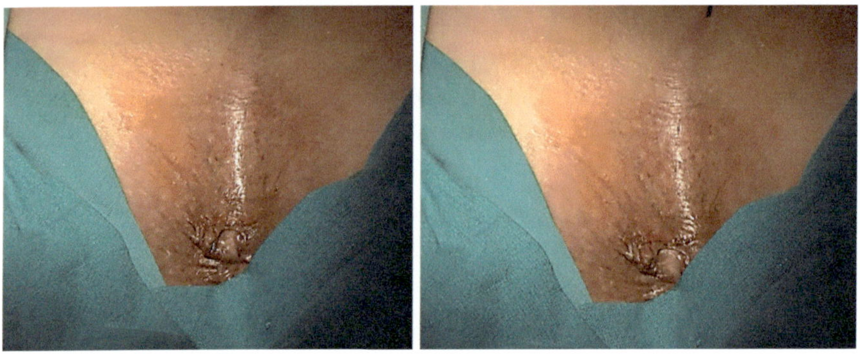

Fig. 7.11 Anal contraction: Deviation to the stimulated side

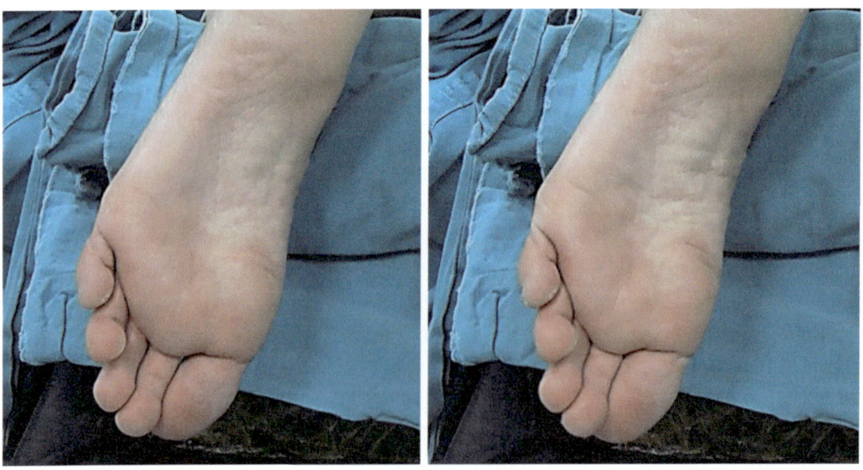

Fig. 7.12 Left plantar flexion (Pay attention to the wrinkles on the soles of the feet, the increase in these wrinkles is an indication of plantar flexion)

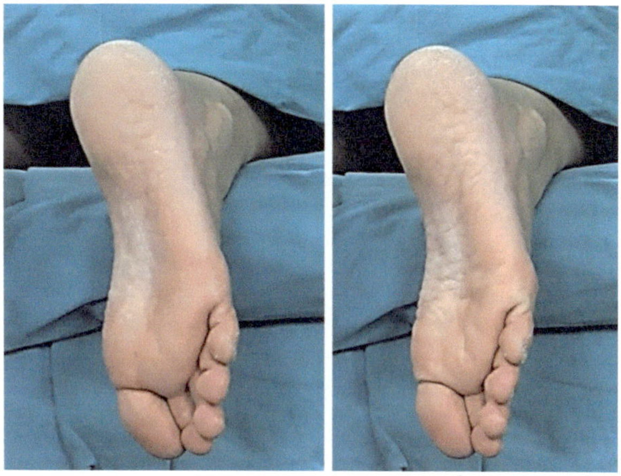

Fig. 7.13 Right plantar flexion (Note the wrinkles on the soles of the feet, the increase in these wrinkles is an indication of plantar flexion)

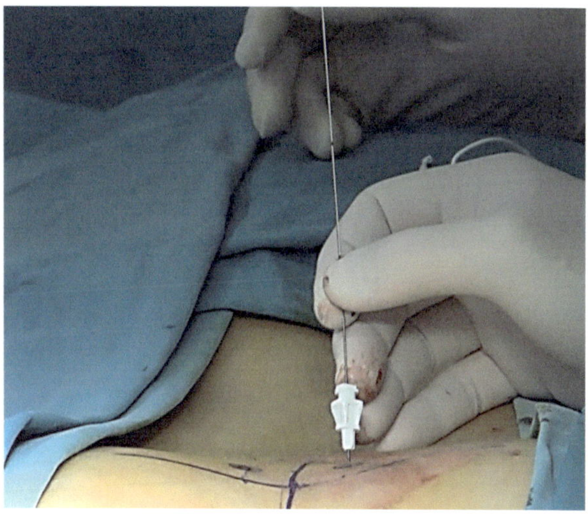

Fig. 7.14 Removing the stylet of the foramen needle and sending the guide. In the meantime, the depth of the guide should be checked and checked with fluoroscopy in the lateral position

At the point where the radiopaque mark is seen in the middle of the sacrum on the scopy, the dilator is held with one hand while the dilator is removed with the guide and only the dilator sheath remains on the patient (Fig. 7.19). After this stage, it should be checked with fluoroscopy that the radiopaque mark is at the midpoint of the sacrum as seen in Fig. 7.18. The level with this mark is the level where the foramen starts.

After removing the guide sheath and dilator on the dilator (Fig. 7.20), the quadripolar tined lead electrode should be pushed through the sheath (Fig. 7.21). In the meantime, it should be checked with fluoroscopy. The leads of the quadripolar electrode are called 0, 1, 2 and 3 numbers from the most distal stimulating part to the proximal. Fluoroscopically, it is aimed that the electrode 0, 1 and 2 remain below the sacrum and the number 3 is usually inside the sacrum (Fig. 7.22).

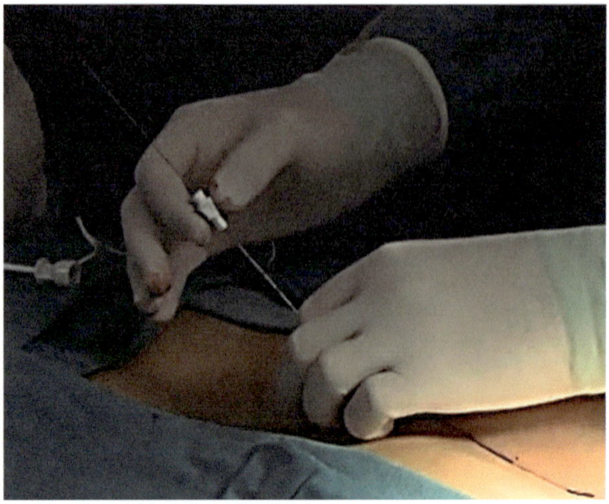

Fig. 7.15 Removal of the foramen needle. It is important that the internal guide does not come off during this time, so the guide guide is held with one hand and the sheath of the foramen needle is pulled with the other hand

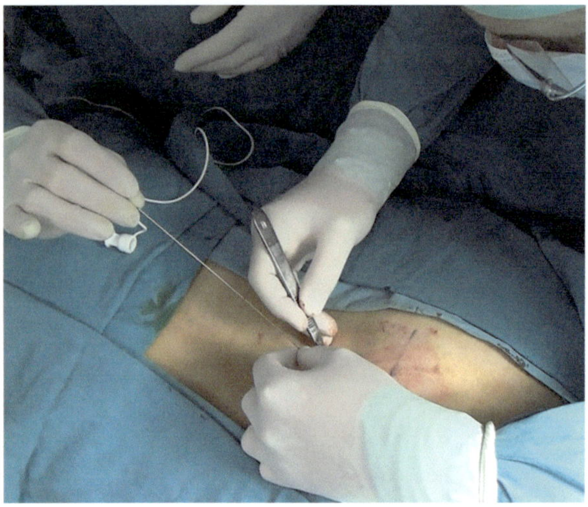

Fig. 7.16 Enlarging the point where the guiding guide enters the skin with the scalpel

After the quadripolar electrode is pushed through the sheath and checked for fluoroscopic position. Just as the foramen needle is stimulated, each pole of the quadripolar electrode should be stimulated and controlled. Stimulation can be rechecked by moving the electrode back and forth to get the lowest voltage and best response (Fig. 7.23). After the stimulation is done, there is the stage of making connections. For this purpose, a 5 cm incision is made on the horizontal axis of the hip, on the side of the entrance and sometimes on the opposite side, under the iliac crest. By making connections, this part will be wrapped in plastic protector and placed just below this incision (Fig. 7.24). In addition, this incision and the created pouch will then be the implantation site of the IPG.

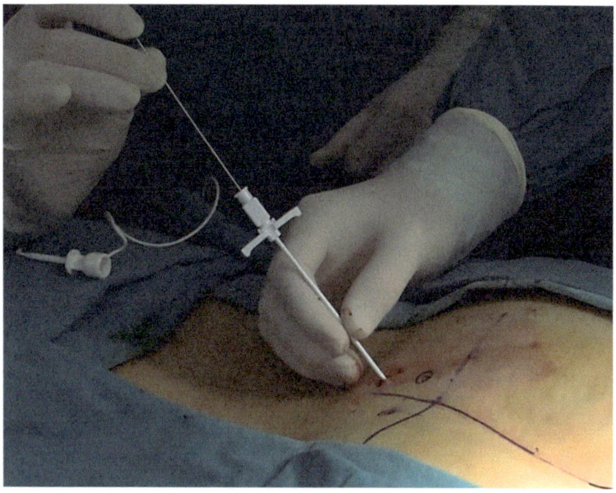

Fig. 7.17 Advencement the dilator and dilator sheath over the guide

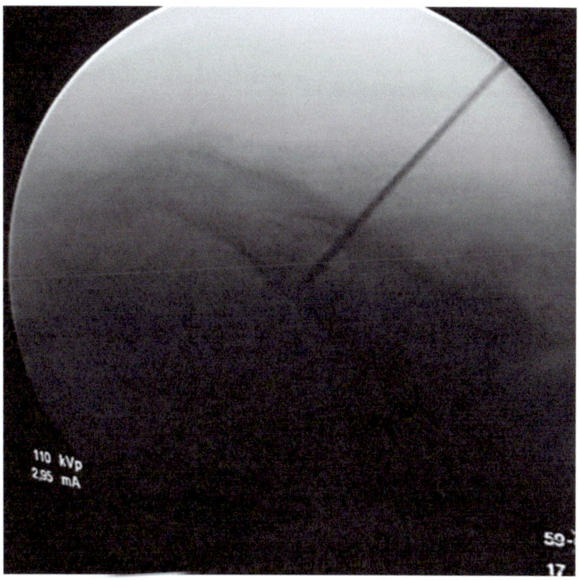

Fig. 7.18 Dilator and sheath pushed over the guide guide. Note that the radiopaque mark is in the middle of the sacrum

At this stage, it is necessary to enter the tunneling tool from the entrance of the foramen needle without damaging the cable, and exit the pouch formed by coming under the iliac crest towards the hip of that side. The tip of the tunneling tool is removed, leaving the plastic part outside, and the quadripolar electrode is passed through this plastic part and removed from the formed pouch. Then, the quadripolar electrode is connected to the extension cable and tightened with the screwdriver included in the kit (Fig. 7.25). After compression, it is placed in a protective sheath and tightly tied on both sides with non-absorbable sutures. It is then placed under the skin.

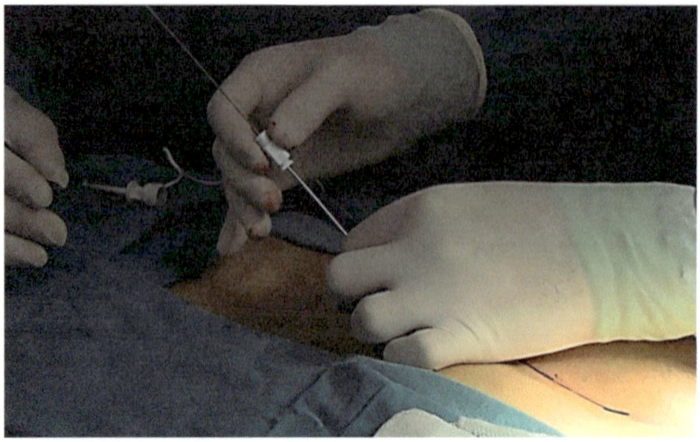

Fig. 7.19 Retraction of dilator and guide leaving the dilator sheath in place

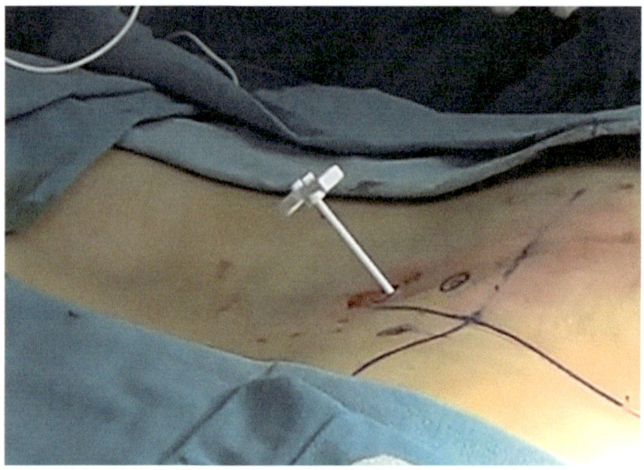

Fig. 7.20 Only the dilator sheath should remain on the patient

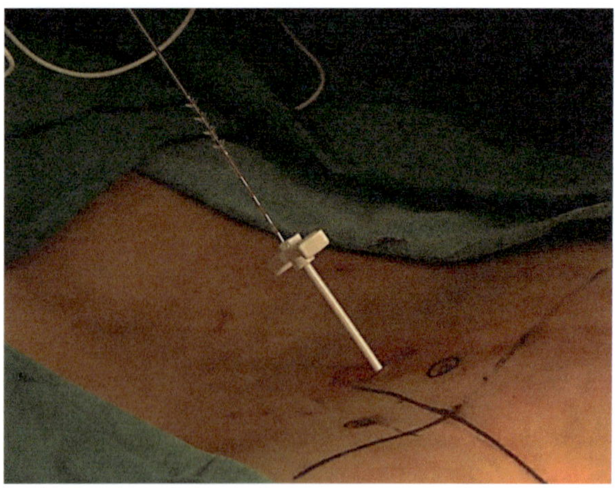

Fig. 7.21 Advencing of the tined lead throught the dilator sheath

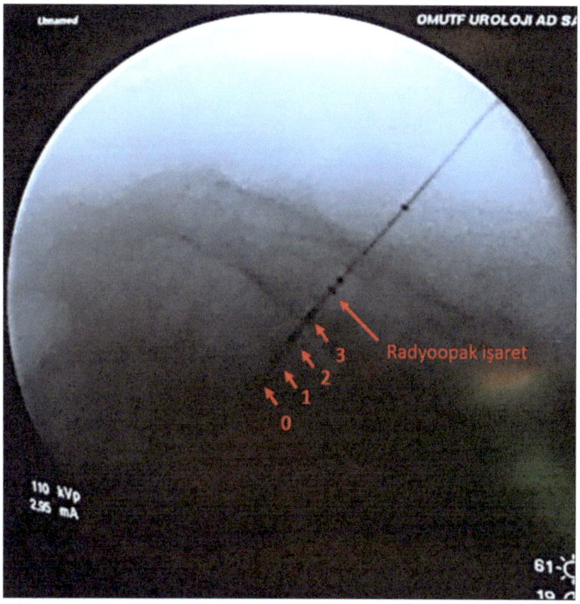

Fig. 7.22 Fluoroscopic lateral view: Quadripolar electrode was advanced through the sheath. Numbers 0, 1 and 2 electrodes are seen under the sacrum while numbers 3 electroda is located inside the sacrum

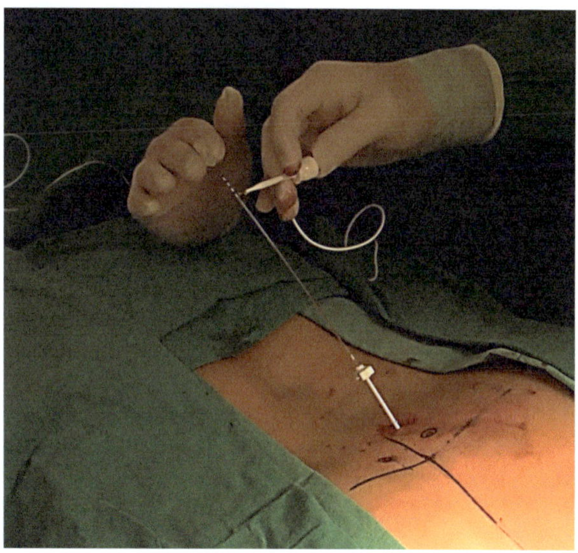

Fig. 7.23 Stimulation of electrodes 0, 1, 2 and 3 after quadripolar electrode placement

After the connection is made, the extension cable is also tested (Fig. 7.26). Then, by entering the subcutaneous pouch with the tunneling device, 7–8 cm above the skin is exited, and an extension cable is sent through the plastic tube and is kept to be connected to the external stimulator by coming out of the skin (Fig. 7.27). After the skin was closed, the procedure is terminated.

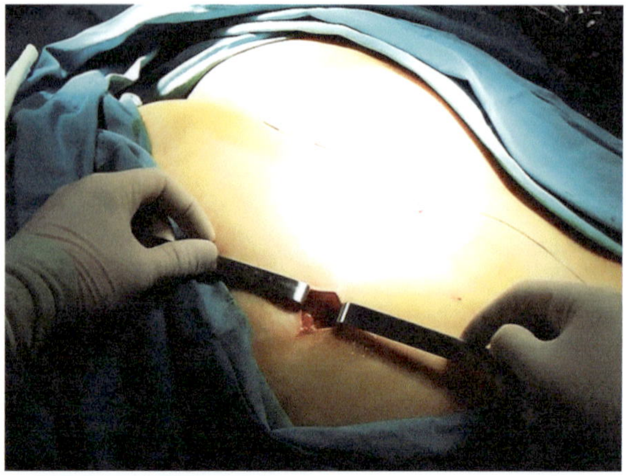

Fig. 7.24 Creation of a subcutaneous pouch with a 4–5 cm incision in the horizontal axis of the hip under the crista iliaca

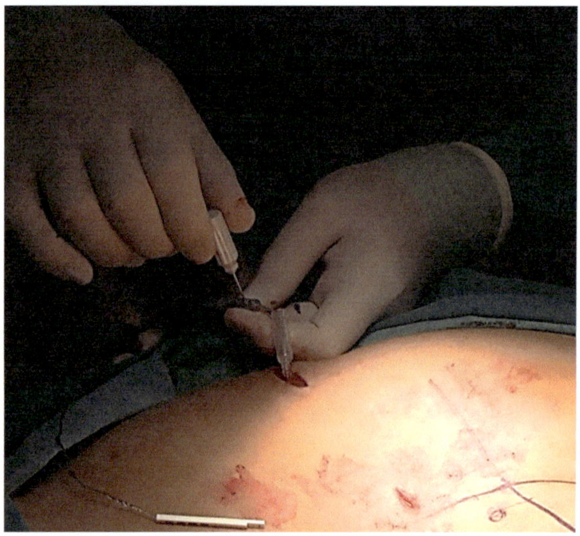

Fig. 7.25 Making the connections of the quadripolar electrode and the extension cable. After being tightened with a screwdriver, it will be placed under the skin by putting it into the sheath seen in the photo

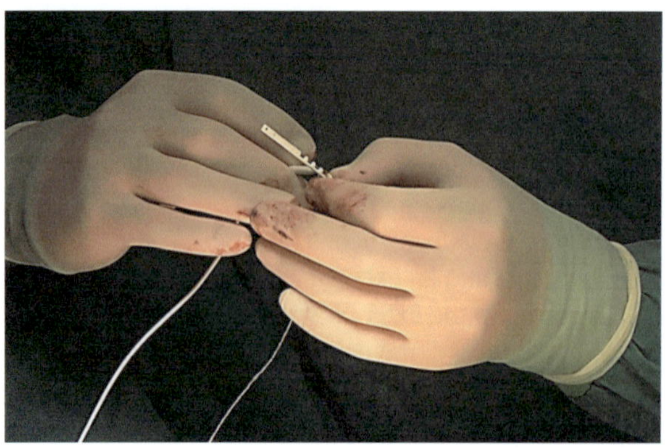

Fig. 7.26 Stimulation and testing of extension cable after connections are made

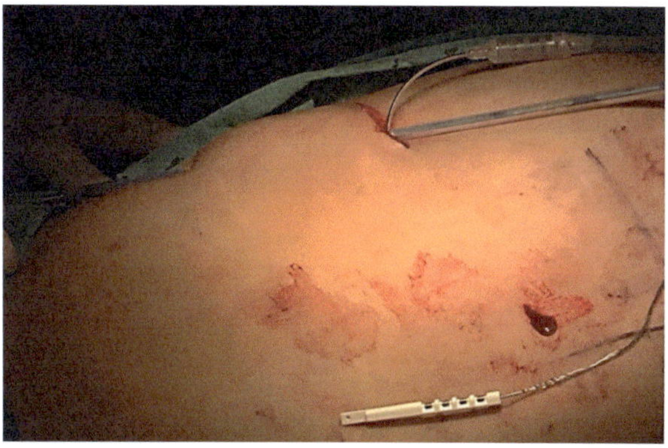

Fig. 7.27 Creation of the second tunnel

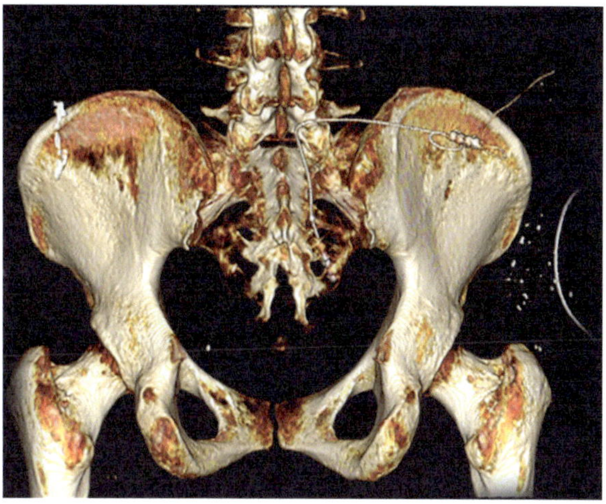

Fig. 7.28 3D computed tomography of a patient who underwent Satage II. The quadripolar electrode entered through the S3 foramen and the connection was made just below the iliac crest as can be seen. Quadripolar electrode is oriented from medial to lateral

Stage II Implantation (IPG Implantation)

After the PNE or Stage I stage, if the patient's clinical improvement is more than 50%, this stage is considered as successful. This period is usually 2 week in PNE and 4 weeks in the quadripolar electrode. If only PNE is performed and response is received in the first stage, a quadripolar electrode and IPG are inserted in Stage II. This is just like stage I, with an additional IPG attached. For a patient who has completed the test phase with the quadripolar electrode, which is the more commonly used method, stage II simply means the insertion of the IPG. Fluoroscopy is not needed for this stage. With only local anesthesia or a light sedation were enought, the pouch created under the iliac crest in the prone position is opened again (Figs. 7.28 and 7.29), and after the connections are removed with a screwdriver, it is connected directly to the IPG and the subcutaneous and skin are closed with the text of the IPG facing the skin. In the meantime, the technical personnel makes the measurements of the electrode and whether the IPG is working. Then the operation is terminated.

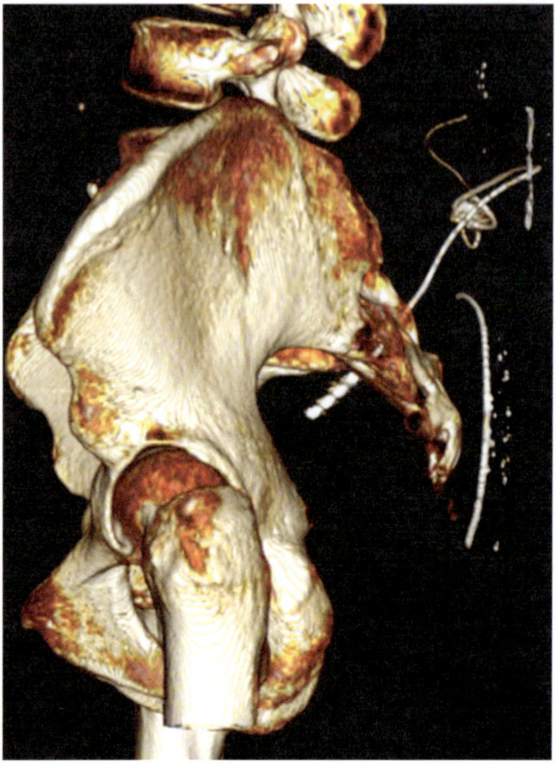

Fig. 7.29 3D computed tomography of a patient who underwent stage II. lateral view

PNE or Two-Stage Implantation

Sacral neuromodulation can be done in two ways. The first is to first perform the testing phase with PNE (no operating room conditions required) for one week and then, if successful (more than 50% symptomatic improvement) from the test, implant the quadripolar electrode and IPG in a single step in operating room conditions. The second method is to attach the quadripolar electrode under operating room conditions and perform the test period. If success is achieved, as in PNE, taking the patient back to the operating room and implanting the IPG is the last step of the two-stage implantation. The temporary monopolar electrode has a disadvantage of 10–15% migration in PNE [19]. Other complications such as pain are seen 2–3% less frequently [20].

In the quadripolar electrode, on the other hand, there is the possibility of testing for a longer period of time, such as two weeks. It is predicted that the probability of migration due to the tined in the electrode is around 16%. But there is this risk, especially in thin patients [21].

In studies where the quadripolar electrode and the monopolar electrode were directly compared, it was observed that these patients went to IPG implantation at a lower rate in the tests performed with the temporary electrode (PNE: 47%,

Quadripolar: 69%). Positive response rate has been reported to be negatively correlated with patient age. When we look at the follow-ups, it was seen that the treatment failure rates (2.9%) of the patients who went to IPG were similar, regardless of the method in the test period [22]. In a similar study, 88% of 17 patients who had Quadripolar electrodes and 6 of 13 patients who had PNE had a positive response ($p = 0.02$). When the patients who underwent IPG implantation were compared among themselves in terms of the method in the test period, no significant difference was found between the improvement parameters. That is, patients who passed the test period achieved similar rates of improvement [23]. The infectious agent in patients whose test period exceeds two weeks is usually staphylococcus strains [24].

In conclusion, although PNE is reasonable, it is a test method to be tried in the first choice. The quadripolar electrode, on the other hand, is an ideal test tool for patients who are at risk of migration, who have an inadequate response due to migration, or who want a long-term test period.

Efficacy and Clinical Results

It is a known fact that urge, urge incontinence and increase in urinary frequency have a negative effect on quality of life. Neuromodulation can be recommended as a treatment that can be used before more invasive surgical procedures for patients who do not respond to medical treatment. Success rates vary between 64% and 88% in patients with urgency and urge incontinence or in refractory cases with a diagnosis of overactive bladder.

In randomized controlled studies, the delayed group was compared with the sacral neuromodulation group. Treatment results in patients with refractory urge incontinence are given in Table 7.2. In Table 7.2, an improvement of 76–100% was reported in the SNM group, while there was only a 5% improvement in the group without SNM implantation, and it was noteworthy that SNM provided a significant improvement compared to the control group. On the other hand, when basal values and sixth month values after SNM are examined in the SNM group, the rate of basal daily incontinence episodes (13.5/day to 1.4/day) and pad use (8.7 pieces/day to 0.7 pieces/day) /day) It is seen that it improved significantly after 6 months.

In addition, Table 7.3 shows that there is a significant improvement in the degree of urinary incontinence, in other words, the amount of urinary incontinence and functional bladder capacity. In the untreated group, symptoms and episodes of urinary incontinence appear to have remained unchanged or worsened. Weil et al. found that there was a significant improvement in the physical health component of quality of life (when evaluated with the SF-36 form) in addition to urinary symptoms and findings in the patients in the SNM group ($p = 0.037$) [25]. Likewise, Schmidt et al. In their study on quality of life, they found a significant improvement in the physical health component of the SNM group ($p = 0.0008$), but they did not detect an improvement in the mental health component [26].

Table 7.2 6-month results in randomized controlled trials. (Cure: More than 90% improvement, Improvement: More than 50% improvement in symptoms)

Study	*n*/total *n* (%)		
SNM group	Cure	İmprovement	Total
Weil et al. [25]	9/16 (56)	5/16 (29)	%85
Schmidt et al. [26]	16/34 (47)	10/34 (29)	%76
Weil et al. [27]	0 (0)	5/5 (100)	%100
Delayed group			
Weil et al. [25]	1/22 (5)	0/22 (0)	%5
Schmidt et al. [26]	0/42 (0)	2/42 (5)	%5
Weil et al. [27]	NR	NR	NR

Table 7.3 Randomized controlled studies: Number of incontinences, amount, bladder capacity

Study	*n*	SNM		*p*	*n*	Control		*p*
Urinary Incontinance episodes per day								
Weil et al. [25]	21	13,5 ± 7,5	1,4 ± 3,3	<0,0005	22	13,5 ± 7,8	11,2 ± 5,6	NS
Schmidt et al. [26]	34	9,7 ± 6,3	2,6 ± 5,1	<0,0001	42	9,3 ± 4,8	11,3 ± 5,9	0,002
PEd us eper day								
Weil et al. [25]	21	8,7 ± 6,8	0,7 ± 1,3	<0,0005	22	8,7 ± 7,1	6,8 ± 4,0	NS
Schmidt et al. [26]	34	6,2 ± 5,0	1,1 ± 2,0	<0,0001	42	5,0 ± 3,7	6,3 ± 3,6	0,003
Degree of incontinence								
Weil et al. [25]	21	2,1 ± 0,6	1,6 ± 1,7	NS	22	2,1 ± 0,6	2,1 ± 0,6	NS
Schmidt et al. [26]	34	2,0 ± 0,7	0,8 ± 0,9	<0,0001	42	1,8 ± 0,6	2,0 ± 0,6	0,006
Bladder capacity ml								
Weil et al. [25]	21	266 ± 112	370 ± 91	0,013	23	X	X	–

X undeclared, *NS* non significant

In case series studies of Urge and Urge incontinence patients, an average of 39% cure rate was reported between 7–64% (Table 7.4). The proportion of patients with more than 50% improvement in their incontinence symptom is 40% on average. Again in the case series, it was observed that 32% of the patients had less than 50% improvement in their incontinence symptoms, and the patients in this group were defined as the unsuccessful group. While daily urinary incontinence episodes vary between 4.5–11.6 times/day before SNM, this number decreases to 0.8–5.0 times/day after SNM (53–92% decrease). It was observed that the average number of daily pad use decreased from 3.0–8.3 pad/day to 0.4–3.4 pad/day (49–94% improvement). When urinary incontinence is classified from mild [1] to severe [3], the mean urinary incontinence episodes per day decreases from 1.4–2.0 to 0.8–1.6 (16–40% reduction). While the mean frequency of urination was 10–15 before implantation, it decreased to 7.0–9.2 after implantation (30–50% reduction). It is observed that the mean voided volume has increased from 99–195 ml to 176–402 (34–288% increase). While the total bladder capacity varies between 122–400 ml on average before implantation, it is seen that these averages increase to 273–596 ml at the sixth month

Table 7.4 SNM case series

Study	Follow-up (mounths)	*n* Cure/total (%)	*n* improvement/total (%)	*n* unresponse/total (%)
Ruiz-Cerda et al. [32]	6,8	14/25 (55)	2/25 (8)	9/25 (36)
Heesakkers et al. [33]	60	X	27/43 (63)	16/43 (37)
Amundsen et al. [29]	7,8	2/12 (17)	10/12 (83)	0/43 (0)
Everaert et al. [34]	12	X	4/5 (80)	1/5 (20)
Groenendijk et al. [35]	6	X	55/84 (65)	29/84 (35)
Hedlund et al. [36]	18	8/14 (57)	5/14 (36)	1/14 (7)
Spinelli et al. [37]		X	3/3 (100)	0/3 (0)
Caraballo et al. [38]	13,4	1/15 (7)	11/15 (73)	3/15 (20)
Janknegt et al. [39]	30,8	25/96 (26)	35/96 (36)	36/96 (38)
Bosch et al. [40]	47	18/45 (40)	9/45 (20)	18/45 (40)
Grunewald et al. [41]	6	6/26 (23)	13/26 (50)	7/26 (27)
Siegel et al. [20]	36	19/41 (46)	5/41 (12)	17/41 (41)
Koldewijn et al. [42]	29	18/28 (64)	3/28 (11)	7/28 (25)
Hohenfellner et al. [32]	13	X	5/5 (100)	0/5 (0)
Shaker et al. [30]	18,8	8/18 (44)	4/18 (22)	6/18 (33)
Weil et al. [43]	37,8	14/24 (58)	3/24 (13)	7/24 (29)
Dijkema et al. [44]	17	6/17 (35)	5/17 (30)	6/17 (35)
Total		139/361 (39)	199/501 (40)	163/501 (32)

after implantation (15–197% increase). When the change in quality of life after implantation was evaluated, it was reported that the quality of life score increased from 34.4 to 83.8 [28]. Amundsen et al. They reported a significant improvement in the quality of life score of SNM (improvement from 250 to 62 $p = 0.03$) [29]. Shaker et al. On the other hand, the effects of BECK depression index and SF-36 quality of life score and SNM on quality of life and depression scores were investigated. They reported an improvement from 10% to 40% on the Beck depression scale. No increase was observed in the SF-36 score, except for the perception of life subgroup [30].

The presence of elderly patients and comorbid factors, namely chronic diseases, are factors that reduce the success of SNM. This finding was discussed in a study in which 105 patients with neurological disorders were evaluated. A 30% improvement in symptoms was observed in patients older than 75 years of age. In patients younger than 45 years of age, 80% response was obtained. No improvement was observed in patients with three or more comorbid diseases [31].

Non-obstructive Urinary Retention

Sacral neuromodulation has been successfully used in idiopathic non-obstructive urinary retention, denervation after hysterectomy, and fowler's syndrome [45, 46]. Factors related to the harvest affect the success rate. In recent years, an increasing number of reports emphasize that sacral neurostimulation will give different results on a patient basis and according to patient characteristics. These conditions are functional obstructions and acontractile bladder. Goh et al. In their study, in patients with non-obstructive urinary retention and clean intermittent catheterization, when SNM separated patients who could urinate more than 50 ml (n: 18) and those who could not (n: 11) before preimplantation, patients who could urinate more than 50 ml were more common reported that it benefited at a rate [47]. In addition, it has been reported that bladder contractility may be predictive for SNM [48].

Jonas et al. In his randomized controlled study, one group of patients with non-obstructive urinary retention underwent SNM implantation and the other group was accepted as the control group as the delayed group. Successful results were obtained in 86% of patients who underwent IPG implantation, while 69% of patients discontinued clean intermittent catheterization. In the remaining 14% patients, more than 50% reduction in clean intermittent catheterization volumes was observed. At the end of the 18-month follow-up, it was noted that 71% of these patients still benefit from the treatment. The improvement in the control group was limited at 9%. It has been reported that the residual volume increases statistically significantly in cases where the IPG is temporarily closed [49].

Datta et al. 60 patients with non-obstructive urinary retention were included in the study. After SNM implantation, it was observed that 72% of the patients were able to urinate spontaneously with an average residual urine volume of 100 ml. 50% of patients discontinued use of clean intermittent catheterization. It has been reported that patients with abnormal sphincteric activity are more successful than patients with normal (43% and 76%). It has also been reported that the average battery life is 7.1 years [50].

White et al. In his study, which included 40 patients with non-obstructive urinary retention, he reported that more than 50% of the symptoms of 70% of the patients were observed during the test. Permanent IPG was placed in these patients and the patients were followed for an average of 40 ± 19 months. At the end of this follow-up, it was reported that 85% of the patients had their symptoms resolved by more than 50%. It was also added to the study that the IPG of 14% of the patients was taken and 21% of them were changed. It was noted that the number of clean intermittent catheterizations and post-void residual volumes were significantly reduced in patients with complete recurrence, and the post-void volumes of patients with incomplete urinary retention were also significantly reduced [51].

Aboseif et al. In the study, 32 patients with non-obstructive urinary retention were tested and IPG implantation was performed in 20 patients. Eighteen patients discontinued clean intermittent catheterization. While the mean voided urine volume increased from 48 ml to 198 ml, the amount of postvoid residual urine decreased from 315 ml to 60 ml.

Test periods of patients with urinary retention should be kept longer than other patients. This period may be 2–3 weeks in PNE and up to 4 weeks in quadripolar electrode. However, bilateral SNM can be recommended in refractory patients after first and unilateral SNM. However, there is not much data on bilateral implantation [52].

Neurogenic Lower Urinary Tract Dysfunction and SNM

Lower urinary tract symptoms and neurogenic bladder are frequently encountered in patients with Parkinson's, stroke, multiple sclerosis and spinal cord trauma.

Peters et al. retrospectively compared the groups of patients who had neurostimulation of neurogenic and non-neurogenic origin in their study and compared the groups with 71 neurological diseases and 269 groups without neurological diseases. In the neurogenic group, there were 17 patients with stroke, 13 with multiple sclerosis, 10 with Parkinson's disease, 4 with incomplete spinal cord trauma, and one with cerebral palsy. Significant improvement in voiding diaries was reported after IPG implantation in both groups. While the mean frequency of urination and urgency of patients with neurogenic bladder were reported as 11.6 ± 4.1 and 4.5 ± 2.9 before implantation, their scores after 24 months were 10.6 ± 2.8 ($p = 0.01$), respectively. It was reported as 3.1 ± 1.9 ($p = 0.02$). No significant improvement was observed in incontinence episodes and incontinence degree (preimplant: 6.7 ± 5.3 and 4.1 ± 2.3, post-24 months-: 5.5 ± 4.8 and 5.0 ± 5.7, p = 0. .06 and $p = 0.2$). In addition, neurogenic bladder patients had overactive bladder scores (preimplant: 68 ± 24, 24. months: 34 ± 16, $p < 0.0001$) and quality of life score (preimplant: 43 ± 23, 24. month: 73 ± 21, p. <0.0001) significant improvement was achieved [53].

Kessler et al. In the study, patients with neurogenic bladder who underwent sacral neuromodulation were compiled [54]. In this review, 43 multiple sclerosis patients, 6 Parkinson's, 4 myelomeningocele, 12 stroke, 2 cerebral pals, 23 pelvic surgeries, 30 disc disease, 31 spinal cord injuries (5 complete, 17 incomplete, 9 unknown) were included in the review. When they are separated clinically; It was classified as 119 chronic urinary retention, 8 urgency-frequency, 77 urge incontinence, and 29 combined symptoms. Positive response was obtained in 68% of the test period. The patients were followed up for an average of 26 months. 87% unilateral 13% bilateral IPG was implanted. A total of 92% post-implant success was achieved (Table 7.5). Electrode migration occurred in 5 patients and pain in one patient. A total of 0% of adverse events were reported during the test phase. In the persistent SNM stage, 69 patients reported adverse events (24%), and 45 of them underwent revision. The most common side effects were electrode migration (15 patients) and pain (12 patients) [54].

SNM does not appear to have a beneficial effect in patients with complete or near-complete spinal cord injury (SCI) [55, 56]. The only exception is bilateral

Table 7.5 NLUTD and SNM success rates

	Test Period		IPG	
	n positive test/total	%	*n* positive test/total	%
Etiology				
Multiple sclerosis	36/43	84	46/52	92
Parkinson	4/6	67	6/6	100
Myelomeningocele	2/4	50	½	50
Stroke	5/12	42	6/10	60
Cerebral palsy	2/2	100	2/2	100
Pelvic surgery	19/23	83	14/23	61
Disc disease	18/30	60	10/18	56
Spinal cord injury	11/31	35	47/61	77
Complete	2/5	40	10/12	83
Incomplete	5/17	29	30/37	81
Unknown	4/9	44	7/12	58
Other	48/80	60	38/52	73
Type of clinical presentation				
Urinary retention	67/119	56	65/89	73
Urgency / frequency	6/8	75	12/14	86
Urge incontinence	46/77	60	62/84	74
Combination	26/29	90	31/37	84

stimulation in the acute phase after spinal cord injury. In four patients with complete SCI, bilateral sacral neuromodulation prevented the development of neurogenic detrusor overactivity with a mean follow-up of 26 months [57]. Since only four patients were studied, these results need to be replicated in a larger study, but if the efficacy of bilateral SNM in the acute phase after SCI is confirmed, it may introduce a new minimally invasive technique to prevent deterioration of the LUS. Positive effects of SNM in patients with incomplete SCI lesions have been reported with success rates ranging from 29% to 40% during the testing phase and 58% to 80% after permanent implantation [54]. Similarly, SNM also improves fecal incontinence in these patients with a success rate ranging from 59% to 92% [58].

Interstitial Cystitis and SNM

Interstitial cystitis is a very distressing condition for both patient and physician, and although treatment strategies have a wide range, they have limited success. In general, sacral neuromodulation is used in patients who are unresponsive to medical treatment and are likely to undergo surgery. Although there is no real FDA approval for interstitial cystitis, it is used because of its urge and urge incontinence component. However, neuromodulation should perhaps be among the multimodal treatment alternatives of interstitial cystitis and should be able to treat a component of interstitial cystitis.

Comiter et al. They placed permanent implants in 17 of 25 patients with interstitial cystitis. As a result of the 14-month follow-up, the daytime urinary frequency of the patients decreased from 17 to 8.7, and their nocturia decreased from 4.5 to 1.1 ($p < 0.001$). The mean voided volume increased from 111 ml to 264 ml ($p < 0.01$). The mean pain score decreased from 5.8 to 1.6 ($p < 0.01$). Interstitial cystitis symptom score and problem scores decreased from 16.5 and 14.5 to 6.8 and 5.4, respectively [59]. Similar findings were obtained by Whitmore et al. in 33 patients with interstitial cystitis [60].

Chai et al. measured the levels of heparin-binding epidermal growth factor-like growth factor (HB-EGF) and antiproliferative factor (APF) in the urine in their SNM study on five interstitial cystitis patients. SNM has been shown to have a reducing effect on these factors [56]. In addition to this analysis, it was reported in the study that clinical symptoms such as urinary frequency and pain were improved [61].

SNM in Pediatric Patients

Clinical conditions associated with lower urinary tract symptoms, which are frequently seen in pediatric patients, can lead to serious adverse outcomes. In these patients, the next treatment step should be applied in the early period before the clinic progresses too much and irreversible changes. Neuromodulation is an alternative treatment modality for overactive bladder, dysfunctional voiding and urinary retention in pediatric patients. Since sacral neuromodulation is a minimally invasive treatment method, it may be more suitable for use in the pediatric patient population. However, it has not yet been approved for use in the pediatric group by the FDA. At this stage, with the growth of the sacral cord and roots, what will happen to the electrode creates a question mark in mind.

Guys et al. performed sacral neuromodulation in a patient with urinary incontinence between the ages of 5 and 21. Most of the patients have been reported to have neurogenic bladder secondary to spina bifida. The patients were divided into two before SNM to obtain a control group and a treatment group. In the study of 21 patients in both groups, the mean age was 11.9 years. It has been reported that urinary incontinence cured in a patient with implantation, but still continued clean intermittent catheterization. In terms of urodynamics, it was reported that compliance was significantly improved in the SNM group, and intestinal transit time was improved in nine patients, and there was no change in the control group [62].

Table 7.6 SNM Complications/Side effects

Complications/side effects	*n*/total (%)
RE-operation	282/855 (33)
IPG replacement	42/279 (15)
Complete removal	44/514 (9)
IPG problems	18/399 (5)
Lead problems	129/785 (16)
Pain	162/653 (25)
Infection	35/727 (5)
Wound problems	19/273 (7)
Bowel dysfunction	20/353 (6)

Complications/Side Effects

Considering the reviews in the literature, it is difficult to talk about side effects for a single patient group. More frequently, there are results that include urge, urge incontinence, and urinary retention. Brazzelli et al. In the review, it is reported that 282 (33%) of 855 sacral implants underwent revision (Table 7.6) [21]. The most common indications for reoperation are stimulator displacement and pain, electrode migration, and infection. Infections can usually be controlled with antibiotics, but severe infections may require removal of the system. Pain at the implantation site is seen in 25% of patients. Electrode migration is seen in 16% and wound site problem in 7% of patients. In addition, changes in bowel functions were found in 6%, infection in 5% and IPG problems in 5% [21]. IPG was changed in 15% of patients. IPG was completely removed in 9% of the patients. Suspected nerve damage was detected in one case and generalized fasciculation of unknown cause in another patient [21].

Conclusion

Urge, urge incontinence, urinary retention and bladder pain syndrome are conditions that reduce the quality of life. Although the treatment of overactive bladder slightly improves the symptoms of the patients, side effects and low efficacy or refractory conditions make medical treatment unsuccessful. After this point, sacral neurostimulation is an effective treatment method with a very high success rate. Despite the significant improvement in the clinic and quality of life of the patients he relatively high SNM side-effect profile and reintervention rates seem to be the disadvantage of SNM.

References

1. Tanagho EA, Schmidt RA, Orvis BR. Neural stimulation for control of voiding dysfunction: a preliminary report in 22 patients with serious neuropathic voiding disorders. J Urol. 1989;142(2 Pt 1):340–5.
2. Sheriff MK, Shah PJ, Fowler C, Mundy AR, Craggs MD. Neuromodulation of detrusor hyperreflexia by functional magnetic stimulation of the sacral roots. Br J Urol. 1996;78(1):39–46.
3. Lavelle JP, Teahan S, Kim DY, Chancellor MB. Medical and minimally invasive treatment of urinary incontinence. Reviews in urology. 1999;1(2):111–9.
4. deGroat WC. Neuroanatomy and neurophysiology: innervation of the lower urinary tract. In: Raz S, editor. Female urology. Philadelphia: WB Saunders Company; 1996. p. 28–42.
5. Van Kerrebroeck PE, Marcelissen TA. Sacral neuromodulation for lower urinary tract dysfunction. World J Urol. 2012;30(4):445–50.
6. Fall M, Lindstrom S. Electrical stimulation. A physiologic approach to the treatment of urinary incontinence. Urol Clin North Am. 1991;18(2):393–407.
7. Amend B, Matzel KE, Abrams P, de Groat WC, Sievert KD. How does neuromodulation work. Neurourol Urodyn. 2011;30(5):762–5.
8. Malaguti S, Spinelli M, Giardiello G, Lazzeri M, Van Den Hombergh U. Neurophysiological evidence may predict the outcome of sacral neuromodulation. J Urol. 2003;170(6 Pt 1):2323–6.
9. Bazeed MA, Thuroff JW, Schmidt RA, Wiggin DM, Tanagho EA. Effect of chronic electrostimulation of the sacral roots on the striated urethral sphincter. J Urol. 1982;128(6):1357–62.
10. Tyagi S, Thomas CA, Hayashi Y, Chancellor MB. The overactive bladder: epidemiology and morbidity. Urol Clin North Am. 2006;33(4):433–8. vii
11. Sarici H, Ozgur BC, Telli O, Doluoglu OG, Eroglu M, Bozkurt S. The prevalence of overactive bladder syndrome and urinary incontinence in a Turkish women population; associated risk factors and effect on quality of life. Urologia 2014;0(0):0.
12. Onur R, Deveci SE, Rahman S, Sevindik F, Acik Y. Prevalence and risk factors of female urinary incontinence in eastern Turkey. Int J Urol. 2009;16(6):566–9.
13. Dursun P, Dogan NU, Kolusari A, Dogan S, Ugur MG, Komurcu O, et al. Differences in geographical distribution and risk factors for urinary incontinence in Turkey: analysis of 6,473 women. Urol Int. 2014;92(2):209–14.
14. Hu TW, Wagner TH. Health-related consequences of overactive bladder: an economic perspective. BJU Int. 2005;96(Suppl 1):43–5.
15. Basra RK, Wagg A, Chapple C, Cardozo L, Castro-Diaz D, Pons ME, et al. A review of adherence to drug therapy in patients with overactive bladder. BJU Int. 2008;102(7):774–9.
16. http://www.sufuorg.com/docs/news/OAB-Amendment-061014.aspx. Available from: http://www.sufuorg.com/docs/news/OAB-Amendment-061014.aspx
17. Cohen BL, Tunuguntla HS, Gousse A. Predictors of success for first stage neuromodulation: motor versus sensory response. J Urol. 2006;175(6):2178 81. discussion 80–1
18. Peters KM, Killinger KA, Boura JA. Is sensory testing during lead placement crucial for achieving positive outcomes after sacral neuromodulation? Neurourol Urodyn. 2011;30(8):1489–92.
19. Koldewijn EL, Rosier PF, Meuleman EJ, Koster AM, Debruyne FM, van Kerrebroeck PE. Predictors of success with neuromodulation in lower urinary tract dysfunction: results of trial stimulation in 100 patients. J Urol. 1994;152(6 Pt 1):2071–5.
20. Siegel SW, Catanzaro F, Dijkema HE, Elhilali MM, Fowler CJ, Gajewski JB, et al. Long-term results of a multicenter study on sacral nerve stimulation for treatment of urinary urge incontinence, urgency-frequency, and retention. Urology. 2000;56(6 Suppl 1):87–91.
21. Brazzelli M, Murray A, Fraser C. Efficacy and safety of sacral nerve stimulation for urinary urge incontinence: a systematic review. J Urol. 2006;175(3 Pt 1):835–41.
22. Leong RK, De Wachter SG, Nieman FH, de Bie RA, van Kerrebroeck PE. PNE versus 1st stage tined lead procedure: a direct comparison to select the most sensitive test method to identify patients suitable for sacral neuromodulation therapy. Neurourol Urodyn. 2011;30(7):1249–52.

23. Borawski KM, Foster RT, Webster GD, Amundsen CL. Predicting implantation with a neuromodulator using two different test stimulation techniques: a prospective randomized study in urge incontinent women. Neurourol Urodyn. 2007;26(1):14–8.
24. Huwyler M, Kiss G, Burkhard FC, Madersbacher H, Kessler TM. Microbiological tined-lead examination: does prolonged sacral neuromodulation testing induce infection? BJU Int. 2009;104(5):646–50. discussion 50
25. Weil EH, Ruiz-Cerda JL, Eerdmans PH, Janknegt RA, Bemelmans BL, van Kerrebroeck PE. Sacral root neuromodulation in the treatment of refractory urinary urge incontinence: a prospective randomized clinical trial. Eur Urol. 2000;37(2):161–71.
26. Schmidt RA, Jonas U, Oleson KA, Janknegt RA, Hassouna MM, Siegel SW, et al. Sacral nerve stimulation for treatment of refractory urinary urge incontinence. Sacral Nerve Stimulation Study Group. J Urol. 1999;162(2):352–7.
27. Chen LM, Wang C, Chen M, Marcello MR, Chao J, Chao L, et al. Prostasin attenuates inducible nitric oxide synthase expression in lipopolysaccharide-induced urinary bladder inflammation. Am J Physiol Renal Physiol. 2006;291(3):F567–77.
28. Cappellano F, Bertapelle P, Spinelli M, Catanzaro F, Carone R, Zanollo A, et al. Quality of life assessment in patients who undergo sacral neuromodulation implantation for urge incontinence: an additional tool for evaluating outcome. J Urol. 2001;166(6):2277–80.
29. Amundsen CL, Webster GD. Sacral neuromodulation in an older, urge-incontinent population. Am J Obstet Gynecol. 2002;187(6):1462–5. discussion 5
30. Shaker HS, Hassouna M. Sacral nerve root neuromodulation: an effective treatment for refractory urge incontinence. J Urol. 1998;159(5):1516–9.
31. Amundsen CL, Romero AA, Jamison MG, Webster GD. Sacral neuromodulation for intractable urge incontinence: are there factors associated with cure? Urology. 2005;66(4):746–50.
32. Hohenfellner M, Schultz-Lampel D, Dahms S, Matzel K, Thuroff JW. Bilateral chronic sacral neuromodulation for treatment of lower urinary tract dysfunction. J Urol. 1998;160(3 Pt 1):821–4.
33. Ho MH, Bhatia NN, Khorram O. Physiologic role of nitric oxide and nitric oxide synthase in female lower urinary tract. Curr Opin Obstet Gynecol. 2004;16(5):423–9.
34. Fu D, Ng YK, Gan P, Ling EA. Permanent occlusion of the middle cerebral artery upregulates expression of cytokines and neuronal nitric oxide synthase in the spinal cord and urinary bladder in the adult rat. Neuroscience. 2004;125(4):819–31.
35. Apostolidis AN, Yiangou Y, Brady CM, Ford AP, Baecker PA, Jacques TS, et al. Endothelial nitric oxide synthase expression in neurogenic urinary bladders treated with intravesical resiniferatoxin. BJU Int. 2004;93(3):336–40.
36. Hedlund H, Schultz A, Talseth T, Tonseth K, van der Hagen A. Sacral neuromodulation in Norway: clinical experience of the first three years. Scand J Urol Nephrol Suppl. 2002;210:87–95.
37. Birder LA, Nealen ML, Kiss S, de Groat WC, Caterina MJ, Wang E, et al. Beta-adrenoceptor agonists stimulate endothelial nitric oxide synthase in rat urinary bladder urothelial cells. J Neurosci Off J Soc Neurosci. 2002;22(18):8063–70.
38. Caraballo R, Bologna RA, Lukban J, Whitmore KE. Sacral nerve stimulation as a treatment for urge incontinence and associated pelvic floor disorders at a pelvic floor center: a follow-up study. Urology. 2001;57(6 Suppl 1):121.
39. Janknegt RA, Hassouna MM, Siegel SW, Schmidt RA, Gajewski JB, Rivas DA, et al. Long-term effectiveness of sacral nerve stimulation for refractory urge incontinence. Eur Urol. 2001;39(1):101–6.
40. Bosch JL, Groen J. Sacral nerve neuromodulation in the treatment of patients with refractory motor urge incontinence: long-term results of a prospective longitudinal study. J Urol. 2000;163(4):1219–22.
41. Gruenewald V, Jonas U. Neurostimulation for lower urinary tract voiding problems. Curr Urol Rep. 2000;1(3):199–203.
42. Behr-Roussel D, Rupin A, Simonet S, Fabiani J, Verbeuren TJ. Urinary nitrate excretion in cholesterol-fed rabbits: effect of a chronic treatment by N-iminoethyl-L-lysine, a selective inhibitor of inducible nitric oxide synthase. Eur J Pharmacol. 2000;388(3):275–9.

43. Weil EH, Ruiz-Cerda JL, Eerdmans PH, Janknegt RA, Van Kerrebroeck PE. Clinical results of sacral neuromodulation for chronic voiding dysfunction using unilateral sacral foramen electrodes. World J Urol. 1998;16(5):313–21.
44. Zhou Y, Ling EA. Nitric oxide synthase--its distribution and alteration in the intramural ganglia of the urinary bladder in normal and urethra-obstructed guinea pigs. Ann Acad Med Singap 1999;28(1):49–61.
45. Dasgupta R, Wiseman OJ, Kitchen N, Fowler CJ. Long-term results of sacral neuromodulation for women with urinary retention. BJU Int. 2004;94(3):335–7.
46. De Ridder D, Ost D, Bruyninckx F. The presence of Fowler's syndrome predicts successful long-term outcome of sacral nerve stimulation in women with urinary retention. Eur Urol. 2007;51(1):229–34. discussion 33–4
47. Goh M, Diokno AC. Sacral Neuromodulation for Nonobstructive Urinary Retention—Is Success Predictable? J Urol. 2007;178(1):197. discussion 9–9.
48. Bertapelle P, Bodo G, Carone R. Detrusor acontractility in urinary retention: detrusor contractility test as exclusion criteria for sacral neurostimulation. J Urol. 2008;180(1):215–6.
49. Jonas U, Fowler CJ, Chancellor MB, Elhilali MM, Fall M, Gajewski JB, et al. Efficacy of sacral nerve stimulation for urinary retention: results 18 months after implantation. J Urol. 2001;165(1):15–9.
50. Datta SN, Chaliha C, Singh A, Gonzales G, Mishra VC, Kavia RB, et al. Sacral neurostimulation for urinary retention: 10-year experience from one UK centre. BJU Int. 2008;101(2):192–6.
51. White WM, Dobmeyer-Dittrich C, Klein FA, Wallace LS. Sacral nerve stimulation for treatment of refractory urinary retention: long-term efficacy and durability. Urology. 2008;71(1):71–4.
52. van Kerrebroeck EV, Scheepens WA, de Bie RA, Weil EH. European experience with bilateral sacral neuromodulation in patients with chronic lower urinary tract dysfunction. Urol Clin North Am. 2005;32(1):51–7.
53. Peters KM, Kandagatla P, Killinger KA, Wolfert C, Boura JA. Clinical outcomes of sacral neuromodulation in patients with neurologic conditions. Urology. 2013;81(4):738–43.
54. Kessler TM, La Framboise D, Trelle S, Fowler CJ, Kiss G, Pannek J, et al. Sacral neuromodulation for neurogenic lower urinary tract dysfunction: systematic review and meta-analysis. Eur Urol. 2010;58(6):865–74.
55. Hohenfellner M, Humke J, Hampel C, Dahms S, Matzel K, Roth S, et al. Chronic sacral neuromodulation for treatment of neurogenic bladder dysfunction: long-term results with unilateral implants. Urology. 2001;58(6):887–92.
56. Schurch B, Reilly I, Reitz A, Curt A. Electrophysiological recordings during the peripheral nerve evaluation (PNE) test in complete spinal cord injury patients. World J Urol. 2003;20(6):319–22.
57. Sievert KD, Amend B, Gakis G, Toomey P, Badke A, Kaps HP, et al. Early sacral neuromodulation prevents urinary incontinence after complete spinal cord injury. Ann Neurol. 2010;67(1):74–84.
58. Worsøe J, Rasmussen M, Christensen P, Krogh K. Neurostimulation for neurogenic bowel dysfunction. Gastroenterol Res Pract. 2013;2013:563294.
59. Comiter CV. Sacral neuromodulation for the symptomatic treatment of refractory interstitial cystitis: a prospective study. J Urol. 2003;169(4):1369–73.
60. Whitmore KE, Payne CK, Diokno AC, Lukban JC. Sacral neuromodulation in patients with interstitial cystitis: a multicenter clinical trial. Int Urogynecol J Pelvic Floor Dysfunct 2003;14(5):305–8; discussion 8–9, 309.
61. Chai TC, Zhang C, Warren JW, Keay S. Percutaneous sacral third nerve root neurostimulation improves symptoms and normalizes urinary HB-EGF levels and antiproliferative activity in patients with interstitial cystitis. Urology. 2000;55(5):643–6.
62. Guys JM, Haddad M, Planche D, Torre M, Louis-Borrione C, Breaud J. Sacral neuromodulation for neurogenic bladder dysfunction in children. J Urol. 2004;172(4 Pt 2):1673–6.

Chapter 8
Starting Robotics, Training and Models

Eyup Veli Kucuk and Alper Kerem Aksoy

Starting Robotics

The use of robots in surgery began in the early 1970s. The actions that could be performed in Laparoscopic practice, which was a common use at the time, were relatively limited compared to the potential of robotic surgery. Robot is minimally invasive technology with wrist capability, tremor filtration and three-dimensional optics advantages compared to laparoscopy. Initially, robotic systems were designed for long-distance trauma surgery in a combat setting [1].

The Stanford Research Institute (SRI) has designed a prototype consisting of 2 separate units: a telepresence surgeon's workstation (TSW) and a remote surgical unit (RSU) [1].

The TWS included an instrument manipulator that transmitted hand movements to the RSU and a stereoscopic video monitör. The RSU, on the other hand, had replaceable tool tips such as forceps, needle drivers, intestinal holders, scalpels, and cautery tips [1].

After a while, SRI moved to the ex vivo and in vivo validation phase.

The SRI system was used for suture incision closure using sections of bovine aorta. The SRI team then moved on to trauma surgery, which included closure of anterior surface gastrotomies, cholecystectomies, repair of liver lacerations, and full-thickness enterotomy.

Next, the SRI team tried urological procedures such as nephrectomy, cystostomy closures, and ureteroureterostomies using the telepresence system [1].

E. V. Kucuk · A. K. Aksoy (✉)
Health Sciences University Umraniye Training and Research Hospital, Istanbul, Turkey

S. Tonyali et al. (eds.), *Current Endourology*,
https://doi.org/10.1007/978-3-032-00010-1_8

Transition to the Private Sector

Computer Motion

In 1994, Computer Motion, supported by NASA, developed the first surgical robot, AESOP (Automatic Endoscopic System for Optimal Positioning). AESOP combined a telemanipulator with footswitch and voice control system. AESOP is the first surgical robot to receive FDA approval [2].

In 1996 Computer Motion created ZEUS, the first full-capacity robotic surgery system. Unlike AESOP, laparoscopic instrumentation was used in ZEUS. ZEUS consisted of two parts, the patient's side and the surgeon's side. The patient side was the side that performed the procedure with laparoscopic instruments. On the surgeon's side, there were two arms that the surgeon used to manage these instruments and a voice-controlled arm that directed the camera. The ZEUS robotic surgery system received FDA approval in 2001 [2].

Intuitive Surgical

The first prototype of Intuitive was Lenny. It was built inspired by SRI's prototype. Its name is an abbreviation of Leonardo da Vinci's name. Lenny had fixed instrumentation and manipulators were attached to the surgical table Lenny was used in animal experiments in 1996. In these experiments, it was determined that it did not provide sufficient quality visualization for surgery [3].

After this failed attempt, Intuitive developed Mona. It was named after Leonardo da Vinci's Mona Lisa. It had a tool interface with 4 rotary ports. The poor visualization and cumbersome setup process were still evident, although it was more comprehensive than Lenny. Lenny is the first robotic surgery system to be put into human trials [3].

The first generation of the da Vinci Surgical System, introduced in 1999, consists of an ergonomically designed surgeon's console, a patient-side cart with four interactive robotic arms, a high-performance vision system and proprietary EndoWrist Instruments [3].

Intuitive's next invention, the most distinctive difference from Da Vinci's predecessors, is the creation of a self-contained car with arms containing instruments on the patient's side. Thus, the necessity of mounting the manipulators on the table is eliminated. This system also eliminated the limitations of patient positioning and balancing problems on the table. Compared to its predecessors, Da Vinci has a revamped stereoscopic viewer [3].

There is a limit to the scope of actions of a human hand, and actions involving smaller movements simply cannot be done.

The 3D immersion technology, together with the 7 degrees of freedom available in DaVinci, has made more sensitive interventions available in surgery that cannot be done simply by human hands [3].

The da Vinci robotic surgery system has become one of the most widely used systems in the world.

Urologic Surgery

The robotic surgery system has been adopted by urologists in minimally invasive surgery, especially since it facilitates access to depth in the pelvis area.

Because of this advantage, urologists became the first practitioners of robotic surgery technology. Robotic surgery has been used in urological oncology for over 20 years [2].

The first robot-assisted prostatectomy was performed at the Vatikuti Institute in Detroit in 2000. Michigan was the first to document this process. It was also noted that robot-assisted prostatectomy is advantageous over laparoscopic prostatectomy [2].

Later, Robotic surgical systems have been used successfully in nephrectomies and adrenalectomies. A case report that underwent robot-assisted nephrectomy for hydronephrotic kidney in 2001 was documented. This study demonstrated that surgical removal of a kidney can be done using a robot [2].

Anderson-Hynes dismembered pyeloplasty was performed on 9 patients between 2001 and 2002 using the daVinci robotic system. The study found that it is possible to perform the procedure robotically [2].

Robotic Training

The use of robotic surgical approaches continues to expand in many surgical fields. In parallel with this expansion, robotics education is becoming more and more important [4].

The use of the robotic surgery system has accelerated the transition to minimally invasive surgery and has led to a completely different skill set for the urology surgeon [4].

The most common approach to training surgical skills is master-apprenticeship training, known as resident's practice on patients under the supervision of a supervisor to develop surgical skills [5].

The development of robotic skills follows the phase of observing, helping, performing under supervision, and finally independent practice [5].

Basic robotic surgery training is divided into two: patient-side training and console training [6].

Patient Side Training

Patient-side training includes patient positioning, pneumoperitoneum creation, port placement, robot placement, and basic laparoscopic skills. Patient-side training.

teaches the steps of the surgical procedure. Meanwhile, it also contributes to the development of assistant-specific skills for the smooth running of procedures on the patient's side. At the same time, the Assistant learns about ergonomics and access restriction created by robotic arms.

Patient positioning and proper port placement are very important for surgical comfort. Appropriate patient positioning ensures that the surgical team (assistant, operating nurse, anesthetist) has adequate access to the patient. Correct port placement also allows convenient access to target organs without any extracorporeal or intracorporeal instrument conflicts.

Basic laparoscopic skills that a robotic surgeon must possess include laparoscopic access and pneumoperitoneum creation, removal of adhesions preventing port entry, clamping, suction and retraction.

Developing basic laparoscopic skills also improves spatial awareness (instruments and organs), the ability to manipulate tissues with precision, and the ability to maneuver and work in a three-dimensional environment.

Learning basic laparoscopic skills has its own learning curve, but the console has been shown to facilitate the development of robotic skills [6].

Console Training

Console training includes dry and wet laboratory simulation and supervised operation.

The current robot system is a master-slave system. The console is the part that controls the mechanical movement. Therefore, knowledge of the console and how to operate the console are very important.

You can master the basic skills on this console such as camera, foot pedal, finger controls relatively easily in virtual reality (VR) simulation or dry lab.

Advanced console skills such as cutting and suturing need to be developed in a supervised simulation environment such as a VR simulator, dry lab, or wet lab.

With the rise of skill-based training and a focus on patient safety in modern surgical practice, simulation not only provides the foundation for initial skill development, but also skill assessment [6].

The need for high capacity application without compromising patient care has been met by surgical simulations and especially virtual reality (VR) surgical simulations. VR simulation is increasingly used in medical education and is considered the first and important step in robotic surgery education. One of the advantages of VR system software is the evaluation and measurement of progress. Simulation exercises start from basic console controls and increase in difficulty toward complex missions [6, 7].

The VR robot simulator provides users with instant and objective performance evaluation without outside observation (Fig. 8.1). Overall, the simulator score corresponds to the user's level of expertise [7].

Surgical simulation is a safe and effective means of training. Most surgical procedures performed by urological trainees such as TURP, TURBT, ureteroscopy are endoscopic and therefore suitable for simulation-based training [7].

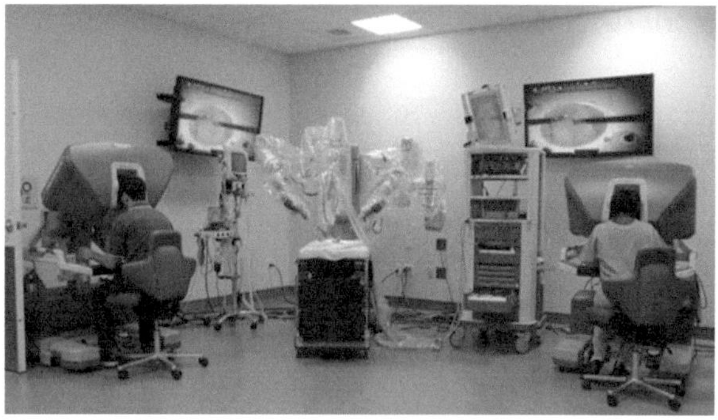

Fig. 8.1 Images of Simulators for Robotic Surgery. The VR robot simulator provides users with instant and objective performance evaluation without outside observation

There are 6 VR simulators for robotic surgery; daVinci Skills Simulator (dVSS), Mimic dV Trainer (MdVT), ProMIS simulator, Simsurgery Education Platform (SEP) simulator, Robotic Surgery Simulator (RoSS) and RobotiX Mentor (RM) [8].

daVinci Skills Simulator

The dVSS was generated by intuitive surgery in 2011 and cost $ 89,000. The practitioners are seated on the console as in traditional direct surgery. If the console is used for surgery, the simulator cannot be used [8].

Mimic dV Trainer

MdVT was created by Mimic Technologies in 2007. it is a standalone simulator and costs 158,000 USD [8].

ProMIS Simulator

The ProMIS laparoscopic simulator was manufactured in Ireland in 2003 by Haptica© and costs 35,000 USD [8].

Simsurgery Education Platform

The SEP simulator was created by SimSurgery in 2005 in Norway. It is a standalone simulator and costs 62,000 USD [8].

Robotic Surgery Simulator

RoSS was created by Simulated Surgical Systems in the USA in 2010 and cost $120,000. It has been shown to determine intraoperative ability [8].

RobotiX Mentor

RM is the newest VR simulator and was created in the USA by 3D systems. It is a standalone simulator and costs 137,000 USD [8].

dVSS and PROMIS require the practitioner to sit on the daVinci console and use the console's main controller to transmit the practitioner's movements to the virtual robotic tools in the environment. In many hospitals, there is practically only one daVinci console, and if used, the practitioner cannot use the dVSS or PROMIS simulator and this is a significant limitation.

The MdVT, RoSS, SEP and RM simulators are "platform independent", meaning that daVinci control panel is not required to use the simulator [8].

Exercises in robotic surgery simulators are given in Table 8.1.

The figures below show images of some exercises taken from the robotic surgery simulator.

Simulator view of intestinal anastomosis in general surgery (Fig. 8.2).

Table 8.1 Exercises available in robotic surgery simulators

Simulator	Exercise
daVinci skills simulator	Needle handling Object manipulation suturing camera movement Tissue handling/clipping Full surgical procedures
Mimic dV trainer	Needle handling Object manipulation suturing camera movement
ProMIS simulator	Needle handling Object manipulation suturing Tissue handling/clipping
Simsurgery educational platform	Needle handling Object manipulation suturing
Robotic surgical simulator	Needle handling Object manipulation suturing camera movement Tissue handling/clipping Full surgical procedures
RobotiX Mentor	Needle handling Object manipulation suturing camera movement Tissue handling/clipping Full surgical procedures

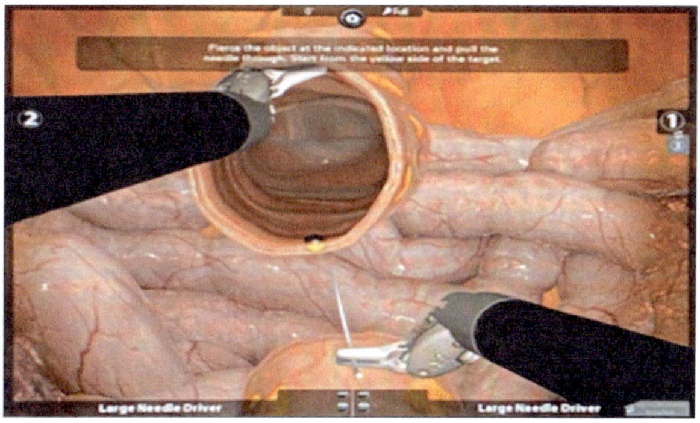

Fig. 8.2 Intestinal anastomosis simulation

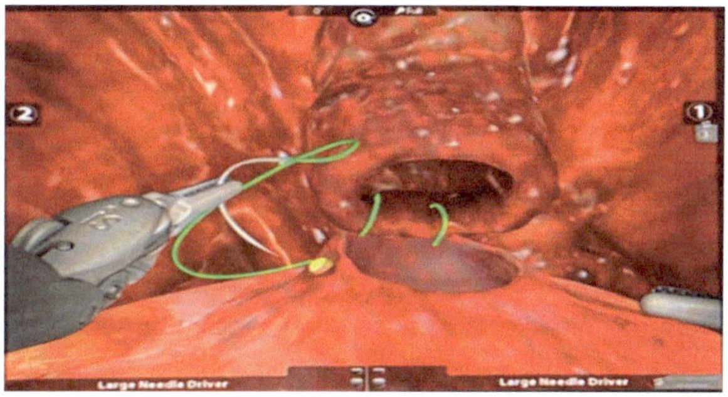

Fig. 8.3 Urethrovesical anastomosis simulation

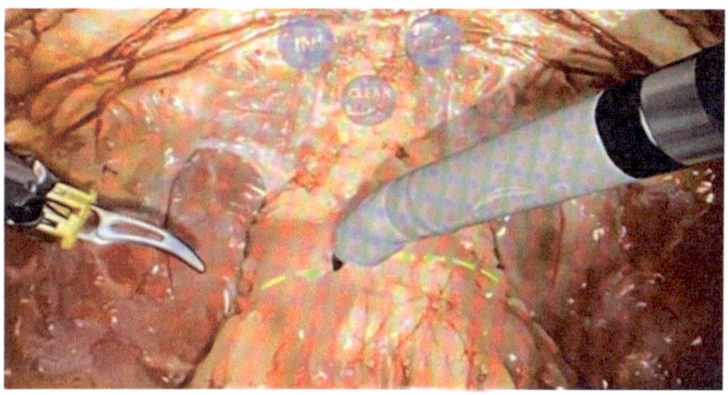

Fig. 8.4 Radical prostatectomy module—guided bladder neck dissection

Simulator image of bladder neck incision and urethrovesical anastomosis, one of the stages of radical prostatectomy where the robot is most commonly used in urological surgery (Figs. 8.3, 8.4, and 8.5).

Despite the many advantages of robotic simulation training, it may not be enough to apply the skills gained in simulation in the operating room. The next step in the correlation between proficiency in laboratories and performance in operating theaters must be established [6].

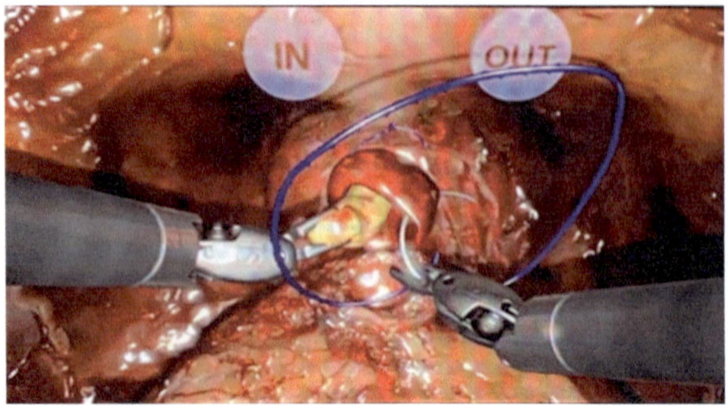

Fig. 8.5 Radical prostatectomy module—urethrovesical anastomosis

Dry Lab

Dry lab simulations safely and clearly simulate cutting, sewing and holding exercises. As the trainee does the exercises sitting at the dVSS console, they complete tasks using robotic instruments. Therefore, the validity of the simulations is very high. Dry laboratory exercises routinely include simple exercises such as ring insertion, needle insertion, suturing, as well as complex exercises such as complex vascular procedures and intestinal anastomoses. It is a good training tool, especially for learning console movements such as camera, foot pedal control, use of hands [6].

Wet Lab

In a dry laboratory, it is impossible to learn to manipulate tissues and understand how they respond to instrument contact. In addition, the use of diathermy and vessel control can only be learned in a wet laboratory. The wet lab experience soon teaches students to recognize the properties of tissues based solely on visual cues.

In wet laboratories; Training can be provided with frozen animal and human body parts or with live animals.

It is an excellent teaching material for learning human and animal body parts, tissue management, anatomy, resection, diathermy and suturing techniques. Robotic wet labs provide learning close to live surgery. It is an excellent educational model for understanding live surgery [6].

Non-technical Skills

Non-technical skills such as teamwork in the operating room, controlling the team during the surgery, risk management and decision making are the characteristics that a surgeon should have. In parallel with the development of technical skills in this multidisciplinary complex environment, non-technical skills also need to be developed. Developing non-technical skills is very important for facilitating the course of surgery and surgical success. Non-technical skills can be developed comfortably in a simulated environment through simulation [6].

Robotic Surgery Training Curricula

Today, robotic surgery has become very common and it has become more important than before for every surgeon candidate to learn this system. This brought up the creation of a programmed education curriculum for students. In the 1990s, with laparoscopic surgery in mind, the Society of Gastrointestinal and Endoscopic Surgeons (SAGES) launched the Laparoscopic Surgery Fundamentals course (FLS) for educational curricula. This is a fully validated and currently used evidence-based skills program.

Although the FLS is useful for developing minimally invasive surgery skills, it does not include specific training for robotic surgery. Therefore, new robotic surgery programs have been tried to be developed. These programs aim to develop procedures similar to FLS to form the robot-assisted surgery curriculum.

While various groups are currently developing the robotics curriculum, there are four prominent groups of curriculums: FRS (Fundamentals of Robotic Surgery), FSRS (Fundamental Skills of Robotic Surgery), BSTC (Basic Skills Training Curriculum) and ERUS (Eau Robotic Urology Section) [9].

Fundamentals of Robotic Surgery Curriculum

In 2012, a group of robotic surgeons developed a new curriculum through a series of courses to create the Fundamentals of Robotic Surgery (FRS) program. The curriculum includes an educational syllabus, psychomotor skills development and team building activities. The FRS program consists of 25 outcome measures that aim to increase trainees' preoperative, intraoperative and postoperative skills through practice [9].

Fundamental Skills of Robotic Surgery Curriculum

The Fundamental Skills of Robotic Surgery curriculum is a simulation-based course developed at the Roswell Cancer Institute in New York. This curriculum consists of 16 tasks divided into four modules. Tasks; It was developed based on input from robotic surgeons and virtual reality simulation engineers and included tasks previously approved in the Fundamentals of Laparoscopic Surgery course. Each task is performed from easy to difficult, followed by an evaluation phase [9].

Eau Robotic Urology Section Fellowship Curriculum

This new curriculum of the European Association of Urology (EAU) was developed by a team of international experts at the EAU Robotics Department Urology Congress (2012) and EAU (2013) congresses. The course begins with an online theoretical training program followed by a week of simulation training in a dry lab, wet lab and virtual reality environment. The student's goal is to perform well in all simulation exercises and skill tasks.

The trainees are then given a modular console training for robotic assisted radical prostatectomy (RARP) under supervision in the operating environment. Students will be trained to gradually perform the surgical steps of the procedure with increasing surgical difficulty. The course takes 3 months to complete. Apprentices will be certified after completing the fellowship phase [9].

Basic Skills Training Curriculum

BSTC curriculum; The first week includes teaching courses and online training modules. Afterwards, a standard 2-hour robot introductory training is given, which includes the practice of basic robot skills on an inanimate model. In the following 3 weeks, students are trained on the Da Vinci Surgery Simulator. In simulation training, skills such as camera use, instrument orientation, third arm functions, coagulation, needle holding and suturing are developed. The course is completed in 4 weeks.

FRS, BSTC and FSRS are designed as an initial qualification that can be included in a centre's training plans. A key benefit of the new ERUS initiative curriculum is that it follows trainees from novice to specialist surgeon by including a fellowship phase in training [9].

The contents of the four main robotics curricula are given in Table 8.2.

Robotic Models

Da Vinci Surgical System

Since the da Vinci system was first approved by the FDA in 2000, it has been the leading robotic surgery system. The components of the robotic surgical system consisted of a robot car with arms, a surgical console, and a vision tower. The system is approved for use in urology, gynecology, general surgery, cardiothoracic surgery, and head and neck surgery [10].

During this period, the four-generation multi-arm da Vinci system with the same concept as da Vinci 2000, S, Si and Xi was launched. A closed surgeon's console with Endowrist technology, a robotic arm in the patient trolley and an

Table 8.2 Four main Curriculum and its features

Name	FRS	FSRS	ERUS	BSTC
Modules included	1. Introduction to robotic systems: Minimally invasive surgery, robotic system advantages and components, system functionality. 2. Didactic instructions e.g. robot docking, trocar placement. 3. Physical model training, on new psychomotor multi-skill device 4. Team training & communication	1. Basic console orientation 2. Psychomotor skills training (ball placement, spatial control) 3. & 4 Intermediate surgical skills	1. Online e-learning 2. Observation of live surgery (bedside/console) 3. Simulation and observation (procedure specific: Dry lab, wet lab, virtual reality) 4. Fellowship: Observation of live surgery, bedside assisting, performing part then full procedure with dual console and mentor.	1. Lecture and online training modules 2. 2-hour introduction to robot 3. 3 weeks of sessions on the Da vinci surgical simulator
Manual skills developed	7 FRS tasks on psychomotor multi-skill device: • Docking/ instrument insertion • Ring tower transfer • Knot tying • Railroad track • Fourth arm cutting • Puzzle piece dissection • Vessel energy dissection	16 tasks on the robotic surgical simulator (RoSS): • Instrument and camera control • 4th arm control • Ball placement • Spatial control • Needle handling • Basic electro-cautery • Tissue cautery • Tissue retraction • Blunt tissue • Vessel dissection • Knot tying	Trainees complete a wide range of manual skills tasks that are either generic or procedure-specific. These occur in simulated, dry lab and wet lab settings before being introduced in the OR.	Da Vinci surgical simulator tasks: • Camera navigation • 3rd arm functionality • Instrument clutching • Endowrist object manipulation • Cautery • Needle handling and driving • Dissection

(continued)

Table 8.2 (continued)

Name	FRS	FSRS	ERUS	BSTC
Skills developed	Didactic & cognitive; psychomotor skills; team training and communications	Didactic & cognitive; technical skills; module 3 & 4	Didactic & cognitive; technical skills, integration of knowledge and skills; application of skills to the OR.	Didactic & cognitive; psychomotor skills
Assessment			Online e-learning exam, simulated assessment and skills tasks. DVD assessment of a procedure, reviewed by 2 experts.	Proficiency is assessed on 2 tasks benchtop models. Performance is based on time to completion and number of errors.

8 mm diameter instrument with 7 degrees of freedom. The latest system, da Vinci Xi, was released in 2014. It is equipped with a thinner robotic arm and newly designed joints, a longer tool shaft and a tip-mounted 8 mm digital camera that can be attached to any arm [11].

Da Vinci intuitive has launched the daVinci™SP 1098, a single-port(SP) surgical system for use in urological procedures [12]. The patient trolley includes three 6 mm wrist instruments and a 12 × 10 mm oval 3DHD articulating camera placed in a 25 mm multi-channel cannula from a single point of entry with a single robotic arm. The instrument connects to the distal (elbow) and proximal (shoulder) joint areas and provides 7 degrees of freedom and intracorporeal triangulation to the target organ in the body. The daVinci™SP 1098 system was approved by the FDA in May 2018 [11, 12].

The surgeon can grasp and rotate the instrument arm around its distal center without having to move each additional instrument.

One instrument may remain stationary in one place, while the remaining instruments are diverted to work in a separate workspace. This improves the usable workspace [12].

Today, in addition to the da Vinci system, there are five other commercial robotic surgery systems: Senhance, Versius, Avatera, Revo-I, and Hinotori.

Senhance has received regulatory approvals for human use in the US, Europe and Japan; Versius and Avatera have been certified with the CE mark (Conformité Européenne) and can be used in Europe; Revo-I is available in Korean market, Hinotori is available in Japanese markets [11].

Senhance

Senhance™ Robotics Platform (TransEnterix, Morrisville, NC, USA), formerly known as Telelap ALFX, is a console recently approved by the FDA for use in minimally invasive surgery [13].

This system includes a 3DHD display combined with infrared eye tracking camera control to focus the surgeon's image. In addition, the Senhance robotic system includes haptic feedback, unlike the Da Vinci robotic system. Haptic feedback refers to the surgeon's ability to sense the degree of force applied to the tissue. In this system, the surgeon feels the sensation coming from the distal end of the instrument that touches the tissue [11].

Initial clinical applications were mainly limited to general surgery and gynecological surgical procedures [13]. Senhance received FDA approval for general surgery and gynecological surgery applications in October 2017. Thus, Senhance became the first new robotic system approved by the FDA after 2000 [11].

Recently, the use of Senhance for radical prostatectomy and various urological procedures has been described in Europe [11].

Versius

The robotic arm of the Versius robotic surgery system is mounted separately on portable trolleys. Each robotic arm has a shoulder, elbow and wrist joint that can mimic the movement of a human arm. The console uses an open design. Polarized glasses are used for 3D HD image. The surgeon can work sitting or standing while using the joystick lever to control the system. The instrument has a diameter of 5 mm and has 7 degrees of freedom. There is also haptic feedback, as in the Senhance system. The system has been used in a preclinical setting where several surgeons have successfully performed prostate surgery, kidney surgery, and pelvic lymph node dissection in cadaver and porcine models. The Versius surgical system (Cambridge Medical Robotics Ltd., Cambridge, UK) received the European CE Mark in March 2019 [11].

Avatera

The Avatera system (avateramedical GmbH, Jena, Germany) is another robotic system approved in Europe in November 2019 for minimally invasive surgery focusing on gynecological and urological surgery. Avatera consists of two parts, surgical robot and console. The patient trolley has three robotic arms for the fully articulated, disposable, 5 mm instruments providing 7 degrees of freedom, and one arm for the 10 mm endoscope. The surgeon sits on the console in an ergonomically designed posture. A microscope-like lens provides 3DHD vision without the need to wrap the surgeon's head to facilitate communication with the surgical team. To date, there are no published data describing the use of the Avatera system and clinical trials are pending [11].

Revo-I

Revoi™ (Meere Company Inc., Yongin, South Korea) is a robotic surgery system that began development in South Korea in 2006. The system is very similar to Da Vinci Si [14].

It includes a four-arm patient trolley, a closed surgeon's console, and an HD vision trolley. The diameter of the 3D endoscope is 10 mm. The instrument is 7.4 mm in diameter, provides 7 degrees of freedom and can be used up to 20 times [11]. This system has demonstrated its safety and feasibility in the clinical practice of Retzius-sparing radical prostatectomy. Received clinical approval from the Korean Food and Drug Administration in 2017 [14].

Hinotori

The Hinotori robotic surgery system (Medicaroid Corporation, Kobe, Japan) is a robotic surgery system made in Japan. Hinotori consists of three parts: the surgeon's cabin, the operating unit and the visual unit. The four robotic arms have multiple joints and can move on eight axes. The console is a semi-closed system. A microscope-like lens creates the 3D image. The instruments are controlled by the surgeon with a ring-shaped handle. It received approval from the Ministry of Health, Labor and Welfare of Japan in August 2020. The results of the first human trials of this robotic system are awaited.

The competition in robotic surgical systems provides an environment for current innovations and high quality product development. In addition, the purchase and maintenance of the Robotic surgery system, instruments and accessories is very expensive for hospitals. A competitive environment can reduce costs and increase the availability of robotic surgery worldwide. Hospitals will be able to choose the most suitable robotic system for their needs and cost [11].

Robotic Ureteroscopy

The first application of robotics in ureteroscopy was discovered in 2011 using the Sensei X™ robotic catheter system (Hansen Medical Inc., Mountain View, CA, USA). It was originally designed for cardiac catheterization.

Desai et al. demonstrated the feasibility of the procedure with this system in 18 patients with an average stone size of 11.8 mm and an average operation time of 91 minutes.

This system was maintained with a robot specially made for ureteroscopy, Roboflex Avicenna™ (Elmed Medical Systems, Ankara, Turkey). This robotic system consists of placing a joystick and a ureteroscope on the robotic deflector controlled at the surgeon's console. A total of 74 patients with an average stone size of 13 mm and an average operation time of 74 minutes were treated with this robotic surgery system.

The two systems above require a standard flexible ureteroscope for insertion into the robotic surgery system. The Auris robotic endoscopy system (ARES™) (Auris Surgical Robotics, Redwood City, CA, USA) is an "all-in-one" system in which the ureteroscope is incorporated into the system. The system includes a multi-channel camera that allows the passage of instruments and irrigation fluid. It also has electromagnetic field generated navigation to control the internal ureteroscope. In 2017, preclinical studies were conducted at the American Urological Association in Boston [14].

Robotic Transurethral Prostate Resection

Aquablation is a new minimally invasive water ablative therapy for resection of prostate tissue. Aquablation system consists of console, robotic arm and resection probe.

After examination of the bladder with the cystoscope, the water probe is inserted into the bladder neck.

The robotic arm is then fixed, followed by transrectal ultrasound to calculate the size of the prostate. Ablation then begins with high-pressure saline delivered to accurately resect the prostate. AquaBeam™ (Procept BioRobotics, Redwood Shores, CA, USA) was approved in December 2017 [14].

The robotic surgery models available today and their contents are given in Table 8.3.

The Da Vinci Surgical System is considered the gold standard of robot-assisted laparoscopic surgery. Newly produced robotic systems must compete with this current gold standard. Each resulting system should be compared to the da Vinci robotic system to evaluate potential effectiveness and safety.

In newly developed robotic surgery systems, it seems that new technologies have been applied by trying to improve the functionality of the old system and have been developed by taking into account the missing features in the installed system. Whether these new features will attract surgeons to adopt and use new robotic systems in clinical practice is a question that needs to be answered in the near future.

Table 8.3 Summary of the robotic surgical systems

Robotic system	Console	Telescope	Robotic arms	Clinical applications
da Vinci™ xi (intuitivesurgical Inc.,Sunnyvale, CA, USA)	3D (three-dimensional) binocular viewing console,Endowrist™ finger controls,foot pedals for clutching andapplication of energy	3DHD (three-dimensional high-definition) 8 mmcamera	Four robotic armshanging from an overheadboom system allowingmultiquadrant access	Pelvic surgery,retroperitonealsurgery, intracorporealreconstruction
da Vinci™ (IntuitiveSurgical Inc.) SP 1098	As aboveadditional foot pedal to allowmovement of robotic arms inunison	3DHD 12 mmarticulating camera	Boom-mounted singlerobotic arm with single25 mm robotic port6 mm articulating roboticinstruments allowingtriangulation	Single-port surgerycadaveric studiesfor prostatectomy,cystectomy, and partialnephrectomy completeUS food and drugadministration-approved
Senhance (TransEnterix surgical Inc., Morrisville, NC, USA)	The surgeon is ergonomically seated in an open console, called the "cockpit," the camera manipulation is controlled by the surgeon's eye movements through an infrared eye-tracking system	3D HD visualization with the use of polarized glasses	Multiport system comprises up to four independent robotic arms in separate carts the available instruments have diameters ranging from 3 to 10 mm	The first clinical applications mainly focused on general surgery and gynecologic surgeries. Recently, the use for radical prostatectomy and various urological procedures was described in Europe
Versius (Cambridge medical Robotics ltd., Cambridge, UK)	The console has an open design. The surgeon can choose to operate in a sitting or a standing position while controlling the system through joystick handles	3D HD visualization with the use of polarized glasses	The robotic arms of this surgical system are individually mounted in portable carts. Each robotic arm has a shoulder, an elbow, and a wrist joint, mimicking the movements of the human arm.	The first clinical series of gynecologic and upper gastrointestinal surgeries using the Versius surgical system in India, the first clinical report of 30 robotic radical hysterectomies was recently published

Avatera (avateramedical GmbH, Jena, Germany)	The surgeon sits at the console in an ergonomically designed position. A microscope-like eyepiece provides 3D full HD vision without enveloping the entire head of the surgeon for easier communication with the surgical team.	3DHD vision microscope-like eyepiece	Three robotic arms for the 5-mm fully articulating instruments and one for the 10-mm endoscope. All the instruments are single-use and disposable.	The publication of clinical studies is awaited.
Hinotori (Medicaroid corporation, Kobe, Japan)	The console is a semi-closed design, and a microscope-like eyepiece provides a 3D view of the surgical field.	3D view microscope-like eyepiece	Four robotic arms, which are mounted in the operative unit, have multiple joints and can move in eight axes.	The results of the first human trials are expected.
Revo-i™ (Meerecompany, Yongin,Republic of Korea)	3D binocular viewing console,wristed instrument control withhand clutchfoot pedal camera clutch	3DHD 10 mmcamera	Four robotic arms mountedto boominstruments are 7.4 mm indiameter	Only clinical study hasbeen with Retzius-sparingradical prostatectomy

(continued)

Table 8.3 (continued)

Robotic system	Console	Telescope	Robotic arms	Clinical applications
Roboflex Avicenna™(Elmed medicalsystems, Ankara,Turkey)	Adjustable seat with armrests forsurgeonjoystick controlstouchscreen to modify speed ofdeflection, adaption to mode ofureterorenoscope, advancementand retraction of laser fiber,adjustment of irrigation flow ratetwo foot pedals control laser andfluoroscopy	Off-the-shelfexisting digitalureteroscope	Robotic manipulator whichholds ureteroscopeendoscope stabilized bytwo holders	Flexible ureteroscopy
Auris roboticendoscopy system(ARES™) (Aurissurgical Robotics,Redwood City, CA,USA)	Video game-like hand controllerwith electromagnetic-generatedreal-time navigation	Remote drivingfully incorporatedflexible digitalendoscope	Three robotic armsincluding camera withmultiple channels allowingthe passage and control oflaser fiber and irrigation	Flexible ureteroscopy
AquaBeam system™(Procept BioRobotics,redwood shores, CA,USA)	Stand-alone with keyboard andtouchscreenan input for transrectalultrasound which maps and planssubsequent prostate resection	22F rigid HopkinsCystoscope	Articulating robotic armthat delivers high-pressuresaline in longitudinal androtational movements	Benign prostatehyperplasia

References

1. George EI, Brand TC, LaPorta A, Marescaux J, Satava RM. Origins of robotic surgery: from skepticism to standard of care. J Soc Laparoskopik Robot Surg. 2018;22(4):e2018.00039.
2. Shah J, Vyas A, Vyas D. The history of robotics in surgical specialties. Am J Robot Surg. 2014;1(1):12–20.
3. DiMaio Mike S, Usha H, Jacob K, Blake R, Richard H, Satava M. Surgical robotics systems applications and visions the da vinci surgical system Springer US Boston MA. 199–217.
4. Mullens CL, Van Horn AL, Marsh JW, Hogg ME, Thomay AA, Schmidt CR, Boone BA. Development of a senior medical student robotic surgery training elective. J Med Educ Curric Dev. 2021;8. https://doi.org/10.1177/23821205211024074.
5. Brinkman WM, Schout BMA, Rietbergen JB, de Vries AH, van der Poel HG, Koldewijn EL, Witjes JA, van Merriënboer JJG. Training robotic surgery in urology: experience and opinions of robot urologists. Int J Med Robot Comp Assis Surg. 201511(3):308–18. https://doi.org/10.1002/rcs.1631.
6. Sridhar AN, Briggs TP, Kelly JD, Nathan S. Training in robotic surgery—an overview. Curr Urol Rep. 2017;18(8). https://doi.org/10.1007/s11934-017-0710-y.
7. Dubin AK, Smith R, Julian D, Tanaka A, Mattingly P. A comparison of robotic simulation performance on basic virtual reality skills: simulator subjective versus objective assessment tools. J Minim İnvaziv Jinekol. 2017;24(7):1184–19. https://doi.org/10.1016/j.jmig.2017.07.019.
8. MacCraith E, Forde JC, Davis NF. Robotic simulation training for urological trainees: a comprehensive review on cost merits and challenges. J Robot Surg. 2019;13(3):371–7. https://doi.org/10.1007/s11701-019-00934-1.
9. Fisher RA, Dasgupta P, Mottrie A, Volpe A, Khan MS, Challacombe B, Ahmed K. An over-view of robot assisted surgery curricula and the status of their validation. Int J Surg. 2015;13:115–123. https://doi.org/10.1016/j.ijsu.2014.11.033.
10. Oleynikov D. Robotic surgery. Surg Clin North Am. 2008;88(5):1121–30 https://doi.org/10.1016/j.suc.2008.05.012.
11. Koukourikis P, Rha KH. Robotic surgical systems in urology: What is currently available? Investig Clin Urol. 2021;62(1):14. https://doi.org/10.4111/icu.20200387.
12. Dobbs RW, Halgrimson WR, Talamini S, Vigneswaran HT, Wilson JO, Crivellaro S. Single-port robotic surgery: the next generation of minimally invasive urology. World J Urol. 2020;38(4):897–905. https://doi.org/10.1007/s00345-019-02898-1.
13. Peters BS, Armijo PR, Krause C, Choudhury SA, Oleynikov D. Review of emerging surgical robotic technology. Surg Endosc. 2018;32(4):1636–55. https://doi.org/10.1007/s00464-018-6079-2.
14. Navaratnam A, Abdul-Muhsin H, Humphreys M. Updates in urologic robot assisted surgery, Version 1. F1000Res. 2018;7:F1000. https://doi.org/10.12688/f1000research.15480.1.

Chapter 9
Robotic/Laparoscopic Radical Nephrectomy/Nephroureterectomy

Ali Yildiz and Murat Arslan

Introduction

Laparoscopic radical nephrectomy (LRN) was first described by Clayman et al. in 1991. Since then, open surgery has increasingly been replaced by laparoscopic approaches [1]. In the early periods, the operative time was 5-8 h, and the estimated blood loss was often over 500 ml [2]. Recent studies have shown that while oncological results and complication rates of open and laparoscopic approaches are similar, laparoscopy is associated with shorter hospital stay and less analgesic requirement, and estimated blood loss [3, 4]. Since the first description of this technique, many modifications have been made to improve surgical outcomes, such as the retroperitoneal approach, hand-assisted, and robotic-assisted technique [5, 6]. The first robotic assisted laparoscopic radical nephrectomy (RLRN) for renal cell cancer (RCC) was described by Klingler et al. in 2000 [7]. However, nowadays LRN remains the gold standard for clinically localized renal mass [1].

In 1991, Clayman firstly also described the technique of laparoscopic nephroureterectomy [8], which was soon replicated by various authors worldwide [9, 10]. However, concerns about the oncological outcome have limited the spread of this technique in the following years. Although many centers perform robotic nephrectomy or partial nephrectomy, very few centers have described the robotic nephroureterectomy [11, 12].

A. Yildiz · M. Arslan (✉)
Department of Urology, Faculty of Medicine, Okan University Hospital, İstanbul, Turkey

S. Tonyali et al. (eds.), *Current Endourology*,
https://doi.org/10.1007/978-3-032-00010-1_9

Laparoscopic Transperitoneal Radical Nephrectomy

Most surgeons favored the transperitoneal approach because of greater working space and familiar anatomical landmarks.

Patient Preparation and Positioning

The patient is first placed supine position. A urethral catheter and nasogastric tube should be inserted after anesthesia induction and intubation. The patient is then carefully placed in a modified lateral decubitus position for a transperitoneal approach. The flank of the patient covers the kidney rest, an axillary roll is placed, and an additional roll is placed longitudinally along the patient's back to support the thoracolumbar spine. Intermittent compression stockings are put on the patient to prevent deep vein thrombosis. Silk or cloth tape is used to fix the patient to the table at a few points for preventing the patient from slipping off the table during the table rotation. Lastly, the abdomen is draped in a sterile fashion.

Access and Trocar Placement

There are several different techniques to exist pneumoperitoneum such as; Veres needle or Hasson cut-down technique. The technique varies depending on the experience and comfort of the surgeon. The abdomen is insufflated to a pressure of 15–20 mmHg. When the abdomen is insufflated adequately, a 10 or 12 mm reusable trocar is inserted into the abdomen at the level of the umbilicus for the camera. A 0^0 or 30^0 lens can be preferred depending on the surgeon's preference. Firstly, it should be checked whether there is any injury of the intraabdominal organs. Although 3 ports are usually sufficient for nephrectomy, a fourth port may be required for liver retraction, especially in right nephrectomies. Other trocars are placed using the triangulation rule. This rule requires a distance of 4 fingers between the optic trocar and the other trocars and 5 fingers between the other working trocars.

Procedure

At the beginning of the operation, firstly Toldt line should be incised with the help of cautery and scissors, and the colon should be medialized. For this, the Toldt line on the right is incised parallel to the ascending colon, and this incision is continued superiorly along the lower surface of the liver medially. The ascending colon is carefully mobilized medially by blunt dissection to expose the hepatic flexure, duodenum, and vena cava inferior. In the meantime, to protect from colon and bowel injuries, one should be very careful when using energy, especially near the organ. The mesenteric fatty tissue, which is brighter than the fatty tissue of the Gerota's fascia, should be recognized and this line should be carefully dissected bluntly, and the Gerota's fascia and adjacent structures should be separated from each other. On the left, the Toldlt line is incised parallel to the descending colon, and the splenocolic, splenorenal, and splenophrenic ligaments are also included in this incision. On this side, the colon and pancreatic tissue are separated from Gerota's fascia and mobilized medially by careful dissection.

After proper medial mobilization of the colon, the psoas muscle and tendon should be defined in the inferior pole of the kidney. At this stage, the gonadal vein first becomes visible. At this point, the ureter is lateral of the gonadal vein. Superiorly, the same dissection continues up to the renal hilum. The ureter should not be cut at this point, as it will help elevate the kidney. During this dissection, the left hand hanging the ureter is slowly shifted towards the hilum and gentle traction is applied so that the lymphatic and vascular structures can be better defined.

Safe dissection of the renal pedicle depends on proper medialization of the colon and intestines and anterolateral retraction of the kidney. When the ureter and lower pole of the kidney are gently hung, the vascular structures can be identified and exposed by blunt-sharp dissection. Since the left gonadal vein drains into the renal vein, the renal vein can be reached when it is followed. At this stage, the renal vein and the renal artery are carefully dissected separately. Dissection can be done bluntly with the aspirator tip or with the help of harmonic cutters or hook electrode cautery. During dissection of the renal vein, attention should be paid to the lumbar veins located posterior to it. After dissection of the artery and vein, the renal artery (first) and the renal vein are ligated and cut using an endovascular gastrointestinal anastomosis (Endo GIA) stapler. If it is difficult to separate the renal artery and vein, both vessels are ligated together with an Endo GIA stapler and cut. In the absence of endo GIA, preferably Hem-o-lok clip can also be used for vessel control. First of all, the renal artery is closed from 3 points with Hem-o-lok clips of appropriate size (preferably large). Then it should be checked that the renal vein is deflated and becomes straight. If the renal vein is still filling, the presence of another artery should be suspected and careful dissection should be continued. After the ligation of the artery, 3 Hem-o-lok clips are placed in the vein.

Finally, the specimen is entrapped in a suitable laparoscopic organ retrieval device. The specimen is taken out from Phannenstiel or Gibson incision. A drain is placed appropriately. The incisions are closed properly and the procedure is completed.

Laparoscopic Retroperitoneal Radical Nephrectomy

Retroperitoneal LRN is a useful approach in patients of prior abdominal surgeries. However, it may be more challenging to perform retroperitoneal LRN in obese patients. Improper orientation and loss of anatomical landmarks can lead to crucial intraoperative complications (such as caval transection etc.) [13].

Patient Preparation and Positioning

In this approach, the patient should be placed in the full flank position. After the axillary roll and anterior/posterior bolster are placed, the table should be flexed. This can provide to extend the space between the 12th rib and the iliac crest. Thick silk or cloth tape is used to fasten up the patient to the operative table. Unlike the transperitoneal LRN, in the retroperitoneal approach, the surgeon and assistant are on the patient's back; the monitor and nurse are located in front of the patient.

Acces and Trocar Placement

In the retroperitoneal approach, the open method (Hasson Technique) should be used to insert the first trocar. Approximately 1.5 cm incision is made off the tip of the 12th rib. After the oblique muscle is divided, the lumbodorsal fascia is reached and the retroperitoneum is entered. Then, a space is created between the psoas muscle and Gerota's fascia with the surgeons' index finger. A balloon dilatator is inserted into the retroperitoneum. Retroperitoneal space is dissected with the help of a balloon dilatator. After adequate space is created, a trocar (preferably with a balloon) is inserted into this area and the retroperitoneal area is carefully observed. The second and third trocars are placed under direct vision, preferably 3–4 cm above the anterior axillary line, and at the junction of the spinal muscles and the 12th rib.

Procedure

After appropriate medial mobilization of intraperitoneal structures, the psoas muscle and tendon should be defined adjacent to the lower pole of the kidney. The ureter is located anteromedial to the tendon. The ureter is traced back to the renal hilum and is used to hang the kidney as with the transperitoneal approach.

The renal hilum is identified with the help of renal artery pulsation. The incision is made off over the pulsation to expose the artery and vein. Firstly, the artery and vein are isolated and dissected separately and they are ligated and cut respectively. After the kidney has been completely freed from the renal fossa and the ureter is ligated and cut, the kidney is entrapped in a laparoscopic organ retrieval bag. The specimen can be removed from the Gibson incision.

Robot-Assisted Laparoscopic Radical Nephrectomy (Transperitoneal)

RLRN was described in 2000. However, it did not become widespread very quickly due to prolonged operation times, increased operation room costs. In addition, RLRN has similar oncologic outcomes to LRN. The docking and undocking of the robot increase the operative time. In the light of this information, RLRN provides no additional benefits and increases the cost. However, it can be considered a useful educational step before performing robotic partial nephrectomy. (22).

Patient Preparation and Positioning

The patient is placed in the modified lateral decubitus position. The robot is docked behind the patient at a 20° angle towards the patients' head.

Access and Trocar Placement

After the pnömoperitoneum is achieved to a pressure of 15–20 mmHg, a 12 mm umblical optic trocar is inserted into the abdomen. For robotic arms, an 8 mm port is placed in the middle of the distance between the anterior superior iliac spine and the umbilicus, and another 8 mm port is placed two fingers medial to the midclavicular line and two fingers below the arcus costarum. The assistant port is placed in the midline, approximately 8 cm inferior to the umbilical trocar. This port is used by the assistant in procedures such as clip placement and aspiration.

Procedure

The surgical steps are performed as described above for transperitoneal LRN.

References

1. Clayman RV, Kavoussi LR, Soper NJ, Dierks SM, Meretyk S, Darcy MD, et al. Laparoscopic nephrectomy: initial case report. J Urol. 1991;146:278–82.
2. Ono Y, Hattori R, Gotoh M, Yoshino Y, Yoshikawa Y, Kamihira O. Laparoscopic radical nephrectomy for renal cell carcinoma: the standard of care already? Curr Opin Urol. 2005;15:75–8.
3. Gratzke C, Seitz M, Bayrle F, Schlenker B, Bastian PJ, Haseke N, et al. Quality of life and perioperative outcomes after retroperitoneoscopic radical nephrectomy (RN), open RN and nephron-sparing surgery in patients with renal cell carcinoma. BJU Int. 2009;104(4):470–5.
4. Wang L, Wang L, Yang Q, Xiao C, Sun Y. Retroperitoneal laparoscopic and open radical nephrectomy for T1 renal cell carcinoma. J Endourol. 2009;23(9):1509–12.
5. Gill IS, Rassweiler JJ. Retroperitoneoscopic renal surgery: our approach. Urology. 1999;54(4):734–8.
6. Nakada SY, Moon TD, Gist M, Mahvi D. Use of the pneumo sleeve as an adjunct in laparoscopic nephrectomy. Urology. 1997;49(4):612–3.
7. Klingler DW, Hemstreet GP, Balaji KC. Feasibility of robotic radical nephrectomy—initial results of single-institution pilot study. Urology. 2005;65(6):1086–9.
8. Clayman RV, Kavoussi LR, Figenshau RS, Chandhoke P, Albala DM. Laparoscopic nephroureterectomy: initial clinical case report. J Laparoendocopic Surg. 1991;1:343–9.

9. Rassweiler J, Henkel TO, Potempa DM, Coptcoat M, Alken P. The technique of transperitoneal laparoscopic nephrectomy, adrenalectomy, and nephroureterectomy. Eur Urol. 1993;23:425–30.
10. Chung HJ, Chiu AW, Chen KK, et al. Retroperitoneoscopy-assisted nephroureterectomy for the management of upper tract urothelial cancer. Min Inv Ther. 1996;5:266–71.
11. Hemal AK, Kumar A, Gupta NP, et al. Retroperitoneal nephroureterectomy with excision of cuff of the bladder for upper urinary tract transitional cell carcinoma: comparison of laparoscopic and open surgery with long-term follow-up. World J Urol. 2008;26:381–6.
12. Park SY, Jeong W, Ham WS, et al. Initial experience of robotic nephroureterectomy: a hybrid-port technique. BJU Int. 2009;104:1718–21.
13. McAllister M, Bhayani SB, Ong A, et al. Vena caval transection during retroperitoneoscopic nephrectomy: report of the complication and review of the literature. J Urol. 2004;172(1):183–5.

Chapter 10
Laparoscopic Live Donor Nephrectomy

Erkan Olcucuoglu, Huseyin Bicer, Mert Ali Karadag, and Muhammed Emin Polat

History

Murray and colleagues performed the first open living donor nephrectomy (OLDN) in 1954, and it has been the standard procedure for living kidney donation for many years since then [37]. However, scarring, postoperative pain, incisional hernia, and other complications were discovered to be caused by a wide flank incision in many donors who underwent OLDN surgery. In order to solve these problems, Ratner and colleagues performed the first laparoscopic living donor nephrectomy (LLDN) to replace the OLDN technique in 1995 [43]. LLDN has been proven to have less postoperative pain, a shorter hospital stay, better cosmetic results, and a faster recovery than OLDN [52].

Techniques and Their Differences

There have been several technical differences and advancements in laparoscopic surgery, including hand-assisted laparoscopic living donor nephrectomy (HALLDN), robotic-assisted laparoscopic living donor nephrectomy (RALLDN), retroperitoneoscopic intervention, laparoscopic single-site surgery (LESS), and natural orifice transluminal endoscopic surgery (NOTES).

HALLDN was first performed in 1998 [53]. The numerous ways in which hands and instruments can be used in this technique make surgical dissection easier and

E. Olcucuoglu (✉) · M. E. Polat
University of Health Sciences, Ankara City Hospital, Clinic of Urology, Ankara, Turkey

H. Bicer · M. A. Karadag
Department of Urology, Kayseri Faculty of Medicine, University of Health Sciences, Kayseri, Turkey

S. Tonyali et al. (eds.), *Current Endourology*,
https://doi.org/10.1007/978-3-032-00010-1_10

more successful, considerably enhancing the technique efficiency and offering a speedier process and shorter operative time. This procedure allows surgeons to have a better feel for the renal tissues and make the most of the OLDN approach [42].

Horgan and colleagues discovered RALLDN in 2002 [25]. This robotic technology, when compared to normal laparoscopic surgery, delivers more precise 3D imaging and increases the surgeons' ability to conduct difficult procedures in a laparoscopic context [19].

When compared to OLDN, LLDN found to be associated with identical rejection rates, graft function, urological complications, and recipient and graft survival. In addition to this analgesic requirement, pain, hospital stay, and time to return to work are significantly better for laparoscopic procedures [20, 42, 47, 55].

According to a meta-analysis, HALLDN was associated with reduced operational time and warm ischemia time, as well as equal safety and overall results when compared to the standard laparoscopic approach [13]. According to this meta-analysis, HALLDN has a shorter operating time and less warm ischemia time than LLDN. However, no significant difference in graft survival or intraoperative complication rates was found between the two groups.

Although there aren't enough reports regarding the robotic method, according to a meta-analysis, this approach has higher complication rates than the laparoscopic method [32, 49].

LESS enables the surgeon to operate from a single incision using multiple access port (usually the umbilicus). The kidney is removed through the same or a different incision. Less pain and better cosmetic results have been discovered in various retrospective and prospective randomized studies alongside equal surgical safety and results [3, 21]. LESS is, however, regarded as a technically more difficult approach than traditional LLDN, and its role in donor operations has not yet been defined.

Transvaginal NOTES-assisted nephrectomy eliminates the need for an abdominal incision for kidney extraction, reducing scarring and suffering. Although preliminary reviews indicate that this procedure is safe, expertise with this technique appears to be limited [1].

LLDN is a unique surgical treatment in which people with no medical issues take surgical risks for patients with end-stage renal failure. It is of great importance to select the best surgical method in order to obtain a living donor kidney. There are two critical aspects to consider: donor mortality and morbidity risks. These risks, which include the transplant facility and operating surgeons, can be reduced via careful selection of surgical abilities and experience, as well as safe surgical practices. It is critical for the donor kidney to operate optimally in order for the receiver to have the greatest results possible after a kidney transplant [13].

In a meta-analysis comparing the surgeries for living donor nephrectomy performed in 2020 [54] was found that the warm ischemia time and operative time in the LLDN and RALLDN groups were longer than those in the HALLDN and OLDN groups, but there was no significant difference in the warm ischemia time and operative time between the LLDN and RALLDN groups. This is probably due to the rapid removal of the kidney from the hand-port after vascular ligation in hand-assisted intervention, whereas the LLDN and RALLDN procedures necessitate skin incision [8].

This meta-analysis found that the estimated blood loss in the HALLDN, LLDN, and RALLDN groups was much lower than that in the OLDN group, which is assumed to be related to the use of thinner instruments, optical magnification and multi-angle vision in laparoscopic surgery [24]. The visual analog scale (VAS) was used to assess pain on the first day following surgery in the studies included in this meta-analysis. Among the four interventions, the RALLDN group got the lowest VAS score. Furthermore, the OLDN group required more morphine than the LLDN group; this demonstrates that donors who had RALLDN and LLDN had less postoperative pain. RALLDN was shown to have the best VAS and morphine uptake values. One probable cause for decreased pain in robotic surgery is that the robotic arms revolve around the port area and move at a set remote center; as a result, there is less pressure around the port, resulting in less injury to the abdominal tissue around the port [4].

According to this, an earlier recovery is achieved with the relief of pain. Therefore, the length of hospital stay was examined, and it was discovered that the OLDN group stayed in the hospital substantially longer than the other three groups. Despite the fact that the RALLDN group had a higher intraoperative complication rate, there was no significant difference in postoperative complications between all groups. Instrument failure, instrument misuse, and organ injury, in addition to vascular injury, can all be considered intraoperative complications [12, 18, 28]. RALLDN technique needs experienced surgeons to be more effective than the LLDN [29].

When evaluated in terms of recipient outcomes, there was no difference in delayed graft function and graft survival in the recipient amongst the four surgical modalities, as prolonged warm ischemia time and operative time had no effect on delayed graft function or 1-year graft survival [54]. In the same study, the OLDN technique was observed to cause more acute rejection (AR) than LLDN and HALLDN, but there was no significant difference in AR between the HALLDN and LLDN groups. It should also be highlighted that the meta-analysis lacked information on immunosuppression and that the HALLDN and LLDN groups may have adopted a more active approach to immunosuppression than other institutions [54]. In summary, no significant differences between the four surgical techniques in terms of donor postoperative complications, recipient delayed graft function, or graft survival were reported in this meta-analysis. While both OLDN and HALLDN methods reduce warm ischemia time and operation time, OLDN increases blood loss. RALLDN and LLDN reduce hospital stay, morphine intake, and VAS, resulting in a faster recovery. Due to its long learning curve, RALLDN, on the other hand, causes higher intraoperative complications. According to the Clavien scale subgroup analysis of intraoperative complications, the rate of intraoperative complications (III-IV) was observed to be greater in the RLLDN group. The majority of intraoperative complications have been found to be due to uncontrollable bleeding caused by intraoperative vascular injury or splenic trauma.

Should the Donor's Left or Right Kidney Be Taken?

According to a meta-analysis conducted in 2015, the surgical feasibility and postoperative graft function of right and left LLDN, were shown to be similar. In the absence of any difference in bilateral renal function, surgeons recommended that either the right or left kidney be transplanted; nevertheless, the longer renal vein of the left kidney may lessen surgical complexity and allow the left kidney to be used in clinical practice [51]. According to the same meta-analysis, right laparoscopic living donor nephrectomy may increase the risk of renal vein thrombosis in the recipient due to the short right renal vein. In a research of 1850 cases completed in 2018 as anti-study, 1682 left and 168 right laparoscopic donor nephrectomies were performed, and no significant difference was identified in terms of operation time, intraoperative blood loss, warm ischemia time, and hospital stay. According to the study, the right kidney can be transplanted safely and indistinguishably from the left kidney with enough laparoscopic experience [31].

Another important issue is the presence of several renal arteries in the kidney to be transplanted. A systemic analysis conducted in 2020 discovered that the right kidney and kidneys with numerous renal arteries are just as safe and feasible as the left kidney and kidneys with a single renal artery [9, 23, 33].

Lldn Step-By-Step Surgical Technique

For this procedure, perioperative single-dose antibiotics are recommended [41]. Preoperative and postoperative hydration must be adjusted to protect graft kidney function. It is recommended that balanced crystalloid solutions (lactated Ringer's solution) be used for intraoperative hydration [40].

This is a procedure that necessitates extensive laparoscopic surgical experience. After inserting a Foley catheter, the patient is put in the flank position. To prevent vascular and nerve compression, the patient's arms and legs are secured with pillows and gel pads.

Following the formation of a pneumoperitoneum with a Veress needle, a 10 mm optical trocar is inserted from the umbilical or paraumbilical region (rectus abdominis laterally) based on the patient's body mass index. To begin the treatment, two 5 mm trocars are placed, under direct vision, in the left iliac fossa and where the anterior axillary line intersects the subcostal region (Fig. 10.1). To exclude the liver on the right side, it is useful to insert a fourth 5 mm trocar 2 cm below the xiphoid.

The Toldt's fascia is initially incised up to the iliac vessels, as is the case with all laparoscopic kidney procedures, and the colon is medialized (Fig. 10.2). To separate the spleen (for the left side) or the liver (for the right side) from the upper pole of the kidney, the posterior peritoneum is incised up to the crus of the diaphragm. The lateral and parietal attachments of the kidney are left in place to prevent the kidney from slipping down and disturbing later the hilar dissection. The colon is

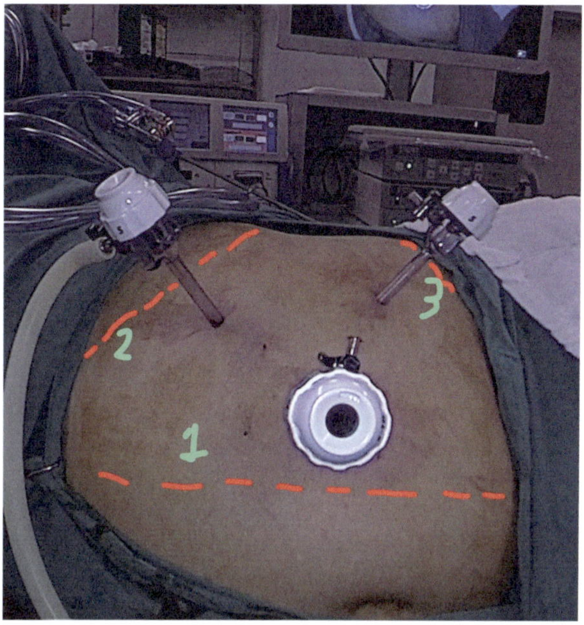

Fig. 10.1 Left laparoscopic live donor nephrectomy patient position (left upper lateral position) and placement of trocars. (1) 10 mm camera port; rectus abdominis lateral at the level of the umbilicus. (2) 5 mm working port; at the midclavicular line in the subcostal region. (3) 5 mm working port; 2 cm medial to the anterior iliac crest

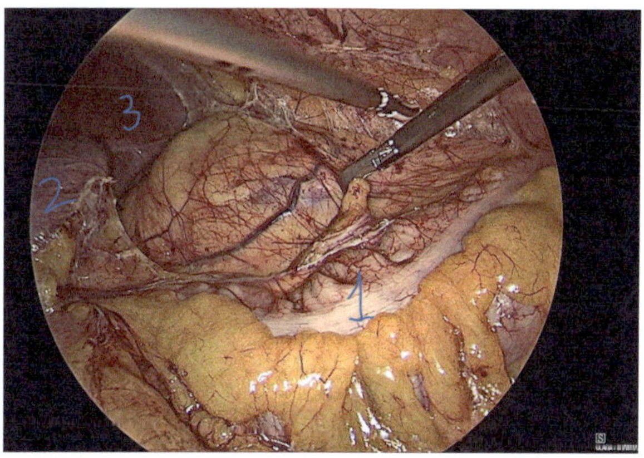

Fig. 10.2 Dropping the descending colon from the Toldt's fascia (1) Descending colon (2) Spleen (3) Diaphragm

medialized, and the gonadal vein, ureter, and psoas muscle are identified (Fig. 10.3). The distal ureter is dissected to the level of the iliac vessels. All periureteral and inferior renal pole fat must be well preserved to keep a well-vascularized ureter. The gonadal vein can be divided proximally and distally and kept with the ureter in order to protect ureteric vascularity.

Then, the spleen and tail of the pancreas are completely mobilized by cutting the splenorenal and splenophrenic ligaments. Care is taken not to injure the pancreas, the splenic artery, and the stomach near the level of the crus of the diaphragm where dissection ends. By achieving this step, the space between the spleen and the kidney is usually widely opened and permits partial mobilization of the upper renal pole. The gonadal

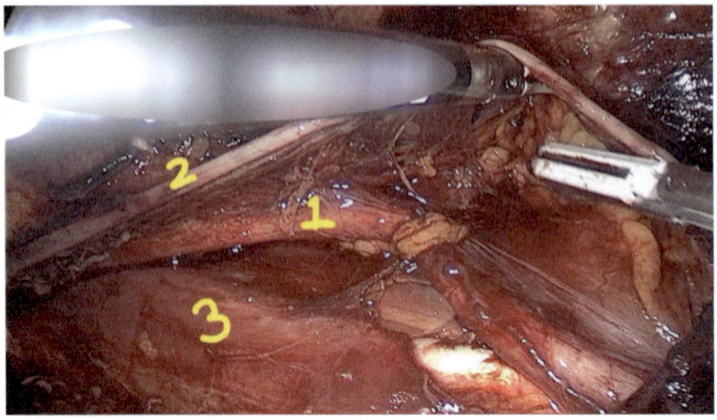

Fig. 10.3 Revealing the ureter and left gonadal vein (1) Ureter (2) Left gonadal vein (3) Psoas muscle

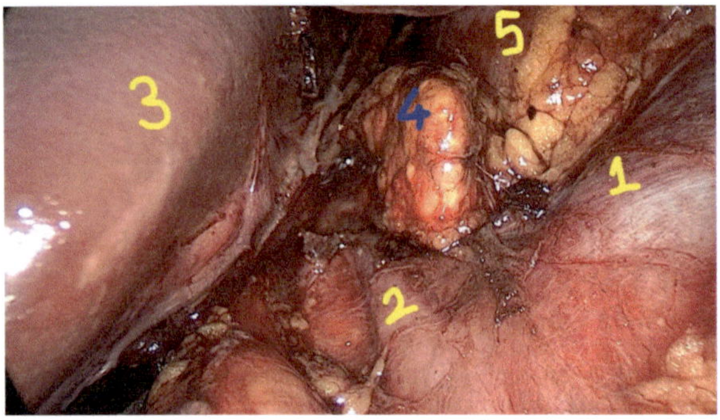

Fig. 10.4 Revealing the renal and suprarenal veins (1) Left renal vein (2) Left suprarenal vein (3) Spleen (4) Suprarenal (5) Renal parenchyma

vein is dissected superiorly in order to locate the renal vein. Then, starting a very careful dissection from the upper border of the renal vein toward the upper pole of the kidney with division of the adrenal vein using vessel sealing device without any clip placement and caring not to injure the anterior branch of the renal artery or small upper pole arteries (Fig. 10.4). The renal artery and vein are separated as far as possible from the kidney and the major vessels. All lymphatics and autonomic nerve plexuses superior to the vein and around the renal artery are sealed and cut. The left renal artery is dissected at its aortic origin. In some cases, retroperitoneal veins (lumbar, ascending lumbar, and hemiazygos) join the left renal vein in up to 75% of individuals, and it must be sealed and cut.

Clips are avoided on all venous branches to prevent their later insertion between the jaws of the stapling device. Very careful dissection is undertaken between the artery and vein to prepare a clear, precise, and secure positioning of the stapling device (Fig. 10.5).

The kidney should be fully separated from the surrounding tissues, leaving only the renal artery, vein, and ureter. For a quicker removal of the kidney, a pfannenstiel incision should be made below the umbilicus (Fig. 10.6). The Hem-o-lok clips are sealed and cut at the level of the common iliac artery from the ureter's most distal end (Fig. 10.7). Before pedicle clamping it is recommended to check the flow of urine from the ureter. After confirming the urine flow, the renal artery and vein are sealed separately using the stapler device (Figs. 10.8 and 10.9). The kidney was removed through a previously made pfannenstiel incision to prepare for the recipient. Before ending the surgery, latero aortic and interaortocaval lymphatics are clipped to prevent chylous leakage.

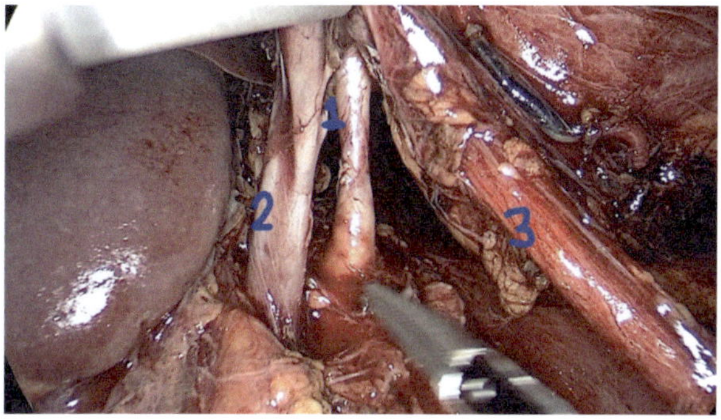

Fig. 10.5 Revealing the renal artery and vein (1) Renal artery (2) Renal vein (3) Ureter

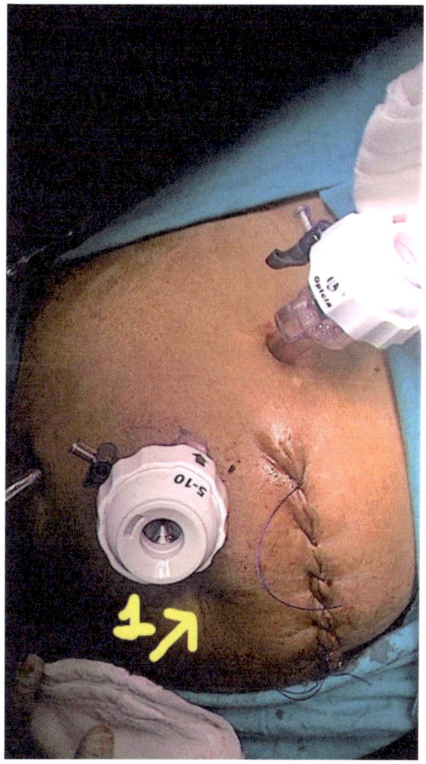

Fig. 10.6 Making a pfannenstiel incision to remove the kidney (1) Umbilicus

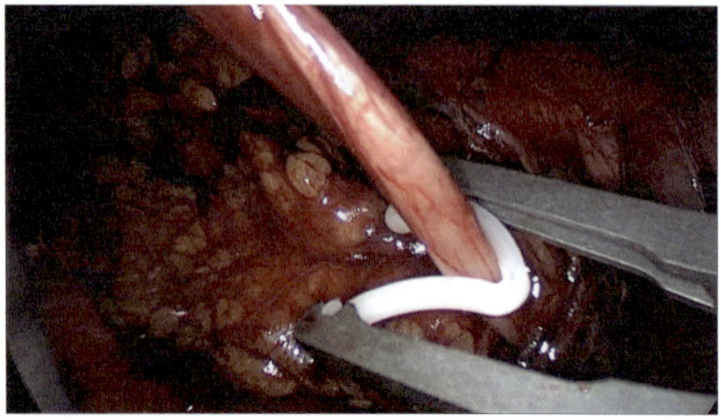

Fig. 10.7 Cutting the ureter at the point where it crosses the common iliac artery by using a distal Hem-o-Lok clip

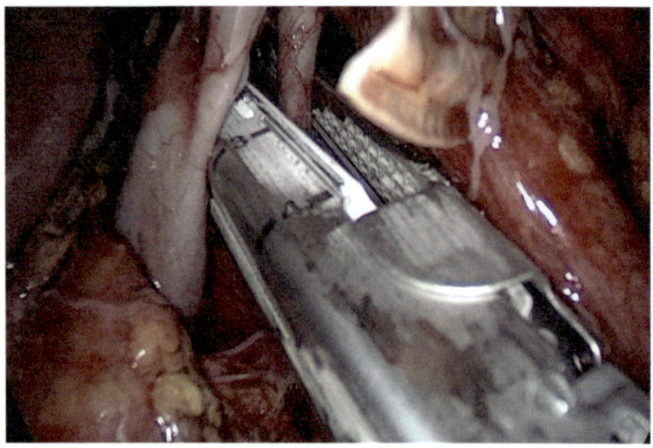

Fig. 10.8 Closing and cutting the left renal artery by stapler

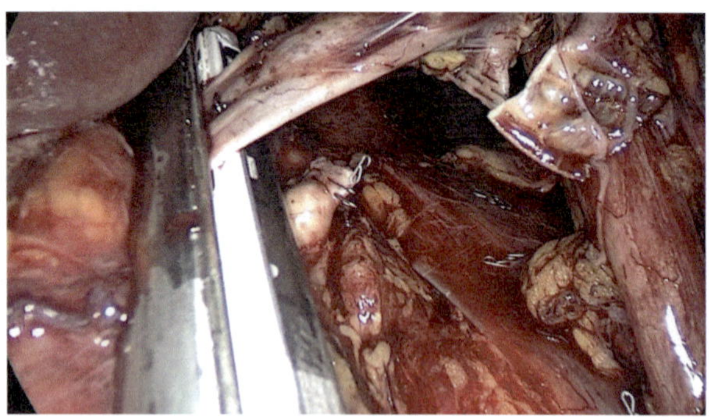

Fig. 10.9 Closing and cutting the left renal vein by stapler

Postoperative Care

The early postoperative period after LLDN is critical in the follow-up of kidney donors. Extubation is performed once the patient has reached a normothermic state. Orogastric tube is removed prior to extubation. Hemoglobin levels are checked every 6 hours following surgery, and if they are normal, they are checked again the next morning along with serum creatinine and electrolytes. Urine output should be closely monitored.

Discomfort and pain in the shoulder area are common complaints following LLDN, possibly related to residual pneumoperitoneum. There is a widespread belief among this category of patients who do not use drugs to aggressively reduce post-operative pain. The treatment of choice for this is "patient-controlled analgesia" (PCA) (PCA; fentanyl or, less usually, morphine). In the absence of PCA, pain is controlled with IV paracetamol and, if necessary, ketoprofen or ketorolac in the first 24 hours [7]. To lessen the risk of nephrotoxicity, the patient should be adequately hydrated. Opiates can also be used to treat pain when morphine-deficient methods are ineffective.

The patient's diet is initiated with fluids on the first postoperative day, and the Foley catheter is removed. The patient should be mobilized as soon as possible, either that day's evening or the following morning.

The advent of early postoperative recovery (ERAS) has resulted in significant changes in the traditional standard of care. Numerous centers in the United States that prevent excess fluid leaking into the third space and intestinal edema, adopt advanced recovery programs that include intraoperative fluid restriction (3 ml/kg/hr), urine output 0.5 ml/kg/hr, use of local subfascial bupivacaine or other anesthetics, and a postoperative drug-free pain control regimen (acetaminophen, ketorolac) [50]. Innovations in this management have been associated to shorter hospital stays, better pain control, and higher patient satisfaction. It has become evident that ERAS will potentially increase the benefits of laparoscopic surgery for kidney donors [45].

Living kidney donors are considered to be "intermediate risk" patients for deep vein thrombosis (DVT) and pulmonary embolism [2]. All living donors should wear compression socks during and after surgery, as well as receive appropriate thromboprophylaxis with low molecular weight heparin for at least one week. The patient is usually discharged on the second day and is checked again after 10 days. If no additional features are included in the follow-up protocol, the patient has 6-month, 1-year, and 2-year controls.

Donors should return to their normal routine as soon as possible, with regular monitoring of their blood pressure and weight. They should be warned to avoid nephrotoxic drugs.

Complications

LLDN appears to be a risk-free method. However, serious complications, including death, can occur. Despite the fact that no deaths were reported in several large series [11, 22, 27, 36], the overall mortality rate is around 0.03% [34]. The majority of these deaths occurred in the postoperative period and were caused by bleeding [16], CO2 gas embolism [5], and pulmonary embolism [34]. The risk of significant intraoperative bleeding during LLDN ranges between 0.6% and 1.6% [11, 36].

Conversion to open surgery has been reported to occur in 0–13% of cases; however, most significant series [2, 11, 22, 27, 36] have documented conversion rates of 1–2%. A recent meta-analysis discovered that conversion to open surgery was 1.1%; half of them were reported due to bleeding and the other half due to harm to other organs. The second surgical intervention was reported to be 0.6%, largely due to bleeding or hematoma drainage attempts [30].

Other intraoperative complications include spleen or liver laceration, ureteral or intestinal injury, and pleural laceration. The overall incidence of surgical complications is 5.46% [22]. All major complications occurred in the first 100 cases in which surgeons performed this surgery [27]. This raises the question of the learning curve and how many laparoscopic nephrectomy procedures should be conducted before the first LLDN. While no precise answer exists, a range of 50 to 100 appears fair for learning this type of operation.

LLDN postoperative complications include hematoma, fever, urinary tract infection, pneumonia, pulmonary embolism, wound infection, incisional hernias, prolonged ileus, chylous ascites, and left testicular pain, which may be caused by disruption of the neural plexus or lymphatic drainage feeding the testis as a result of gonadal vein division or excessive mobilization of the left colon. Chylous leakage is a rare complication of LLDN. Prevention is accomplished by meticulously and thoroughly closing the lymphatic vessels throughout the dissection area [10, 48].

Long-term complications include arterial hypertension, renal failure, and proteinuria, which are more common in high-risk donors such as older or younger donors with obesity, hypertensive donors, and those who have kidney stones [39, 44]. Donors with isolated abnormalities, such as obesity, can make a donation nowadays. Aside from the technical difficulties of positioning and instrumentation, surgeons may encounter lengthier operating times, more anesthetic, and post-operative complications. According to studies, laparoscopic donor nephrectomy is generally safe in obese donors. Obese donors have a higher baseline cardiovascular risk and the risk endanger their own long-term health [23].

The remaining kidney's function improves as a result of the kidney donation. At three months, clearance of the remaining kidney has increased to an average GFR of 65–75% of renal function previous to kidney donation [2]. The average decrease in GFR after donation was 26 mL/min/1.73 m2 (range 8–50) [2, 15].

Despite a decrease in GFR, the incidence of end-stage renal disease (ESRD) in living kidney donors appears to be similar to or lower than that observed in the general population [2, 35, 46]. The estimated lifetime risk of ESRD among donors is 90 per 10,000, 326 per 10,000 in the general population, and 14 per 10,000 in matched healthy non-donor controls [38]. This could be due to the fact that kidney donors get more frequent check-ups than the general population, and because they are aware that they have only one kidney, they alter their fluid consumption and nutrition accordingly. Living donor nephrectomy alone does not lead to renal failure [26].

In terms of hypertension, a large meta-analysis found that donors raised their systolic blood pressure by 5 mmHg 5–10 years after donation [6]. Donors have the same rate of hypertension as the general population [17]. Finally, it is worth mentioning that living donors have a higher life expectancy than the general population [14, 26, 46].

Tips and Tricks

- The donor should keep the functionally better kidney; however, this criterion may change if both the donor and receiver have multiple renal arteries and veins that are at high risk of developing surgical complications.
- For the closure of renal artery and vein, a vascular stapler should be used. Hem-o-lok clip should not be used.
- Dissection should not be performed between the lower pole of the kidney and the proximal ureter in order to preserve the ureter feeding. The golden triangle zone should be protected.
- The ureteral serosa and surrounding tissues should be preserved and dissected.

References

1. Alcaraz A, Musquera M, Peri L, Izquierdo L, García-Cruz E, Huguet J, Alvarez-Vijande R, Campistol JM, Oppenheimer F, Ribal MJ. Feasibility of transvaginal natural orifice transluminal endoscopic surgery-assisted living donor nephrectomy: is kidney vaginal delivery the approach of the future? Eur Urol. 2011;59(6):1019–25. https://doi.org/10.1016/j.eururo.2011.03.021.
2. Andrews PA, Burnapp L. British transplantation society/renal association UK guidelines for living donor kidney transplantation 2018: summary of updated guidance. Transplantation. 2018;102(7):e307. https://doi.org/10.1097/tp.0000000000002253.
3. Autorino R, Brandao LF, Sankari B, Zargar H, Laydner H, Akça O, De Sio M, Mirone V, Chueh SC, Kaouk JH. Laparoendoscopic single-site (LESS) vs laparoscopic living-donor nephrectomy: a systematic review and meta-analysis. BJU Int. 2015;115(2):206–15. https://doi.org/10.1111/bju.12724.
4. Bhattu AS, Ganpule A, Sabnis RB, Murali V, Mishra S, Desai M. Robot-assisted laparoscopic donor nephrectomy vs standard laparoscopic donor nephrectomy: a prospective randomized comparative study. J Endourol. 2015;29(12):1334–40. https://doi.org/10.1089/end.2015.0213.
5. Boghossian T, Henri M, Dubé S, Bendavid Y, Morin M. Laparoscopic nephrectomy donor death due to cerebral gas embolism in a specialized transplant center: risk zero does not exist. Transplantation. 2005;79(2):258–9. https://doi.org/10.1097/01.tp.0000141757.64379.8f.
6. Boudville N, Prasad GV, Knoll G, Muirhead N, Thiessen-Philbrook H, Yang RC, Rosas-Arellano MP, Housawi A, Garg AX. Meta-analysis: risk for hypertension in living kidney donors. Ann Intern Med. 2006;145(3):185–96. https://doi.org/10.7326/0003-4819-145-3-200608010-00006.
7. Breda A, Bui MH, Liao JC, Schulam PG. Association of bowel rest and ketorolac analgesia with short hospital stay after laparoscopic donor nephrectomy. Urology. 2007;69(5):828–31. https://doi.org/10.1016/j.urology.2007.01.083.
8. Broe MP, Galvin R, Keenan LG, Power RE. Laparoscopic and hand-assisted laparoscopic donor nephrectomy: a systematic review and meta-analysis. Arab J Urol. 2018;16(3):322–34. https://doi.org/10.1016/j.aju.2018.02.003.
9. Broudeur L, Karam G, Chelghaf I, De Vergie S, Rigaud J, Perrouin Verbe MA, Branchereau J. Feasibility and safety of laparoscopic living donor nephrectomy in case of right kidney and multiple-renal artery kidney: a systematic review of the literature. World J Urol. 2020;38(4):919–27. https://doi.org/10.1007/s00345-019-02821-8.
10. Capocasale E, Iaria M, Vistoli F, Signori S, Mazzoni MP, Dalla Valle R, De Lio N, Perrone V, Amorese G, Mosca F, Boggi U. Incidence, diagnosis, and treatment of chylous leakage

after laparoscopic live donor nephrectomy. Transplantation. 2012;93(1):82–6. https://doi.org/10.1097/TP.0b013e31823b2d8e.
11. Chin EH, Hazzan D, Herron DM, Gaetano JN, Ames SA, Bromberg JS, Edye M. Laparoscopic donor nephrectomy: intraoperative safety, immediate morbidity, and delayed complications with 500 cases. Surg Endosc. 2007;21(4):521–6. https://doi.org/10.1007/s00464-006-9021-y.
12. Cohen AJ, Williams DS, Bohorquez H, Bruce DS, Carmody IC, Reichman T, Loss GE Jr. Robotic-assisted laparoscopic donor nephrectomy: decreasing length of stay. Ochsner J. 2015;15(1):19–24.
13. Elmaraezy A, Abushouk AI, Kamel M, Negida A, Naser O. Should hand-assisted retroperitoneoscopic nephrectomy replace the standard laparoscopic technique for living donor nephrectomy? A meta-analysis. Int J Surg. 2017;40:83–90. https://doi.org/10.1016/j.ijsu.2017.02.018.
14. Fehrman-Ekholm I, Nordén G, Lennerling A, Rizell M, Mjörnstedt L, Wramner L, Olausson M. Incidence of end-stage renal disease among live kidney donors. Transplantation. 2006;82(12):1646–8. https://doi.org/10.1097/01.tp.0000250728.73268.e3.
15. Fenton A, Montgomery E, Nightingale P, Peters AM, Sheerin N, Wroe AC, Lipkin GW. Glomerular filtration rate: new age- and gender-specific reference ranges and thresholds for living kidney donation. BMC Nephrol. 2018;19(1):336. https://doi.org/10.1186/s12882-018-1126-8.
16. Friedman AL, Peters TG, Jones KW, Boulware LE, Ratner LE. Fatal and nonfatal hemorrhagic complications of living kidney donation. Ann Surg. 2006;243(1):126–30. https://doi.org/10.1097/01.sla.0000193841.43474.ec.
17. Garg AX, Prasad GV, Thiessen-Philbrook HR, Ping L, Melo M, Gibney EM, Knoll G, Karpinski M, Parikh CR, Gill J, Storsley L, Vlasschaert M, Mamdani M. Cardiovascular disease and hypertension risk in living kidney donors: an analysis of health administrative data in Ontario, Canada. Transplantation. 2008;86(3):399–406. https://doi.org/10.1097/TP.0b013e31817ba9e3.
18. Geffner S, Klaassen Z, Tichauer M, Chamberlain RS, Paragi PR. Robotic-assisted laparoscopic donor nephrectomies: early experience and review of the literature. J Robot Surg. 2011;5(2):115–20. https://doi.org/10.1007/s11701-011-0245-z.
19. Giacomoni A, Concone G, Di Sandro S, Lauterio A, De Carlis L. The meaning of surgeon's comfort in robotic surgery. Am J Surg. 2014;208(5):871–2. https://doi.org/10.1016/j.amjsurg.2014.04.012.
20. Greco F, Hoda MR, Alcaraz A, Bachmann A, Hakenberg OW, Fornara P. Laparoscopic living-donor nephrectomy: analysis of the existing literature. Eur Urol. 2010;58(4):498–509. https://doi.org/10.1016/j.eururo.2010.04.003.
21. Gupta A, Ahmed K, Kynaston HG, Dasgupta P, Chlosta PL, Aboumarzouk OM. Laparoendoscopic single-site donor nephrectomy (LESS-DN) versus standard laparoscopic donor nephrectomy. Cochrane Database Syst Rev. 2016;2016(5):Cd010850. https://doi.org/10.1002/14651858.CD010850.pub2.
22. Harper JD, Breda A, Leppert JT, Veale JL, Gritsch HA, Schulam PG. Experience with 750 consecutive laparoscopic donor nephrectomies—is it time to use a standardized classification of complications? J Urol. 2010;183(5):1941–6. https://doi.org/10.1016/j.juro.2010.01.021.
23. Heimbach JK, Taler SJ, Prieto M, Cosio FG, Textor SC, Kudva YC, Chow GK, Ishitani MB, Larson TS, Stegall MD. Obesity in living kidney donors: clinical characteristics and outcomes in the era of laparoscopic donor nephrectomy. Am J Transplant. 2005;5(5):1057–64. https://doi.org/10.1111/j.1600-6143.2005.00791.x.
24. Horgan S, Benedetti E, Moser F. Robotically assisted donor nephrectomy for kidney transplantation. Am J Surg. 2004;188(4A Suppl):45s–51s. https://doi.org/10.1016/j.amjsurg.2004.08.028.
25. Horgan S, Vanuno D, Benedetti E. Early experience with robotically assisted laparoscopic donor nephrectomy. Surg Laparosc Endosc Percutan Tech. 2002;12(1):64–70. https://doi.org/10.1097/00129689-200202000-00011.
26. Ibrahim HN, Foley R, Tan L, Rogers T, Bailey RF, Guo H, Gross CR, Matas AJ. Long-term consequences of kidney donation. N Engl J Med. 2009;360(5):459–69. https://doi.org/10.1056/NEJMoa0804883.

27. Jacobs SC, Cho E, Foster C, Liao P, Bartlett ST. Laparoscopic donor nephrectomy: the University of Maryland 6-year experience. J Urol. 2004;171(1):47–51. https://doi.org/10.1097/01.ju.0000100221.20410.4a.
28. Janki S, Klop KWJ, Hagen SM, Terkivatan T, Betjes MGH, Tran TCK, Ijzermans JNM. Robotic surgery rapidly and successfully implemented in a high volume laparoscopic center on living kidney donation. Int J Med Robot. 2017;13(2) https://doi.org/10.1002/rcs.1743.
29. Khajeh E, Nikbakhsh R, Ramouz A, Majlesara A, Golriz M, Müller-Stich BP, Nickel F, Morath C, Zeier M, Mehrabi A. Robot-assisted versus laparoscopic living donor nephrectomy: superior outcomes after completion of the learning curve. J Robot Surg. 2023;17(5):2513–26. https://doi.org/10.1007/s11701-023-01681-0.
30. Kortram K, Ijzermans JN, Dor FJ. Perioperative events and complications in minimally invasive live donor nephrectomy: a systematic review and meta-analysis. Transplantation. 2016;100(11):2264–75. https://doi.org/10.1097/tp.0000000000001327.
31. Kumar A, Chaturvedi S, Gulia A, Maheshwari R, Dassi V, Desai P. Laparoscopic live donor nephrectomy: comparison of outcomes right versus left. Transplant Proc. 2018;50(8):2327–32. https://doi.org/10.1016/j.transproceed.2018.03.034.
32. Lentine KL, Lam NN, Axelrod D, Schnitzler MA, Garg AX, Xiao H, Dzebisashvili N, Schold JD, Brennan DC, Randall H, King EA, Segev DL. Perioperative complications after living kidney donation: a national study. Am J Transplant. 2016;16(6):1848–57. https://doi.org/10.1111/ajt.13687.
33. Lim EJ, Fong KY, Li J, Chan YH, Aslim EJ, Ng LG, Gan VHL. Single versus multiple renal arteries in living donor kidney transplantation: a systematic review and patient-level meta-analysis. Clin Transpl. 2023;37(11):e15069. https://doi.org/10.1111/ctr.15069.
34. Matas AJ, Bartlett ST, Leichtman AB, Delmonico FL. Morbidity and mortality after living kidney donation, 1999-2001: survey of United States transplant centers. Am J Transplant. 2003;3(7):830–4.
35. Mjøen G, Hallan S, Hartmann A, Foss A, Midtvedt K, Øyen O, Reisæter A, Pfeffer P, Jenssen T, Leivestad T, Line PD, Øvrehus M, Dale DO, Pihlstrøm H, Holme I, Dekker FW, Holdaas H. Long-term risks for kidney donors. Kidney Int. 2014;86(1):162–7. https://doi.org/10.1038/ki.2013.460.
36. Mjøen G, Øyen O, Holdaas H, Midtvedt K, Line PD. Morbidity and mortality in 1022 consecutive living donor nephrectomies: benefits of a living donor registry. Transplantation. 2009;88(11):1273–9. https://doi.org/10.1097/TP.0b013e3181bb44fd.
37. Murray G, Holden R. Transplantation of kidneys, experimentally and in human cases. Am J Surg. 1954;87(4):508–15. https://doi.org/10.1016/0002-9610(54)90411-0.
38. Muzaale AD, Massie AB, Wang MC, Montgomery RA, McBride MA, Wainright JL, Segev DL. Risk of end-stage renal disease following live kidney donation. JAMA. 2014;311(6):579–86. https://doi.org/10.1001/jama.2013.285141.
39. Nogueira JM, Weir MR, Jacobs S, Breault D, Klassen D, Evans DA, Bartlett ST, Cooper M. A study of renal outcomes in obese living kidney donors. Transplantation. 2010;90(9):993–9. https://doi.org/10.1097/TP.0b013e3181f6a058.
40. O'Malley CMN, Frumento RJ, Hardy MA, Benvenisty AI, Brentjens TE, Mercer JS, Bennett-Guerrero E. A randomized, double-blind comparison of lactated Ringer's solution and 0.9% NaCl during renal transplantation. Anesth Analg. 2005;100(5):1518–24. https://doi.org/10.1213/01.Ane.0000150939.28904.81.
41. Orlando G, Manzia TM, Sorge R, Iaria G, Angelico R, Sforza D, Toti L, Peloso A, Patel T, Katari R, Zambon JP, Maida A, Salerno MP, Clemente K, Di Cocco P, De Luca L, Tariciotti L, Famulari A, Citterio F, Tisone G, Pisani F, Romagnoli J. One-shot versus multidose perioperative antibiotic prophylaxis after kidney transplantation: a randomized, controlled clinical trial. Surgery. 2015;157(1):104–10. https://doi.org/10.1016/j.surg.2014.06.007.
42. Özdemir-van Brunschot DM, Koning GG, van Laarhoven KC, Ergün M, van Horne SB, Rovers MM, Warlé MC. A comparison of technique modifications in laparoscopic donor nephrectomy: a systematic review and meta-analysis. PLoS One. 2015;10(3):e0121131. https://doi.org/10.1371/journal.pone.0121131.

43. Ratner LE, Ciseck LJ, Moore RG, Cigarroa FG, Kaufman HS, Kavoussi LR. Laparoscopic live donor nephrectomy. Transplantation. 1995;60(9):1047–9.
44. Reese PP, Feldman HI, McBride MA, Anderson K, Asch DA, Bloom RD. Substantial variation in the acceptance of medically complex live kidney donors across US renal transplant centers. Am J Transplant. 2008;8(10):2062–70. https://doi.org/10.1111/j.1600-6143.2008.02361.x.
45. Rege A, Leraas H, Vikraman D, Ravindra K, Brennan T, Miller T, Thacker J, Sudan D. Could the use of an enhanced recovery protocol in laparoscopic donor nephrectomy be an incentive for live kidney donation? Cureus. 2016;8(11):e889. https://doi.org/10.7759/cureus.889.
46. Segev DL, Muzaale AD, Caffo BS, Mehta SH, Singer AL, Taranto SE, McBride MA, Montgomery RA. Perioperative mortality and long-term survival following live kidney donation. JAMA. 2010;303(10):959–66. https://doi.org/10.1001/jama.2010.237.
47. Serrano OK, Kirchner V, Bangdiwala A, Vock DM, Dunn TB, Finger EB, Payne WD, Pruett TL, Sutherland DE, Najarian JS, Matas AJ, Kandaswamy R. Evolution of living donor nephrectomy at a single center: long-term outcomes with 4 different techniques in greater than 4000 donors over 50 years. Transplantation. 2016;100(6):1299–305. https://doi.org/10.1097/tp.0000000000001251.
48. Shafizadeh SF, Daily PP, Baliga P, Rogers J, Baillie GM, Rajagopolan PR, Chavin KD. Chylous ascites secondary to laparoscopic donor nephrectomy. Urology. 2002;60(2):345. https://doi.org/10.1016/s0090-4295(02)01743-0.
49. Wang H, Chen R, Li T, Peng L. Robot-assisted laparoscopic vs laparoscopic donor nephrectomy in renal transplantation: a meta-analysis. Clin Transpl. 2019;33(1):e13451. https://doi.org/10.1111/ctr.13451.
50. Wang J, Ma H, Fu Y, Wang N. Comparison of postoperative morphine requirements in renal donors and patients with renal carcinoma undergoing laparoscopic nephrectomy. Transplant Proc. 2016;48(1):31–4. https://doi.org/10.1016/j.transproceed.2015.12.032.
51. Wang K, Zhang P, Xu X, Fan M. Right versus left laparoscopic living-donor nephrectomy: a meta-analysis. Exp Clin Transplant. 2015;13(3):214–26.
52. Wilson CH, Sanni A, Rix DA, Soomro NA. Laparoscopic versus open nephrectomy for live kidney donors. Cochrane Database Syst Rev. 2011;11:Cd006124. https://doi.org/10.1002/14651858.CD006124.pub2.
53. Wolf JS Jr, Tchetgen MB, Merion RM. Hand-assisted laparoscopic live donor nephrectomy. Urology. 1998;52(5):885–7. https://doi.org/10.1016/s0090-4295(98)00389-6.
54. Xiao Q, Fu B, Song K, Chen S, Li J, Xiao J. Comparison of surgical techniques in living donor nephrectomy: a systematic review and Bayesian network meta-analysis. Ann Transplant. 2020;25:e926677. https://doi.org/10.12659/aot.926677.
55. Yuan H, Liu L, Zheng S, Yang L, Pu C, Wei Q, Han P. The safety and efficacy of laparoscopic donor nephrectomy for renal transplantation: an updated meta-analysis. Transplant Proc. 2013;45(1):65–76. https://doi.org/10.1016/j.transproceed.2012.07.152.

Chapter 11
Cardiovascular Effects of Laparoscopic and Robotic Surgery

Ekrem Bilal Karaayvaz

Laparoscopic (LS) and Robotic Surgery or Robotic Assisted Surgery (RAS) is fundamentally is same technic where RAS enables precise remote control of the laparoscopic and surgical equipment in the procedures more than human hand can do. If these two technics used correctly, patients have less tissue manipulation leading fast recovery, less scar, less pain, less blood loss with less complication and can mobilize earlier.

One should know that no doctor can use these devices without proper training. And every doctor can learn these procedures with training in time. But experience and doctor's capabilities are also key factor. The operation type is also a key factor for the cardiovascular effect because different type of LS and RAS operations need different position and technic. Usually the positioning and technic itself determines the risk.

Changes in the Physiological State During the Laparoscopic and Robotic Surgery

LS and RAS require the patient in a selected position with insufflating inert gas which causes increased intra-abdominal pressure. Therefore regulatory adaptations and changes in the physiology are usually due to patient positioning, carboperitoneum and increased intra-abdominal pressure (IAP). If these changes in physiological state is not followed and controlled, they may lead some pathological and even life threatening situations.

E. B. Karaayvaz (✉)
Department of Cardiology, İstanbul University, İstanbul Faculty of Medicine, Istanbul, Türkiye

S. Tonyali et al. (eds.), *Current Endourology*,
https://doi.org/10.1007/978-3-032-00010-1_11

Patient Positioning

In a normal surgery patient may have different positions but LS surgeries and especially RAS surgeries have exaggerated positions. In RAS surgeries once the robotic system is replaced patient position could not change and access to the patient during the procedures becomes harder in LS and RAS procedures.

Different procedures may need different positions. Trendelenburg position may favor for hemodynamic state because blood can easily return to heart but may not be so good for respiration because with the increased abdominal pressure and elevated abdomen, inspiration and expiration may become harder [1]. Lower limb supports may cause compression to the veins and may decrease the venous return. Trendelenburg position increases intra-cranial and intra-ocular pressures. Steep Trendelenburg position, which is usually used in urologic LS and RAS operations, increases intra-cranial pressure and intra-abdominal pressure even more and also can cause acid reflux, oral ulcerations and conjunctival burns. If the steep Trendelenburg position state prolongs, patient may have laryngeal edema and a dangerous complication called 'Well Leg Compartment Syndrome' may develop which is combination of reduced arterial blood supply and reduced venous return due to carboperitoneum and angles of blood vessels in this position [1]. In the reverse Trendelenburg position while respiration is easy, hemodynamic state especially due to venous return may compromise. Also decreased venous return and increased pressure in lower limbs may cause deep vein thrombosis and even pulmonary emboli [1].

Letar M et al. has studied the RAS radical prostatectomy in 45° Trendelenburg position and discovered that during the operation central venous pressure increased three-fold, mean pulmonary artery pressure and pulmonary capillary wedge pressure increased two-fold. Mean arterial blood pressure increased by 35%. Mixed venous oxygen saturation with stroke volume, heart rate, and cardiac output were unaltered [2]. Comorbidities, hydration state and periprocedural medications alters cardiac output in Trendelenburg position but in most healthy cases hemodynamic changes can be covered and cardiac output does not change.

Gas Insufflation

The ideal gas insufflated during LS and RAS operations must be non-toxic, non-inflammatory, highly diffusible and can be easily ventilated through lungs. Carbondioxide is the choice of inert gas during LS and RAS because its highly diffusible, easily excreted therefore has minimal risk of emboli. When carbondioxide is absorbed by lymphatic and venous system the result is hypercarbia and respiratory asidosis. This causes vasoconstriction in the pulmonary system and vasodilatation in cerebrovascular system. But simply increasing ventilation rate, normocarbia can be easily achieved [3]. But with pulmonary compromised patients having longer procedures may cause acidosis and hypercarbia [4]. In mild hypercarbia, with sympathetic stimulation tachycardia, increased cardiac output and increased systemic resistance can be seen. But with severe hypercarbia myocardial contractility decreases and arrhythmia occurrence may increase. Studies showed that in healthy individuals within 5 min of abdominal insufflation, SVR and MAP suddenly increases while cardiac index declines % 50 to its preoperative value. Abdominal aortic compression and neuroendocrine system is suspected to cause this event [5–7].

Increased Abdominal Pressure

Insufflating abdomen with carbondioxide increases the intra-abdominal pressure (IAP). Elevated IAP can lead to inferior vena cava compression, aortic compression, decreased splanchnic blood flow, decreased renal blood flow, and diaphragmatic displacement [8]. Central Venous Pressure (CVP) may be misleading because increased IAP interferes with preload and with its indices [9]. Normally intra-abdominal pressure is kept between 8 and 12 mmHg during operations. Up to 12 mm Hg hemodynamic changes are minimal and cardiac output may even increase. After 15 mmHg, while preload decreases, systemic vascular resistance and afterload increases even more. This results in diminished cardiac output and elevated mean arterial pressure. In reverse Trendelenburg position with carboperitoneum, cardiac output may reduce considerably [7].

Because increased intra-abdominal pressure means increased vagal stimulation, it may even lead to bradycardia if not controlled [10]. Increased intra-abdominal pressure may also cause atelectasis, gastric regurgitation with aspiration and decreased urinary output. Usually decreased urinary output does not affect renal function in patients with normal renal function. With steep Trendelenburg position and longer operation times, urinary retention and urinary tract infections may happen.

In obese patients, the ventilation due to increased abdominal pressure can be troublesome and for this reason increasing PEEP during ventilation may also diminish cardiac output [11, 12].

Grailey K. et al. compared laparoscopic versus open colorectal resection where the results of this pooled analysis demonstrated the potential short-term advantages of laparoscopic colorectal resection in the elderly population [13].

Even though nearly every physiological change during LS and RAS operations can be tolerable in patients with normal physiological state, longer procedure times, larger trocars, high gas inflow rate, higher pressure and difficult trocar placement may cause problems and complications.

Laparoscopic and Robotic Surgery in Patients with Established Cardiovascular Disease (CVD)

The physiological changes during LS and RAS are usually tolerated but in patients with cardiac diseases, congenital heart diseases and obese patients these procedures may be challenging. But with prepared and careful assist laparoscopy can be advantageous even in patients with cardiovascular diseases (CVD) [14]. Even though the methods used in LS and RAS seems harmless, they can cause problems so that with carboperitoneum, increased abdominal pressure and Trendelenburg position; increased mean arterial pressure, central venous pressure, mean pulmonary artery, pulmonary capillary wedge pressure, and systemic vascular resistance may impair cardiac function [2, 15, 16]. With longer procedure times and having CVD, this impairement can lead hemodynamic instability more rapidly and can cause severe consequences. The most important reason for hemodynamic instability in LS is increased intra-abdominal pressure [17].

Having CVD alter the response time and mechanism of the heart. In some cases cardiac performance stays nearly normal like several months later after a very early performed successful primary PCI to an acute coronary syndrome. But in some cases cardiac tolerance is nearly zero where even an upper track respiratory infection can cause cardiac decompensation and hospitilazation. Therefore in LS or RAS patients with cardiovascular diseases, the induction of anaesthesia and release of carboperitoneum shoud be slow and should let the cardiovascular system to catch up. Also gradual positioning helps to improve hemodynamic status [18]. This catching up changes patient to patient and must be individualized with careful attention of anesthesiologist and operator.

During LS and RAS operations, there are a couple of conditions that have to be intervened to the patients with CVD. These are hypotension, hypertension, cardiac ischemia and arrhythmia.

Blood loss or bleeding is usually the main reason of hypotension after or during the operations. It usually presents with sinus tachycardia. But severe cardiac pump failure and pulmonary embolism should always be kept in mind. Trochar misplacement in a major artery can cause blood loss and CO_2 gas embolism. Transesophageal echocardiography (TEE) can be use to monitorize the cardiac chambers for this kind of instances [19] post and intraoperative.

Hypertension mostly seen due to stress and uncontrolled hypertension disease (undiagnosed before or missed medication). When LS, RAS and their physiological changes are evaluated, hypertension can be seen more than usual. Hypertension can also be the indicator of serebrovascular disease or myocardial infarction (MI). Therefore, it should be interpreted carefully. The hypertensive response should not be corrected with opioids or inhalation agents since they will delay recovery, but should be managed pharmacologically with a β-blocker (esmolol or metoprolol) or an α-agonist (dexmedetomidine) [18].

Hypertension or hypotension, the hemodynamic instability should suggest myocardial infarction (MI) as one of the reasons. If not considered, patient can end up with cardiac arrest. In LS and RAS operations increased SVR can cause extra ischemia to a patient having MI than a patient having MI in non-LS or non-RAS operation, with increasing the afterload.

As heart failure advances cardiac devices like left ventricular asist devices (LVAD) can help the patients to maintain normal life outside the hospital. Vigneswaran et al. analyzed laparoscopic operations in patients with left ventricular assist device (LVAD). Their observation is laparoscopic abdominal procedures are safe and feasible in patients with LVADs. Despite bleeding, thrombotic risks, placement of ports and perioperative management; the presence of a LVAD itself should not be considered a contraindication for laparoscopic surgery and may in fact be the preferred method for access in these patients [20].

During LS and RAS arrhythmia is not usually seen in normal population. And not all cardiac diseases predisposed to arrhythmia. But in patients with CVD carboperitoneum, increased abdominal pressure, Trendelenburg position and increased procedure times can increase sympathetic activity. And in patients who were predispose to arrhythmia like severe systolic heart failure, this increased sympathetic activity can cause arrhythmias and distrups the hemodynamic state. Because of that if a patient with CVD disease have a predisposition to arrhythmia, he or she should carefully be evaluated and perioperative preparations must be made for medications and cardioversion/defibrillation if needed.

References

1. Sood J. Advancing frontiers in anaesthesiology with laparoscopy. World J Gastroenterol. 2014;20(39):14308–14.
2. Lestar M, Gunnarsson L, Lagerstrand L, Wiklund P, Odeberg-Wernerman S. Hemodynamic perturbations during robot-assisted laparoscopic radical prostatectomy in 45° Trendelenburg position. Anesth Analg. 2011;113(5):1069–75.
3. Wahba RW, Mamazza J. Ventilatory requirements during laparoscopic cholecystectomy. Can J Anaesth. 1993;40(3):206–10.
4. Wittgen CM, Andrus CH, Fitzgerald SD, Baudendistel LJ, Dahms TE, Kaminski DL. Analysis of the hemodynamic and ventilatory effects of laparoscopic cholecystectomy. Arch Surg. 1991;126(8):997–1000, discussion -1
5. Hirvonen EA, Nuutinen LS, Vuolteenaho O. Hormonal responses and cardiac filling pressures in head-up or head-down position and pneumoperitoneum in patients undergoing operative laparoscopy. Br J Anaesth. 1997;78(2):128–33.
6. O'Leary E, Hubbard K, Tormey W, Cunningham AJ. Laparoscopic cholecystectomy: haemodynamic and neuroendocrine responses after pneumoperitoneum and changes in position. Br J Anaesth. 1996;76(5):640–4.
7. Joris JL, Noirot DP, Legrand MJ, Jacquet NJ, Lamy ML. Hemodynamic changes during laparoscopic cholecystectomy. Anesth Analg. 1993;76(5):1067–71.
8. O'Malley C, Cunningham AJ. Physiologic changes during laparoscopy. Anesthesiol Clin North Am. 2001;19(1):1–19.
9. Koliopanos A, Zografos G, Skiathitis S, Stithos D, Voukena V, Karampinis A, et al. Esophageal Doppler (ODM II) improves intraoperative hemodynamic monitoring during laparoscopic surgery. Surg Laparosc Endosc Percutan Tech. 2005;15(6):332–8.

10. Motew M, Ivankovich AD, Bieniarz J, Albrecht RF, Zahed B, Scommegna A. Cardiovascular effects and acid-base and blood gas changes during laparoscopy. Am J Obstet Gynecol. 1973;115(7):1002–12.
11. Almarakbi WA, Fawzi HM, Alhashemi JA. Effects of four intraoperative ventilatory strategies on respiratory compliance and gas exchange during laparoscopic gastric banding in obese patients. Br J Anaesth. 2009;102(6):862–8.
12. Talab HF, Zabani IA, Abdelrahman HS, Bukhari WL, Mamoun I, Ashour MA, et al. Intraoperative ventilatory strategies for prevention of pulmonary atelectasis in obese patients undergoing laparoscopic bariatric surgery. Anesth Analg. 2009;109(5):1511–6.
13. Grailey K, Markar SR, Karthikesalingam A, Aboud R, Ziprin P, Faiz O. Laparoscopic versus open colorectal resection in the elderly population. Surg Endosc. 2013;27(1):19–30.
14. Hekmat M, Taghipoor HR, Nobahar MR, Monfared MB, Tehrani MM, Arabnia MK, et al. Laparoscopic cholecystectomy and open-heart surgery at the same time. J Card Surg. 2005;20(6):557–9.
15. Hirvonen EA, Nuutinen LS, Kauko M. Hemodynamic changes due to Trendelenburg positioning and pneumoperitoneum during laparoscopic hysterectomy. Acta Anaesthesiol Scand. 1995;39(7):949–55.
16. Members ATF, Kristensen SD, Knuuti J, Saraste A, Anker S, Bøtker HE, et al. 2014 ESC/ESA Guidelines on non-cardiac surgery: cardiovascular assessment and management: The Joint Task Force on non-cardiac surgery: cardiovascular assessment and management of the European Society of Cardiology (ESC) and the European Society of Anaesthesiology (ESA). Eur Heart J. 2014;35(35):2383–431.
17. Dexter SP, Vucevic M, Gibson J, McMahon MJ. Hemodynamic consequences of high- and low-pressure capnoperitoneum during laparoscopic cholecystectomy. Surg Endosc. 1999;13(4):376–81.
18. Sood Jayashree JAK. Anaesthesia in laparoscopic surgery. In: Sood Jayashree JAK, editor. Sir Ganga Ram Hospital. 1st ed. New Delhi: Jaypee Brothers Medical Publishers; 2007. p. 282.
19. Schmandra TC, Mierdl S, Bauer H, Gutt C, Hanisch E. Transoesophageal echocardiography shows high risk of gas embolism during laparoscopic hepatic resection under carbon dioxide pneumoperitoneum. Br J Surg. 2002;89(7):870–6.
20. Vigneswaran Y, Wang V, Krezalek M, Prachand V, Wyers S, Juricek C, et al. Laparoscopic procedures in patients with cardiac ventricular assist devices. Surg Endosc. 2019;33(7):2181–6.

Chapter 12
Laparoscopic Radical Prostatectomy

Mehmet Gurkan Arikan and Orcun Celik

Prostate cancer is the cancer most commonly detected in males over the age of sixty and the second cancer causing highest number of deaths after lung cancer [1]. Although different treatment options are available for prostate cancer, radical prostatectomy (RP) is the golden standard and in localized diseases and nerve sparing open RP was defined by Walsh and Donker in 1982 [2]. Laparoscopic radical prostatectomy (LRP) has come up again thanks to the improvements in minimal invasive surgery. Although positive results were not reported in first LRP applications, a new era began after the introduction of the technique published by Guillonneau et al. in 1998 [3]. The main aim was to achieve maximum accordance of LRP to oncological principles as in open RP, the preservation of continence and erection among the important parameters for the quality of life is also important [4, 5]. Lower postoperative pain compared to open surgery and less intracorporal pressure related bleeding were reported [6, 7]. Catheterization duration also decreased thanks to the application of vesico-urethral anastomosis through direct view and optical magnification [8].

Patient Selection

Regardless of open or laparoscopic surgery, localized prostate cancer and life expectancy over 10 years in suitable patients constitute the primary criteria for radical prostatectomy decision.

M. G. Arikan
Edirne Sultan Murat 1. State Hospital, Urology Clinic, Edirne, Türkiye

O. Celik (✉)
İzmir Ekol Hospital, Urology Clinic, İzmir, Türkiye

S. Tonyali et al. (eds.), *Current Endourology*,
https://doi.org/10.1007/978-3-032-00010-1_12

In addition to common contraindications such as abdominal wall infection, peritoneal inflammation, intestinal obstruction, coagulation disorders, severe cardiac or pulmonary co-morbidity, surgeon experience and patient anatomy related contraindications should also be regarded in patient selection [9, 10]. Especially in cases with recently onset disease, patients with high body mass index, high prostate volume and endurance or patients who had androgen deprivation treatment, multi prostate biopsy or TURP/open prostatectomy should be avoided. Success of recovery LRP following radiotherapy is disputed and thus radiotherapy can be considered as a certain contraindication for LRP [9–11].

Patient Preparation

Following general endotracheal anesthesia induction, the patient's arms are stabilized adjacent to the body and the patient is laid supine in Trendelenburg position. If perineal or rectal intervention is required, the legs are opened to each side or the patient is taken in low lithotomy position to be able to access and pressure points are supported by pads. The surgical area is shaved from the coastal margin to the femur and following the skin preparation through standard povidone iodine, sterile cover is located. Orogastric tube is inserted to decrease stomach distension. Balloon catheter to be inflated (70 cm^3) is inserted in the rectum and then 16-French Foley catheter is inserted under sterile conditions. Surgery team is positioned as the surgeon on the left of the patient and two assistants on the other side [9, 12, 13].

Operative Technique

As in open retropubic radical prostatectomy, technical modifications including ascendant and descendant were also developed in addition to trans-peritoneal and extraperitoneal approach in LRP [13].

Trans-Peritoneal Approach

The first 10/12 mm trocar was inserted from the periumbilical area with pneumoperitoneum formation through Veress needle or open Hasson technique. After locating the other four trocars (two 10 mm and two 5 mm) under laparoscopic view, the procedure is started with a maximum pressure of 15 mmHg and maximum flow of 30 mL (Figs. 12.1, 12.2 and 12.3) [9].

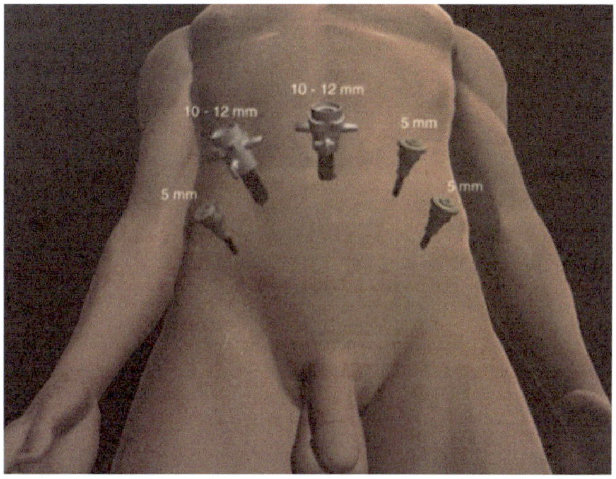

Fig. 12.1 Trochar configuration. (Campbell-Walsh Urology, 10th Edition, Page 2834)

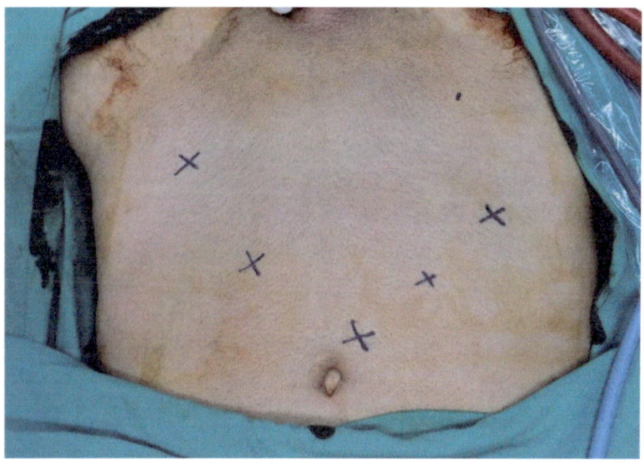

Fig. 12.2 Trochar configuration. (Taken from the archieve of Prof. Dr. Orçun Çelik)

Trochar insertion has different variations based on different centers;

- **Montsouris Variation:** After the formation of pneumoperitoneum through Veress needle, the first 10 mm trocar is inserted under the umbilicus, the second 10 mm trocar through McBurney point and another 5 mm trocar is inserted in the supero-medial of the second trocar in right pararectal area at umbilicus level. The fourth trocar (5 mm) is inserted right in the middle of antero-superior iliac spine and umbilicus line. Finally, a 5 mm trocar is inserted between umbilicus and symphysis pubis [14].
- **Creteil Variation:** Following the insertion of a 12 mm trocar under the umbilicus through open Hasson technique, a second 12 mm trocar is inserted at the level of this port in the lateral of rectus sheath on the side of the surgeon, again another 10 mm trocar is inserted at the same level on assistant side and two 5 mm trocars are inserted on both sides at antero-superior iliac spine level [15].
- **Cleveland Variation:** After inserting a 12 mm trocar below umbilicus through open Hasson technique, two 10 mm trocars at the lateral of rectus muscle and

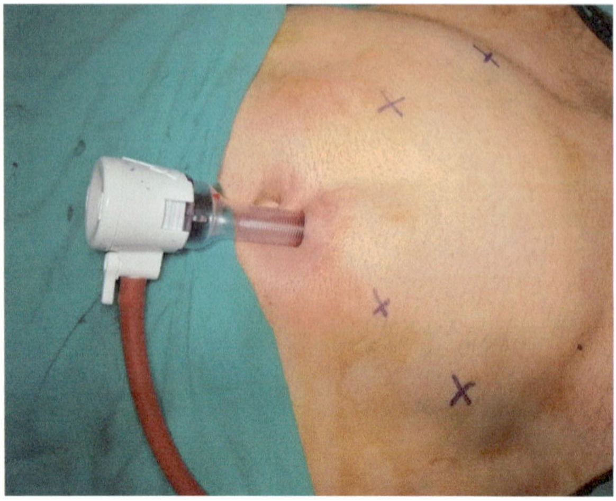

Fig. 12.3 Trochar configuration. (Taken from the archieve of Prof. Dr. Orçun Çelik)

nearly two fingers below umbilicus and 5 mm trocars at both sides in the middle of umbilicus and antero-superior iliac spine in left iliac fossa are inserted [16].

- **Heilbronn Variation:** After inserting a 12 mm trocar below umbilicus through open Hasson technique, at both sides, 10 mm trocars at the lateral of rectus muscle and nearly two fingers below umbilicus and 5 mm trocars are inserted over both frontal axillary lines at umbilicus level. Sixth 5 mm port is inserted in right lower abdomen following the cutting of uracus and both lateral umbilical ligaments [17].

Pelvic area is investigated for injury, bleeding and adhesions carefully. Peritoneum is incised from the uracus superior from peritoneum abdominal wall to access retzius space and bladder dissection is enlarged from lateral up to medial umbilical ligament in trans-peritoneal approach. Avascular retrius area is enlarged through traction application from uracus posterior. Peri-prostatic adipose tissues are removed and the superficial branches of dorsal venous plexus are checked with bipolar cautery. Key anatomic structures at this stage are bladder and prostate, puboprostatic ligaments, endopelvic fascia, pubis and external illiac artery and vein at the lateral [13].

Extra-Peritoneal Approach

The layers are separated through a 1.5 cm medial line cut between periumbilical area and anterior rectus fascia. Following the horizontal incision of anterior rectus fascia, blunt dissection is conducted through index finger right before peritoneum along posterior rectus sheath. Then a balloon dilatator is inserted in preperitoneal space and is advanced towards pubis in the direction of median line. Retzius space is enlarged with 500 ml air-filled balloon under laparoscopic view [12]. Then trocars are inserted under laparoscopic view as previously explained in trans-peritoneal approach. .

In 3-port eLRP technique defined by Akın et al., balloon trocar is inserted through sub-umbilicus incision. The first port is inserted in the area after enlarging retzius area. Bilateral 10 mm study trocars are then inserted nearly four fingers away from the incision [18].

Latter stages of the procedure are continued through trans-peritoneal approach.

Deep Dorsal Venous Complex Control

Following the traction of bladder towards the cranial, the adipose tissue covering the upper part of endopelvic fascia is swept and fascia is made visible. While the prostate is pushed towards the medial with the help of a nut and is incised at the area where fascia is weak, attention should be paid to the lateral branches of Dorsal Venous Complex (DVC) below. Incision in endopelvic fascia is enlarged up to puboprostatic ligaments towards anteromedial [19]. After cutting puboprostatic ligaments, superficial branches of DVC are easily seen from the median line over bladder neck. Levator ani muscle adjacent to this area is eliminated to the lateral. DVC is bound through laparoscopic suture technique following the cutting of puboprostatic ligaments and is cut with bipolar scissors. Conducting the stage far away from prostate apex as much as possible would minimize apical prostate injury possibility [9].

Apical Dissection

Prostate apex is the area where surgery margin is the most strict in postoperative histopathological results. The intensity of anatomic structures providing the reservation of continence and erection increases the importance of apical dissection. Both neurovascular bundles become visible in rectum lateral through blunt dissection following DVC. At this stage, the process will be continued considering whether the neurovascular bundle would be preserved or not.

If nerve-sparing technique is not going to be applied, striated sphincter fibers surrounding the membraneous urethra in the form of a horseshoe are cut with bipolar forceps and scissors after the DVC is cut and urethral smooth muscle becomes visible [13]. When the prostate is mildly tractioned towards the cranial, anterior wall of urethra becomes apparent. Leaving maximum urethral lenght from prostate-urethral junction, it is cut with a scissors without any use of energy. Prostate is pulled towards the cranial after cutting Foley catheter together with the urethra. Attention should be paid not to separate recto-urethral muscle while cutting the rear wall of urethral truncation. After separating from the rectum through blunt dissection in apex medial, distal prostate pedicles are cut using Hem-O-Lok clips [9, 13].

Neurovascular bundles are located in the triangle including medial, lateral, posterolateral prostatic margin and anterior Denonvilliers' fascia in Neuroprotective

Technique [20]. Lateral pelvic fascia is incise without urethral transaction and right-angle clamp is advanced below lateral pelvic fascia. This maneuver separates neurovascular bundle from the prostate. Vascular branches entering the prostate are checked with 5 mm titanium clips. Bipolar and monopolar energy use is avoided at this stage. Lateral side of striated sphincter should be dissected up to the lateral of urethral smooth muscle not to damage neurovascular bundle while cutting the urethra [9].

Bladder Neck Cut

After separating prostate from rectum, the gland is mildly pulled towards the ventral through applying traction on intra-abdominal Foley catheter. Balloon helps to determine vesico-prostatic commissure. The transition zone of the prevesical adipose tissue to the anterior surface of the prostate can also be a touchstone. The junction can also be seen through taking bladder done in traction in cranial direction through forceps. Vesico-prostatic junction is cut starting from the median line but incision should not be extensively advanced to the lateral to avoid bleeding from bladder pedicles. Lowering the catheter balloon, the catheter is hanged inside the abdomen from the opening and thus the prostate is lifted [9, 12, 13].

Control of Seminal Vesicles and Prostatic Pedicles

After the prostate is raised to the anterior, superficial and deep sections of both lateral pedicles are gradually cut through two or three 10 mm Hem-O-Lok clipses. Clipses should be placed close to prostate base in neuroprotective technique. Vas deferences are separately dissected and cut following the separation of pedicles. Seminal vesicles are completely freed and cut [9, 13].

Then specimen is put in laparoscopic bag and is kept away from sight inside the abdomen until the anastomosis is completed.

Pelvic Lymphadenectomy

Obturator fossa access is quite comfortable thanks to bladder mobilization and thus it is generally applied at this stage. Lymphadenectomy decision can be taken thanks to nomograms covering PSA, clinical phase and Gleason score as suggested in EAU guidelines.

Bladder Neck Reconstruction

Bladder neck reconstruction through some posterior and even tennis racket shaped sutures before anastomosis in 10–15% of the cases but reconstructed bladder neck diameter should be a little longer than urethral diameter [10].

Vesicourethral Anastomosis

The main objectives in vesicourethral anastomosis stage are keeping intrinsic sphincter mechanism protected, water-tight, tension-free and non-obstructed. Anastomosis is accepted as a standard application with six different sutures in open radical prostatectomy [13]. Methods differing in suture types (barbed, monofilament, etc) and suture techniques (continuous, separated, etc) with no superiorities among one another were reported [21–23]. The selected method should be based on the experience and personal preference of the surgeon in application. Van Velthoven technique commonly preferred for shortening anastomosis duration in recent years was explained in this section [24].

Two 14 cm 3-0 Vicryl 5/8 sutures are prepared through knotting them back-to-back. The first suture is started as bladder neck outer-inner and urethra inner-outer at 4 o'clock level. The knot is tied behind bladder neck and the needle is located on the right-hand side of operation area. Using the needle at the other hand, a symmetrical suture is made on the first located at 5 o'clock level. After posterior anastomosis is completed from right to the left, from outside towards inside in bladder and from inside towards outside in urethra, each consecutive suture is pulled mildly. Anterior anastomosis is continued the same way through inserting a Foley catheter in the bladder. Both continuous sutures are ended at 10 o'clock level and are knotted outside the bladder. Leakage is checked through 120 cc saline and catheter balloon is inflated.

Removal of Specimen

With the help of laporoscop, drainage catheter is inserted and fastened in operation area. Then periumbilical trocar incision is widened and the specimen is taken out.

Complications

Complication rates following laparoscopic radical prostatectomy change between 18.5% and 39.2% as shown in Table 12.1 [7, 25, 26]. Long and difficult nature of learning curve has caused a high range of complication rates. When the series in literature were evaluated, it was observed that complication rate significantly decreased with increased experience [13, 27, 28].

Table 12.1 LRP complications and prevalence

Complication	%
Bladder neck obstruction	0.7–4.6
Urinoma/anastomotic leakage	1.4–10
Lymphocele	0.2–5.4
Ileus	0.3–2.1
Venous thromboembolism	0.3–2
Wound site infection	0.5–3.8
Cardiac problems	0.1–0.7
Urethral injury	0.1–0.5
Rectal injury	0.4–2.1
Bleeding requiring transfusion	<2
Total	18.5–39.2

Table 12.2 Continence rates following LRP

References	Continence ratio
Hoznek et al. [29]	86%
Olasson et al. [30]	78.4%
Salomon et al. [31]	90%
Eden et al. [32]	90%
Guillonneau et al. [25]	82.3%
Anastasiadis et al. [33]	71.6%
Rassweiler et al. [34]	83.6%
Rozet et al. [35]	98%
Stolzenburg et al. [36]	92%

Results

Functional Results

Continence and erection are the most important criteria when the functional results of open surgery and LRP are compared. Surgeon experience and improved surgical techniques are directly related to these criteria. Following radical prostatectomy, urinary incontinence emerges as stress incontinence. In terms of urinary incontinence, acquisition of a good angle of view through magnifying operation area, minimal bleeding during operation and the better anastomosis give superiority to LRP over open surgery. However, it did not detect any difference in continence rates between surgical techniques [7]. Although the continence rate changes between 71.6% and 98% in patients who had LRP, a significant decrease in urinary incontinence is observed 6 months after the operation (Table 12.2) [13].

Erection quality is another criteria of postoperative functional results of LRP. Erection quality is affected by variables such as patient age, comorbidities, post-operative potency level and the preservation of neurovascular bundle at operation margin.

Table 12.3 Potency rates following LRP

References	Potency percentage
Salomon et al. [31]	58.8%
Eden et al. [32]	62%
Anastasiadis et al. [33]	<53
Roumeguere et al. [37]	65.3%
Su et al. [38]	76%
Rassweiler et al. [34]	67%
Wagner et al. [39]	72%
Gill et al. [40]	88%
Stolzenburg et al. [36]	67.7%

Potency rates in literature showed no difference between surgical techniques and post-LRP potency rates were found as 53–88% (Table 12.3) [13].

Although laparoscopic series reported good erectile dysfunction results, its superiority could not be proven [13].

Oncological Results

Surgical margin positivity and biochemical recurrence are the most important parameters in postoperative oncological assessment. Stage and surgeon experience are the main effects in surgical margin positivity [41, 42]. As peripheral zone is the originating point of prostate adenocarcinomas, dissections close to the prostate due to the surgical technique effect oncological results. Surgical margin positivity is mostly seen in apex of the prostate and posterolateral area. In largest LRP series, surgical margin positivity rates based on stage were reported as 7.4–15.5% in stage T2 and around 21.1–31.8% in stage T3 [13, 42, 43].

Despite all these, open and laparoscopic RP were compared in the series of experienced surgeons and no superiority was shown in terms of surgical margin positivity among them [13].

Biochemical recurrence can be a more objective evaluation than surgical margin in terms of postoperative oncological control. Literature reported a general biochemical recurrence rate of 0–11.4% following LRP [43]. Three-year biochemical recurrence-free general survival rate was reported as 90.5% [43].

References

1. Boring CC, Squires TS, Tong T, Montgomery S. Cancer statistics, 1994. CA Cancer J Clin. 1994;44(1):7–26.
2. Walsh PC, Donker PJ. Impotence following radical prostatectomy: insight into etiology and prevention. J Urol. 1982;128(3):492–7.

3. Guillonneau B, Cathelineau X, Barret E, Rozet F, Vallancien G. Laparoscopic radical prostatectomy. Preliminary evaluation after 28 interventions. Presse Med. 1998;27(31):1570–4.
4. Jacobsen NE, Moore KN, Estey E, Voaklander D. Open versus laparoscopic radical prostatectomy: a prospective comparison of postoperative urinary incontinence rates. J Urol. 2007;177(2):615–9.
5. Miller J, Smith A, Kouba E, Wallen E, Pruthi RS. Prospective evaluation of short-term impact and recovery of health related quality of life in men undergoing robotic assisted laparoscopic radical prostatectomy versus open radical prostatectomy. J Urol. 2007;178(3 Pt 1):854–8. discussion 9
6. Bhayani SB, Pavlovich CP, Hsu TS, Sullivan W, Su L. Prospective comparison of short-term convalescence: laparoscopic radical prostatectomy versus open radical retropubic prostatectomy. Urology. 2003;61(3):612–6.
7. Ficarra V, Novara G, Artibani W, Cestari A, Galfano A, Graefen M, et al. Retropubic, laparoscopic, and robot-assisted radical prostatectomy: a systematic review and cumulative analysis of comparative studies. Eur Urol. 2009;55(5):1037–63.
8. Rassweiler J, Seemann O, Schulze M, Teber D, Hatzinger M, Frede T. Laparoscopic versus open radical prostatectomy: a comparative study at a single institution. J Urol. 2003;169(5):1689–93.
9. Rassweiler J, Erdogru T, Sugiono M, Hrutza M, Teber D. Transperitoneal laparoscopic radical prostatectomy: technical variations, oncologic and functional results, and training. In: Gill IS, editor. Laparoscopic urology. New York: Informa Healthcare; 2006.
10. Spaliviero M, Gill IS. Laparoscopic radical prostatectomy. In: Novick AC, editor. Operative urology. New Jersey: Humana Press; 2006.
11. Vallancien G, Gupta R, Cathelineau X, Baumert H, Rozet F. Initial results of salvage laparoscopic radical prostatectomy after radiation failure. J Urol. 2003;170(5):1838–40.
12. Abbou C, Hoznek A, Salomon L, Gettman MT, Sebe P. Laparoscopic radical prostatectomy: extraperitoneal technique. In: Gill IS, editor. Laparoscopic urology. New York: Infrorma Healthcare; 2006.
13. Su L, Smith JA. Laparoscopic and robot-assisted laparoscopic radical prostatectomy and pelvic lymphadenectomy. In: Wein A, editor. Campbell-Walsh urology. 3rd and 10th ed. Philadelphia: Elsevier; 2012.
14. Guillonneau B, Vallancien G. Laparoscopic radical prostatectomy: the Montsouris technique. J Urol. 2000;163(6):1643–9.
15. Gill IS, Zippe CD. Laparoscopic radical prostatectomy: technique. Urol Clin North Am. 2001;28(2):423–36.
16. Jacob F, Salomon L, Hoznek A, Bellot J, Antiphon P, Chopin DK, et al. Laparoscopic radical prostatectomy: preliminary results. Eur Urol. 2000;37(5):615–20.
17. Rassweiler J, Sentker L, Seemann O, Hatzinger M, Rumpelt HJ. Laparoscopic radical prostatectomy with the Heilbronn technique: an analysis of the first 180 cases. J Urol. 2001;166(6):2101–8.
18. Akin Y, Kose O, Gulmez H, Leon Mar R, Erturhan S, Nuri Gorgel S, et al. A novel surgical technique for extraperitoneal radical prostatectomy with using 3 trocars: results after 154 cases. Arch Esp Urol. 2021;74(2):231–8.
19. Myers RP. Practical surgical anatomy for radical prostatectomy. Urol Clin North Am. 2001;28(3):473–90.
20. Tewari A, Peabody JO, Fischer M, Sarle R, Vallancien G, Delmas V, et al. An operative and anatomic study to help in nerve sparing during laparoscopic and robotic radical prostatectomy. Eur Urol. 2003;43(5):444–54.
21. Kowalewski KF, Tapking C, Hetjens S, Nickel F, Mandel P, Nuhn P, et al. Interrupted versus continuous suturing for Vesicourethral anastomosis during radical prostatectomy: a systematic review and meta-analysis. Eur Urol Focus. 2019;5(6):980–91.
22. Li H, Liu C, Zhang H, Xu W, Liu J, Chen Y, et al. The use of unidirectional barbed suture for Urethrovesical anastomosis during robot-assisted radical prostatectomy: a systematic review and meta-analysis of efficacy and safety. PLoS One. 2015;10(7):e0131167.

23. Matsuyama H, Matsumoto H, Nagao K, Harada N, Hara T, Sakano S. Running suture versus interrupted suture for vesicourethral anastomosis in retropubic radical prostatectomy: a randomized study. Int J Urol. 2015;22(3):271–7.
24. Van Velthoven RF, Ahlering TE, Peltier A, Skarecky DW, Clayman RV. Technique for laparoscopic running urethrovesical anastomosis: the single knot method. Urology. 2003;61(4):699–702.
25. Guillonneau B, Rozet F, Cathelineau X, Lay F, Barret E, Doublet JD, et al. Perioperative complications of laparoscopic radical prostatectomy: the Montsouris 3-year experience. J Urol. 2002;167(1):51–6.
26. Hruza M, Weiss HO, Pini G, Goezen AS, Schulze M, Teber D, et al. Complications in 2200 consecutive laparoscopic radical prostatectomies: standardised evaluation and analysis of learning curves. Eur Urol. 2010;58(5):733–41.
27. Akdere H, Aktoz T, Arikan MG, Atakan IH, Veneziano D, Gozen AS. Embarking with laparoscopic radical prostatectomy and dealing with the complications and collateral problems: a single-center experience. Turk J Urol. 2020;46(1):37–43.
28. El-Feel A, Davis JW, Deger S, Roigas J, Wille AH, Schnorr D, et al. Positive margins after laparoscopic radical prostatectomy: a prospective study of 100 cases performed by 4 different surgeons. Eur Urol. 2003;43(6):622–6.
29. Hoznek A, Antiphon P, Tomasz Borkowski Matthew T, Ran G, Laurent K, Safwat S, Alexandre Z, de la Taille Clment-Claude, Abbou. Assessment of surgical technique and perioperative morbidity associated with extraperitoneal versus transperitoneal laparoscopic radical prostatectomy. Urology. 2003;61(3):617–22. https://doi.org/10.1016/S0090-4295(02)02415-9.
30. Eric Olsson L, Salomon L, Andràs AN, Anthony H, Fabien C, Dominique S, Claude CC, Abbou. Prospective patient-reported continence after laparoscopic radical prostatectomy. Urology. 2001;58(4):570–2. https://doi.org/10.1016/S0090-4295(01)01261-4.
31. Salomon L, Anastasiadis AG, Alexandre RK, La Taille D, Fabien SD, Anthony V, Andras C, Dominique H, Clement-Claude C, Abbou. Urinary continence and erectile function: a prospective evaluation of functional results after radical laparoscopic prostatectomy. Eur Urol. 2002;42(4):338–43. https://doi.org/10.1016/S0302-2838(02)00360-3.
32. Eden CG, Cahill D, Vass JA, Adams TH, Dauleh MI. Laparoscopic radical prostatectomy: the initial UK series. BJU Int. 2002;90(9):876–82. https://doi.org/10.1046/j.1464-410X.2002.03049.x.
33. Anastasiadis AG, Salomon L, Hoznek RKA, Clement-Claude DC, Abbou. Radical retropubic versus laparoscopic prostatectomy: a prospective comparison of functional outcome. Urology. 2003;62(2):292–7. https://doi.org/10.1016/S0090-4295(03)00352-2.
34. Rassweiler J, Schulze M, Teber D, Seemann O, Frede T. Laparoscopic radical prostatectomy: functional and oncological outcomes. Curr Opin Urol. 2004;14(2):75–82. https://doi.org/10.1097/00042307-200403000-00005.
35. Rozet F, Galiano M, Cathelineau X, Barret E, Cathala N, Vallancien G. Extraperitoneal laparoscopic radical prostatectomy: a prospective evaluation of 600 cases. J Urol. 2005;174(3):908–11. https://doi.org/10.1097/01.ju.0000169260.42845.c9.
36. Stolzenburg J-U, Truss MC. Technique of laparoscopic (endoscopic) radical prostatectomy SUMMARY. BJU Int. 2003;91(8):749–57. https://doi.org/10.1046/j.1464-410X.2003.04206.x.
37. Roumeguere T, Bollens R, Vanden M, Dan B, David R, Paul B, Thierry H, Amir Q, Eric D, Wespes CC, Schulman AR, Zlotta. Radical prostatectomy: a prospective comparison of oncological and functional results between open and laparoscopic approaches. World J Urol. 2003;20(6):360–6. https://doi.org/10.1007/s00345-002-0306-z.
38. Li-Ming S, Link RE, Sam B, Wendy B, Sullivan CP, Pavlovich. Nerve-sparing laparoscopic radical prostatectomy: replicating the open surgical technique. Urology. 2004;64(1):123–7. https://doi.org/10.1016/j.urology.2004.02.010.
39. Wagner A, Link R, Pavlovich C, Sullivan W, Su L. Use of a validated quality of life questionnaire to assess sexual function following laparoscopic radical prostatectomy. Int J Impot Res. 2006;18(1):69–76. https://doi.org/10.1038/sj.ijir.3901376.

40. Gill IS, Ukimura O, Mauricio R, Alireza AF, Dinesh M, Jihad S, Tsuneharu K, Mihir Desai M. Lateral pedicle control during laparoscopic radical prostatectomy: refined technique. Urology. 2005;65(1):23–7. https://doi.org/10.1016/j.urology.2004.10.045.
41. Ahlering TE, Eichel L, Edwards RA, Lee DI, Skarecky DW. Robotic radical prostatectomy: a technique to reduce pT2 positive margins. Urology. 2004;64(6):1224–8.
42. Rassweiler J, Schulze M, Teber D, Marrero R, Seemann O, Rumpelt J, et al. Laparoscopic radical prostatectomy with the Heilbronn technique: oncological results in the first 500 patients. J Urol. 2005;173(3):761–4.
43. Guillonneau B, el-Fettouh H, Baumert H, Cathelineau X, Doublet JD, Fromont G, et al. Laparoscopic radical prostatectomy: oncological evaluation after 1,000 cases a Montsouris institute. J Urol. 2003;169(4):1261–6.

Chapter 13
Robot Assisted Radical Prostatectomy

H. Cihan Demirel and John W. Davis

Modern radical retropubic prostatectomy (RRP) technique is often attributed to the 1980 description by Walsh et al. and considered a standard treatment for clinically localized prostate cancer [1]. Later in 1992, Schuessler et al. described the laparoscopic radical prostatectomy (LRP) method, which they stated had better oncological, functional, and cosmetic results despite a long and challenging learning curve [2]. Then, with the development of the da Vinci Robotic System (Intuitive, Sunnyvale, CA, USA) in 1999, robotic surgery found its own use in urology. In 2001, Binder and Kramer published the first "Robot Assisted Laparoscopic Radical Prostatectomy" (RaRP) series with 10 patients [3]. The use of robotic systems in urology gained momentum and in 2002, as Menon et al. published a series describing the benefits of RaRP and surgical anastomosis techniques [4] and since then, despite the lack of comparative publications in the literature regarding the superiority of the method over open surgery and its higher cost, its use has increased considerably in recent years to more than 80% of radical prostatectomy in the USA [5].

With the gradual development of minimally invasive methods like laparoscopic and robotic surgeries, functional success has gained importance as well as oncological control, and the concept of "Trifecta" (1-continence, 2-potency and 3-cancer control) was first introduced by Salomona in 2003. In early studies, trifecta success was reported in approximately 53–62% of patients who underwent radical retropubic prostatectomy (RRP) and 91% of patients who underwent robot-assisted radical

H. C. Demirel (✉)
Department of Urology, Division of Surgery, Istanbul Aydin University Medical Faculty, VM Medical Park Florya Hospital, İstanbul, Turkey

J. W. Davis
Department of Urology, Division of Surgery, The University of Texas MD Anderson Cancer Center, Houston, TX, USA

Urosurgical Prostate Program, Department of Urology, The University of Texas MD Anderson Cancer Center, Houston, TX, USA

S. Tonyali et al. (eds.), *Current Endourology*,
https://doi.org/10.1007/978-3-032-00010-1_13

prostatectomy (RaRP) [6]. Due to the advances in minimally invasive surgery, Rocco and his team in 2011 introduced the concept called "Pentafecta" because patients are in demand and expectation not only with the trifecta result, but also with an "uncomplicated procedure" and "low surgical margin positivity (PSM)". they have posed [7].

Pre-operative Patient Preparation

As a clinical principle, the patient's disease, its biological significance, and all the treatment options available should be explained in detail to the patient. The advantages, disadvantages, risks and possible complications of all methods should be clearly explained to the patient, knowing that some patients want more or less detailed information. While advising on treatment options to the patient, key variables include the age, general condition, body habitus, comorbidities, previous surgeries, and treatments (chemotherapies and/or abdominal-pelvic radiotherapies, etc.).

Oncological and functional expectations and complications should be shared with the patient, and it should be emphasized that the main goal is to ensure oncological control, and it should be reminded that robotic surgery can be switched to open surgery if necessary.

Final treatment decisions conclude with informed consent and a pivot to instructions and expectations for completing a treatment. While preparing for surgery, the patient's hematocrit level and metabolites should be at appropriate levels, and the urine should be sterile. If the patient is using anticoagulants and/or antiplatelets, the relevant departments should be consulted to discontinue the agents or replace them with short-acting ones. Traditionally, patients who will undergo robotic surgery would undergo bowel preparation before the surgery, in order not to experience problems due to intestinal distension during the surgery, and in order for the patient to have a more comfortable recovery period in the postoperative period. Many surgeons have simplified this to a lighter prep and/or enema. Antibiotic prophylaxis should be administered preoperatively as deemed appropriate by the surgical team. The risk of deep vein thrombosis development increases in pelvic surgeries. In order to prevent this situation, low molecular weight heparin prophylaxis, wearing compression stockings during the operation and early mobilization in the postoperative period are other important and must-do preparations.

Patient Position and Placement of the Robotic Arms

The most important and first step in robot-assisted radical prostatectomy is the correct adjustment of the operating table, the placement of the patient on the table in accordance with the surgery, and the proper adjustment of the robot and its arms. Robot arms should reach the surgical area easily, should not complicate the operation, should not collide with each other and the surrounding objects, and should not allow the development of complications due to impact. Modern "Xi" systems have additional functionality such as targeting, and a rotational boom for the arms—these allow options such as side docking and positioning supine rather than using lithotomy with stirups.

If single port robotic surgery is not performed, the operating table must be in the trendelenburg position for both extraperitoneal and transperitoneal radical prostatectomy to remove the intestines from the field. While extreme trendelenburg (30° or 45° angle according to the surgeon's preference) position is required in the transperitoneal approach, there is no need for such extreme tension in extraperitoneal methods. Recently, we find that 15° is sufficient for extraperitoneal and 25° for transperitoneal. In order to prevent the patient from slipping, both shoulders should be supported by the support pieces attached to the table, and gel supports should be placed between the table and the shoulders to prevent pressure-related damage to the shoulders. Commercial products are available that add padding to the pressure points and anti-slip substance to keep the patient from moving.

The table should be broken from the hip level to define the pelvis. If the leg parts of the table can be broken, slight flexion should be created at the knee level. As in the shoulder, gel supports should be placed on the back of the knee and on the heels against compression lesions (Fig. 13.1).

The placement of the ports in robotic surgery shows some differences according to the method to be applied. The first port to be placed is the camera port. In the transperitoneal approach, an entrance is made approximately 1 cm above the umbilicus from the left of the midline. Access can be made with a "Veress needle" directly in people who have not undergone abdominal surgery, or a 12 mm port is placed by entering the peritoneal cavity under direct vision with the "Hasson technique". In the extraperitoneal approach, the entrance should be from the left lateral under the umbilicus, and after the extraperitoneal distance is dilated with a finger and a balloon, a 12 mm camera port is placed. Other ports should be placed under direct view

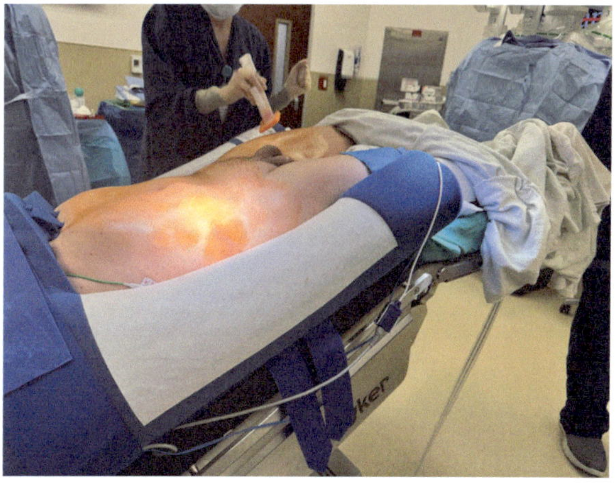

Fig. 13.1 Patient positioning for robot-assisted radical prostatectomy

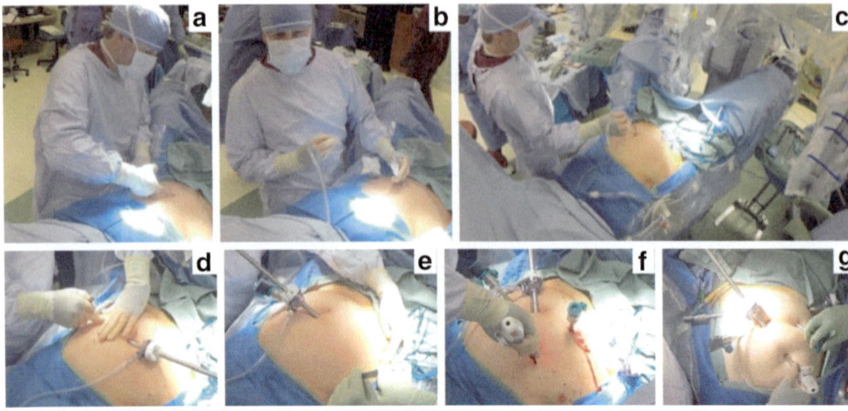

Fig. 13.2 Port placements of robot-assisted radical prostatectomy

with the 30° telescope in the upward facing position. Here are some advantages of the DaVinci Xi® system. These are that since it has an 8 mm camera, the smaller port can be used and the camera can be adjusted to face up or down from the console without having to take it out [8–11]. Port placements in transperitoneal and extraperitoneal techniques are shown in Fig. 13.2 in detail.

Surgical Techniques

To date, many techniques have been described by many surgeons for RARP, considering oncological, functional and cosmetic needs. These techniques can be listed as multi-port extraperitoneal, intraperitoneal, retzius sparing technique, perineal, single port extraperitoneal, transperitoneal, transperineal, and transvesical approaches. The best-described, long-running technique with many results in the literature, which has become the cornerstone of robotic prostatectomy, is the anterior approach RaRP, which is similar to open radical prostatectomy. In this section, some of these techniques will be discussed in terms of surgical techniques and outcomes. Lymph node dissection will not be covered in this chapter as it is described in another chapter.

Multi-port RaRP Methods

Anterior Approach RaRP

It can be performed with an extraperitoneal or transperitoneal approach, depending on the surgeon's preference. The main difference in these approaches is port layouts. After the port placements and the first stages, both methods are completed in the same way. In the extraperitoneal approach, the space between the rectus abdominis muscle and the posterior layer of this muscle is enlarged with a dilatation balloon. Ports are placed in the extraperitoneal space and the Retzius space is further developed. The next steps are similar to those of the transperitoneal anterior approach. In transperitoneal prostatectomy, ports are placed in the peritoneal cavity.

After the ports are placed, the parietal peritoneum lateral to the lateral umbilical ligaments is incised first. The bladder is released and the Retzius space is exposed, then the adipose tissue surrounding the prostate is cleared. The bilateral endopelvic fascia is cleared of fat and opened. The puboprostatic ligaments are cut and the dorsal venous complex (DVC) is controlled athermally (attached by suture) [12]. Then, the bladder neck (BN) is cut from the prostate-bladder junction by protecting the situation and the dissection is continued posteriorly. The retrotrigonal space is opened until seminal vesicles and vas deferens are visible. The vas deferens are cut and the distal portion is used to lift the prostate. This maneuver facilitates the isolation and dissection of seminal vesicles. Denonvilliers' fascia is then incised. The prostate is then dissected posterolaterally and the dissection is advanced towards the apex. After checking the prostatic pedicles and DVC, the urethra is cut.

Some tips that will facilitate surgery and provide better functional results during these methods are described below.

Endopelvic Fascia Dissection

As in open RRP, after the bladder is released from surrounding adhesions and connective tissues, the endopelvic fascia is usually opened and then the prostate is released anterolaterally [13]. The increased prostate motility as a result of release may aid in the dissection of the neurovascular bundles (NVB) when greater countertension is applied to the prostate. There are also methods by which the endopelvic fascia can be preserved, but these methods reduce prostate mobility and may make dissection very difficult in larger prostates.

Bladder Neck Dissection

After revealing the junction of the prostate and bladder, the bladder neck can be dissected and cut in the midline with a gentle athermal dissection, and the muscle fibers can be preserved. If the bladder neck is not preserved, the bladder can also be cut with cautery and the neck is circumferentially excised [14].

Protection of Neurovascular Bundles (NVB)

Two techniques are available for dissection and preservation of NVB: antegrade or retrograde approach. After seminal vesicle release and transection of the vas deferens, the prostate is lifted and Denonvilliers' fascia is opened using sharp dissection. The prostate is dissected posteriorly from Denonvilliers' fascia. The dissection is continued posterolaterally until the NVB becomes evident. The next step is the release of NVB from the posterolateral prostate surface. During **antegrade** dissection, after gentle traction on the bundle and countertraction of the prostate, the triangle between the pedicle and the prostatic pseudocapsule is determined. Once the desired plane for the NS has been determined, dissection is performed by moving from the anteromedial to the prostatic apex [15].

The **retrograde** approach involves peeling the lateral prostatic fascia (LPF) from the prostatic pseudocapsule. Gentle dissection of the LPF is performed at the mid-prostate level to avoid pseudocapsule infringement. If present, one of the markers at this step may be the prostatic artery, which can help define the course of NVB retrogradely until the prostatic pedicle is encountered. Once the desired plane has been determined, the dissection is advanced caudally, thus defining the space created during the posterior dissection and releasing the NVB at this point. The dissection of the bundle is advanced towards the pedicle in a retrograde fashion. The pedicle is identified, clipped, and dissected at its entrance at the posterolateral angle of the base of the prostate [16].

The neurovascular bundle can be preserved completely (**intrafascial dissection**) or partially (**interfascial dissection**) or completely dissected (**extra-fascial dissection**) [17]. In order to determine the level of dissection, to facilitate and standardize the dissection, the authors have defined various grading systems.

The initial description was made in 2011 by Tewari et al., as a 1–4 rating system for NVB protection. According to this definition, grade 1; described an approach, which they graded as corresponding to complete intrafascial dissection (with complete preservation of NVB), while grade 4 to complete extrafacial dissection (with no preservation of NVB). Grade 2 corresponds to an interfascial dissection performed by first cutting the venous plane of the bundle and then the adipose tissue of the bundle [18]. A year after Tewari explained this scale, Schatloff et al. developed this scale further. Accordingly, they made the definition of Tewari in reverse and graded them from one to five. They used an artery lying at the lateral border of the prostate as a "touchpoint" for dissection. Grade 5 corresponds to a complete intrafascial dissection (full NVB preservation), while grades 4 and 3 correspond to a dissection just medial and just lateral to the pointing artery, respectively. Grade 2 represents a dissection lateral to the artery in adipose tissue with embedded vessels. In grade 1, extrafacial dissection (NVB is not preserved at all) is performed. According to this system, NVB is >95% preserved at grade 5, while the probability of protection decreases as it approaches grade 1 (75%, >50%, 50%) and is not protected at all at grade 1 [19, 20].

Control of Dorsal Venous Complex (DVC) and Puboprostatic Ligaments

When cutting anterior of the prostate, a plane may develop between the anterior fibromuscular stroma and the detrusor apron. With this dissection technique, the structures located in front of the prostate, also known as the pubovesical complex, are fully preserved [21].

Apical Dissection

Dissection of the prostate apex can be accomplished by sharp and direct cutting of the membranous urethra at the level of the urethroprostatic junction. Alternatively, it can be performed by progressively dissecting three different muscle layers at the level of the urethral sphincter complex (rhabdosphincter, circular smooth muscle, longitudinal smooth muscle, and mucosa) as described in the "Veil of Aphrodite" technique. Rotation of the prostate during this phase assists in laterally and posteriorly dissection and identification of the apex. The technique of higher nerve relaxation, also called the veil of Aphrodite, has been suggested to improve functional outcomes [22, 23].

This procedure suggests intrafacial/interfacial dissection between the 1 o'clock and 5 o'clock positions for the right side and between the 6 o'clock and 11 o'clock positions for the left side. Gani et al. later modified this technique and suggested that tissues, including the pubovesical ligaments, be preserved between the 11 o'clock and 1 o'clock positions [24]. This procedure (super veil) is more demanding than the standard procedure, therefore it is recommended for patients in the low risk group.

Posterior-Retzius Sparing RaRP

Another technique is Retzius sparing RaRP, performed with a transperitoneal posterior approach, first described by Bocciardi et al. in 2010 [25, 26]. The anatomical rationale of this technique is the preservation of anterior structures such as pubovesical ligaments, puboprostatic fascia, NVBs, accessory pudendal artery and DVC, which are involved in maintaining continence and potency. There is no significant difference in port placements compared to the standard technique. However, it is often necessary to use 30° optics facing upwards. So the DaVinci Xi® platform is advantageous here and will save time. The narrow working area and the upward direction of the operation field, as opposed to the usual, require a learning curve. This approach involves incision of the parietal peritoneum on the anterior surface of the vesicorectal sac at the level of the seminal vesicles (Fig. 13.3). After the vas

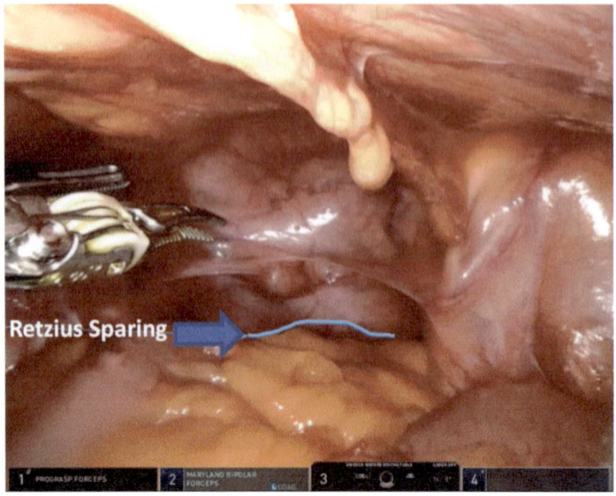

Fig. 13.3 The anatomic plain of retzius sparing surgery

deferens and seminal vesicles have been dissected and retracted with two transabdominally placed sutures, the prostate dissection is performed antegradely. Denonvilliers' fascia is separated by the posterolateral surface of the prostate and the prostatic apex is reached. This technique allows intrafascial anterograde nerve-sparing surgery to be performed if it is oncologically safe. Conversely, in the case of more advanced disease, interfascial or extrafacial antegrade dissection is performed. The surgeon should then return to determine the vesicoprostatic plane and examine the bladder neck. Two short sutures can be placed at the 6 and 12 o'clock positions to easily identify the ureteral orifices during the first steps of anastomosis. The anterior surface of the prostate is then antegradely dissected without cutting the Santorini plexus. Prostate dissection is completed by cutting the urethra [27–29].

Uretrovesical Anastomosis

If the bladder neck is smooth and of appropriate width after dissections, anastomosis can be made directly to the urethra. If the bladder neck is wide, it should be narrowed with separate sutures and made suitable for anastomosis.

V-Loc(TM) [Covidien, New Haven, Conn.] sutures facilitate the procedure in anastomosis. Before the urethrovesical anastomosis, posterior to the bladder, the remnants of Denonvilliers' fascia and tissues posterior to the urethra can be brought closer together (Rocco Suture) [30]. With this approximation, the tension of the anastomosis is reduced. It is also thought to contribute to continence. Similar to the "Rocco Suture", posterior repair can be performed for early recovery of continence or the Van-Velthoven Suture Technique can be used [31]. Athermal ligation of the Santorini vein complex/DVC is also a useful method to increase the length of the obtained urethra. After the anastomosis is completed, the bladder should be filled with saline solution and checked for leakage.

Single Port RaRP (SP-RaRP)

One of the natural processes of minimally invasive surgery is the need to reduce the number of ports and the overall incision length. Because of this need, the search for surgeons continued and, as in some other operations, trials were conducted using a single port in radical prostatectomy. However, the necessity of placing a single port with a larger incision and the difficulty of placing the instruments used, constantly colliding during the operation, making the operation difficult and taking too long prevented the development of the technique. With the industry constantly experimenting with surgeons, the Da Vinci SP® platform was licensed by the US Drug Administration (FDA) in 2018. This platform is an innovative technology as all instruments work in the same port. Three independent arms with two joints of 6 mm diameter in a 25 mm trocar manufactured according to the platform share the same space with an oval camera (10 mm × 12 mm) with different deflection angles. This platform also has an extra pedal, called the displacement pedal, which is used to direct the robot to work in different quadrants.

Single port-RaRP implementation requires a serious learning curve for the whole team. This learning process requires dry laboratory, animal and cadaver work for the whole team. Port placement, use of levers without colliding, and lever change pedal operation should be carefully learned.

Initial setup and positioning for single-port-RaRP is broadly similar to multi-port RaRP, with some critical changes. Preoperative preparation is done as described at the beginning of my section. The patient position should be adjusted as with the multiport RaRP. Well; If the transperitoneal method is preferred, extreme Trendelenburg should be in the supine position, the arms should be bent and the shoulders should be supported with padded pads. If it is to be done with the extraperitoneal method, there is no need to give Trendelenburg position. Thus, side effects such as difficulty in ventilation due to Trendelenburg position, and increases in intraocular, intracranial and intrathoracic pressure can be prevented. Overall, this platform and using the extraperitoneal method is an effective way to reach the prostate, despite hostile abdomen risks from prior surgery.

Extraperitoneal Anterior SP-RaRP

The ideal location for port placement should be in the midline below the umbilicus, 25 cm from the target (prostate). In addition, the port should be placed at a distance of at least 10 cm from the surgical area in order for the articulated arms to work comfortably. If an extra instrument is to be used, the trocar should be placed at a location so that it does not collide with the SP arms. A 2–3 cm infraumbilical incision is made approximately one finger under the umbilicus. The anterior rectus sheath is determined and cut sharply. After developing the Retzius space, the surgical balloon system is incision and placed under the pubic bone. Then, the balloon is inflated with 400 cc of air to create a sufficient working area.

Port Layout

The wound retractor/protective component (Alexis®) of the GelPOINT system (Applied Medical, Rancho Santa Margarita, CA, USA) is secured to the wound. More recently, Intuitive has its own adatable docking system call Access Port that allows additional laparoscopic access to the field and more space for the arms to deploy into their working postitions before reaching the target organ (single port arms much extend 10 cm before the elbow joints can flex outward and creat triangulation). The inner ring is fixed under the rectus fascia and the outer ring is held above the skin to provide 360° atraumatic wound retraction. A 25 mm SP® cannula with a 12 mm laparoscopic port as well as a multi-channel guide port is inserted into the GelSeal cap. The GelSeal cap is then attached to the wound retractor, insufflation is set up, and the SP® robot is clamped to the multichannel port.

Floating Technique

Unlike traditional single port surgery, the Alexis® wound retractor is not fixed to the skin. Instead, it acts as a conduit between the robotic arm and the patient's body. The GelPOINT® system is placed "floating" during surgery and the robotic cannula is above the patient's body. This allows the maximum working area of the robotic tools.

After placement, the procedure can be followed step by step according to the standard anterior dissection technique [8]. After the prostatic fatty tissue is cleaned, the endopelvic fascia is exposed and opened by incising it left and right. The Dorsal vein complex (DVC) is then athermal ligated. After dividing the anterior and posterior aspects of the bladder neck (BN), both the vas deferens and bilateral LV are exposed and dissected. After controlling the prostate pedicles with clips, they are cut. The posterior surface of the prostate is then separated from the rectum. The apical dissection is completed by controlling and cutting the dorsal vein complex, and then the urethra is cut with a sharp dissection and the prostate is completely separated. Finally, the urethrovesical anastomosis is completed with a continuous suture over an 18 Fr catheter. The tightness of the anastomosis is checked, all specimens are taken out and the abdominal wall is closed in layers.

Comparison of Surgical Techniques

When the techniques are compared in terms of advantages-disadvantages; The advantages of extraperitoneal multiport RaRP operations can be listed as not needing excessive Trendelenburg position, early recovery of bowel functions and development of ileus, and low incidence of intestinal injury during the operation. The disadvantages are that the technique does not allow insufflation with a Veress needle, the working area is quite narrow (especially in bulky patients), and it is not suitable for patients who have previously undergone laparoscopic inguinal hernia repair (with mesh). The most important advantage of Retzius-sparing RaRP (RS-RaRP) operations is the early recovery of incontinence (92% of patients are continent from the start). Other advantages are that the incidence of inguinal hernia formation is reduced after the operation and that it is safer in patients who have had laparoscopic hernia repair before. Although there was no statistically significant difference in many studies, its disadvantages are that the surgical margin positivity (PSM) is relatively high and the learning curve is long and laborious even for surgeons experienced in transperitoneal RaRP.

Although there are no large series yet, faster recovery of the patient, less postoperative pain (therefore also reduced need for opioids) and early discharge can be counted among the advantages of SP-RaRP. One of the largest series, Kaouk et al. In the current SP-RaRP series of 200 patients, >90% of patients were discharged on the same day. In addition, the fact that Trendelenburg is not needed during extraperitoneal SP-RaRP is an advantage, especially for obese patients. There are no multicenter studies with a large population that can provide clear information about surgical margin positivity and long-term oncologic outcomes. The main disadvantages are high cost, longer operation time, requiring a serious dry laboratory and cadaver experience, and difficulty in learning curve.

Comparison of Results

Many techniques have been described for robotic surgery, which have been in use since the beginning of the twenty-first century. The most common of these techniques is the anterior approach extraperitoneal RaRP, which is performed in steps similar to open RRP. However, in recent years, especially with the introduction of the concept of "pentafecta", other techniques have also been tried and among these techniques, the popularity of the posterior approach has been Retzius Sparing RaRP (RS-RaRP). There are many meta-analyses comparing multiport RaRP techniques in the literature.

One of the most recent of these, Checcucci et al. S-RaRP and RS RaRp techniques were compared in terms of many parameters. As a result; that was reported that the operation time was significantly lower in RS-RaRP ($p = 0.003$), and there was no significant difference between the groups in terms of estimated mean blood loss ($p = 0.93$) and complication rates ($p = 0.71$). They also stated that the rate of surgical margin positivity was significantly lower in S-RaRP ($p = 0.01$). When both techniques are compared in terms of continence rates, it was reported that continence rates were better in RS-RaRP at 1st, 3rd, 6th and 12th months ($p = 0.02$, $p < 0.001$, $p = 0.001$, and $p = 0.004$, respectively) [32].

In 2020 Saidan et al. published a study with 95 patients. In this study multi-port and single-port RaRP were compared and they stated that no significant difference was found in terms of blood loss, average operation time, number of days of hospitalization, perioperative complication rates (Clavien-Dindo >2) and surgical margin positivity [33]. In addition, in a study by Kaouk, multi-port and single-port robotic surgeries were compared in terms of cost. And although the cost of SP-RaRP surgery was found to be higher than multi-armed RaRP, it was stated that there was no difference between the total cost due to the short hospital stay [34].

One of the most recent meta-analyses on this subject, the European Department of Robotic Urology (ERUS) evaluated four studies involving a total of 610 patients comparing SP-RaRP and MP-RaRP, and 1- in terms of cost, although SP-RaRP is more expensive than MP-RaRP but there was not statistically significant difference ($p = 0.3$), 2- also the need for painkillers was found to be less in the SP-RaRP arm, 3- the same day discharge rates were significantly higher in SP-RaRP with 70% compared to MPRaRP (5%) ($p = 0.001$). However the short hospitalization period is initially advantageous in terms of cost reduction and the superiority of a new technique. But it is not easy to find an answer to the question "Are patients prepared to be discharged on the same day after such a major surgery?" [35].

In a recent study of Moschovas SP-RaRP, again emphasizing the learning curve, attention should be paid to the prostate weight <80 g and the patient's BMI <35 kg/m^2 in the first patients, and the use of an extra assistant port while performing nerve-sparing surgery reduces unnecessary electrocautery use. and that it will facilitate the surgeon's work and shorten the operation time during aspiration and traction (Hybrid-SP approach). The use of the assistant port is recommended to surgeons during the learning process during the transition from MP-RaRP to SP-RaRP [36].

In addition, as Jihad Kaouk stated in his studies, the invention of the SP-RaRP console also allows for more comfortable application of narrower area surgeries such as transperineal and transvesical RaRP [37].

RaRP Trends Across the United States and MDACC Experience

RaRP in the United States and the MD Anderson Cancer Center Experience is a standard, curative treatment for localized prostate cancer and highly selected cases of locally advanced/regional lymph node disease. The patient selection derives from a process of optimizing diagnostic testing, followed by risk classification, and concluding with a mutually agreed treatment plan with the patient. Low grade prostate cancer is mostly excluded in favor of active surveillance, and extremes of age/co-morbidity that predict a shorter survival less than 5 years may also settle on an observation plan. Many patients with clinically significant disease have overlapping selection criteria for surgery or radiation, although there are occasional difficult recommendations to offer when age is >75 but health is good and Gleason score is 4 + 3 or higher. Most patients will undergo MRI staging, and high risk cases may add PSMA PET staging.

The surgical plan for RARP includes three key planning choices, and a 5 step consideration of potential barriers to the prostate. For key planning choices, the topics include (a) selection for a lymph node dissection using nomograms, (b) selection for nerve sparing using appropriate nomograms, and (c) surgical approach considerations based upon tumor location and surgeon preference. For the latter, an anterior tumor may indicate the need for a traditional anterior surgical approach, whereas more typical tumor locations in the peripheral zone may be approached by novel retzius-sparing or "hood" approaches. For the consideration of barriers to the prostate, they include: (a) extremes of patient weight (BMI >45), (b) prior abdominal surgery that may complicate port placement, (c) history of pelvic surgeries such as implant reservoirs, kidney transplant, or hernia mesh, (d) anatomic variants of the prostate itself (size, median lobe, prior TURP, close ureters to the trigone, pubic arch interference), and (e) staging studies indicating extraprostatic disease and/or early lymph node metastases. Based upon these assessments, the surgeon can plan for safe port access, major approach difference such as extraperitoneal versus transperitoneal, single port versus multiport, and traditional resection versus anterior fascia sparing (hood or retzius sparing).

Conclusion

In recent years, when technological progress has been shaped according to the course of minimally invasive surgery, many new systems have come into use with the efforts of the industry and surgeons. The use of these systems, which were expensive in the beginning, has become increasingly widespread and has almost become the gold standard in the surgical treatment of prostate cancers. The most important factors in this are that the functional results are quite good compared to open surgery, the learning curve is shorter than laparoscopy, and it is comfortable for the patient and the surgeon. Innovations in technology have enabled the SP-RaRP platform and radical prostatectomy, one of the most complicated surgeries in urology, has become almost day surgery. It is early to say this since there are no large comparative series in the literature, but the current series tell us that there is no difference between the old platforms and SP-RaRP platforms in terms of oncological and functional results and cost, and that SP-RaRP is more advantageous in terms of cosmetic and patient comfort. Large-scale, multicenter, comparative studies are needed to reach a definitive conclusion.

References

1. Walsh PC. Radical prostatectomy for the treatment of localized prostatic carcinoma. Urol Clin North Am. 1980;7(3):583–91.
2. Schuessler WW, Schulam PG, Clayman RV, Kavoussi LR. Laparoscopic radical prostatectomy: initial short-term experience. Urology. 1997;50(6):854–7. https://doi.org/10.1016/S0090-4295(97)00543-8.

3. Binder J, Kramer W. Robotically-assisted laparoscopic radical prostatectomy. BJU Int. 2001;87(4):408–10. https://doi.org/10.1046/j.1464-410x.2001.00115.x.
4. Menon M, Shrivastava A, Tewari A, Sarle R, Hemal A, Peabody JO, Vallancien G. Laparoscopic and robot assisted radical prostatectomy: establishment of a structured program and preliminary analysis of outcomes. J Urol. 2002;168(3):945–9. https://doi.org/10.1097/01.ju.0000023660.10494.7d.
5. Preisser F, Nazzani S, Mazzone E, Knipper S, Bandini M, Tian Z, Haese A, Saad F, Zorn KC, Montorsi F, Shariat SF, Graefen M, Tilki D, Karakiewicz PI. Regional differences in total hospital charges between open and robotically assisted radical prostatectomy in the United States. World J Urol. 2019;37(7):1305–13. https://doi.org/10.1007/s00345-018-2525-y. Epub 2018 Oct 12
6. Salomon L, Saint F, Anastasiadis AG, Sebe P, Chopin D, Abbou CC. Combined reporting of cancer control and functional results of radical prostatectomy. Eur Urol. 2003;44(6):656–60. https://doi.org/10.1016/j.eururo.2003.09.009.
7. Patel VR, Sivaraman A, Coelho RF, Chauhan S, Palmer KJ, Orvieto MA, Camacho I, Coughlin G, Rocco B. Pentafecta: a new concept for reporting outcomes of robot-assisted laparoscopic radical prostatectomy. Eur Urol. 2011;59(5):702–7. https://doi.org/10.1016/j.eururo.2011.01.032. Epub 2011 Jan 25
8. Taşçı Aİ. Robotik Yardımlı Laparoskopik Radikal Prostatektomi. Güncel Üroloji 2. Baskı, Editörler: Yaman MÖ, Kadıoğlu A, Taşçı Aİ, Türk Üroloji Dernegi/ Turkish Association of Urology Yayını No:18 sy: 859-872 ISBN: 978-605-68063-1-5, İstanbul 2018.
9. Davis JW, editor. Robot-assisted radical prostatectomy beyond the learning curve. Springer International Publishing Switzerland; 2016. https://doi.org/10.1007/978-3-319-32641-2. ISBN 978-3-319-32639-9 ISBN 978-3-319-32641-2 (eBook). Library of Congress Control Number: 2016936375.
10. Huynh LM, Ahlering TE. Robot-assisted radical prostatectomy: a step-by-step guide. J Endourol. 2018;32(S1):S28–32. https://doi.org/10.1089/end.2017.0723. PMID: 29421921; PMCID: PMC6071518.
11. Arenas-Gallo C, Shoag JE, Hu JC. Optimizing surgical techniques in robot-assisted radical prostatectomy. Urol Clin North Am. 2021;48(1):1–9. https://doi.org/10.1016/j.ucl.2020.09.002.
12. Guru KA, Perlmutter AE, Sheldon MJ, Butt ZM, Zhang S, Tan W, Wilding G, Kim HL, Mohler JL. Apical margins after robot-assisted radical prostatectomy: does technique matter? J Endourol. 2009;23(1):123–7. https://doi.org/10.1089/end.2008.0398.
13. Albisinni S, Dasnoy C, Diamand R, Mjaess G, Aoun F, Esperto F, Porpiglia F, Fiori C, Roumeguere T, DE Nunzio C. Anterior vs. Retzius-sparing robotic assisted radical prostatectomy: can the approach really make a difference? Minerva Urol Nephrol. 2022;74(2):137–45. https://doi.org/10.23736/S2724-6051.21.04623-1. Epub 2021 Oct 29. . PMID: 34714037
14. Gu X, Araki M, Wong C. Continence outcomes after bladder neck preservation during robot-assisted laparoscopic prostatectomy (RALP). Minim Invasive Ther Allied Technol. 2015;24(6):364–71. https://doi.org/10.3109/13645706.2015.1027711. Epub 2015 Mar 22. PMID: 25797687
15. Sridhar AN, Abozaid M, Rajan P, Sooriakumaran P, Shaw G, Nathan S, Kelly JD, Briggs TP. Surgical techniques to optimize early urinary continence recovery post robot assisted radical prostatectomy for prostate cancer. Curr Urol Rep. 2017;18(9):71. https://doi.org/10.1007/s11934-017-0717-4. PMID: 28718165; PMCID: PMC5514172.
16. Kumar A, Patel VR, Panaiyadiyan S, Seetharam Bhat KR, Moschovas MC, Nayak B. Nerve-sparing robot-assisted radical prostatectomy: current perspectives. Asian J Urol. 2021;8(1):2–13. https://doi.org/10.1016/j.ajur.2020.05.012. Epub 2020 Jun 11. PMID: 33569267; PMCID: PMC7859364
17. Shikanov S, Woo J, Al-Ahmadie H, Katz MH, Zagaja GP, Shalhav AL, Zorn KC. Extrafascial versus interfascial nerve-sparing technique for robotic-assisted laparoscopic prostatectomy: comparison of functional outcomes and positive surgical margins characteristics. Urology.

2009;74(3):611–6. https://doi.org/10.1016/j.urology.2009.01.092. Epub 2009 Jul 18. PMID: 19616830

18. Tewari AK, Srivastava A, Huang MW, Robinson BD, Shevchuk MM, Durand M, Sooriakumaran P, Grover S, Yadav R, Mishra N, Mohan S, Brooks DC, Shaikh N, Khanna A, Leung R. Anatomical grades of nerve sparing: a risk-stratified approach to neural-hammock sparing during robot-assisted radical prostatectomy (RARP). BJU Int. 2011;108(6 Pt 2):984–92. https://doi.org/10.1111/j.1464-410X.2011.10565.x.
19. Schatloff O, Chauhan S, Sivaraman A, Kameh D, Palmer KJ, Patel VR. Anatomic grading of nerve sparing during robot-assisted radical prostatectomy. Eur Urol. 2012;61(4):796–802. https://doi.org/10.1016/j.eururo.2011.12.048. Epub 2012 Jan 4. PMID: 22230713.
20. Schatloff O, Kameh D, Giedelman C, Samavedi S, Abdul-Muhsin H, Coelho RF, Kang SG, Palmer KJ, Patel VR. Proposal of a method to assess and report the extent of residual neurovascular tissue present in radical prostatectomy specimens. BJU Int. 2013;112(4):E301–6. https://doi.org/10.1111/bju.12038. Epub 2013 Apr 19. PMID: 23601173.
21. Reiner WG, Walsh PC. An anatomical approach to the surgical management of the dorsal vein and Santorini's plexus during radical retropubic surgery. J Urol. 1979;121(2):198–200. https://doi.org/10.1016/s0022-5347(17)56718-x.
22. Lunacek A, Schwentner C, Fritsch H, et al. Anatomical radical retropubic prostatectomy 'curtain dissection' of the neurovascular bundle. BJU Int. 2005;95:1226–31.
23. Kaul S, Savera A, Badani K, et al. Functional outcomes and oncological eficacy of Vattikuti institute prostatectomy with Veil of Aphrodite nerve-sparing: an analysis of 154 consecutive patients. BJU Int. 2006;97:467–72.
24. Ghani KR, Trinh QD, Menon M. Vattikuti institute prostatectomy-technique in 2012. J Endourol. 2012;26:1558–65.
25. Galfano A, Ascione A, Grimaldi S, Petralia G, Strada E, Bocciardi AM. A new anatomic approach for robot-assisted laparoscopic prostatectomy: a feasibility study for completely intrafascial surgery. Eur Urol. 2010;58(3):457–61. https://doi.org/10.1016/j.eururo.2010.06.008. Epub 2010 Jun 16. PMID: 20566236.
26. Urkmez A, Ranasinghe W, Davis JW. Surgical techniques to improve continence recovery after robot-assisted radical prostatectomy. Transl Androl Urol. 2020;9(6):3036–48. https://doi.org/10.21037/tau.2020.03.36. PMID: 33457277; PMCID: PMC7807332.
27. Egan J, Marhamati S, Carvalho FLF, Davis M, O'Neill J, Lee H, Lynch JH, Hankins RA, Hu JC, Kowalczyk KJ. Retzius-sparing robot-assisted radical prostatectomy leads to durable improvement in urinary function and quality of life versus standard robot-assisted radical prostatectomy without compromise on oncologic efficacy: single-surgeon series and step-by-step guide. Eur Urol. 2021;79(6):839–57. https://doi.org/10.1016/j.eururo.2020.05.010. Epub 2020 Jun 11. PMID: 32536488.
28. Stonier T, Simson N, Davis J, Challacombe B. Retzius-sparing robot-assisted radical prostatectomy (RS-RARP) vs standard RARP: it's time for critical appraisal. BJU Int. 2019;123(1):5–7. https://doi.org/10.1111/bju.14468. Epub 2018 Jul 27. PMID: 29959814.
29. Rosenberg JE, Jung JH, Edgerton Z, Lee H, Lee S, Bakker CJ, Dahm P. Retzius-sparing versus standard robot-assisted laparoscopic prostatectomy for the treatment of clinically localized prostate cancer. BJU Int. 2021;128(1):12–20. https://doi.org/10.1111/bju.15385. Epub 2021 May 6. PMID: 33686742.
30. Rocco B, Gregori A, Stener S, Santoro L, Bozzola A, Galli S, Knez R, Scieri F, Scaburri A, Gaboardi F. Posterior reconstruction of the rhabdosphincter allows a rapid recovery of continence after transperitoneal videolaparoscopic radical prostatectomy. Eur Urol. 2007;51(4):996–1003. https://doi.org/10.1016/j.eururo.2006.10.014. Epub 2006 Oct 23. PMID: 17079070.
31. Van Velthoven RF, Ahlering TE, Peltier A, Skarecky DW, Clayman RV. Technique for laparoscopic running urethrovesical anastomosis:the single knot method. Urology. 2003;61(4):699–702. https://doi.org/10.1016/s0090-4295(02)02543-8.

32. Checcucci E, Veccia A, Fiori C, Amparore D, Manfredi M, Di Dio M, Morra I, Galfano A, Autorino R, Bocciardi AM, Dasgupta P, Porpiglia F. Retzius-sparing robot-assisted radical prostatectomy vs the standard approach: a systematic review and analysis of comparative outcomes. BJU Int. 2020;125(1):8–16. https://doi.org/10.1111/bju.14887. Epub 2019 Aug 26. PMID: 31373142.
33. Saidian A, Fang AM, Hakim O, Magi-Galluzzi C, Nix JW, Rais-Bahrami S. Perioperative outcomes of single vs multi-port robotic assisted radical prostatectomy: a single institutional experience. J Urol. 2020;204(3):490–5. https://doi.org/10.1097/JU.0000000000000811. Epub 2020 Feb 24. PMID: 32091305.
34. Lenfant L, Sawczyn G, Kim S, Aminsharifi A, Kaouk J. Single-institution cost comparison: single-port versus multiport robotic prostatectomy. Eur Urol Focus. 2021;7(3):532–6. https://doi.org/10.1016/j.euf.2020.06.010. Epub 2020 Jul 4. PMID: 32631777.
35. Bertolo R, Garisto J, Bove P, Mottrie A, Rocco B, EAU Robotic Urology Section (ERUS) Working Group on Science. Perioperative outcomes between single-port and "Multi-Port" robotic assisted radical prostatectomy: where do we stand? Urology. 2021;155:138–43. https://doi.org/10.1016/j.urology.2021.06.005. Epub 2021 Jun 18. PMID: 34153366.
36. Moschovas MC, Seetharam Bhat KR, Onol FF, Rogers T, Ogaya-Pinies G, Roof S, Patel VR. Single-port technique evolution and current practice in urologic procedures. Asian J Urol. 2021;8(1):100–4. https://doi.org/10.1016/j.ajur.2020.05.003. Epub 2020 May 22. PMID: 33569276; PMCID: PMC7859361.
37. Kaouk JH, Ferguson EL, Beksac AT, Zeinab MA, Kaviani A, Weight C, Haywood S, Eltemamy M, Purysko A, McKenney JK, Klein E. Single-port robotic Transvesical partial prostatectomy for localized prostate cancer: initial series and description of technique. Eur Urol. 2022;82(5):551–8. https://doi.org/10.1016/j.eururo.2022.07.017. Epub 2022 Aug 13. PMID: 35970657.

Chapter 14
Robotic Radical Cystectomy

Cagri Akpinar, Evren Suer, and Kadir Turkolmez

Bladder cancer is the tenth most common cancer in the worldwide when both genders are considered and the seventh most common cancer in the male population [1]. While approximately 75% of patients with BC present with disease confined to the mucosa or submucosa, 25% of patients present as muscle invasive bladder cancer (MIBC). The standard treatment for patients with urothelial MIBC and MIBC with variant histologies is radical cystectomy (RC) [2]. Also, to improve these results in patients with cN0M0 disease, cisplatin-based neoadjuvant chemotherapy has been used since the 1980s [3, 4].

Traditionally, RC is recommended in patients with T2–T4a, N0–Nx, M0 disease [5]. In addition, RC is recommended for recurrent high-risk non-muscle invasive bladder cancer (NMIBC), BCG-resistant, BCG-relapsed, and BCG-unresponsive NMIBC, as well as extensive papillary disease uncontrolled by TURB and intravesical therapy alone [6]. Patients scheduled for RC should be treated without delays to maximize survival [7]. This surgical procedure can be performed as open or robot-assisted radical cystectomy (RARC) after the advantages or disadvantages of both techniques are informed to the patient [8].

RARC was first described in 2003 [9]. Unlike open surgery, RARC has been developing over the last 15 years due to the multiple technologic advances in robotic platforms, instrumentation, and endoscopic training in residency are quickly evolving. The goal in RARC, is to reduce pre-procedural morbidity and provide earlier return of normal activity while maintaining oncological equivalance [10, 11].

All patients scheduled for RARC should undergo a complete metastatic and staging evaluation. Currently, there is no need for routine bowel preparation prior to surgery. For most patients it is recomended to use an enema immediately prior to

C. Akpinar (✉) · E. Suer · K. Turkolmez
Department of Urology, Ankara University School of Medicine, Ankara, Turkey

S. Tonyali et al. (eds.), *Current Endourology*,
https://doi.org/10.1007/978-3-032-00010-1_14

surgery. Also, all patients are marked for the potential urostomy site and they are educated for regarding care and maintenance of the chosen urinary diversion. *(himman).*

Step-by-Step Surgical Technique

Operating Room Equipment and Port Placement

In a robot assisted approach, a daVinci 3 or 4 arm system may be used. A 0 and 30-degree lens is required. The required robotic instruments are monopolar robotic scissors, maryland bipolar, forceps, and two needle drivers. In addition, an endovascular GIA stapler, Hem-o-lok clips a suction-irrigator, and an atraumatic grasper are needed. The primary assistant operates from the patient's right (Fig. 14.1).

The patient is placed in a supine position with a Foley catheter inserted in the bladder. Pneumoperitoneum of 15 mmHg is established for port placement. Access and establishment of the pneumoperitoneum can be performed with a Veress or Hassan technique. The pressure is then lowered to 12 mmHg for the rest of the procedure. Port points to be entered are marked. The patient is marked approximately 15 cm superior to the pubic symphysis which is distance from the symphysis pubis to the umbilicus. The camera port is placed 5 cm superior the umbilicus in the midline. Two 8-mm trocars are placed level with the umbilicus, pararectally, on the left and right sides. The left port are placed 8 cm from the midline, and the right port is placed 10 cm from the midline to enable more space for the assistant's port. A third robotic port is placed a 8 cm lateral from the left port. A 15-mm assistant port is placed approximately 3–4 cm superomedial to anterior superior iliac spine. Lastly a 5-mm assistant port is placed approximately 4 cm superior to a line drawn between the umbilicus and the 8-mm port on the right side. The patient is then placed in the steep trendelenburg position and the robot is docked. Patient positioning and port placement for the robotic radical cystectomy portion are shown in Fig. 14.2. In the right, left and left lateral port a monopolar scissors, bipolar Maryland and a ProGrasp are placed respectively. Care is taken to advance the instruments under direct vision aiming towards the pubic bone in order not to damage central structures, such as bowel and vessels.

Identificiation, Mobilization, Division and Clipping of the Ureters

The surgeon should orient himself/herself to the pelvic anatomy by identifying specific landmarks. Also the relationship of the iliac vessels to the internal ring and umbilical ligaments is identified. The procedure is begun by incising peritoneum

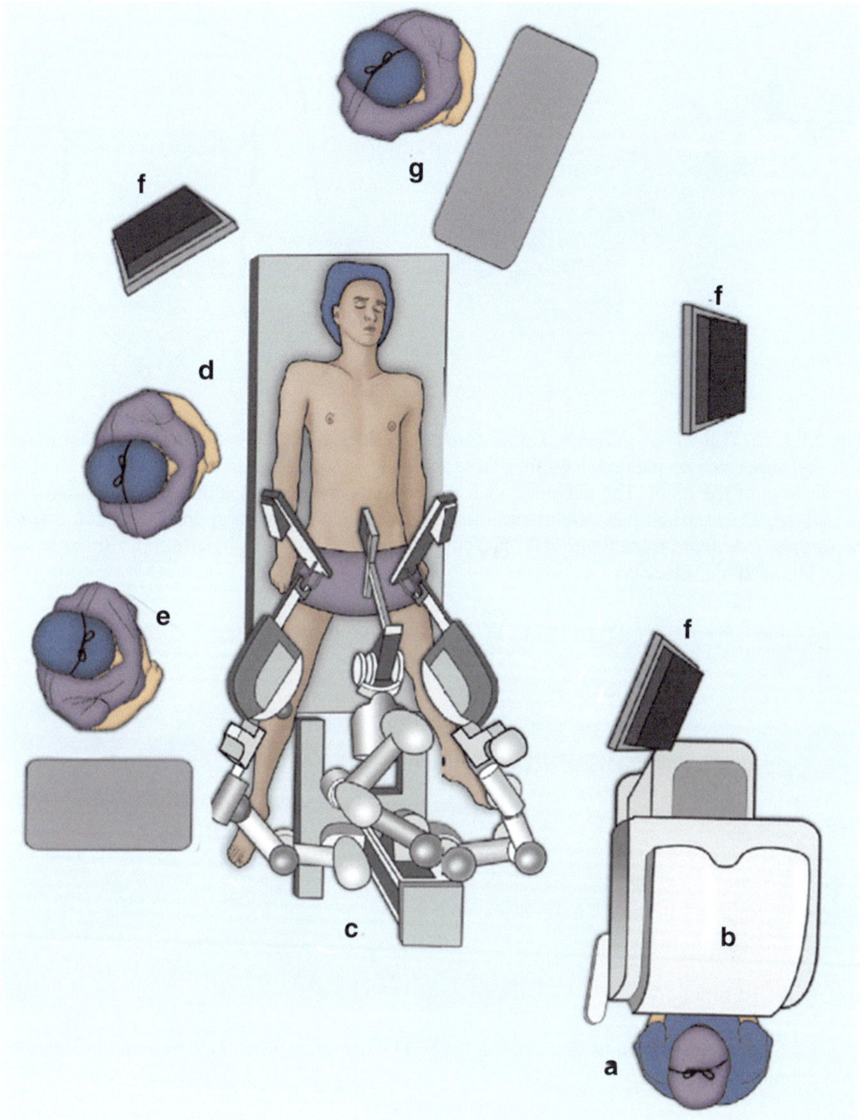

Fig. 14.1 Operating room setup for robotic cystectomy. A, Surgeon; B, console; C, da Vinci system; D, assistant; E, scrub nurse; F, high-definition monitors; G, anesthesia

lateral to the left colon. The left colon and sigmoid colon should be released from the left side wall to allow access to the left ureter.

First left and then right ureter are identified at the level where they cross the common iliac arteries (Fig. 14.3a). The peritoneum is carefully opened and the ureters dissected as far as the level of the bladder, proximally and distally. Adequate

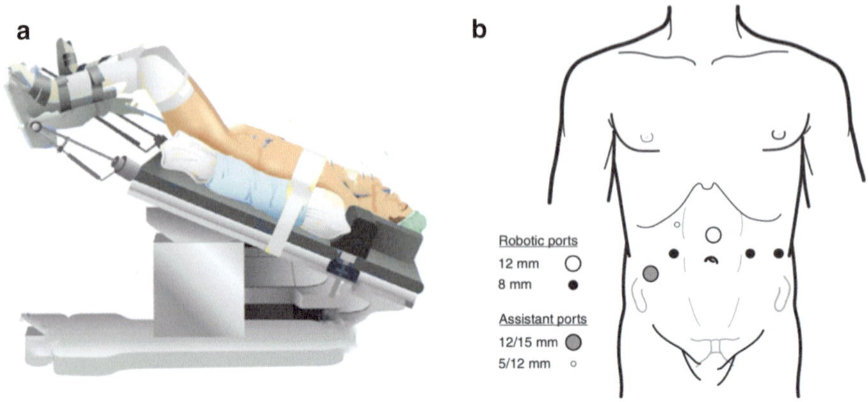

Fig. 14.2 (**a**) *Patients positioning*; Under general anesthesia, the patient's arms were laid to one side and supported by padded, legs are placed in venodynes, knees flexed and seperated to allow for docking of the robot. The patient is then placed in the steep trendelenburg position. (**b**) *Port placement*; The assistant ports are placed on the opposite side if intracorporeal diversion is to be performed. (Modified from Bishoff JT, Kavoussi LR. [2007]. Atlas of laparoscopic urologic surgery. Philadelphia: Elsevier)

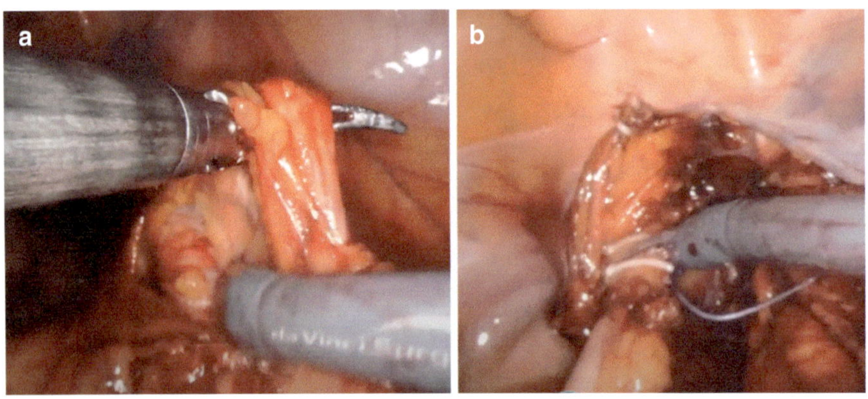

Fig. 14.3 (**a**) Identification of the ureter at the level where they cross the common iliac arteries. (**b**) Clipping the ureter

periureteral tissue is preserved during the dissection as possible. The ureters are dissected to the ureterovesical junction where they are clipped with two Hem-o-Lok clips and then transected Fig. 14.3b. A stay suture is placed on both proximal clips for easier identification of the ureters. One may use a different color suture for the left and right sided clips. Frozen section is sent from the both distal ureteric margine.

Pelvic Lymph Node Dissection

Pelvic lymph node dissection (PLND) can be performed before or after cystectomy, according to the surgeon's preference. The surgeon may prefer to perform PLND before cystectomy, as anatomical landmarks are still in place.

Incision is made of the peritoneum lateral to the medial umbilical ligament just above the vas deferens, which is divided. The incision is continued up along the medial aspect of the external iliac vessels up to the ureter. A space is created in the preperitoneal plane down to the endopelvic fascia sweeping the lymphatic tissue away towards the obturator vessels. In this way, the medial aspect of the specimen is defined. Then a release of the lymphatic tissue over the external iliac vessels using the split-and-roll technique down to the obturator fossa is performed. It is mandatory to correctly identify the obturator nerve and remove all the lymphatic tissue in this area. The previous release lateral to the vessels easier this dissection. Proximal attachments at the level of the ureter or at the aortic bifurcation are clipped and divided. Followed by the presacral nodes are removed with care not to cause any damage to the crossing left common iliac vein, which is quite thin and vulnerable in this area.

Posterior Dissection and Identification of the Anterior Rectal Space

Before starting the posterior dissection, the surgeon can orient himself by determining the level of the vas deferens.The assistant retracts the peritoneum and then the dissection starts with an incision in the peritoneum right under the seminal vesicles in the pouch of Douglas (Fig. 14.4a). This approach facilitates the dissection of the pedicles. The bladder is lifted with the ProGrasp and with the incision, seminal vesicles and vas deferens are exposed. The denonvillier's fascia is exposed by a

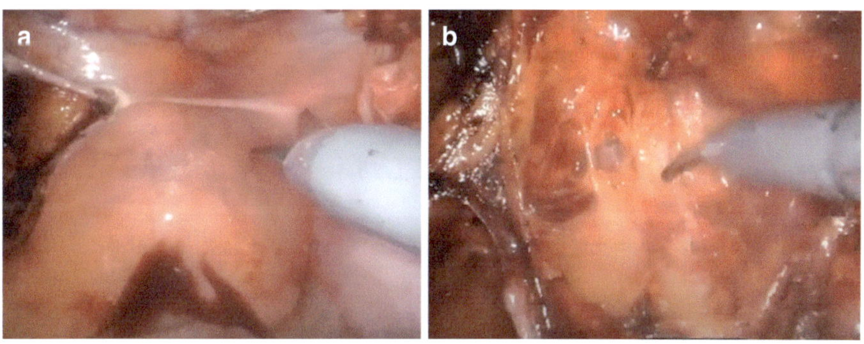

Fig. 14.4 (**a**) Visualization of area to be incised. (**b**) Incising for posterior dissection and prerectal space

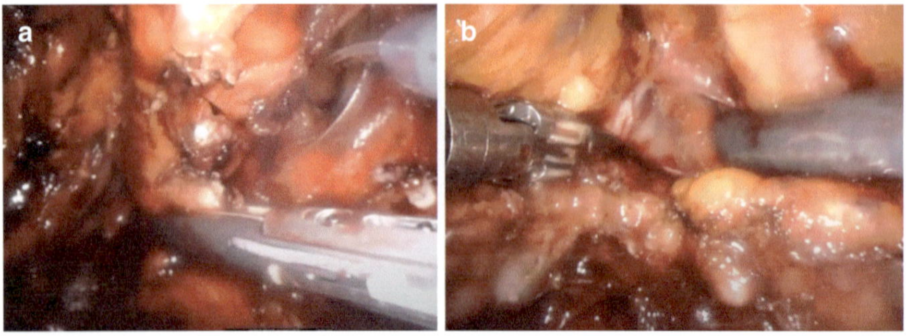

Fig. 14.5 (**a**) Division of the lateral pedicles by Ligasure/Bipolar instrument. (**b**) Lateral dissection extending through the endopelvic fascia

blunt and careful dissection posterior to the seminal vesicle, and a prerectal surgical plane is developed between denovillier's fascia and rectum (Fig. 14.4b). The recto-prostatic dissection should proceed on anterior surface to the yellow prerectal fat tissue to avoid rectal injury. The dissection continues between the rectum and the prostate all the way to the apex.

In female patients, dissection is performed along the anterior vaginal mucosa in a vaginal sparing procedure. If the anterior vaginal wall will not be preserved, the vaginal cuff is identified with a sponge-stick in the vagina and the vaginal apex incision is performed with monopolar cautery.

After dissection is completed on the posterior surface of the bladder, the incision is lateralised on both sides towards the bladder and prostate pedicles. Lateral dissection is continued to isolate the pedicles. The bladder pedicles are thinned and the superior vesical artery, inferior vesical artery and vesicoprostatic arteries are exposed and are taken on the both sides with an endovascular stapler, Ligasure/Vessel Sealer or Hem-o-Lok clips (Fig. 14.5a). Depending on the disease, it may be chosen to remove the neurovascular bundles or to perform a nerve-sparing procedure. T1 or unilateral T2 disease may be appropriate for a nerve-sparing procedure, but the goal of negative surgical margins should not be compromised. The lateral dissection extends through the endopelvic fascia thereby bladder is completely relased from the lateral attachments and rectum (Fig. 14.5b).

Lateral and Apical Dissection, and Transected of the Urethra

Medial umbilical ligament are identified. The peritoneum just lateral to the ligaments and medial to the external iliac artery is incised. The space of retzius is developed. Using sharp and blunt dissections, the space between lateral wall of the bladder and the pelvic side wall is developed up to the endopelvic fascia. Then, the endopelvic fascia is opened, lateral aspect of the prostate is seperated from the levator ani muscle and prostate apex is isolated. Using the fourth arm, the bladder is retracted towards the umbilicus. After retraction, the lateral pedicles are identified and divided with a the LigaSure or Hem-o-Lok clips. In a non-nerve-sparing procedure, the dissection is continued the LigaSure. The urachus and the median umbilical ligaments are coagulated with bipolar cautery and cut. The bladder is then taken down, staying in the correct plane by following the areolar tissue. The apical dissection of the prostate is completed. The dorsal vein complex is isolated, and then cut with monopolar robotic scissors or ligated with a 1 Vicryl suture. Maximum sparing of the urethra is performed, and prior to cutting, a suture or Hem-o-Lok clip is placed on the prostatic apex to avoid spilling tumour cells. If the previous posterior dissection is sufficient, only minimal posterior tissue residues, and the specimen is completely released. A frozen section is taken from the proximal portion of the divided urethra prior to creation of a neobladder. When the specimen is totally freed, it is placed in an 15-mm Endocatch retrieval bag.

Tips and Tricks

We recommend that this surgery be performed with a four arm system. In terms of secondary assistant requirement, We leave ample room for a second assisted area on the left side of the patient in the operating room setup. We prefer to perform extendend PLND before cystectomy as the anatomical landmarks are still in place.

References

1. Ferlay J, Colombet M, Soerjomataram I, Parkin DM, Piñeros M, Znaor A, et al. Cancer statistics for the year 2020: an overview. Int J Cancer. 2021;149:778–89.
2. Stein JP, Lieskovsky G, Cote R, Groshen S, Feng AC, Boyd S, et al. Radical cystectomy in the treatment of invasive bladder cancer: long-term results in 1,054 patients. J Clin Oncol. 2001;19(3):666–75. Epub 2001/02/07. https://doi.org/10.1200/jco.2001.19.3.666. PubMed PMID: 11157016.
3. David KA, Milowsky MI, Ritchey J, Carroll PR, Nanus DM. Low incidence of perioperative chemotherapy for stage III bladder cancer 1998 to 2003: a report from the National Cancer Data Base. J Urol. 2007;178(2):451–4. Epub 2007/06/15. https://doi.org/10.1016/j.juro.2007.03.101. PubMed PMID: 17561135.
4. Porter MP, Kerrigan MC, Donato BM, Ramsey SD. Patterns of use of systemic chemotherapy for Medicare beneficiaries with urothelial bladder cancer. Urol Oncol. 2011;29(3):252–8. Epub 2009/05/20. https://doi.org/10.1016/j.urolonc.2009.03.021. PubMed PMID: 19450992.
5. Hautmann RE, Abol-Enein H, Hafez K, Haro I, Mansson W, Mills RD, et al. Urinary diversion. Urology. 2007;69(1 Suppl):17–49. Epub 2007/02/07. https://doi.org/10.1016/j.urology.2006.05.058. PubMed PMID: 17280907.
6. Babjuk M, Böhle A, Burger M, Compérat E, Kaasinen E, Palou J. EAU guidelines on non-muscle invasive (Ta, T1, CIS) bladder cancer. EAU guidelines 2020.
7. Russell B, Liedberg F, Khan MS, Nair R, Thurairaja R, Malde S, et al. A systematic review and meta-analysis of delay in radical cystectomy and the effect on survival in bladder cancer

patients. Eur Urol Oncol. 2020;3(2):239–49. Epub 2019/11/02. https://doi.org/10.1016/j.euo.2019.09.008. PubMed PMID: 31668714.
8. Witjes JA, Bruins HM, Cathomas R, Compérat EM, Cowan NC, Gakis G, et al. European association of urology guidelines on muscle-invasive and metastatic bladder cancer: summary of the 2020 guidelines. Eur Urol. 2021;79(1):82–104.
9. Menon M, Hemal AK, Tewari A, Shrivastava A, Shoma AM, El-Tabey NA, et al. Nerve-sparing robot-assisted radical cystoprostatectomy and urinary diversion. BJU Int. 2003;92(3):232–6. Epub 2003/07/31. https://doi.org/10.1046/j.1464-410x.2003.04329.x. PubMed PMID: 12887473.
10. Tan WS, Khetrapal P, Tan WP, Rodney S, Chau M, Kelly JD. Robotic assisted radical cystectomy with extracorporeal urinary diversion does not show a benefit over open radical cystectomy: a systematic review and meta-analysis of randomised controlled trials. PLoS One. 2016;11(11):e0166221. Epub 2016/11/08. https://doi.org/10.1371/journal.pone.0166221. PubMed PMID: 27820855; PubMed Central PMCID: PMCPMC5098822.
11. Tan WS, Lamb BW, Kelly JD. Evolution of the neobladder: a critical review of open and intracorporeal neobladder reconstruction techniques. Scand J Urol. 2016;50(2):95–103. Epub 2016/02/18. https://doi.org/10.3109/21681805.2016.1141318. PubMed PMID: 26882458.

Chapter 15
Minimally Invasive Adrenalectomy: The Technical Steps of the Laparoscopic and Robotic Approaches

Murat Sambel, Sahin Kilic, and Mutlu Ates

Introduction

Minimally invasive adrenalectomy (laparoscopic and robotic) offers advantages such as earlier recovery, a shorter hospital stay, less postoperative pain, lower transfusion requirements, and fewer wound site complications compared with open surgery [1, 2].

Laparoscopic adrenalectomy was first described by Gagner et al. in 1992 [3]. This minimally invasive surgical approach has now almost entirely replaced open adrenalectomy in the management of small and medium-sized adrenal lesions, and it is regarded as the standard treatment for benign adrenal masses. Laparoscopic adrenalectomy can be performed by the transperitoneal or retroperitoneal routes. The transperitoneal approach provides a wide operating field and direct access to the adrenal vessels. However, this approach carries a greater risk of intraperitoneal organ injury. The advantage of the retroperitoneal approach is that there is no relationship with the intra-abdominal organs, whereas the narrow working space and the lack of clear anatomical landmarks during surgery are disadvantages. Nonetheless, the two approaches are in terms of morbidity, operative time, length of hospital stay, and return to normal activities [4].

Surgical techniques, patient positioning, and trocar placement differ depending on the laparoscopic approach used. The first laparoscopic adrenalectomy was performed with a lateral transperitoneal approach (LTA) and with the patient in the lateral decubitus position [5]. Laparoscopic adrenalectomy can also be performed using anterior transperitoneal, posterior retroperitoneal, and lateral retroperitoneal approaches [3, 5–8].

Irrespective of which method is used, the preparation stage before the operation is highly important. Depending on the preliminary diagnosis, various issues should

M. Sambel (✉) · S. Kilic · M. Ates
Antalya Training and Research Hospital, Antalya, Turkiye

S. Tonyali et al. (eds.), *Current Endourology*,
https://doi.org/10.1007/978-3-032-00010-1_15

be considered on the operating table after the recommended medical treatments. Antibiotic prophylaxis is essential, and nasogastric or orogastric tube placement is beneficial. In addition, the insertion of a urethral Foley catheter before the operation commences is important for urine output monitoring during anesthesia.

Clinical Indications for Adrenalectomy

Clinical indications for adrenalectomy [9, 10]:

1. Functional adrenal mass identified at preoperative work-up:
   - Primary aldosteronism
   - Pheochromocytoma
   - Adrenal Cushing syndrome
   - Cushing disease refractory to pituitary targeted therapy
   - Ectopic Cushing syndrome with an unknown or inoperable primary site
   - Adrenocortical adenoma
2. Adrenal mass >4 cm in size at preoperative imaging
3. Adrenal incidentalomas growing more than 1 cm at follow-up imaging
4. Adrenocortical carcinoma or metastatic tumor

Contraindications and Patient Selection for Adrenalectomy

Severe coagulopathy and poor cardiopulmonary performance status represent absolute contraindications to adrenalectomy, regardless of the technique used. Contraindications to a minimally-invasive approach include large tumor size (>6 cm) and adrenocortical carcinoma. Based on preoperative imaging, open adrenalectomy is recommended in cases showing local invasion to adjacent tissues and organs, associated lymph node metastases, or suspected venous thrombus, in order to achieve negative surgical margins [11]. The National Comprehensive Cancer Network (NCCN) guidelines recommend open adrenalectomy with lymphadenectomy for adrenocortical carcinoma, regardless of size [10].

The European Society of Endocrine Surgeons (ESES) and the European Network for the Study of Adrenal Tumors (ENSAT) guidelines strongly recommend open adrenalectomy and locoregional lymphadenectomy as the first-line approach. However, laparoscopic adrenalectomy may be considered with a weak recommendation in high-volume and experienced centers for adrenocortical carcinomas smaller than 6 cm, provided there is no radiologic suspicion of local invasion and lymph node metastasis [12]. Although laparoscopic surgery is the preferred approach for pheochromocytomas, open surgery is recommended for large or locally invasive tumors and for cases in which adequate metabolic control cannot be achieved [13].

Tumor size, obesity, and a history of previous abdominal surgery are relative contraindications to laparoscopic surgery. Although there is no clear limit in terms of lesion size, open surgery is recommended for masses larger than 12 cm because of the high risk of malignancy and technical difficulty they entail [14].

Preoperative Preparation

A comprehensive preoperative endocrinological evaluation is required for patients scheduled to undergo laparoscopic adrenalectomy. It is crucial that the patient be endocrinologically optimized before surgery, and that management of potential postoperative endocrine disorders be planned in collaboration with an endocrinologist to minimize perioperative mortality and morbidity. In patients with pheochromocytoma, phenoxybenzamine, a long-acting α-adrenergic blocker, should be initiated at least two weeks before surgery to control blood pressure, and a β-blocker may be added subsequently in patients with tachycardia. Preoperative hydration and electrolyte repletion should be achieved through a high-sodium diet, and fluid intake should be increased during the week preceding surgery. Intraoperative blood pressure should also be carefully monitored.

Hypokalemia should be corrected aggressively in patients with aldosteronoma. Serum potassium should be maintained above 3.5 mEq/L, and treatment with spironolactone or amiloride should be initiated if necessary. In patients with Cushing's syndrome, electrolyte imbalances and hyperglycemia should be corrected before surgery. It should also be noted that these patients have an increased susceptibility to infection and a tendency toward hypercoagulability. Postoperatively, these patients should be closely monitored in collaboration with the endocrinology department for appropriate hydrocortisone replacement therapy [15–17].

Minimally Invasive Adrenalectomy Techniques

The choice of surgical approach depends on the size and characteristics of the lesion, the patient's overall condition, and the surgeon's experience [18, 19].

Laparoscopic Adrenalectomy

The Anterior Transperitoneal Approach (ATA)

ATA, which is more familiar to general surgeons, is a sub-mesocolic approach and the least commonly used technique. A greater number of ports are needed for successful surgery with this approach.

The procedure is performed under general anesthesia with the patient placed in the supine position. The first assistant and the camera operator stand on the patient's right side, while the surgeon stands on the left. Pneumoperitoneum is established at the level of the umbilicus using a "Veress" needle or by the open (Hasson) technique. After insertion of the initial 10–12 mm umbilical trocar, three additional 5–10 mm trocars are placed under laparoscopic guidance (Fig. 15.1).

A 30° is typically used. The operation begins by lifting the transverse meso colon to expose the Treitz ligament and identify the inferior mesenteric vein. The posterior peritoneum is incised lateral to the inferior mesenteric vein, near the inferior border of the pancreas. This maneuver allows visualization of the left renal vein. The left adrenal vein is then isolated and clipped. The left adrenal gland is then bluntly dissected using electro-cautery or an ultrasonic scalpel. The freed gland is placed in an endoscopic retrieval bag and extracted through the umbilical port.

The sub-mesocolic approach is associated with significantly shorter operative times and hospital stays. Early identification and ligation of the adrenal vein, with minimal dissection and gland manipulation, are the main advantages of this approach [5].

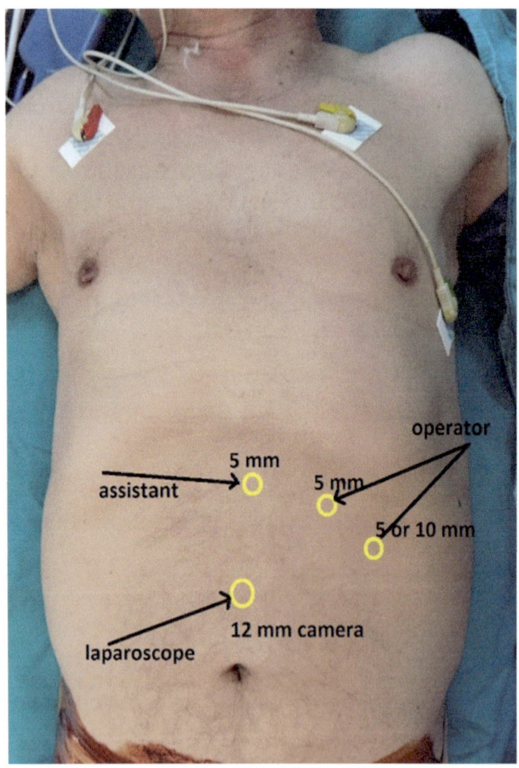

Fig. 15.1 Patient position and trocar placement in left laparoscopic adrenalectomy with ATA

Posterior Retroperitoneal Approach (PRA)

PRA was first performed in humans by Walz in 1996. This technique provides direct access to the adrenal gland while avoiding entry into the intra-abdominal cavity, and it may be particularly advantageous in patients with a history of previous abdominal surgery [20].

The procedure is performed with the patient under general anesthesia and in the prone position with moderately bent hip joints. Initially, a 1.5 cm incision is made immediately below the 12th rib. The thoracolumbar fascia is perforated with a hemostat or with the help of the index finger to permit access to the retroperitoneal space. The psoas muscle and the lower pole of the kidney are palpated with a finger. Careful finger dissection creates a potential space for the placement of a balloon dilator. After the balloon dilatator has been inserted into the retroperitoneal area approximately 800 mL of air is inflated into the balloon to create the working space. Following retroperitoneal balloon dilatation, two 5-mm trocars are inserted with internal finger guidance 5 cm laterally and medially to the initial incision. A 10–12 mm trocar is then inserted from initial incision and pneumoperitoneum achieved, through which a 30-degree endoscope is passed (Fig. 15.2).

Pneumoretroperitoneum allows blunt dissection of the area underneath the diaphragm and the fatty tissue overlying the kidney. The perinephric fat is dissected from the posterior aspect of the kidney. The superior pole of kidney can be seen cranially, the paraspinal muscles medially, and the posterior surface of the liver or spleen laterally. The adrenal tumor can often be identified and mobilized from the superior pole of the kidney together with the adrenal gland. Adrenalectomy is completed by detaching the gland from surrounding structures. The specimen is retrieved through the initial incision [20].

Bilateral procedures can also be performed using PRA. However, PRA has several limitations, including difficulty in removing large tumors, challenges in obese patients, and a limited working space [21].

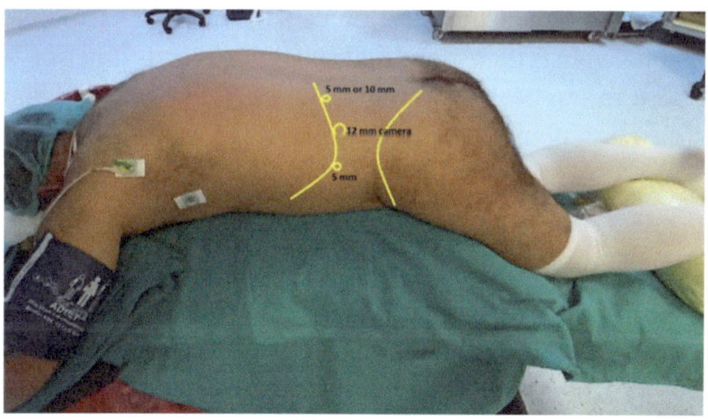

Fig. 15.2 Patient position and trocar placement in left laparoscopic adrenalectomy with PRA

Lateral Transperitoneal Approach (LTA)

LTA was the first described and remains the most commonly used technique in minimally invasive adrenalectomy. This technique is also frequently employed in our clinic. LTA offers several advantages over retroperitoneal approaches, including straightforward trocar placement, a wider working area, prominent anatomical landmarks, and excellent exposure due to gravity displacing the abdominal contents from the operating field. Consequently, it is particularly preferred in obese patients and for large adrenal masses.

The procedure is performed under general anesthesia with the patient in a 60–90° lateral decubitus position, with the tumor facing side upward. The operating table is flexed to increase the space between the 12th rib and the iliac crest. Although three trocars are generally sufficient for left adrenalectomy, an additional trocar may be required for liver retraction during right adrenalectomy (Figs. 15.3 and 15.4). All trocars are inserted through the peritoneum [22].

The procedure begins with the creation of pneumoperitoneum using a "Veress" needle, followed by placement of a 10–12 mm camera trocar in the pararectal region, superolateral to the umbilicus. Working trocars are typically inserted at the superior pararectal and subcostal regions along the anterior axillary and midclavicular lines. For right adrenalectomy, an additional 5 mm trocar is placed in the epigastric area for liver retraction. Trocar placement may be modified according to the surgeon's preference.

During left adrenalectomy, the splenic ligaments are detached from the retroperitoneum to mobilize the spleen and rotate it medially. The splenic flexure of the colon is medialized, and the avascular plane between the tail of the pancreas and the kidney is carefully dissected. The left adrenal vein is then identified and divided as it entry into the left renal vein (Fig. 15.5), [23].

During right adrenalectomy, the triangular ligament and retroperitoneal attachments of the right hepatic lobe are dissected. The liver is elevated using a fan or snake retractor, and right colonic flexure is mobilized with a Kocher maneuver. The lateral border of the inferior vena cava (IVC) is carefully dissected, and the right adrenal vein is then identified and divided at its junction with the IVC (Fig. 15.6), [23].

Elevation of the liver is maintained by a locked laparoscopic grasper fixed to the side abdominal wall throughout surgery to facilitate the exposure of the right

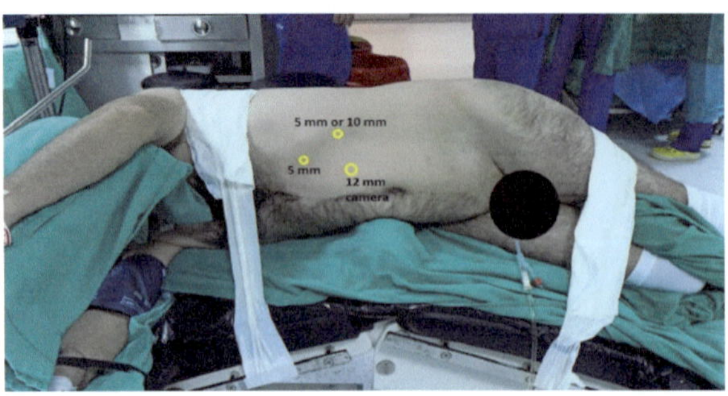

Fig. 15.3 Patient position and trocar placement in left laparoscopic adrenalectomy with LTA

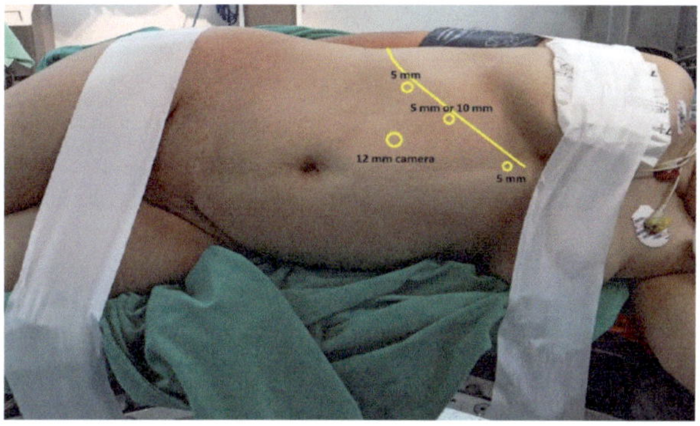

Fig. 15.4 Patient position and trocar placement in right laparoscopic adrenalectomy with LTA

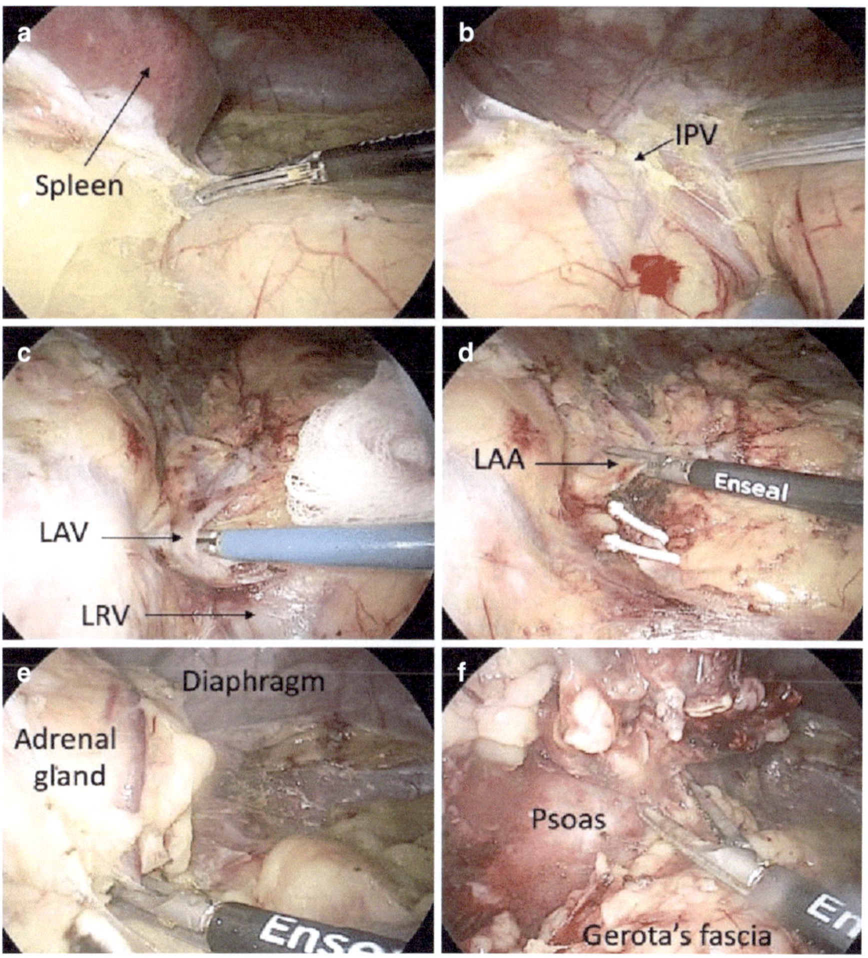

Fig. 15.5 Steps for left laparoscopic adrenalectomy with LTA [23]. (**a**) Mobilization of the left colonic flexure, (**b**) Exposure of the left inferior phrenic vessels, (**c**) Dissection of the left adrenal vein (LAV), (**d**) Adrenal vein transection, (**e**) Inferior and lateral dissection of the left adrenal gland, (**f**) Posterior dissection of the left adrenal gland. (IPV-inferior phrenic vessels, LAV-left adrenal vein, LRV-left renal vein, LAA-left adrenal artery)

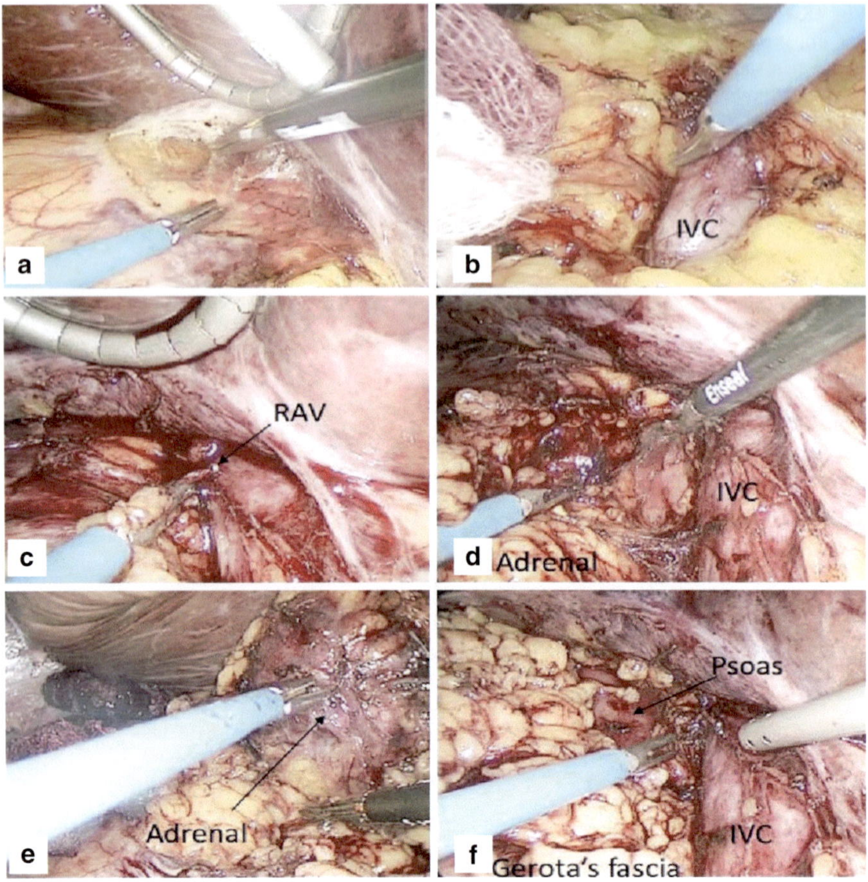

Fig. 15.6 Steps for right laparoscopic adrenalectomy with LTA [23]. (**a**) Mobilization of the right colonic flexure, (**b**) Exposure of the right side of the inferior vena cava, (**c**) Right adrenal vein clipping, (**d**) Dissection of the medial border of the right adrenal gland, (**e**) Inferior, lateral and posterior dissection of the right adrenal gland, (**f**) View of the resection bed (IVC-inferior vena cava, RAV-right adrenal vein)

adrenal gland. Early ligation of the adrenal vein may be necessary in cases of hormone-secreting adenomas. Once the surrounding vessels, including the adrenal vein, have been divided, the adrenal gland is placed in a specimen retrieval bag and retracted through a port site.

Lateral Retroperitoneal Approach (LRA)

Urologists are the surgeons with the greatest familiarity with the retroperitoneal anatomy and the urinary system organs. LRA is therefore commonly used by urological surgeons for adrenalectomy. LRA is particularly favorable in patients with prior histories of abdominal surgery, since it avoids the peritoneal cavity, similarly to PRA [7, 8]. Although the operative time is longer than in LTA, fewer bowel complications are observed in LRA, and it is also slightly less invasive than LTA [24]. While a large mass size is restrictive for LRA, this is not as important as for PRA [25].

The patient is placed in the 90° angle lateral decubitus position with the tumor side up. The table is flexed to open the space between the 12th rib and the iliac crest. An open (Hasson) technique is used for the initial trocar placement. A 1.5 cm incision is made in the lumbar (Petit's) triangle below the 12th rib at the lateral border of the paraspinalis muscles. The muscle fibers are carefully separated, and the retroperitoneum is entered by piercing the thoracolumbar fascia with the tip of a forceps. The retroperitoneal fat tissue is removed from the front of the psoas muscle by palpation with the index finger. The peritoneum is felt and medialized. A balloon dilator is then inserted to create a working space. Subsequently, two 5 mm trocars are placed immediately under the 12th rib with finger guidance, with a distance of approximately four fingers between them. A 12 mm assistant trocar is then inserted into the first incision (Fig. 15.7).

Following pneumoretroperitoneum, perinephric fatty tissue is dissected from the posterior aspect of the kidney. The superior pole of the kidney can be seen cranially, the paraspinal muscles laterally, and the ureter and main vascular structures medially. Gerota's fascia is incised and, following the psoas muscle and the ureter, the adrenal gland is identified superiorly to the renal veins.

The learning curve in the laparoscopic adrenalectomy procedure involves up to 30–40 cases, and the duration of surgery becomes shorter as the surgeon's experience increases [26]. Laparoscopic adrenalectomy techniques are summarized in Table 15.1.

Robotic Adrenalectomy

Laparoscopic adrenalectomy remains the standard surgical approach for adrenalectomy. Robotic systems offer several advantages over conventional laparoscopy, including improved ergonomics, magnified three-dimensional imaging, and enhanced ease of instrument rotation. These features make it ideal for adrenal

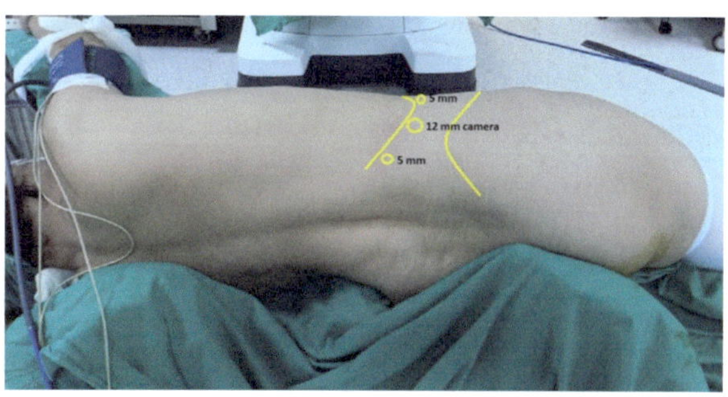

Fig. 15.7 Patient position and trocar placement in right laparoscopic adrenalectomy with LRA

Table 15.1 Summary of laparoscopic adrenalectomy techniques

Laparoscopic Adrenalectomy	Advantages	Disadvantages
Lateral transperitoneal approach	Sufficient working space Good visualization of the upper retroperitoneal region Easy retraction of adjacent organs under the effect of gravity, and good exploration of the peritoneal space Short operation time Less trocar requirement compared to anterior approach	Repositioning required for bilateral adrenalectomy Entry is into the peritoneal cavity, and this may therefore involve adhesions from previous procedures and the possibility of being affected by intraperitoneal diseases CO_2 pneumoperitoneum-induced hemodynamic and respiratory effects
Anterior transperitoneal approach	A wider surgical field Excellent view of the operative site and surrounding structures Well-known and conventional anatomical orientation Bilateral laparoscopic adrenalectomy without the need for repositioning	Additional trocar required for traction of adjacent structures Entry into the peritoneal cavity, and this may therefore entail adhesions from previous procedures and the possibility of being affected by intraperitoneal diseases CO_2 pneumoperitoneum-induced hemodynamic and respiratory side-effects
Posterior retroperitoneal approach	The procedure is not affected by adhesions rom previous operations or intraperitoneal diseases because of the extraperitoneal approach Beneficial in obese patients in terms of protection from hemodynamic and respiratory side-effects caused by CO_2-pneumoperitoneum Bilateral laparoscopic adrenalectomy without the need for repositioning	The learning process is challenging High probability of disruption of surgeon orientation Limited working space Manipulation is more difficult in large tumors
Lateral retroperitoneal approach	The procedure is not affected by adhesions from previous operations or intraperitoneal diseases because of the extraperitoneal approach Beneficial in obese patients in terms of protection from hemodynamic and respiratory side effects caused by CO_2-pneumoperitoneum Ability to return to the flank transperitoneal approach	The learning process is challenging High probability of disruption of surgeon orientation Limited working space Manipulation is more difficult in large tumors

surgery performed in tight spaces with many vital structures surrounding the fragile gland. Robotic adrenalectomy can provide potential advantages including a shorter hospital stay, less blood loss, and lower occurrence of postoperative complications.

These factors seem to support the use of robotics for the minimally invasive surgical management of adrenal masses [27]. The four laparoscopic adrenalectomy approaches can also be applied to the robotic system. The first robotic adrenalectomy was performed in 2000 with LTA and is often applied using LTA [28]. Retroperitoneal approaches in robotic surgery entail various difficulties compared to the transperitoneal approaches, such as relative port placement and a small working space. Although we use both methods in our clinic, we often decide to perform LTA. In the robotic approach, patient surgical preparation and basic surgical steps are similar to those involved in laparoscopic adrenalectomy. However, the number of trocars and their location may differ slightly from those in laparoscopic adrenalectomy.

Robotic Lateral Transperitoneal Approach

This procedure is performed under general anesthesia with the patient positioned in a 60–90° lateral decubitus position, with the tumor side facing upward, similar to laparoscopic LTA (see the Laparoscopic Adrenalectomy section). We use the Da Vinci Xi (Intuitive Surgical, Sunnyvale, CA, USA) robotic surgery system with five trocars (four robots, one assistant) for robotic adrenalectomy. In contrast to left adrenalectomy, we also insert one additional 5 mm trocar in the epigastric region in right adrenalectomy.

After establishing pneumoperitoneum with a “Veress” needle, we place an 8 mm robotic camera trocar in the pararectal area, superolateral to the umbilicus. Three additional 8 mm robotic working trocars are then inserted under direct visualization. We place the first robotic working trocar below the costal border of the rectus muscle, and the second in the pararectal area in the midclavicular line. The third robotic trocar is placed at a distance of 7–8 cm from the second trocar in a half-moon form. All trocars are placed 7–8 cm apart from each other to avoid contact between them. We place the 12 mm assistant trocar between the robotic camera trocar and the upper robot arm trocar at the midline of the abdomen (Fig. 15.8). During left robotic adrenalectomy, all the trocars are placed symmetrically to the right adrenalectomy over the anterior abdominal wall, except for the 5 mm liver elevation trocar, which is not needed. We insert the robotic scissors into the first (upper) trocar, the robotic Maryland dissector into the second trocar, and the robotic prograsper into the third trocar.

All the steps in robotic adrenalectomy are similar to those in laparoscopic adrenalectomy. During right adrenalectomy with robotic LTA, the triangular ligament and retroperitoneal attachments of the liver are dissected to mobilize the liver. The liver is then elevated using a snake or fan retractor, and the inferior vena cava (IVC) is identified. Gerota’s fascia is opened to expose the upper pole of right kidney. Dissection is continued along the superior pole of the right kidney until the right adrenal gland is visualized. The medial aspect of the adrenal gland is carefully dissected to locate the adrenal vein, which is ligated using polimer clips. Adrenalectomy is complated by finishing the peripheral dissection of the gland (Fig. 15.9) [22].

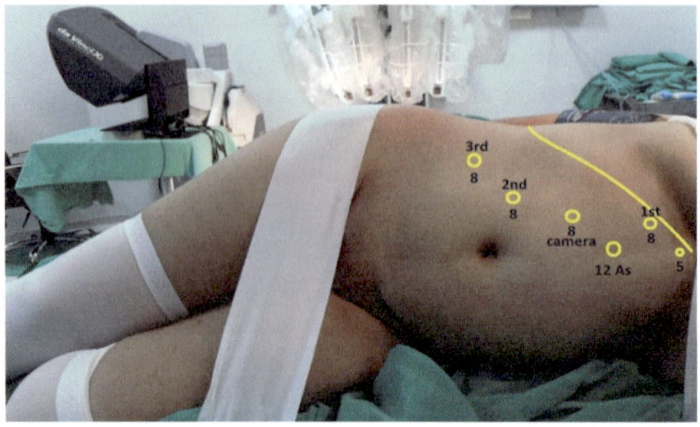

Fig. 15.8 Patient position and trocar placement in right robotic adrenalectomy with LTA

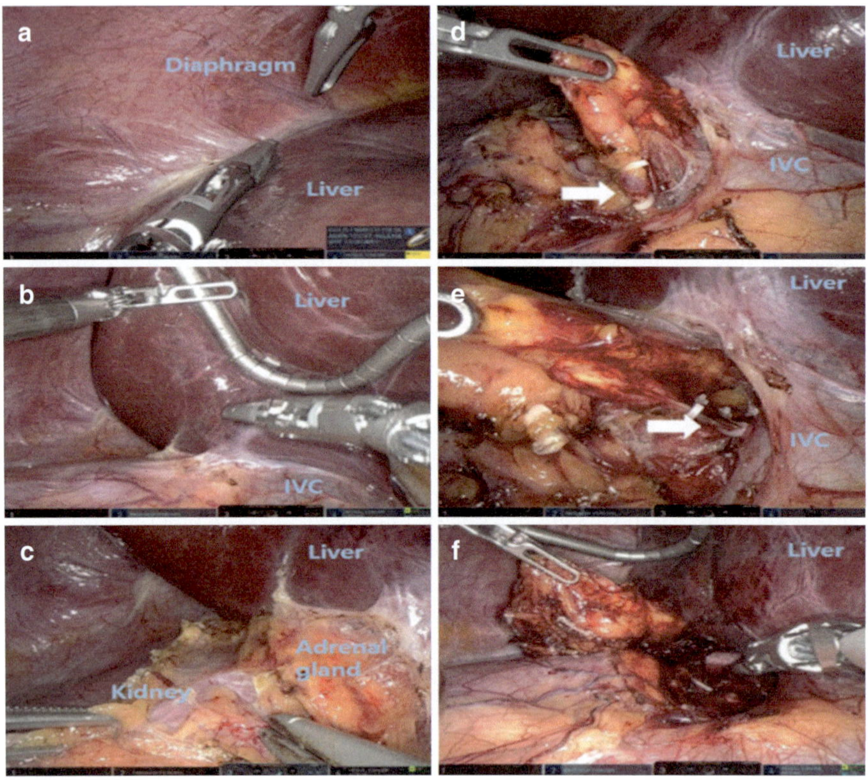

Fig. 15.9 The steps in right robotic adrenalectomy with LTA [22]. (**a**) Liver mobilization, (**b**) Liver retraction and inferior vena cava identification, (**c**) Gerota's fascia dissection and adrenal gland identification, (**d**) Adrenal vein identification, (**e**) Clipping of the adrenal vein, (**f**) Adrenalectomy completion

The descending colon is medialized by dissecting the splenocolic and splenophrenic ligaments during left adrenalectomy with robotic LTA. The avascular plane is dissected between the tail of the pancreas and kidney, and the location of the left adrenal gland and left renal vein is established. After opening Gerota's fascia, carefully dissection is performed around the left renal vein to locate the adrenal vein. Once the adrenal vein has been identified it is ligated using hem-o-lock clips. The remaining soft tissue around the adrenal gland is detached, and the adrenalectomy is completed (Fig. 15.10) [22].

Robotic Lateral Retroperitoneal Approach

The patient is positioned in a 90° lateral decubitus position with the tumor side facing upward, similar to laparoscopic LRA (see the Laparoscopic Adrenalectomy section). The operating table is flexed to increase the space between the 12th rib and the iliac crest. The open (Hasson) technique is used for the initial trocar placement. A 1.5 cm incision is made to the lumbar (Petit's) triangle below the 12th rib at the

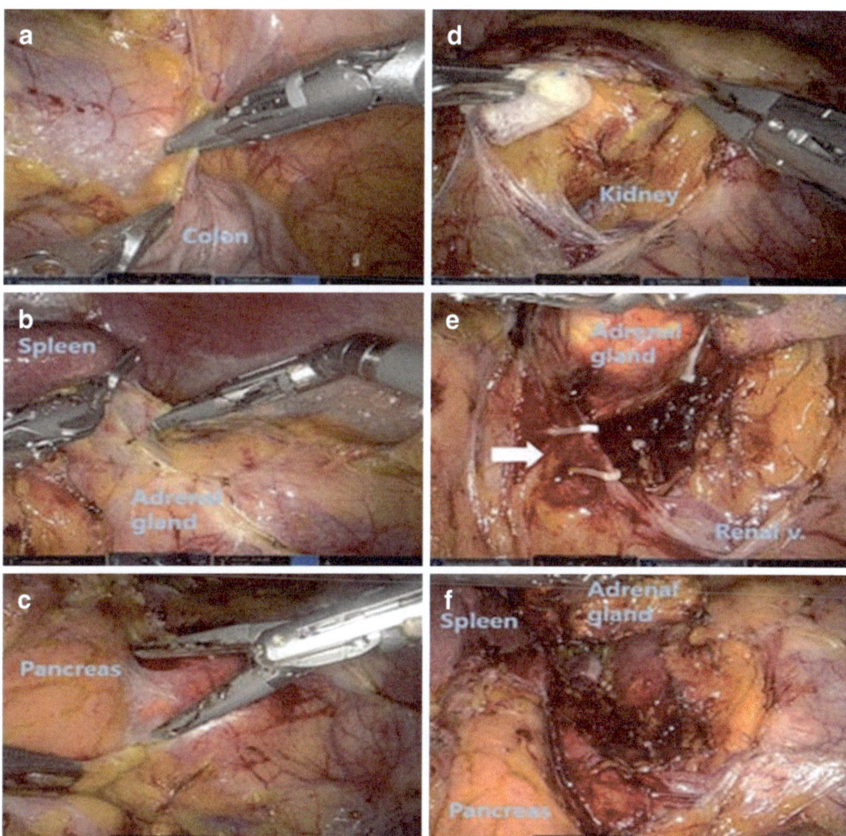

Fig. 15.10 The steps for left robotic adrenalectomy with LTA [22]. (**a**) Left colon mobilization, (**b**) Spleen mobilization, (**c**) Pancreas and Gerota's fascia dissection, (**d**) Exposure of the left kidney, (**e**) Adrenal vein identification and ligation, (**f**) Adrenalectomy completion

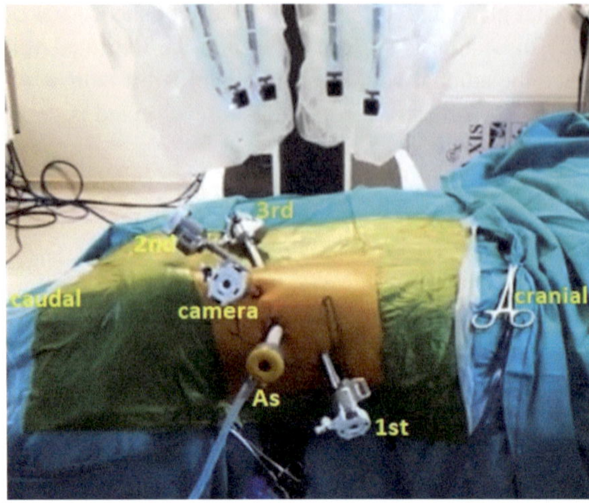

Fig. 15.11 Patient position and trocar placement in left robotic adrenalectomy with LRA

lateral border of the paraspinal muscles. The muscle fibers are carefully separated, and the retroperitoneum is entered by piercing the thoracolumbar fascia with the tip of a forceps. The retroperitoneal fat tissue is removed from the front of the psoas muscle by palpation with the index finger. The peritoneum is felt and medialized, after which a balloon dilator is inserted and a working space is created. Subsequently, the first 8 mm robotic trocar is inserted immediately under the 12th rib with finger guidance. The other two 8 mm robotic trocars are installed in a half-moon form with finger guidance, approximately four fingers' width apart. A 12 mm assistant trocar is inserted into the first incision. Following docking of the three robotic arms, the peritoneum is medialized, and the last 8 mm robotic trocar is inserted under direct visualization. We insert the robotic scissors into the first (upper) trocar, the robotic Maryland dissector into the second trocar, and the robotic prograsper into the third trocar (Fig. 15.11). The other steps of the procedure are similar to those involved in laparoscopic LRA [29].

Partial Adrenalectomy

Partial adrenalectomy has been increasingly applied in recent years. It is performed in order to prevent adrenal insufficiency in cases of solitary adrenal gland, bilateral disease, and familial cancer syndromes (von Hippel Lindau, multiple endocrineneoplasia type 2, neurofibromatosis type I, or cuccinate dehydrogenase enzyme mutations).

Several studies have reported that Addisonian crisis can be seen in up to 35% of patients who have undergone bilateral adrenalectomy, with a 3% mortality rate [30]. In addition, the need for steroids after adrenalectomy is associated with decreased quality of life, increased fatigue, stress, decreased resistance to infection, and weight gain [31].

One crucial stage in partial adrenalectomy involves preparing the gland for total adrenalectomy during the operation and revealing its condition (Fig. 15.12). The location of the mass is the most important feature in deciding whether to perform a partial adrenalectomy [32].

In addition, although there are no clear size criteria for partial adrenalectomy, a mass smaller than 4 cm is a widely accepted indication, since this represents the threshold value with the best ability to differentiate benign and malignant masses in several studies [33].

It is sufficient for 15–30% of the adrenal tissue to be left in situ following partial adrenalectomy, while the adrenal vein must be protected to ensure the continuation of the gland's activity [34].

The use of intraoperative ultrasound is useful for mass identification. Intraoperative indocyanine green (ICG) in either conventional or robot-assisted laparoscopic partial adrenalectomy may help identify vascular structures and partial adrenalectomy margins.

In conclusion, numerous studies have shown that partial adrenalectomy is a viable and safe procedure. The procedure has now become an accepted alternative in the treatment of adrenal tumors in patients with hereditary syndrome or a solitary adrenal gland. In addition, since cortical insufficiency may develop even in patients

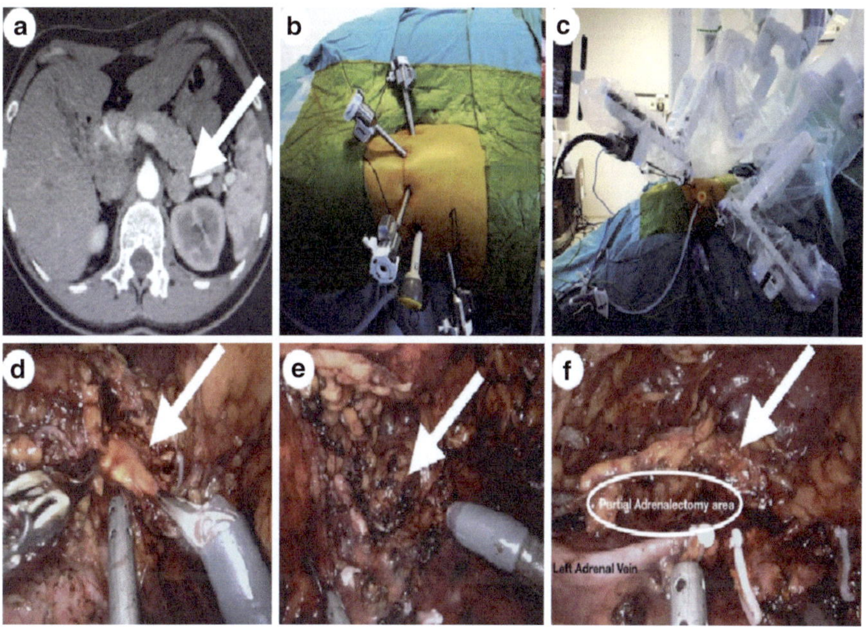

Fig. 15.12 Summary of left robotic partial adrenalectomy with LRA [35]. (**a**) A left adrenal mass at enhanced computed tomography, (**b**) Trocar placement for LRA, (**c**) Placement of the robotic arms after docking, (**d**) An adrenal mass in the left adrenal gland, (**e**) Left adrenal mass after dissection, (**f**) Residual left adrenal gland (white arrow), left adrenal vein, and the area of the resected adrenal mass

with a normal gland, it appears very probable that partial adrenalectomy will play an even more important role in the future. The perioperative results are similar to those of total adrenalectomy, and it can be safely performed with open or minimally invasive methods.

Conclusion

Patient positioning and proper port placement before laparoscopic or robot-assisted laparoscopic surgery are two extremely important steps that can have a direct impact on the overall success of the procedure. Preoperative planning is of the greatest importance as the robot is docked to the patient once the positioning process is completed. Predefined templates are very useful. However, it is important to adapt to the specific situation according to the planned operation site and the patient's individual anatomy.

References

1. Turner DJ, Miskulin J. Management of adrenal lesions. Curr Opin Oncol. 2009;21:34–40.
2. Brunt LM, Doherty GM, Norton JA, Quasebarth MA, Moley JF, et al. Laparoscopic adrenalectomy compared to open adrenalectomy for benign adrenal neoplasms. J Am Coll Surg. 1996;183:1–10.
3. Gagner M, Lacroix A, Bolte E. Laparoscopic adrenalectomy in Cushing's syndrome and pheochromocytoma. N Engl J Med. 1992;327:1033.
4. Constantinides VA, Christakis I, Touska P, et al. Systematic review and meta-analysis of retroperitoneoscopic versus laparoscopic adrenalectomy. Br J Surg. 2012;99:1639–48.
5. Lezoche E, Guerrieri M, Crosta F, et al. Flank approach versus anterior sub-mesocolic access in left laparoscopic adrenalectomy: a prospective randomized study. Surg Endosc. 2008;22:2373–8.
6. Brunt LM, Molmenti EP, Kerbl K, et al. Retroperitoneal endoscopic adrenalectomy: an experimental study. Surg Laparosc Endosc. 1993;3:300–6.
7. Lin Y, Li L, Zhu J. Experience of retroperitoneoscopic adrenalectomy in 195 patients with primary aldosteronism. Int J Urol. 2007;14:910–3.
8. Sasagawa I, Suzuki Y, Itoh K, et al. Posterior retroperitoneoscopic partial adrenalectomy: clinical experience in 47 procedures. Eur Urol. 2003;43:381–5.
9. Li AY, Dream S. Adrenalectomy. In: StatPearls [Internet]. Treasure Island (FL): StatPearls Publishing; 2022; Available from: https://www.ncbi.nlm.nih.gov/books/NBK559093/.
10. Shah MH, Goldner WS, Benson AB, et al. Neuroendocrine and adrenal tumors, NCCN clinical practice guidelines in oncology. J Natl Compr Cancer Netw. 2021;19:839–68.
11. Mihai R. Open adrenalectomy. Gland Surg. 2019;8:28–35.
12. Gaujoux S, Mihai R. Joint working group of Ensat. European Society of Endocrine Surgeons (ESES) and European Network for the study of adrenal tumors (ENSAT) recommendations for the surgical management of adrenocortical carcinoma. Br J Surg. 2017;104:358–76.
13. Lenders JW, Duh QY, Eisenhofer G, et al. Pheochromocytoma and paraganglioma: an Endocrine Society clinical practice guideline. J Clin Endocrinol Metab. 2014;99:1915–42.

14. Alemanno G, Bergamini C, Prosperi P, et al. Adrenalectomy: indications and options for treatment. Updat Surg. 2017;69:119–25.
15. Bornstein SR, Allolio B, Arlt W, et al. Diagnosis and treatment of primary adrenal insufficiency: an Endocrine Society clinical practice guideline. J Clin Endocrinol Metab. 2016;101:364–89.
16. Funder JW, Carey RM, Mantero F, et al. The Management of Primary Aldosteronism: case detection, diagnosis, and treatment: an Endocrine Society clinical practice guideline. J Clin Endocrinol Metab. 2016;101:1889–916.
17. Romero DG, Yanes Cardozo LL. Clinical practice guideline for Management of Primary Aldosteronism: what is new in the 2016 update? Int J Endocrinol Metab Disord. 2016;2:3.
18. Lal G, Clark OH. Thyroid, parathyroid and adrenal. In: Brunucardi FC, Andersen DK, Billiar TR, et al., editors. Schwartz's principles of surgery. 11th ed. New York: McGraw Hill; 2019. p. 1625–704.
19. Madani A, Lee JA. Surgical approaches to the adrenal gland. Surg Clin North Am. 2019;99:773–91.
20. Walz MK, Peitgen K, Hoermann R, et al. Posterior retroperitoneoscopy as a new minimally invasive approach for adrenalectomy: results of 30 adrenalectomies in 27 patients. World J Surg. 1996;20:769–74.
21. Dickson PV, Jimenez C, Chisholm GB, et al. Posterior retroperitoneoscopic adrenalectomy: a contemporary American experience. J Am Coll Surg. 2011;212:659–65.
22. Choi YS, Lee JS, Yi JW. Comparative analysis of laparoscopic and robotic Transperitoneal Adrenalectomy performed at a single institution. Medicina (Kaunas). 2022;29(58):1747.
23. Makkai-Popa ST, Pascotto B, Arru L, et al. Minimally invasive Adrenalectomy: technical aspects of the laparoscopic and the robotic approach. Chirurgia (Bucur). 2020;115:80–8.
24. Suzuki K, Kageyama S, Hirano Y, et al. Comparison of 3 surgical approaches to laparoscopic adrenalectomy: a nonrandomized, background matched analysis. J Urol. 2001;166:437–43.
25. Wang B, Ma X, Li H, et al. Anatomic retroperitoneoscopic adrenalectomy for selected adrenal tumors >5 cm: our technique and experience. Urology. 2011;78:348–52.
26. Guerrieri M, Campagnacci R, De Sanctis A, et al. The learning curve in laparoscopic adrenalectomy. J Endocrinol Invest. 2008;31:531–6.
27. Brandao LF, Autorino R, Laydner H, et al. Robotic versus laparoscopic adrenalectomy: a systematic review and meta-analysis. Eur Urol. 2014;65:1154–61.
28. Bentas W, Wolfram M, Bräutigam R, et al. Laparoscopic transperitoneal adrenalectomy using a remote-controlled robotic surgical system. J Endourol. 2002;16:373–6.
29. Ates M, Kilic S, Ozsoy C, et al. Robot-assisted laparoscopic retroperitoneal partial adrenalectomy: the first case in the literature. Cent Eur J Urol. 2020;73:238–9.
30. Telenius-Berg M, Ponder MA, Berg B, et al. Quality of life after bilateral adrenalectomy in MEN 2. Henry Ford Hosp Med J. 1989;37:160–3.
31. van Heerden JA, Sizemore GW, Carney JA, et al. Surgical management of the adrenal glands in the multiple endocrine neoplasia type II syndrome. World J Surg. 1984;8:612–21.
32. Kok KY, Yapp SK. Laparoscopic adrenal-sparing surgery for primary hyperaldosteronism due to aldosterone-producing adenoma. Surg Endosc. 2002;16:108–11.
33. Angeli A, Osella G, Alì A, et al. Adrenal incidentaloma: an overview of clinical and epidemiological data from the National Italian Study Group. Horm Res. 1997;47:279–83.
34. Ikeda Y, Takami H, Niimi M, et al. Laparoscopic partial or cortical-sparing adrenalectomy by dividing the adrenal central vein. Surg Endosc. 2001;15:747–50.
35. Ates M, Akin Y. Re: Giuseppe Simone, Umberto Anceschi, Gabriele Tuderti, et al. Robot-assisted Partial Adrenalectomy for the Treatment of Conn's Syndrome: Surgical Technique, and Perioperative and Functional Outcomes. Eur Urol 2019;75:811–816. Eur Urol. 2020;78:e83–4.

Chapter 16
Endourology and Robotic Surgery in Andrology

Ahmet Halil Sevinc, Turgay Kacan, Murat Dursun, and Ates Kadioglu

Endourology in Andrology

It is aimed to explore the role of endourology in the field of andrology, highlighting key advancements, techniques, and their clinical applications. This is a review of how endourological approaches are being utilized to address andrological conditions, and to discuss their efficacy, safety, and potential future developments. Endourological procedures play a crucial role in the management of male infertility, particularly in cases involving anatomical obstructions or abnormalities. The minimally invasive nature of these techniques, combined with their high success rates and safety profiles, makes them an invaluable component of modern andrological practice. Transurethral resection of the ejaculatory duct and laparoscopic varicocelectomy are two of these procedures.

Transurethral Resection of the Ejaculatory Duct (TURED)

Introduction

Azoospermia (the lack of sperm in the ejaculate) is found in 15% of infertile men; in 40% of these patients, obstructive azoospermia is the reason. An obstruction at the level of the epididymis or further distal to the vas deferens can be surgically reconstructed and is therefore a surgically reversible cause of male infertility. Obstructions more distal to the vas deferens are uncommon and rarely diagnosed,

A. H. Sevinc · T. Kacan · M. Dursun · A. Kadioglu (✉)
Division of Andrology, Department of Urology, Istanbul University Istanbul School of Medicine, Istanbul, Turkiye

S. Tonyali et al. (eds.), *Current Endourology*,
https://doi.org/10.1007/978-3-032-00010-1_16

but they can still be treated using endoscopic surgical techniques [1]. There is a possibility of transurethral correction of the narrow segment at the terminal end of the vas where the ejaculatory ducts enter the urethra [2].

Ejaculatory duct obstruction (EDO) is rare and is diagnosed in 1–5% of infertile men [3]. The availability of high-resolution transrectal ultrasonography (TRUS) has led to an increase in the diagnosis of this disorder in symptomatic or asymptomatic men [4–6]. In most men, EDO is treated using transurethral resection of the ejaculatory ducts (TURED), and there have been several reports of successful pregnancies after surgery [3, 7–10].

EDO is one of the few surgically correctable causes of male infertility [8, 10]. EDO can be categorized as complete or incomplete, anatomical, functional, congenital or acquired. Complete obstruction of both ducts and functional obstructions result in low-volume ejaculate, whereas partial or unilateral obstruction may be associated with normal or low seminal volumes. Although most patients with any type of EDO may present with postejaculatory pain or hematospermia, most are asymptomatic except for infertility. Patients with unilateral or partial EDO may have severe oligoasthenospermia [11].

Diagnosis of EDO requires a high level of suspicion, therefore, the clinician should consider this in the differential diagnosis of men presenting with nonspecific complaints of sexual dysfunction, such as periejaculatory pain, low ejaculate volume, and hematospermia, which may be related to underlying EDO.

Although TRUS is most commonly used in urology to visualize the prostate for prostate biopsy, it is also a method to evaluate obstructive azoospermia. SVs are identified at the posterior base of the prostate. The vas deferens may be located medial to the ipsilateral LV. ED is a hypoechoic structure on transrectal ultrasonography [12]. If TRUS shows SV width > 1.5 cm or ED diameter >2.3 mm, EDO should be suspected. Diagnosis is more likely if observed in conjunction with a cyst or duct calcification [13].

Surgical Technique

First described by Farley and Barnes in 1973 for the treatment of ejaculatory duct stenosis, TURED remains the mainstay of EDO treatment [14]. The procedure can be performed under general or regional anesthesia, and the standard surgical setup is the same as for transurethral resection of the prostate (TURP) and is draped to allow digital rectal examination to aid palpation and expression of the seminal vesicles. TURED is performed using cystourethrosocopy to inspect the verumontanum, urethral sphincter, and the position of the bladder neck [15]. Careful examination is performed for midline cysts, extension of the ejaculatory ducts, bulbous or bilobed verumontana, and inflammatory calcifications. Resection should be carried out with using a pediatric resectoscope (with a smaller resection loop) or a conventional resectoscope in the midline near the verumontanum (for complete occlusion) or laterally (hemi TURED for unilateral occlusion) with pure cut to minimize further cauterization of the ejaculatory ducts that could lead to restenosis. The level of resection is guided by synchronous TRUS, especially when the obstruction is in the proximal ducts, the surgeon must always be alert to potential injuries to the rectum, bladder neck and external urethral sphincter to avoid inadvertent injury to the rectum. HemiTURED can be used to substitute resection of the entire verumontanum in patients with partial EDO. At the correct level of resection, cloudy, milky fluid is often seen flowing through the opened ducts. Adjunctive studies such as vasography or SV chromotubation may be used simultaneously to confirm patency. Patients will typically require urinary catheterization for 24 h post-operatively. After the TURED procedure, ejaculation may begin again after 7–10 days. A semen analysis may be performed up to 2 weeks after TURED and repeated at regular intervals thereafter until semen parameters stabilize [16].

Possible complications of TURED include epididymo-orchitis, gross hematuria, acute urinary retention, urinary reflux into EDs and SVs, retrograde ejaculation due to bladder neck damage, urinary incontinence due to external urinary sphincter resection, and secondary obstruction of EDs due to scarring. Secondary obstruction of EDs is a feared complication in men presenting with oligoasthenospermia resulting from partial obstruction, which can lead to azoospermia. Complication rates have been reported from 4% to 26% [7, 17–19]. If urinary reflux in the ED or SV is suspected because of watery ejaculates, seminal creatinine can be checked. Terminal incontinence can even be severe enough to require the use of incontinence pads. Goluboff performed a voiding cystourethrography on a patient 2 years after TURED and showed unilateral urinary reflux with delayed drainage of contrast after voiding [20].

Early complications are less common. After catheter removal, acute urinary retention may occur, especially in patients with preexisting voiding dysfunction. Reinsertion of the catheter for 24–48 h is required [20]. Patients should be counseled about the potential outcomes of TURED. Approximately 4% of patients treated with TURED for partial EDO become azoospermic, possibly due to postoperative fibrosis of the ejaculatory ducts [21].

Evaluation

Popken et al. showed that TURED eliminated painful ejaculation and hematospermia associated with EDO in all patients [22]. A similar study by Weintraub et al. using TURED as the preferred treatment modality for patients with radiologically proven EDO also showed relief of perijaculatory pain as well as hematospermia and perineal and/or testicular pain in the majority of patients [8]. Long-term relief of postcoital or perineal pain following TURED can be expected in 60% of patients [14, 23]. Yurdakul et al. demonstrated a 100% response rate in achieving normal ejaculatory volumes after TURED in a retrospective review of 12 azoospermic men with complete EDO [24]. In their 10-year series, Smith et al. showed that men treated for low-volume azoospermia or low-volume oligoasthenospermia had a similar (65–70%) improvement in semen quality after TURED [25]. One study has shown that the underlying etiology of EDO is an important factor for successful symptom relief after TURED. The authors showed that patients with congenital EDO had superior success rates with 100% improvement in semen parameters (motility and volume), 83% improvement in sperm count, and 66% successful conception rate. On the other hand, only 37.5% improvement in semen parameters was seen in acquired EDO group, and only 12.5% of them were able to conceive [26]. In a smaller series of 16 patients, EDO due to cysts was shown to respond better to TURED. The same study showed that patients with partial EDO responded better to TURED (94% of patients improved) compared to men with complete EDO (59% of patients showed improvement) in postoperative semen analysis [7].

In selected patients, TURED can result in significant improvements in semen parameters and subsequent successful conception rates, offering a safe and minimally invasive technique to resolve EDO. As with all surgical cases, careful patient selection, adequate patient counseling, and the surgeon's operative experience are essential for optimal results. Patients should be made aware of the long follow-up periods required to evaluate the long-term effects of the procedure. The chances of success are minimal in patients with evidence of concomitant testicular dysfunction; Overall spontaneous pregnancy rates in these men are low (20–30%) and patients should be informed of the potential adverse outcomes prior to the procedure to ensure realistic patient expectations. With this in mind, a high index of suspicion should always be maintained for the diagnosis of factor infertility when EDO is presented with male patients.

Laparoscopic Varicocelectomy

Introduction

Varicocele is described as dilated and tortuous veins of the pampiniform plexus of the scrotal veins. Varicocele occurs in approximately 15% of the male population [27] and 21–39% of infertile men [28].

Despite the wide knowledge about varicocele and many studies on different surgical methods, the ideal varicocele ligation method is still debated. The ideal technique should have low recurrence and complication rates [29]. Different approaches have been used in the treatment of varicocele, including open surgery, sclerotherapy and currently laparoscopy [30–32]. The Palomo technique was associated with a relatively high incidence of postoperative recurrence and therefore the modified Palomo procedure was often preferred [33, 34].

Ivanissevich described a procedure in which the testicular vein was ligated through the inguinal ring and the testicular artery was preserved [34]. In 1991, Aaberge and colleagues introduced laparoscopic varicocelectomy as a new and less invasive treatment for varicocele [35].

In recent years, laparoscopic varicocele ligation (LV) has gained popularity and acceptance. The laparoscope's internal magnification helps in identifying the spermatic veins and artery, which can potentially decrease the risk of varicocele recurrence and ischemic damage to the testicle. Additionally, this technique allows the surgeon to preserve the lymphatics and genital branches of the genitofemoral nerve that run alongside the spermatic vessels, thereby reducing the formation of lymphoceles and postoperative pain [36].

Laparoscopic management of varicoceles in adults may reflect the excellent visibility of the posterior abdominal wall achieved using the laparoscope, allowing comprehensive exploration of areas known to be responsible for recurrent varicoceles, namely the renal, vas-associated, pelvic and retropubic crossed veins [36]. The traditional laparoscopic technique of varicose vein ligation is to ligate the veins with clips and then intersect them between the clips [37, 38]. Sasagawa successfully dissected the internal spermatic vessels using a completely harmonic scalpel [39].

Current guidelines recommend that treatment for varicocele should be considered in patients with clinically palpable disease and abnormal semen parameters. However, clinicians often struggle with deciding whether to treat varicocele in patients with testicular pain or low testosterone levels. Moreover, varicocele is highly associated with DNA fragmentation due to oxidative stress, and surgical repair of varicocele has been shown to improve markers of oxidative stress and consequently sperm DNA integrity [40].

The American Urological Association suggests that varicocele treatment should be offered to the male partner of a couple who are trying to conceive when the following conditions are met: the varicocele can be felt, the couple has been diagnosed with infertility, the woman has normal fertility or potentially treatable infertility, and the male partner has one or more abnormal semen parameters. In adolescents treatment may beconsidered if there is significant testicular asymmetry (>20%) observed in repeated examinations, testicular pain, or abnormal semen analysis results. Repairing very large varicoceles is also possible; however, the for this is relative and controversial if there is no atrophy present.

It is important to take an appropriate history from the onset of symptoms to their appearance. A general physical examination should be followed by an appropriate clinical examination of the external genitalia, groin and testicle.

Routine preoperative examinations were performed after the clinical diagnosis of varicocele was made to ensure suitability for general anesthesia. Ultrasonographic examination can be performed to evaluate enlarged veins along the spermatic cord and epididymis, the diameter of the largest vein when the patient is performing the Valsalva maneuver while standing, reflux in the veins during the Valsalva maneuver, and other pathologies that may cause varicocele, especially in the right retroperitoneum.

Surgical Technique

The procedure is usually performed using general anesthesia. A prophylactic intravenous antibiotic is during induction before to the incision. The patient is positioned in supine position. An urethral catheter is placed to empty the bladder, and a Veress needle is inserted at the umbilicus to inflate the peritoneal cavity with carbon dioxide. Alternatively, Hasson's technique can be performed at the lower edge of the umbilicus, and the trocar can be inserted into the peritoneum under direct vision. Pneumoperitoneum is created with CO_2 at 2–3 liters per minute and an intra-abdominal pressure of 10–12 mmHg is achieved. Three laparoscopic ports are placed for varicocelectomy according to baseball diamond concept. Trocars; 5 mm or 10 mm supra-umbilical trocar for camera and insufflation, 5 mm trocar halfway to two-thirds between the umbilicus and pubic symphysis in the midline (for unilateral case), 5 mm trocar on ipsilateral side of the varicocele, lateral to the epigastric vessels around the line of the umbilicus (for bilateral cases two 5 mm trocars on each side) should be placed. The intraabdominal vas deferens can be identified as structure joining the spermatic cord above the internal inguinal ring. The gonadal vessels are visualized easily in the retroperitoneum. The posterior peritoneum is incised with cautery, laser, or endoscopic scissors. The gonadal vessels are then mobilized; however, it is sometimes difficult to reliably identify the spermatic artery and its branches through the laparoscope. Therefore, many surgeons prefer to use the laparoscopic Doppler probe to facilitate the identification of the spermatic artery during laparoscopic varicocele ligation. After identifying the gonadal artery, the surgeon isolates the gonadal vein or veins using blunt dissection with atraumatic graspers. The testicular veins are sealed with suture, clips or a harmonic scalpel (depending on the surgeon 's preference). Hemostasis is secured and confirmed. Laparoscopic ligation is an effective and safe approach to achieving pain relief in varicocele patients [41].

Evaluation

After in 1991, Aaberge and colleagues introduced laparoscopic varicocelectomy then laparoscopic varicocele ligation has been performed by many urologists and reports have been published from various medical centers. Data show that laparoscopic varicocele ligation is therapeutically comparable to open surgical and radiographic (embolization) techniques [42].

In a systematic review consisted of 1021 patients, compared to microsurgical group laparoscopic could significantly increase the risk of hydrocele, significantly increase the recurrence rate and no significant difference in spontaneous pregnancy between patients in both groups [43].

Wu et al., found that sperm concentration parameters increased significantly in microsurgery than in laparoscopic surgery. In this review compared to the laparoscopy group, the microsurgery group had lower postoperative incidence of hydrocele and recurrence rate, but longer in the operation time [44].

Pajovic et al. stated that although laparoscopic surgery could spare both the spermatic artery and lymphatic channel, identification and preservation of both was better and more reliable on the microsurgical approach [45].

In a meta-analysis indicated that compared with open varicocelectomy, microsurgery had a higher pregnancy rate, while there was no significant difference between microsurgical and laparoscopic varicocelectomies or between laparoscopic and open varicocelectomies [46].

Robotic Surgery in Andrology

Robot assisted surgery has been utilized in various fields of medical practice since the first approach into robotic systems in 1985 [47]. In urology, the use of robotic procedures began in the year 2000, particularly in the radical surgery of the prostate, as the prostate is located in a challenging area to access [48]. In 2004, robotic surgery applied to the ex vivo vaso-vasostomy model, as demonstrated by Kuang and colleagues, proved to be feasible in terms of application [49]. This study highlighted the applicability of robotic surgical technology for andrological procedures, pioneering robotic surgical applications in andrology. Subsequently, successful use of robotic surgery has been demonstrated in in vivo vaso-vasostomy, microsurgical varicocelectomy, denervation of the spermatic cord in chronic testicular pain, and microTESE procedures in non-obstructive azoospermic patients [50].

With technological advancements, robotic surgery can mitigate the hand tremors of the surgeon and assist in performing precise maneuvers by mimicking wrist movements. Additionally, it provides the capability to perform surgeries easily in hard-to-reach areas. Its minimally invasive nature can expedite the recovery process, reduce pain, and shorten hospital stays. Three-dimensional and 10–15 times magnified imaging contribute to a clearer view of the surgical field.

Robot-Assisted Microsurgical Vasovasostomy and Vasoepididymostomy

Introduction

Obstructive azoospermia refers to the absence of sperm in the ejaculate due to blockage in the reproductive ducts despite normal sperm production within the testis [51]. This condition affects 20–40% of azoospermic males [52]. Obstruction can manifest as functional blockage in intratesticular, epididymal, vas deferens, ejaculatory duct, or distal seminal channels.

In cases of intratesticular obstruction, sperm retrieval can only be achieved through the testicular sperm extraction (TESE) method. For males with epididymal or vasal obstruction, microsurgical vaso-vasostomy or epididymovasostomy are preferred methods, provided that the female partner has sufficient ovarian reserve.

Microsurgery is a technically challenging procedure that demands the surgeon's precise manual skills, sustained concentration, and the capability to operate under a microscope. To address these challenges, the robot-assisted microsurgery technique has been introduced. Models have demonstrated a rapid learning curve, reduced operation durations, and decreasedoccurrence of sperm granulomas at the vaso-vasostomy anastomosis site compared to conventional microsurgery.

Vasectomy reversal (VR) surgeries have two indications: the desire to achieve natural fertilization again and the development of post-vasectomy pain syndrome.

Various reasons may lead to the desire for natural conception after a vasectomy. Additionally, although the underlying mechanism is not well understood, pain can develop post-vasectomy. VR can help alleviate pain by restoring flow and reducing pressure in the epididymis.

All patients presenting for VR should undergo a systematic evaluation that begins with a detailed history, physical examination, and laboratory assessment. For patients desiring fertility, it is important to determine the presence of impaired spermatogenesis before or after vasectomy to make a decision regarding VR. Since post-vasectomy semen analysis will be azoospermic, it cannot provide adequate evaluation. Therefore, other methods such as assessing environmental toxin exposure, history of other scrotal and inguinal surgeries, testicular size, epididymal dilatation, gynecomastia, presence of sperm granuloma, and hormonal laboratory measurements should be used in decision-making.

Surgical Technique

In VR, regardless of whether a macroscopic, microscopic, or robot-assisted technique is used, the operation consists of six basic steps: incision, scrotal exploration, proximal vasal/epididymal dissection, distal vasal dissection, and vasovasostomy/vasoepididymostomy. At the beginning, the proximal and distal ends of the vas deferens are palpated under the scrotum and secured with a towel clip. An incision of approximately 1–2 cm is made over the fixed area. It is crucial that the anastomosis is tension-free and that the ends consist of non-fibrotic, well-vascularized viable tissue. If necessary, the incision can be extended to the internal ring of the inguinal canal to gain an additional 3–4 cm of vas deferens length. If there are adhesions to the tunica of the epididymis, releasing these adhesions can also provide an additional 3–4 cm of length. When the vas deferens is cut, the anastomosis should be performed with viable tissue that has sufficient blood supply. If not, segments of the vas should be removed until viable tissue is encountered. To confirm proper localization, fluid from the proximal cut end on the testicular side of the vas is placed on a slide and examined under a microscope. If sperm is observed under the microscope, vasovasostomy is continued; otherwise, a decision is made to perform vasoepididymostomy. To achieve a tension-free anastomosis, the adventitia of both ends is approximated with a 3-0 Prolene suture. After this step, the robot is positioned on the right side of the patient. For the anastomosis, two 5-mm micro forceps along with a 30 or 0-degree optic are used. Micro scissors can also be added to this setup. The anastomosis can be performed either as a single layer using 9-0 nylon sutures or as a double layer using both 9-0 and 10-0 nylon sutures. After similar procedures are performed on the other side, the robot is removed from the surgical field. The vas deferens is placed back into the scrotum, and the subcutaneous tissues and skin are closed with absorbable sutures.

In vasoepididymostomy, the vas deferens is prepared for anastomosis similar to the vasovasostomy technique. Subsequently, the tunica vaginalis is opened for inspection of the epididymis. The epididymal tunica is grasped with microsurgical forceps and suspended, and a circular segment approximately the diameter of the vas deferens lumen is excised to create a window. The vas deferens is brought close to the epididymal opening, and positioned for anastomosis. To reduce tension at the anastomosis, the adventitia of the vas deferens is sutured to the epididymal tunica using 6/0 Prolene sutures. The muscle and adventitial layers of the vas deferens posterior wall are then approximated to the epididymal tunica using double-armed 9/0 nylon sutures. Next, a selected dilated epididymal tubule is incised parallel to the tunical opening using a 15-degree microknife or microscissors, and the epididymal fluid is examined under a light microscope for the presence of sperm. If sperm are not observed, another tubule more proximal is selected for anastomosis, and the procedure is repeated. Double-armed 10/0 nylon sutures are placed from the inside out at the 3, 6, 9, and 12 o'clock positions along the incision edges of the epididymal tubule, and anastomosis is performed with the mucosa of the vas deferens. After tying the mucosal sutures, the muscle and adventitial layers of the vas deferens anterior wall are approximated to the epididymal tunica using 9/0 nylon sutures, completing the anastomosis.

Evaluation

In humans, the first in vivo study of vaso-vasostomy assisted by a robot was conducted by Fleming in 2004 [53]. This study emphasized that robot-assisted vaso-vasostomy could be an alternative to microscopic vaso-vasostomy. De Neayer, in 2007, demonstrated successful outcomes with robot-assisted vaso-vasostomy, showing no intraoperative and postoperative complications [54]. Parekattil and colleagues achieved successful results in vasectomy reversal surgeries performed 7, 18, and 19 years after vasectomy in 2009 [55]. The same group, in 2010, compared 20 cases of robot-assisted vaso-vasostomy performed by a single microsurgeon with 7 cases of microscopic vaso-vasostomy [56]. It was shown that the operative time significantly decreased after the first nine cases. Gudeloglu and colleagues demonstrated a patency rate of 97% in the Robot-Assisted Microsurgical Vasectomy Reversal (RAVV) group and 55% in the Robot-Assisted Microsurgical Vasoepididymostomy (RAVE) group among 180 patients (106 RAVV and 74 RAVE patients) undergoing the procedure [57]. Additionally, during surgery, the TilePro software is utilized to project three different image inputs onto the surgeon console. These inputs include a microscopic image of sperm analysis in the fluid from the epididymal tubule and an additional optical magnification image obtained from the Video Telescopic Operating Monitor (VITOM). The 15–20× extra optical magnification provided by a different telescope during robot-assisted vasoepididymostomy can eliminate the need for the surgeon to manually zoom in and out, potentially enhancing the success of the procedure.

After bilateral open mesh inguinal hernia repair, a patient was identified with iatrogenic vasal obstruction at the level of the internal inguinal ring. In order to perform tension-free microscopic vaso-vasostomy repair, robot-assisted vas deferens dissection was conducted. The portion of the vas deferens up to the ampulla was dissected and extracted through a window created in the medial umbilical ligament via the inguinal canal. This successful Microscopic Vaso-Vasostomy (MVV) was performed by Najari and colleagues [58]. Trost and colleagues, in cases of iatrogenic vasal obstruction following bilateral mesh inguinal hernia repair, successfully applied robot-assisted intracorporeal dissection and robot-assisted intracorporeal microscopic vaso-vasostomy [59]. No intraoperative or postoperative complications were observed, and it was noted that the mesh was preserved with minimal incisions thanks to RAVV.

In the meta-analysis conducted by Seth et al., which included 95 studies of different designs between January 1901 and June 2023, it was shown that the best patency results for vasovasostomy were obtained with the robot-assisted microsurgical technique (94,4%), followed by pure microsurgical vasovasostomy (87,5%) and macroscopic vasovasostomy (83,7%) [60]. While the pregnancy rate following microsurgical vasovasostomy is higher than macroscopic vasovasostomy (47,4 vs. 43,7%), exact pregnancy rates with robotic vasovasostomy have not yet been determined.

Robot-Assisted Microsurgical Varicocelectomy

Introduction

Varicocele is a commonly encountered condition associated with andrological issues such as male subfertility, impairment in ipsilateral testicular growth, pain, discomfort, and hypogonadism [61, 62]. The prevalence of varicocele is approximately 15% in the general population, 25% in individuals with abnormal sperm analysis, 35–44% in those presenting with primary infertility, and 45–81% in men with secondary infertility [63]. Varicocelectomy has been shown to improve semen parameters. In a study comparing varicocelectomy methods, the subinguinal microsurgical technique demonstrated higher rates of spontaneous pregnancy, lower recurrence, and lower complication rates compared to other approaches [64].

Indications for varicocelectomy are the effects on fertility due to damage to sperm, testicular structural disorder, and pain.

Surgical Technique

The procedure starts with a subinguinal incision made over the external inguinal ring. The spermatic cord can be lifted using a penrose drain or a retractor. If the present on both sides, the other side is also prepared. The robot is then positioned on the right side of the patient. Micro forceps are loaded into the right robotic arm, micro bipolar forceps into the left arm, and curved monopolar scissors into the fourth arm. A zero degree optical telescope is used. In the first step, the cremasteric sheath is incised and the vas deferens is isolated, followed by the testicular artery.

All enlarged vessels are identified and ligated at both ends using 3-0 silk sutures or titanium clips. The vessels are cut with curved monopolar scissors. The cremasteric sheath is sutured and the spermatic cord is placed back in its original position. Subcutaneous tissues and skin are then closed.

Evaluation

The first study evaluating robot-assisted bilateral abdominal varicocelectomy cases was reported by Corcione and colleagues in 2005 [65]. This study encompasses two patients from a series of 32, focusing on the feasibility and safety of robotic surgery. Subsequently, in 2008, the first case series comparing subinguinal Robot-Assisted Microsurgical Varicocelectomy (RAVx) with microsurgical varicocelectomy (Vx) found similar operative durations (73.9 min vs. 71.1 min) [66]. Although both groups experienced no difficulties in identifying and dissecting vascular structures and vas deferens, a short learning curve for suturing was noted due to the absence of tactile sensation. Additionally, the elimination of the surgeon's normal physiological tremor was emphasized. No complications or varicocele recurrences were observed in both groups during the intraoperative and postoperative periods.

In a series of 238 patients who underwent the RAVx method, a significant improvement in sperm count and motility was observed in 76% of patients with oligospermia. Furthermore, 28% of patients with azoospermia showed a conversion to oligospermia in semen analysis [57]. Moreover, 92% of patients with testicular pain reported adecrease in pain scores. Additionally, robot-assisted targeted microsurgical denervation of the spermatic cord was performed on 84% of these patients.

The robot-assisted laparoscopic artery-preserving varicocelectomy procedure, performed using indocyanine green fluorescence angiography, was carried out on a total of 45 varicocelectomies in 27 patients [67]. The testicular artery was successfully visualized 47.2 s after ICG injection. Upon evaluation, a single artery was identified in 68.9% of all 45 spermatic cords, while two arteries were found in 31.1%. Within 6 months post-surgery, a significant improvement in semen concentration and motility was observed, and no complications such as recurrence, hydrocele, or testicular atrophy were noted.

Robot-Assisted Microsurgical Denervation of the Spermatic Cord

Introduction

Chronic inguinal or scrotal content pain (CISCP), also known as testicular pain syndrome or orchialgia, is defined as periodic or constant testicular pain lasting more than 3 months, which can be unilateral or bilateral [68]. The etiology, pathophysiology, and progression of CISCP are not fully understood. Etiological factors may include hydrocele, varicocele, post-vasectomy pain, infection, referred pain, autoimmune diseases, tumors, and idiopathic reasons [69]. Sensory and sympathetic nerve fibers are more densely concentrated around the vas deferens in the spermatic cord. Chronic neuropathy developing through the two-hit theory of Wallerian degeneration in these nerves may be a contributing factor to prolonged pain.

In the initial management of orchialgia, conservative interventions such as scrotal support, observation, nonsteroidal anti-inflammatory drugs, antibiotics, and antidepressants are employed. When conservative treatments fail to yield satisfactory results, spermatic cord block is recommended. Microsurgical denervation of the spermatic cord (MDSC) has emerged as an alternative treatment to orchiectomy and epididymectomy. MDSC allows for testicular preservation and offers high success rates.

Surgical Technique

The procedure is performed through a subinguinal incision. The spermatic cord is accessed, the ilioinguinal and genitofemoral nerves are dissected and ligated. The robot is positioned on the patient's right side. The right arm is equipped with microforceps, the left arm is equipped with a bipolar gripper, and the fourth robotic arm is equipped with monopolar curved scissors. Optimal visualization is achieved with a zero degree optical telescope. The anterior cremasteric muscle is incised. The presence of a testicular artery is identified. The posterior cremasteric fibers and the posterior fat component are removed. The vas deferens is isolated and typically the artery and vein leading to the vas are removed from the vas deferens. Then the perivasal tissue is also removed. The robot is withdrawn from the surgical field. The spermatic cord is placed back in its anatomical position. Subcutaneous tissues and skin are closed.

Evaluation

Parekattil and his team developed a target-specific approach incorporating robot-assisted microsurgical denervation of the spermatic cord (RMDSC) and shared their results through seven updates [70]. Patient selection criteria included chronic testicular pain (lasting more than 6 months), ineffectiveness of conservative pain treatments, absence of neurological and urological examination findings, and incomplete resolution of pain after spermatic cord block with local anesthetic agents. The group examined 860 RMDSC cases in their latest published clinical database report. The average robotic console time was 20 min (range: 15–80). Complete resolution of pain was observed in 462 cases (49%), while more than a 50% reduction in PIQ-6 and VAS scores was achieved in 292 cases (34%). Pain persisted in 142 cases (17%). A significant observation was a meaningful reduction in pain during follow-up; 67% of patients at 6 months, 68% at 1 year, 77% at 2 years, 86% at 3 years, and 83%

at 4 years. The average surgery duration decreased from 41 min in the initial cases to 20 min in the latest update. Complete resolution of pain was significantly lower in the latest update (49%) compared to previous reports (70.5–75%). Complications included testicular artery injury in 2 cases, testicular ischemia in 1 case, vasal injury in 1 case, seroma in 4 cases, hematoma in 23 cases, wound infection and dehiscence in 24 cases, penile swelling/pain in 2 cases, pulmonary embolism in 1 case, hydrocele in 1 case, urinary retention in 1 case, port site pain in 1 case, reflected leg pain in 1 case, and port site bleeding in 1 case. Testicular artery injuries were detected during the surgery and successfully repaired; long-term testicular atrophy was not identified. Testicular ischemia was recorded in a case that had undergone previous pelvic and inguinal surgeries. This study demonstrates the feasibility and effectiveness of targeted RMDSCs in the treatment of chronic testicular and scrotal pain.

Additionally, Parekattil and Cohen performed robotic microsurgical ligation of the genitofemoral and lower hypogastric nerve fibers above the internal inguinal ring in 30 patients experiencing persistent pain after microsurgical denervation of the spermatic cord and phantom groin pain following orchiectomy [71]. The surgery was conducted using an abdominal approach, with five cases performed using the single-port method. After 1 month of follow-up, complete pain resolution was observed in 60% of cases (18/30), and more than a 50% reduction was seen in 13% of cases (4/30). The average surgical duration was 10 min (range: 5–30).

Robot-Assisted Microscopic Testicular Sperm Extraction

Introduction

Non-obstructive azoospermia (NOA) refers to the absence of sperm in the ejaculate after centrifugation in two consecutive sperm analyses [51]. Azoospermia is observed in approximately 1% of the male population and 10–15% of infertile males, with NOA constituting the majority of azoospermic cases [72]. NOA may result from either primary testicular dysfunction or a dysfunction in the hypothalamic-pituitary-gonadal axis. For individuals suitable for assisted reproductive technology protocols, obtaining sperm is considered. The gold standard surgical approach for sperm retrieval is TESE. Microscopic TESE (mTESE) is performed under surgical microscopy and has a 50% higher sperm retrieval rate compared to traditional TESE.

Surgical Technique

A vertical incision is made to the scrotal median raphe. The testicle is reached through the incision. The robot is placed on the patient's right side. The right arm is loaded with microforceps, the left arm is loaded with a bipolar gripper, and the fourth robotic arm is loaded with monopolar curved scissors. After the testicle is isolated, a longitudinal incision is made into the tunica albuginea. Then, the tunica albuginea is inverted and horizontal slides are obtained and the surface area is expanded. In this way, it is aimed to reach full seminiferous tubules. Sampling is done from these targeted areas and the samples are examined immediately by an experienced embryologist. After sufficient sperm is obtained or sufficient sampling is performed, the tunica albuginea is closed with 6-0 Prolene suture. The testicle is placed in its anatomical position within the scrotum and the tissues are closed.

Evaluation

Parekattil and Gudeloglu performed 12 robot-assisted microsurgical testicular sperm extractions (ROTESE) between 2009 and 2012 [73]. It is emphasized that the triple image obtained from the andrology laboratory microscope through video linkage during surgery provides an advantage in evaluating the tissue and enhances efficiency. No complications were encountered in these procedures. Although there is a lack of information about the success of sperm retrievability in ROTESE, the authors mentioned that the use of robotics in tissue manipulation and dissection is slightly easier and more ergonomic compared to conventional microsurgical TESE.

References

1. Modgil V, Rai S, Ralph DJ, Muneer A. An update on the diagnosis and management of ejaculatory duct obstruction. Nature Publishing Group; 2016. https://doi.org/10.1038/nrurol.2015.276.
2. Wein AJ, Kavoussi LR, Novick AC, Partin AW, Peters CA. Campbell-Walsh urology. Elsevier; 2021.
3. Pryor JP, Hendry WF. Ejaculatory duct obstruction in subfertile males: analysis of 87 patients. Fertil Steril. 1991;56(4):725–30. https://doi.org/10.1016/S0015-0282(16)54606-8.
4. Jarow JP. Transrectal ultrasonography of infertile men. Fertil Steril. 1993;60(6):1035–9. https://doi.org/10.1016/S0015-0282(16)56406-1.
5. Belker AM, Steinbock GS. Transrectal prostate ultrasonography as a diagnostic and therapeutic aid for ejaculatory duct obstruction. J Urol. 1990;144(2 Pt 1):356–8. https://doi.org/10.1016/S0022-5347(17)39455-7.
6. Littrup PJ, Lee F, McLeary RD, Wu D, Lee A, Kumasaka GH. Transrectal US of the seminal vesicles and ejaculatory ducts: clinical correlation. Radiology. 1988;168(3):625–8. https://doi.org/10.1148/radiology.168.3.3043543.
7. Kadioğlu A, Cayan S, Tefekli A, Orhan I, Engin G, Turek PJ. Does response to treatment of ejaculatory duct obstruction in infertile men vary with pathology? Fertil Steril. 2001;76(1):138–42. https://doi.org/10.1016/S0015-0282(01)01817-9.
8. Weintraub MP, De Mouy E, Hellstrom WJG. Newer modalities in the diagnosis and treatment of ejaculatory duct obstruction. J Urol. 1993;150(4):1150–4. https://doi.org/10.1016/S0022-5347(17)35711-7.
9. Hellerstein DK, Meacham RB, Lipshultz LI. Transrectal ultrasound and partial ejaculatory duct obstruction in male infertility. Urology. 1992;39(5):449–52. https://doi.org/10.1016/0090-4295(92)90245-R.
10. Meacham RB, Hellerstein DK, Lipshultz LI. Evaluation and treatment of ejaculatory duct obstruction in the infertile male. Fertil Steril. 1993;59(2):393–7. https://doi.org/10.1016/S0015-0282(16)55683-0.

11. Avellino GJ, Lipshultz LI, Sigman M, Hwang K. Transurethral resection of the ejaculatory ducts: etiology of obstruction and surgical treatment options. Fertil Steril. 2019;111:427–43. https://doi.org/10.1016/j.fertnstert.2019.01.001.
12. Jurewicz M, Gilbert BR. Imaging and angiography in male factor infertility. Fertil Steril. 2016;105(6):1432–42. https://doi.org/10.1016/J.FERTNSTERT.2016.04.009.
13. Schroeder-Printzen I, Ludwig M, Köhn F, Weidner W. Surgical therapy in infertile men with ejaculatory duct obstruction: technique and outcome of a standardized surgical approach. Hum Reprod. 2000;15(6):1364–8. https://doi.org/10.1093/HUMREP/15.6.1364.
14. Farley S, Barnes R. Stenosis of ejaculatory ducts treated by endoscopic resection. J Urol. 1973;109(4):664–6. https://doi.org/10.1016/S0022-5347(17)60510-X.
15. Paick JS. Transurethral resection of the ejaculatory duct. Int J Urol. 2000;7(Suppl 1):42–7. https://doi.org/10.1046/J.1442-2042.2000.00170.X.
16. Conlin M. Glenn's urologic surgery Graham S.D., Keane T.E. and Glenn J.F.: Glenn's urologic surgery. Philadelphia: Lippincott Williams & Wilkins 2004. 1098 pages. J Urol. 2006;175(4):1579. https://doi.org/10.1016/S0022-5347(05)01058-X.
17. El-Assmy A, El-Tholoth H, Abouelkheir RT, Abou-El-Ghar ME. Transurethral resection of ejaculatory duct in infertile men: outcome and predictors of success. Int Urol Nephrol. 2012;44(6):1623–30. https://doi.org/10.1007/S11255-012-0253-6.
18. Turek PJ, Magana JO, Lipshultz LI. Semen parameters before and after transurethral surgery for ejaculatory duct obstruction. Accessed 4 Feb 2024. [Online]. Available: https://pubmed.ncbi.nlm.nih.gov/8632556/
19. Tu XA, et al. Transurethral bipolar plasma kinetic resection of ejaculatory duct for treatment of ejaculatory duct obstruction. J Xray Sci Technol. 2013;21(2):293–302. https://doi.org/10.3233/XST-130377.
20. Goluboff ET, Kaplan SA, Fisch H. Seminal vesicle urinary reflux as a complication of transurethral resection of ejaculatory ducts. J Urol. Accessed 4Feb 2024. [Online]. Available: https://pubmed.ncbi.nlm.nih.gov/7869511/
21. Xu B, et al. Novel methods for the diagnosis and treatment of ejaculatory duct obstruction. BJU Int. 2011;108(2):263–6. https://doi.org/10.1111/J.1464-410X.2010.09775.X.
22. Popken G, Wetterauer U, Schultze-Seemann W, Deckart A, Sommerkamp H. Transurethral resection of cystic and non-cystic ejaculatory duct obstructions. Int J Androl. 1998;21(4):196–200. https://doi.org/10.1046/J.1365-2605.1998.00111.X.
23. Purohit RS, Wu DS, Shinohara K, Turek PJ. A prospective comparison of 3 diagnostic methods to evaluate ejaculatory duct obstruction. J Urol. 2004;171(1):232–6. https://doi.org/10.1097/01.JU.0000101909.70651.D1.
24. Yurdakul T, Gokce G, Kilic O, Piskin MM. Transurethral resection of ejaculatory ducts in the treatment of complete ejaculatory duct obstruction. Int Urol Nephrol. 2008;40(2):369–72. https://doi.org/10.1007/S11255-007-9273-Z.
25. Smith JF, Walsh TJ, Turek PJ. Ejaculatory duct obstruction. Urol Clin North Am. 2008;35(2):221–7. https://doi.org/10.1016/J.UCL.2008.01.011.
26. Netto NR, Esteves SC, Neves PA. Transurethral resection of partially obstructed ejaculatory ducts: seminal parameters and pregnancy outcomes according to the etiology of obstruction. J Urol. 1998;159(6):2048–53. https://doi.org/10.1016/S0022-5347(01)63243-9.
27. Hopps CV, Lemer ML, Schlegel PN, Goldstein M. Intraoperative varicocele anatomy: a microscopic study of the inguinal versus subinguinal approach. J Urol. 2003;170(6 Pt 1):2366–70. https://doi.org/10.1097/01.JU.0000097400.67715.F8.
28. Greenberg SH. Varicocele and male fertility. Fertil Steril. 1977;28(7):699–706. https://doi.org/10.1016/S0015-0282(16)42669-5.
29. Hassan JM, Adams MC, Pope JC IV, Demarco RT, Brock JW. Hydrocele formation following laparoscopic varicocelectomy. J Urol. 2006;175(3 Pt 1):1076–9. https://doi.org/10.1016/S0022-5347(05)00402-7.
30. Kočvara R, Dvořáček J, Sedláček J, Dítě Z, Novák K. Lymphatic sparing laparoscopic varicocelectomy: a microsurgical repair. J Urol. 2005;173(5):1751–4. https://doi.org/10.1097/01.JU.0000154357.72837.43.

31. Misseri R, Gershbein AB, Horowitz M, Glassberg KI. The adolescent varicocele. II: the incidence of hydrocele and delayed recurrent varicocele after varicocelectomy in a long-term follow-up. BJU Int. 2001;87(6):494–8. https://doi.org/10.1046/J.1464-410X.2001.00110.X.
32. Palomo A. Radical cure of varicocele by a new technique; preliminary report. J Urol. 1949;61(3):604–7. https://doi.org/10.1016/S0022-5347(17)69113-4.
33. Link BA, Kruska JD, Wong C, Kropp BP. Two trocar laparoscopic varicocelectomy: approach and outcomes. JSLS. 2006;10(2):151. Accessed 13 Feb 2024. [Online]. Available: pmc/articles/PMC3016114/
34. Ivanissevich O. Left varicocele due to reflux; experience with 4,470 operative cases in forty-two years. J Int Coll Surg. 1960;34:742–55. Accessed 13 Feb 2024. [Online]. Available: https://pubmed.ncbi.nlm.nih.gov/13718224/
35. Donovan JF, Winfield HN. Laparoscopic varix ligation. J Urol. 1992;147(1):77–81. https://doi.org/10.1016/S0022-5347(17)37138-0.
36. Franco I. Laparoscopic varicocelectomy in the adolescent male. Curr Urol Rep. 2004;5(2):132–6. https://doi.org/10.1007/S11934-004-0026-6.
37. Matsuda T, Ogura K, Uchida J, Fujita I, Terachi T, Yoshida O. Smaller ports result in shorter convalescence after laparoscopic Varicocelectomy. J Urol. 1995;153(4):1175–7. https://doi.org/10.1016/S0022-5347(01)67542-6.
38. Hüscher CGS, et al. Laparoscopic cholecystectomy by ultrasonic dissection without cystic duct and artery ligature. Surg Endosc. 2003;17(3):442–51. https://doi.org/10.1007/S00464-002-9068-3.
39. Sasagawa I, Yazawa H, Suzuki Y, Tateno T, Takahashi Y, Nakada T. Laparoscopic varicocelectomy in adolescents using an ultrasonically activated scalpel. Arch Androl. 2000;45(2):91–4. https://doi.org/10.1080/014850100418765.
40. Vakalopoulos I, et al. Should we expand the indications for varicocele treatment? Transl Androl Urol. 2017;6(5):93142–942. https://doi.org/10.21037/TAU.2017.08.01.
41. Maghraby HA. Laparoscopic varicocelectomy for painful varicoceles: merits and outcomes. J Endourol. 2002;16(2):107–10. https://doi.org/10.1089/089277902753619627.
42. Ouanes Y, et al. Functional outcomes of surgical treatment of varicocele in infertile men: comparison of three techniques. Ann Med Surg. 2022;78:103937. https://doi.org/10.1016/J.AMSU.2022.103937.
43. Warli SM, Nabil RA, Kadar DD, Prapiska FF, Siregar GP. A comparison between the efficacy and complication of laparoscopic and microsurgical varicocelectomy: systematic review and meta-analysis. Urol Ann. 2024;16(2):113–9. https://doi.org/10.4103/ua.ua_3_23.
44. Wu X, Liu Q, Zhang R, Wang W, Gao Y. Therapeutic efficacy and safety of laparoscopic surgery versus microsurgery for varicocele of adult males. Medicine. 2017;96(34):e7818. https://doi.org/10.1097/MD.0000000000007818.
45. Pajovic B, Radojevic N, Dimitrovski A, Radovic M, Rolovic R, Vukovic M. Advantages of microsurgical varicocelectomy over conventional techniques. Eur Rev Med Pharmacol Sci. 2015;19(4):532–8.
46. Yuan R, Zhuo H, Cao D, Wei Q. Efficacy and safety of varicocelectomies: a meta-analysis. Syst Biol Reprod Med. 2017;63(2):120–9. https://doi.org/10.1080/19396368.2016.1265161.
47. Kwoh YS, Hou J, Jonckheere EA, Hayati S. A robot with improved absolute positioning accuracy for CT Guided stereotactic brain surgery. IEEE Trans Biomed Eng. 1988;35(2):153–60. https://doi.org/10.1109/10.1354.
48. Franco A, Ditonno F, Manfredi C, Johnson AD, Mamgain A, Feldman-Schultz O, Feng CL, Pellegrino AA, Mir MC, Porpiglia F, Crivellaro S, De Nunzio C, Chow AK, Autorino R. Robot-assisted surgery in the field of urology: the most pioneering approaches 2015–2023. Res Rep Urol. 2023;15:453–70. https://doi.org/10.2147/RRU.S386025.
49. Kuang W, Shin PR, Matin S, Thomas AJ. Initial evaluation of robotic technology for microsurgical vasovasostomy. J Urol. 2004;171(1):300–3. https://doi.org/10.1097/01.ju.0000098364.94347.02.

50. Douroumis K, et al. Robotic-assisted microsurgery in andrology: a systematic review. Asian J Androl. 2023;25(4):454–61. https://doi.org/10.4103/aja202295. Wolters Kluwer Medknow Publications
51. WHO laboratory manual for the examination and processing of human semen Sixth Edition.
52. Wosnitzer MS, Goldstein M. Obstructive azoospermia. Urol Clin N Am. 2014;41(1):83–95. https://doi.org/10.1016/j.ucl.2013.08.013.
53. Fleming C. Robot-assisted vasovasostomy. Urol Clin N Am. 2004;31(4 SPEC ISS):769–72. https://doi.org/10.1016/j.ucl.2004.07.001. W.B. Saunders.
54. De Naeyer G, Van Migem P, Schatteman P, Carpentier P, Fonteyne E, Mottrie A. Robotic assistance in urological microsurgery: Initial report of a successful in-vivo robot-assisted vasovasostomy. J Robot Surg. 2007:161–2. https://doi.org/10.1007/s11701-007-0025-y. Springer London
55. Parekattil SJ, Cohen MS, Vieweg JW. Human robotic assisted bilateral vasoepididymostomy and vasovasostomy procedures: initial safety and efficacy trial. In: Photonic therapeutics and diagnostics V. SPIE; 2009. p. 71611L. https://doi.org/10.1117/12.808624.
56. Parekattil SJ, Atalah HN, Cohen MS, Video technique for human robot-assisted microsurgical vasovasostomy*. 2007. [Online]. Available: www.liebertpub.com.
57. Gudeloglu A, Brahmbhatt JV, Parekattil SJ. Robotic microsurgery in male infertility and urology-taking robotics to the next level. Transl Androl Urol. 2014;3(1):102–12. https://doi.org/10.3978/j.issn.2223-4683.2014.01.08. AME Publishing Company.
58. Najari BB, Li PS, Mehta A, Green D, Tewari A, Goldstein M. V1593 Robotic-Assisted laparoscopic mobilization of the vas deferens for correction of obstructive azoospermia induced by mesh herniorrhaphy. J Urol. 2013;189(4S) https://doi.org/10.1016/j.juro.2013.02.3143.
59. Trost L, Parekattil S, Wang J, Hellstrom WJG. Intracorporeal robot-assisted microsurgical vasovasostomy for the treatment of bilateral vasal obstruction occurring following bilateral inguinal hernia repairs with mesh placement. J Urol. 2014;191(4):1120–5. https://doi.org/10.1016/j.juro.2013.11.107.
60. Seth I, et al. Vasovasostomy: a systematic review and meta-analysis comparing macroscopic, microsurgical, and robot-assisted microsurgical techniques. Andrology. 2024;12(4):740–67. https://doi.org/10.1111/andr.13543.
61. Damsgaard J, et al. Varicocele is associated with impaired semen quality and reproductive hormone levels: a study of 7035 healthy young men from six European countries. Eur Urol. 2016;70(6):1019–29. https://doi.org/10.1016/j.eururo.2016.06.044.
62. Dursun M, Beşiroğlu H, Aydın R, Kaçan T, Sevinç AH, Kadıoğlu A. Is varicocoelectomy indicated in infertile men with isolated teratozoospermia? A systematic review and meta-analysis. Andrology. 2024; https://doi.org/10.1111/andr.13602.
63. Jensen CFS, Østergren P, Dupree JM, Ohl DA, Sønksen J, Fode M. Varicocele and male infertility. Nat Rev Urol. 2017;14(9):523–33. https://doi.org/10.1038/nrurol.2017.98. Nature Publishing Group.
64. Çayan S, Shavakhabov S, Kadioğlu A. Treatment of palpable varicocele review in infertile men: a meta-analysis to define the best technique. J Androl. 2009;30(1):33–40. https://doi.org/10.2164/jandrol.108.005967.
65. Corcione F, et al. Advantages and limits of robot-assisted laparoscopic surgery: preliminary experience. Surg Endosc Other Interv Tech. 2005;19(1):117–9. https://doi.org/10.1007/s00464-004-9004-9.
66. Shu T, Taghechian S, Wang R. Initial experience with robot-assisted varicocelectomy. Asian J Androl. 2008;10(1):146–8. https://doi.org/10.1111/j.1745-7262.2008.00354.x.
67. Teng J, et al. Robotic-assisted laparoscopic artery-sparing varicocelectomy using indocyanine green fluorescence angiography: initial experience. Andrologia. 2020;52(11) https://doi.org/10.1111/and.13774.
68. Davis BE, Noble MJ, Weigel JW, Foret JD, Mebust WK. Analysis and management of chronic testicular pain. J Urol. 1990:936–9. https://doi.org/10.1016/S0022-5347(17)40143-1.

69. Sun HH, Tay KS, Jesse E, Muncey W, Loeb A, Thirumavalavan N. Microsurgical denervation of the spermatic cord: a historical perspective and recent developments. Sex Med Rev. 2022;10(4):791–9. https://doi.org/10.1016/j.sxmr.2021.11.005.
70. Calixte N, et al. Targeted robotic assisted microsurgical denervation of the spermatic cord for the treatment of chronic Orchialgia or groin pain: a single center, large series review. J Urol. 2018;199(4):1015–22. https://doi.org/10.1016/j.juro.2017.10.030.
71. Parekattil SJ, Cohen MS. Robotic microsurgery 2011: male infertility, chronic testicular pain, postvasectomy pain, sports hernia pain and phantom pain. Curr Opin Urol. 2011;21(2):121–6. https://doi.org/10.1097/MOU.0b013e3283435ac4.
72. Aziz N. The importance of semen analysis in the context of azoospermia. Clinics. 2013;68(Suppl. 1):35–8. https://doi.org/10.6061/clinics/2013(Sup01)05. Universidade de Sao Paulo. Museu de Zoologia.
73. Parekattil SJ, Gudeloglu A. Robotic assisted andrological surgery. Asian J Androl. 2013;15(1):67–74. https://doi.org/10.1038/aja.2012.131.

Chapter 17
Posterior Uretral Valve Ablation

R. Cankon Germiyanoglu and Gokhan Demirtas

Introduction

Posterior Urethral Valve (PUV) is a pathology that causes infravesical obstruction in infants and mostly causes irreversible problems in kidney and bladder functions secondary to obstruction. PUV is a fibrous membrane located in the posterior urethra, covered with uroepithelium on both sides, without a muscle layer. (Picture put) It is seen in 1/5000–1/8000 in boys. It is the most common cause of chronic kidney disease and end-stage kidney disease in children. The course of the disease is directly related to the severity of the obstruction and the degree of kidney and bladder damage that develops depending on the time of intrauterine formation. Although it is not possible to reverse the kidney damage in general, the main aim of the treatment is to restore the bladder dynamics as much as possible and to minimize the additional burden on the kidneys. Despite all advanced treatment approaches, approximately one-third of patients develop long-term renal failure.

History

PUV was first described by Hugh Hampton Young in 1919. The effects of this disease, whose anatomical features were understood before, on kidney development?, kidney physiology, bladder development and function were understood later.

R. C. Germiyanoglu (✉) · G. Demirtas
Ankara, Türkiye

S. Tonyali et al. (eds.), *Current Endourology*,
https://doi.org/10.1007/978-3-032-00010-1_17

Classification

In PUV classification, the classification defined by Young in the 1900s is still used today. Young defined PUV types in three different classes.

Type I PUV (90–95%)

In the most common type there is a ridge lying on the floor of the urethra, continuous with the verumontanum, which takes an anterior course and divides into two fork-like processes in the region of the bulbomembranous junction. These processes are continued as thin membranous sheets, direct upward and forward which may be attached to the urethra throughout its entire circumference. It is generally supposed that the valves have complete fusion anteriorly, leaving only an open channel at the posterior urethral wall. Yet, the fusion of the valves anteriorly may not be complete in all cases, and at this point a slight separation of the folds exists.

Type 2 PUV

When first described, folds originating from the posterolateral aspect of the verumontanum were considered as structures that progressed towards the bladder neck. However, these structures are not accepted as obstructive valves today. For this reason, type 2 PUV is not used much in classification other than historical meaning.

Type 3 PUV

This type accounts for 5% of PUV cases. The valve is located at the level of the membranous urethra, distal to the verumontanum. The valve structure allows the passage of urine from the middle through a transverse space and extends downward during voiding, causing an obstruction mostly at the level of the bulbar urethra.

Embryology

The development of PUV has not been fully explained embryologically. 9–14 days in the intrauterine period. As a result of the defect in the development of the posterior urethra, a membrane development that causes obstruction in this region is considered. Abnormal urethral drainage and abnormal integration of Wolfian ducts into the urethra are the most common causes for the continuity of the urogenital membrane. Type 1 valves are thought to be embryologically formed by an anomaly at the entrance of the mesonephric ducts into the fetal cloaca. Due to this entrance anomaly, fibrous stromal structures that cause obstruction are formed where the plicae colliculi should be. Type 3 valves are thought to be caused by the incomplete regression of the urogenital part of the cloacal membrane. In both types, valves can be thin or thick. It has been proven in some studies that different types of valves actually represent different variations of the posterior urethral membranes that are congenital obstructing.

Clinic

Clinical presentation varies depending on age. Although the average age at diagnosis was around 8 years in the first publications about this disease, nowadays, the diagnosis is made in the womb in a very high proportion of patients (40–60%) due to the much more common use of ultrasonography during pregnancy. In this way, many patients have the chance to intervene in the early period. However, diagnosis during pregnancy is not sufficient on its own due to the inadequacy of health services to reach every part of the society and because only half of the cases can be diagnosed before the 24th week in prenatal ultrasonography. In addition, most of the cases diagnosed before the 24th week are high. Despite intrauterine interventions, death or renal failure develops in approximately half of these patients.

In infants diagnosed in the neonatal period, physical examination may reveal a palpable abdominal mass and ascites (urinary acid) due to distended bladder or hydronephrosis. Severely affected infants may present with urosepsis or a general condition disorder. Respiratory distress may be observed due to pulmonary hypoplasia resulting from intrauterine oligohydramnios. During delivery, these patients may have a cyanotic appearance and low APGAR scores. Today, the causes of mortality in posterior urethral valve patients are respiratory rather than renal or infectious. Most children diagnosed at older ages present with voiding dysfunction or urinary tract infection. In a series of patients diagnosed at a late stage, where the mean age at diagnosis was 7 years, complaints at presentation were; Nocturnal enuresis was reported in 67% of patients, frequent urination in 60%, diurnal enuresis in 47%, hematuria in 16%, urinary tract infection in 12%.

Diagnosis

The presence of bilateral ureterohydronephrosis, a thick-walled non-emptying bladder and an enlarged posterior urethra (keyhole sign) in the boys, especially after the 24th antenatal week, are diagnostic findings. PUV should be suspected in the presence of dry diapers, palpable bladder, hydronephrotic kidneys, and other non-specific findings in the neonatal period. In the infant period, weak urine flow and recurrent urinary tract infection are the most common presentation forms. In older children, frequent urinary tract infections, secondary enuresis nocturna, dysfunctional voiding, and decreased urinary flow rate can be seen. Prune-belly syndrome, bilateral vesicoureteral reflux, bilateral ureteropelvic and ureterovesical stenosis should be considered in the differential diagnosis of bilateral hydronephrosis.

Ultrasonography is the first evaluation and diagnostic tool in patients diagnosed in the antenatal or neonatal period. All urinary system and intra-abdominal pathologies should be carefully investigated in ultrasonography. Hydroureteronephrosis is the most common ultrasonographic finding in PUV. In addition, other identified findings include perinephric urinoma or ascites, impaired corticomedullary separation as an indicator of dysplasia, and an increase in bladder wall thickness. In a study evaluating USG as a diagnostic tool in PUV screening, 74% of the cases had bilateral, 14% unilateral hydronephrosis, and 87% had abnormal bladder (thickened, distant or trabeculated) findings. In the same study, it is reported that while the sensitivity of kidney USG is 88% in PUV patients, this rate increases to 95% when kidney and bladder USG are combined.

The gestational age at which hydronephrosis is first detected is very important for prognosis. In one study, fetuses with normal renal anatomy before 24 weeks had a better prognosis than fetuses with hydronephrosis at the same weeks. A meta-analysis revealed that the most reliable parameter for predicting postnatal renal functions was the ultrasonographic view of the fetal renal cortex. If the amniotic fluid volume is normal in fetuses with suspected PUV, repeated fetal US is recommended to evaluate the degree of hydronephrosis and the amount of amniotic fluid. Amniotic fluid is vital to the normal development of the lungs. Therefore, oligohydramnios causes pulmonary hypoplasia, which is an important life-threatening problem. If oligohydramnios develops in fetuses with PUV, bladder drainage can restore amniotic fluid and normal pulmonary development. Pre-interventional karyotype analysis reveals both male sex and chromosomal anomalies in approximately 12% of cases. It is recommended to put Since the presence of renal dysplasia is an irreversible condition, fetuses with good renal function should be identified before intrauterine intervention. In order to determine good renal prognosis, fetal urine samples are taken on three different days between the 20th and 32nd weeks in fetuses considered to have PUV, and the following parameters are evaluated. The parameters used to predict postnatal renal functions in fetuses with PUV and their normal values are shown in Table 17.1.

Elevated electrolyte and beta 2-microglobulin levels in fetal urine indicate irreversible renal dysfunction. If fetal urine is hypotonic and oligohydramnios is present, fetal intervention is recommended. The main purpose of this intervention is primarily to prevent life-threatening pulmonary hypoplasia by increasing amniotic fluid. If the fetus is younger than 32 weeks of gestation, vesicoamniotic shunt (VAS) is recommended, while if the gestational age is greater than 32 weeks, preterm delivery is recommended. Although this intervention improves the perinatal

Table 17.1 Parameters used to predict renal function in fetuses with posterior urethral valves

Variable	Good predicted renal function	Poor predicted renal function
Amniotic fluid volume	Normal or mildly decreased	Moderately or severely decreased
Sonographic appearance of renal parenchyma	Normal or mildly increased echogenicity	From markedly increased echogenicity to a clearly cystic appearance
Fetal urine biochemistry		
Sodium(mEq/L)	<100	>100
Chloride (mEq/L)	<90	>90
Osmolality (mEq/L)	<200	>200
β_2-microglobulin (mg/L)	<6	>6

survival chances of the fetus and bladder outlet obstruction. There is no evidence that it improves bladder and kidney function. The complication rate of VAS procedure is 21–59%, shunt dislocation is 44%, mortality is 33–43%, and renal failure rate is over 50%. The rate of fetal loss due to the procedure is also 5%. When oligohydramnios is corrected, the risk of pulmonary hypoplasia is reduced. In the PLUTO (Percutaneous Shunting in Lower Urinary Tract Obstruction) study, which is an international randomized controlled study, it was not proven that VAS insertion provided any benefit on kidney and bladder functions. In recent years, fetal cystoscopic valve ablation has also been performed experimentally.

PUV is one of the most common genitourinary system pathologies diagnosed today and constitutes approximately 10% of all fetal uropathies. Although ultrasonography (USG) is a reliable diagnostic method in fetal hydronephrosis, it is very difficult to make a specific diagnosis of PUV alone.

Voiding Cystourethrography (VCUG) is the most important method in the definitive diagnosis because it provides information about the anatomy and functions of the bladder, bladder neck and urethra in the diagnosis of PUV. VCUG should be performed as soon as possible in cases with suspected valve. Neurogenic bladder, urethral stricture, anterior urethral upper urinary tract infections in children with obstruction and PUV Since tract images are similar to each other,

For the correct diagnosis, the urethra image during voiding is absolutely necessary. Posterior the urethra is dilated and elongated. Resim The bladder neck is prominent and the bladder is thick, trabeculated and diverticular appearance due to muscular hypertrophy. VCUG is often extensive bladder diverticulum and high-grade vesicoureteral reflux (VUR) in half of the cases.

In cases with high-grade reflux and/or on USG, thinning or suggestive of scarring with nuclear imaging using mercapto-acetyltriglycine (MAG3) or 99mTc-Dimercaptosuccinic acid (DMSA) radiopharmaceutical in patients with abnormal renal parenchyma split renal functions and renal scar status can be revealed. During this procedure, the bladder should be emptied with a catheter. To complete renal maturation, this procedure must be performed as soon as possible after birth.

It should be done at 6–8 weeks. Effective for determining basal differential renal functions is a method. Visualization of the kidneys in cases of poor kidney function is not optimal. Dynamic contrast magnetic resonance urography (MRU) as an alternative to renal scintigraphy. This method provides high resolution renal images as well as differential. It can also evaluate renal functions, but the need for anesthesia limits its use.

Treatment

The bladder of every newborn with PUV diagnosis or suspected PUV in antenatal USG should be decompressed with a feeding tube of appropriate thickness (5 FR-8FR) after the birth immediately. The prostatic urethra is severely dilated due to valvular obstruction and the bladder neck is hypertrophied. Therefore, urethral catheterization may be difficult as the catheter may be inserted in the prostatic urethra. It is recommended to check with USG whether the catheter has passed into the bladder. The inflated catheter balloon may cause obstruction in the ureteral orifices in the thick-walled bladder, and may also cause spasm in the bladder, which may adversely affect urinary drainage. Therefore, it is not recommended to use a Foley catheter in the first attempt.

Electrolytes, BUN, creatinine and fluid balance should be closely monitored. It should be noted that when serum creatinine is measured in the newborn immediately after birth, it shows the renal functions of the mother. To consider the neonatal renal function adequate, the creatinine value should be gradually increased to 0.3-0. It should go down to 4 mg/dL. However, if renal function is impaired, creatinine remains the same or rises despite bladder decompression. If renal functions are inadequate, important complications such as metabolic acidosis and hyperkalemia occur. Renal tubular acidosis (RTA), renal failure, end-stage renal disease, and somatic growth abnormalities are common in these patients.

In patients with poor general condition, the diagnosis should be confirmed by performing VCUG as soon as the patient is stable after appropriate treatment. Valve ablation should also be performed when the patient is able to receive anesthesia following VCUG.

Transurethral Valve Ablation

The next treatment step in the postnatal patient whose bladder was drained and medically stabilized is the removal of the valve. A patient who diagnosed with PUV,cystoscopic valve ablation should be the first surgical procedure of choice in the newborn. The miniaturization of endoscopes, rapid changes in fiberoptic and digital technology played an important role in this choice. The aim of treatment is to restore normal urine flow to the urethra and to ensure that the bladder is filled and emptied frequently. The reason why endoscopic valve ablation is superior to urinary diversion and passive urinary drainage is that the bladder provides this circadian rhythm.

The most commonly used minimally invasive treatment option for PUV treatment is endoscopic transurethral ablation by using cold knife or heat energy. Other options for PUV surgical treatment, Whitaker-Sherwood hook fulguration, different types of venous urethral valve ablation using a valvulotome, use of a fogarty or foley balloon catheter, Neodymium:YAG or Holmium:YAG laser ablation and valve via suprapubic approach antegrade resection.

The operating room should be prepared before patient enters and the room temperature should be made suitable. The patient is placed in the lithotomy position and the extremities are wrapped with cotton or bandage to minimize possible body heat loss.

6 Fr, 7.5 Fr, or 8.5 Fr cystoscope in neonates and a 10 Fr cystoscope in older children can be used for transurethral endoscopic valve ablation. Before starting cystoscopy, the navicular fossa and distal urethra should be gently dilated with dilators. The endoscope is lubricated using a lubricant gel. Cystoscopy is performed and the valve in the posterior urethra is visualized and type classification is made. An endoscopic examination of the bladder is then performed. Diverticulum in the bladder and the presence or absence of trabeculation, ureteral orifice localizations are recorded. With the bladder full and the endoscope just distal to the veru montanum, the valve is made visible by gentle suprapubic pressure. The aim of valve ablation is to eliminate the resistance to the urine flow by making an incision rather than removing these visible leaves completely.

The PUV can be incised at 5, 7, and 12 o'clock using a hook-shaped cold blade or loop electrode using a small pediatric resectoscope under direct vision with the endoscope. In addition, valve ablation can be performed by using a wire connected with a bugbee catheter or electrocautery, and using a cutting current under sufficient power current according to the device used at the valves at 5 and 7 o'clock. If the diameter of the endoscope used is not suitable with the urethra, endoscopic valve ablation can be tried again after 1–2 weeks for treatment purposes. In infants with a normal caliber urethra, the 9.5 Fr resectoscope Collins knife can be used with the working element. The valves in the posterior urethra are thin and minimal. Because of their vascularity, aggressive resection should be avoided.

The Whitaker-Sherwood hook is in the form of lace crochet and has been used successfully as a method for cutting valves blindly or under scope. The hook is placed from the urethra to the bladder and touch the valv membrane at 12 o'clock, and valve ablation is performed by means of diathermy. The bladder was full in all process.

An alternative method is the use of Nd:YAG laser. Neonatal cystoscopes as thin as 6 and 9 Fr can be used in premature or very small newborns, but their visualization is not good. Some pediatric urologists prefer incision with a cold knife because urethral stricture may develop due to electrocoagulation. Complete resection of the valve during this procedure is unnecessary, because when the thin membrane was cut, the valve was observed to be absorbed in the following days. In recent years, it has been reported that these valves are also ablated with holmium:YAG laser. Mandal et al. They listed the advantages of using Ho:YAG laser in 3 items. First of all, it causes less edema and inflammation with the effect of limited tissue penetration, causes less irritative voiding symptoms in the postoperative period, has better vision compared to other laser treatment methods, and lastly, the use of a small cystoscope in the treatment is sufficient for the use of laser probe and larger diameter emphasized that there is no need for the use of a resectoscope.

Mohan's valvutom is an instrument used in newborns with a diameter of 2 mm and in older children with a diameter of 3 mm. After filling the bladder under general anesthesia, the valvutom placed into the bladder through the urethra is gently withdrawn, first associated with the valve, and then completely retracted and valve ablation is performed. The process is repeated at 3, 9, 12 or 5, 7, 12 o'clock.

To perform ablation with the aid of a Fogarty or Foley balloon catheter, the bladder is filled with an opaque solution with the aid of a 6 fr catheter while the baby is under anesthesia until the posterior urethra is visible. The catheter is removed and a 4 Fr fogarty catheter or equivalent Foley catheter is inserted into the bladder and the balloon is inflated with 0.75 cc of saline. The surgeon gently pulls the catheter back up to the valve level. With a sudden and sharp retraction, the valve membrane is ruptured. It is recommended that the procedure be performed under fluoroscopic control in order not to cause urethral injury.

In developed world countries and clinics where endoscopic surgery can be performed, treatment options other than endoscopic valve ablation have taken their place in history as methods that are no longer used. The bladder is left catheterized for 24–48 h after PUV ablation. Although the best time for control VCUG removal after valve ablation is controversial, 2 or 3 months after the operation. Urethral anatomy, bladder capacity, presence and degree of reflux should be checked by taking VCUG. Decreased bladder trabeculation, reduced reflux degree, and a 2.5–3 ratio of posterior urethra to anterior urethra in control VCUG are findings suggesting a successful ablation.

Extravasation, hematuria, anuria, urethral stricture and incontinence are complications that may develop due to PUV treatment. The overall complication rate seen after PUV ablation varies between 5% and 25%. Prevention of urethral stricture development after PUV ablation depends on many factors. Appropriate and gentle surgical approach, avoiding the use of large instruments in the small diameter urethra, keeping the fulguration time short, avoiding deep and excessive fulguration, performing the fulguration under direct vision, using a preoperative small diameter non-reactive catheter, and keeping the catheterization time short reduce the risk of complications. The use of modern surgical technique and appropriate size of cystoscopic equipment and the restriction of electrosurgery have reduced the frequency of urethral injury to 5%. Bladder neck hypertrophy and high placement of the bladder neck make the bladder incomplete may cause discharge. In these patients, a transurethral incision into the bladder neck can be performed simultaneously with valve ablation or later. However, while this intervention facilitates the emptying of the bladder, it may cause retrograde ejaculation and delay in healing.

Vesicostomy

An alternative to primary valve ablation is cutaneous vesicostomy. This initiative; Hydroureteronephrosis despite valve ablation or urethral catheterization in infants with very low birth weight, premature neonates with a pediatric cystoscope too thick for the urethra.

It may be necessary in the elderly and in patients with progressively deteriorating renal function.

Vesicostomy has some advantages as a urinary diversion method. It decompresses the bladder and upper urinary system and does not affect bladder growth in this process. It allows the continuation and growth of the bladder cycle by allowing urination with low pressure through vesicostomy and allowing the bladder to contact with urinary system growth factors. Another advantage is that it allows antegrade valve ablation. Open or percutaneous vesicostomy has been reported that it is at least as effective as valve ablation in the initial treatment.

Diversion

The high diversion option is used in very few patients. Among the treatment options in this group are percutaneous nephrostomy, cutaneous pyelostomy and ureterostomy techniques. Primary valve ablation is the best treatment option because the bladder cycle is preserved, but it is a good treatment alternative for valve patients with high urinary diversion complex and unsuitable for primary treatment. Indication is believed to occur in patients with PUV when drainage at the bladder level is inadequate or fails to prevent infections. Insufficient bladder drainage, serum.

It should also be considered as a treatment option in clinical situations where creatinine level does not fall below 2 mg/dl or hydroureteronephrosis does not regress.

Follow-Up

At our centre following the second check cystoscopy, the patients are followed up closely by the nephrologists and also in a dedicated posterior urethral valve clinic. The protocol includes regular evaluation of both upper and lower urinary tract anatomy ad function along with periodic monitoring of renal function, GFR estimation is carried out after 1 year of age and videourodynamics performed at age 5 years.

The incidence of renal and bladder dysfunction varies, and a recent systematic review by Hennus et al. confirmed these findings. They found that only the nadir creatinine was a predictor of renal dysfunction. Hennus pml van der heıjden a systematic review on renal and bladder dysfunction.

Conclusion

Primary valve ablation is the preferred modality of treatment. It is physiological as it allows the bladder to continue cycling. The miniaturization of pediatric endoscopes allows for majority of valves to be ablated primarily.

In premature babiesthe urethra may not accommodate the smallest cystoscope, and catheter drainage may be required for a few weeks before ablation can be safely performed.

Check cystoscopy within 3 months of primary valve ablation ensures adequacy of treatment and allows residual obstruction to be treated early. Significant complications like urinary incontinence due to sphincter damage are uncommon, and ensuring good visualization of important landmarks during the procedure will minimize problems.

Short Brief

Endoscopic Valve Management

(Step by Step)

- Place the infant in supine lithotomy position.
- Warm the infant.
- Calibrate the meatus (narrowest point of the urethra).
- Dilate the meatus gently to. 9 Fr.
- Insert the 8.5-Fr instrument under vision into the urethra.
- Incise the valves with the hook knife at the 12, 5, 7 o'clock positions.
- Place a transurethral catheter (24–48 h).

Tips and Tricks

- Do not insert an endoscope in a male newborn or young infant's urethra without calibrating or dilating the meatus in advance.
- Keep the suprapubic tube open during the entire procedure.
- Visualize the valves endoscopically by pressing the bladder suprapubic.
- Leave the valve remnants behind and do not fulgurate the remaining tissue in order to prevent strictures.
- Perform a vesicostomy if the caliber of the urethra in a small premature newborn is less than 8 Fr.

Complications

- Balloon-catheter placement in the prostatic urethra.
- Urethral strictures.
- Meatal stenosis.

Chapter 18
Anesthesia in Endourology

Meltem Savran Karadeniz, Emre Sertac Bingul, and Kamil Mehmet Tugrul

Introduction

Today, endourological interventions are minimal invasive surgeries covering majority of the urological operations. Endoscopy refers to optic examination of luminal cavities and it is named after the examined organ such as urethroscopy, cystoscopy, ureteroscopy, ureterorenoscopy (rigid/ flexible URS). Endoscopic methods are used as therapeutic interventions for such pathologies like transurethral bladder tumor or benign prostate hyperplasia resections (TUR-T, TUR-P), and percutaneus nephrolithotomies (PCNL). Most of these surgeries are performed under local or regional anesthesia whereas some requires general anesthesia depending on the patients' comorbidities and personal choices.

An efficient sedation covering anxiolysis, analgesia and amnesia provides a good comfort for both the surgeon and the patient undergoing endourological interventions with local/regional anesthesia. Sedation may alter consciousness in a wide spectrum from "awake" to "unconscious" depending on the drug amounts used.

Minimal sedation: Patient answers to verbal commands. Cardiopulmonary system is not affected.

Moderate sedation: Response to verbal commands is minimal. Mild cardiovascular depression may occur.

Deep sedation: Patients do not answer to verbal or tactile stimuli but a weakened response to painful stimuli is observed. Spesific attention should be paid for airway security. Oxygen support may be needed [1].

M. Savran Karadeniz (✉) · E. S. Bingul
Istanbul University Istanbul Faculty of Medicine, Department of Anesthesiology, Istanbul, Turkey

K. M. Tugrul
Liv Vadistanbul Hospital, Department of Anesthesiology, Istanbul, Turkey
e-mail: mtugrul@istanbul.edu.tr

S. Tonyali et al. (eds.), *Current Endourology*,
https://doi.org/10.1007/978-3-032-00010-1_18

Various scales are present to evaluate sedation depth. The Observer Assessment of Alertness/Sedation Scale (OAA/S scale) and Ramsey Sedation Scale (RSS) are the most preferred scales to evalute patients' consciousness and sedation level. Sedation procedures have several risks including respiratory depression, hemodynamic instability, and unintentional motor activities during the surgery.

It has been suggested that diagnostic and therapeutic interventions supported by local or regional anesthesia techniques should be under monitorized anesthesia care (MAC). As a definition by American Society of Anesthesiologists; "MAC" is to apply moderate sedation and analgesia with a proper preparation of necessary equipment and experienced healthcare professionals in case of urgent general anesthesia need. Nowadays, in many institutions, Healthcare and medical support services have obliged the companion of anesthesiologists for such sedation procedures. Standard monitorization covering oxygenation, ventilation, hemodynamics and temperature should be provided for the patients and the target is to obtain a moderate sedation to control the anxiety, which is caused by the operating room environment, and also sufficient amnesia and analgesia [2].

Analgesia may not be provided with local anesthesia as desired. Sedo-analgesia is the most appropriate approach in such situations whereas sedation alone is generally appropriate in patients under spinal or epidural anesthesia since the analgesia is complete. An "ideal" sedative is defined to be a fast-acting and easily titrated agent that has a high rate of clearence. Benzodiazepines (e.g., midazolam), propofol, opioids (e.g., fentanyl, remifentanyl), and dexmedetomidine are the most common used drugs.

Benzodiazepines and barbiturates bind to Gamma amino butyric acid (GABA) receptors which leads opening of chlor ion channels to inhibit neural activation. Midazolam is the most chosen drug among the benzodiazepines. It provides retrograde/anterograde amnesia, anxiolysis and hypnosis with a fast-acting feature after IM or IV administration. The efficacy lasts about 30 min. Geriatric population represents high risk due to the hypoalbuminemia and diminished hypoxic neural ventilatory response which leads to hypoventilation, apnea and hypoxemia. Standard dosage for midazolam is 0.01 mg/kg and it can be used either alone or with propofol IV.

Propofol is a hypnotic agent which again shows its effect via GABA receptor related inihibitory neurotransmission. It should be used by experienced physicians since it may cause respiratory depression quite easily. Depending on the administered dose; sedation, anxiolysis, hypotension and respiratory depression are the most common effects of propofol.

A 1–2 mg/kg midazolam IV generally provides relief for simple interventions such as 15-minute-long cystoscopy performed under local anesthesia. Occasionally, fentanyl 1 μgr/kg IV (a synthetic opioid) may be added to sedation procedure. An absent motor activity represents great importance during the endoscopic interventions which requires moderate to deep sedation [3]. Intermittent boluses of midazolam 0.01 mg/kg IV might be sufficient for geriatric and frail patients under regional anesthesia in such interventions like TUR-P, TUR-T, rigid/flexible URS. If the regional block is appropriately performed, opioids may not be needed.

Dexmedetomidine is a selective alpha-2 receptor agonist which has been gaining popularity, lately. It has sedative, anxiolytic, and analgesic features and its symphatolytic effect; leads to a mild hypotension and bradicardia. These spesific effects might be quite useful for geriatric and hypertensive patients since it prevents reflex tachycardia, causes a balanced hypotension, and lowers myocardial oxygen consumption for endourologic interventions. It should be administered via IV infusion due to its short half-life. Standard dosage is 0.4–0.5 μg/kg/h IV infusion following a 0.5 μg/kg IV loading [4].

Spesific Anesthesia Techniques for Different Endourological Operations

Transurethral Resection of Prostate (TURP)

Transurethral resection is performed using high-frequency diathermy. However, nowadays, laser resection is preferred as a minimally invasive technique as it reduces bleeding and prevents the occurrence of TUR syndrome. Resection often performed via bipolar cauterization using isotonic saline which causes less complication in comparison with unipolar cauterization. Electrolyte-free solutions (Mannitol, sorbitol, glycine) are chosen to prevent electric current during unipolar tissue resection which has now become formal technique and is preferred less [5]. Among the electrolyte-free solutions; mannitol is the most common used one with the lowest adverse effect. The most important complication that may occur during the operation is TUR syndrome, which is caused by the perforation of the prostate capsule adjacent to the deep venous structure, and the suction of a large amount of fluid into the bloodstream due to the pressure gradient. Clinical findings generally appear within 15 min of perforation. Caused by hyperhidration and hyponatremia; cardiac output elevates and bradicardia, cardiac decompensation, hypotension, pulmonary edema may be observed. Central nervous system is generally affected leading agitation, restlesness, confusion, convulsion and even coma. Therefore, chosen anesthesia technique is quite important because regional techniques allow clinicians to monitorize the consciousness during the surgery. In general, these operations last relatively short (About 60 min) and single-shot spinal anesthesia with bupivacaine/ropivacaine is adequate. The chosen local anesthetics should be hyperbaric, and considering the accompanying comorbidities, total dose should be titrated (Around 10–15 mg) to cover T10 dermatomal level. Preferably, block level should not exceed this level since it may help early recognition of bladder perforation causing sudden abdomen and shoulder pain. Table 18.1 summarizes spinal regions of urologic organ innervations.

Intraoperative standard monitorisation with electrocardiogram, pulse oxymetry, and noninvasive blood pressure is adequate unless there is not any accompanying cardiac condition which require further invasive arterial catheterization. Patients may

Table 18.1 Urologic system innervation

Organ	Symphatic	Parasymphatic	Pain
Kidney	T8-L1	N. Vagus	T8-L2
Ureter	T8-L2	N. Vagus S2-S4	T8-L2
Bladder	T11-L2	S2-S4	*
Prostate	T11-L2	S2-S4	*

*Prostate and bladder mucosa pain fibers are originated from S2-S4, whereas tension feeling of the bladder arise from T11-L2

represent cardiac pathologies and should be questioned for antiaggregant or anticoagulant usage that requires cessation before the surgery. If used for prophylactic purposes, low molecular weight heparin (LMWH) should be discontinued 12 h before the intervention, and 24 h before the surgery if given for thereupatic purposes. Low dose aspirin treatment is not a contraindication for neuroaxial blocks. Fondaparinux (Arixtra™) 36–42 h, Apixaban (Eliquis™) 3 days, Rivaroxaban (Xarelto™) 3 days, Dabigatran (Pradaxa™) 5 days, Clopidogrel (Plavix™) 7 days, Ticlopidine (Ticlocard™) 10 days, Ticagrelor (Brilinta™) 5–7 days, and Cilostazol (Pletal™) should be discontinued 42 h prior to regional blocks [6, 7]. In cases where spinal anesthesia is contraindicated (sepsis, bacteremia, severe hypovolemia, coagulopathy, anticoagulant medication, increased intracranial pressure, and patient's refusal), general anesthesia should be preferred as the second option. Supraglottic airways can be used for operations that take approximately 1 h, but for longer surgeries, endotracheal intubation is the best method for general anesthesia and ventilation.

Transurethral Resection of Tumor (TURT)

Bladder tumors are resected transurethrally for diagnosis and treatment. As a general principle, it is similar to the transurethral resection of the prostate. Spinal or general anesthesia techniques may both be preferred [8]. It is important for anesthesiologist to know the localisation and the spread of the tumor before the operation. Laterally located tumors may be adjacent to the obturator nerve and stimulation of this nerve causes adductor muscle group contractions which can lead to iatrogenic bladder perforation. Abdominal distention, shoulder pain, nausea, vomiting, bradycardia, and hypotension may be the possible symptoms and findings, after perforation. Spinal anesthesia alone does not prevent adductor contraction; therefore, it is needed to add obturator nerve block. Obturator nerve originates from L2–4 and moves along adjacent to the pelvis lateral wall. After passing through obturator foramen, it divides to posterior and anterior branches. Then splits into several branches which reach hip and knee joints also innervating adductor muscles. Anterior branch motor fibres are located in the fascia between pectineus and adductor brevis muscles; and posterior ones are located between adductor brevis and magnus muscles. To block the obturator nerve, the position should be supine, and the thigh is positioned a little abducted and laterally rotated. Afterwards, a linear USG probe (5–13 MHz) is placed on the inguinal region to visualize femoral artery and vein, and then the probe is moved 1–3 cm inferomedially to observe adductor muscle trio. Two separate injections are made; first into the fascia between *m. adductor brevis* and *m. adductor longus* to block the anterior branch, and second into the fascia between *m. adductor brevis* and *m. adductor magnus* to block the posterior branch using in-plane technique and 10 ml 0.025% bupivacaine for each [9]. One should note, this block may be applied by the surgical team transvesically during the surgery [10].

Considering the operation duration, airway control can be provided via supraglottic airway devices. Adequate neuromuscular blockade is also necessary, occassionally. Otherwise, bladder perforation might occur due to adductor muscle contractions.

Ureterorenoscopy (URS)

URS is a both therapotic and diagnostic intervention for ureter and pelvicalicial system diseases. Generally, the intervention is made retrogradely through bladder and ureters. However, it is possible through percutaneous nephrostomy which is called "anterograde" technique. Today, using flexible devices increases endoscopic techniques' success. Nephrolithiazis and ureterolithiazis are the most common indications for URS (30–40%). Diagnostic URS is the second common indication with a ratio of 20%. The rest are upper urinary tract malignities (15–20%) and ureteral stricture dilatation (5%) [11].

General anesthesia with supraglottic airway devices is the primary method for URS surgeries. Spinal anesthesia may be chosen, but block level must reach T8 level to obtain ideal analgesia. Of note, higher block levels can cause sympathetic system depression and hypotension which is an issue, especially for geriatric patients. In comparison with general anesthesia, longer recovery times and postoperative anesthesia care unit stay was observed afterwards. T9-T11 level epidural anesthesia may be considered for high-risk cardiac patients which is not a routine clinical practice.

For very short diagnostic procedures, deep sedation with remifentanyl and propofol should be chosen, which however again requires experienced physicians to obtain optimum depth of anesthesia and motor inactivity. Sudden movements like coughing are not wanted. Main aim is to provide comfort for both the patient and the surgeon.

Percutaneus Nephrostomy (PCNS) and Percutaneus Nephrolytotomy (PCNL)

PCNS is applied via transcutaneus punction of kidney pelvicaliceal system and basicly is an alternative to retrograde URS.

PCNL is a well-chosen approach for extraction of ureter or kidney stones bigger than 2–3 cm. It is a minimal invasive technique with a quite low complication incidence. Excessive fluid irrigation is required during PCNL which occassionally causes hemoglobine drop. However, the literature does not report TUR with the technique. The most common complication is hypothermia due to the cold irrigation fluids. Other complications are kidney pelvis perforation, bleeding, infection and near organ lacerations. Bleeding generally occurs due to the several percutaneus punctions made or large stones prolonging surgical duration. Transfusion is reportedly needed in 4–6% of cases. Positioning is quite important since the operation is done in prone position, and lomber lordosis must be stabilized using soft-gel pillows around chest and abdomen. Special attention should be paid on face and eye protection from compression. The recommended anesthesia technique for PCNL is general anesthesia with orotracheal intubation. However, regional techniques may be used if needed (Spinal, combined spinal/epidural anesthesia). Regional blocks can be supported with moderate sedation if the surgery prolongs, and the position becomes disturbing.

Local anesthesia is adequate for PCNS. Sedoanalgesia may provide better comfort for the patients. But spesific patient groups such as children or mentally retarded patients require general anesthesia [12, 13].

Cystoscopy

Often indicated for diagnostic purposes (Such as lower urinary track originating macrohematuria) or control follow-ups of the none-muscle invasive bladder tumors, cystoscopy is a common short procedure. There are two types of cystoscopes which are rigid and flexible. Both can be safely used under local anesthesia which is applied through urethra.

Minor Interventions via Cystoscopy

Cystoscopy is a diagnostic method; however some therapeutic interventions are also performed with it as well. These interventions may be biopsy of a suspicious formation in the bladder (punch biopsy) performed via a forceps or removal of a double-J catheter and can be performed under sedation and general anesthesia. But local anesthesia may also be preferred due to the short duration of the procedure. Single-use gels containing 2% lidocaine HCl and 0.05% clorhexidine 2HCl (Antiseptic) are commonly used. This lubricant gel is injected through urethra's external meatus slowly, and 4–5 min settling time is waited. Some specific factors belonging to patient are important and effect the choice of anesthesia technique. Gender is one of these decisive factors. For example, double-J catheter removal is well-tolerated with women whereas it becomes relatively difficult for men considering the strong sphyncter tonus and longer urethral track. Therefore, local anesthesia might not be sufficient. For these cases, moderate to deep sedation or general anesthesia can be chosen in order provide comfort for both the patient and the surgeon. Another factor is having comorbidities which occassionally contraindicate anesthesia. Emphasizing the short duration of the procedure, patient should be informed in detail about the intervention which may cause small pain that is preferred rather than the adverse effects of general anesthesia. An informed consent should be taken from the patient and just before the intervention intravenous analgesics should be administered such as opioids or non-steroidal antiinflamatory drugs. During the intervention, a good cooperation with the patient is necessary. The same management is also valid for urgent double-j catheter placement due to the lower urinary system obstruction caused by stones. Informing the patient is the most important step before proceeding to the intervention under local anesthesia.

Anesthesia Techniques in Laparoscopic and Robot Assisted Surgeries

Laparoscopic procedures are preferred for their less tissue trauma, length of hospital stay and postoperative pain, and better surgical view features in urologic surgeries. Robotic-assisted surgeries are now widely used due to being more precise and still being minimal invasive techniques, even it has been put into practice in the early 2000s. Recent literature displays more advantages in cystectomy, prostatectomy, and pelvic lymph adenectomy when compared to laparoscopic techniques [14]. However, both surgical techniques require special anesthetic considerations taking the physiological changes into account due to pneumoperitoneum and surgical position [15].

Physiologic Effects of Pneumoperitoneum

Cardiovascular effects With the start of insufflation, intraabdominal pressure elevation results in cardiac output increase due to venous return which was already pooled in the splanchnic circulation. Cardiac output may decrease 30% because of the vena cava inferior occlusion in the later phases. Along with the dropped output, insufflation caused hypercarbia lead cathecolamin decharge that increases systemic vascular resistance. Thereby, elevated blood pressure and pulmonary vascular resistance, tachycardia, myocardial strain, and dropped renal, portal, and splanchnic perfusion occur. Profound hypercarbia and acidosis cause myocard depression and cardiovascular collapse. Considering all these conditions, it is extremely important to preserve hemodynamic stability intraoperatively [16].

Respiratory effects Functional residual capacity (FRC) decreases due to intraabdominal pressure increase and upward shift of the diaphragma. This is also enhanced by trendelenburg position. As FRC drops, increased airway pressure, reduced pulmonary compliance, ventilation-perfusion mismatch, atelectasis, hypoxia, and hypercarbia may be observed. Intraoperative protective ventilation strategies, positive end-expiratory pressure and intermittant recruitment maneuvers of the lung are chosen in order to lessen detrimental effects of pneumoperitoneum [15, 17].

Renal effects Glomerular and medullar blood flow decrease due to perirenal pressure increase. Plasma renin, angiotensin, aldosteron, and antidiuretic hormone levels elevate. Intraabdominal pressure exceeding 20 mmHg results in approximate 25% decrease of glomerular filtration which eventually causes in urinary output decrease. Literature represents an increased risk of acute kidney injury if there is accompanying chronic hypertension in laparoscopic and robotic surgery patients [18].

Neurologic effects Intraabdominal pressure increase also reduces cerebral blood flow and intracranial pressure increase. Hypercarbia contributes serebral edema development. Fluctuation in consciousness is common in the postoperative period, and especially delirium may be present in the elderly. Retroperitoneal surgeries are known to be associated with hypercarbia, and intraoperative goal should be based on preserving carbondioxyde levels between normal limits (40–45 mmHg).

Other complications include subcutaneus emphysema, pneumothorax, pneumopericardium, and venous gas embolism. Sudden $EtCO_2$ drop and hypotension are generally associated with venous gas embolism. In such situations, intraabdominal gas should be drained away immediately, and the patient should be taken trendelenburg and left lateral decubitus position. Inotropes (norepinephrine, epinephrine) may be chosen to prevent hypotension. If cardiovascular collapse occurs, cardiopulmonary resuscitation should be started immediately [19, 20].

Physiologic Effects of the Surgical Position

Generally, 20–30° of trendelenburg is adequate for laparoscopic surgeries, whereas robotic prostatectomies require a steeper trendelenburg (45°) for better surgical visualisation. However, considering pneumoperitoneum, this situation causes low FRC, reduced compliance, ventilation-perfusion mismatch, and even pulmonary edema. Prolonged steep trendelenburg results in cephalad shift of diaphragma which occassionally leads intubation tube displacement. In addition, edema in the upper airways and face, and also cerebral and intraocular pressure elevation may be present [21–23].

Exaggerated positions (as in robotic surgeries) may harm peripheral nerves by stretching or occluding. Extremities and the face should be protected, shoulders should be supported using gel pads while positioning.

Preoperative Anesthesia Evaluation

In addition to routine anesthesia preparation, further examinations such as echocardiography may be required for patients with severe cardiovascular or cerebrovascular diseases. In case of cardiac failure or valvular diseases, open surgical indications may convert to more minimal invasive techniques. Antihipertensives should not be ceased preoperatively. For example, beta-blocker agent cessation provokes rebound symphatetic activity, so patients are recommended to take these drugs early in operation morning. Antiplatelet cessation should be decided based on common opinion of anesthesiology and cardiology physicians for patients with coronary stent. Generally, acetyl salicylic acid is continued until the surgery day. While laparoscopic and robotic surgery is more advantageous in patients with respiratory system disorders, open surgical techniques are more appropriate in patients with glaucoma since intraocular pressure may increase [17].

Premedication

Benzodiazepines are used for anxiolysis except for geriatric patient population. H_2 receptor antagonists and proton pump inhibitors are recommended for fastening gastric emptying. Patients should wear compression stockings for tromboembolism prophylaxis, and in case of increased risk, low molecular weight heparins should be administered before the day of surgery.

Anesthetic Management

In addition to standard monitorization, invasive arterial monitoring, bispectral index (especially for robotic surgery) for depth of anesthesia, near infrared spectroscopy (NIRS) for cerebral perfusion, and train-of-four for muscle relaxation are recommended. General anesthesia is applied via using volatile or intravenous anesthetics [24]. Nitrous oxide should be avoided in such surgeries to prevent bowel distension. Profound muscle relaxation should be provided because of the need for complete stabilization of the patient due to fixed surgical ports in robotic surgery. Rocuronium and cis-atracurium are used for neuromuscular blockade and sugammadex can be used to reverse neuromuscular blockade at the end of the operation. Lung protective ventilation should be applied using volume controlled or pressure-controlled ventilation–volume guaranteed modes. Tidal volume is set to 6–8 ml/kg, and PEEP is set to 5–10 cmH_2O, generally. Due to insufflated gas, peak pressure may be allowed up to 35 cmH_2O which should not be exceeded [17].

Both pneumoperitoneum and prolonged trendelenburg position complicate intraoperative fluid management from anesthesiologic aspect. Implementation of personalized fluid protocols will be beneficial in preventing postoperative complications. Therefore, it is important to estimate stroke volume. Advanced hemodynamic monitoring methods (stroke volume variation, pulse pressure variation, pleth variability index etc. examination) are not very valuable in such cases because of the pneumoperitoneum and steep trendelenburg position. However, there is also one study showing that these parameters are superior to other standard hemodynamic variables in robotic radical prostatectomy [25]. On the other hand, laparoscopy and pneumoperitoneum can reduce glomerular filtration and urine output within hours following insufflation. In laparoscopic surgeries, 3–5 ml/kg crystalloid should be given if advanced hemodynamic monitorization is not used.

Liberal fluid replacement may complicate vesicourethral anastomosis due to excessive urination in robotic surgeries. Intravenous fluid should be kept to minumum (<2 liter) in the intraoperative period. Liberal therapy also aggravates facial, pharyngeal, and laryngeal edema formation which may result in dyspnea after extubation. Considering these, restrictive fluid regimen (zero balance) seems to be the most convenient approach to prevent such complications [26, 27]. Noradrenaline infusion use is a good option to provide blood pressure regulation. If blood loss exceeds 500 ml, erythrocyte suspension and fresh frozen plasma should be transfused.

Once the position is brought back to supine, fluid deficit should be provided with balanced electrolyte solutions. Of note, correcting anemia prior to surgery reduces the acute kidney injury development. Blood pressure regulation is also very important in hypertensive patients to prevent akut kidney injury prior to surgery. Insufflation pressure should not exceed 10–12 mmHg and ischemia duration must be shorter than 25 min in partial nephrectomies.

Emergence and Recovery

Main goal is to provide a quick, comfortable, and complication-free recovery. Pre-extubation recruitment maneuver is reported to reduce postoperative respiratory complications by preventing hypoxia and hypercarbia. Postoperative nausea-vomiting is a common complication after laparoscopic surgery. Thereby, reducing gastric content and administering anti-emetics may be beneficial. Postoperative intensive care follow-up may be necessary occassionally, and dexamethasone may be administered to prevent edema related complications. Patients with comorbidities should be admitted to intensive care unit and taken into monitorized care.

Postoperative Analgesia Management

Compared with the open techniques, laparoscopic and robotic surgeries reduce postoperative pain and analgesic requirement, yet the pain characteristic is still complex. Incision, port and drainage related somatic pain, peritoneal and diaphragmatic irritation related shoulder pain, and tissue trauma related inflamator pain should be intervened with multimodal analgesic therapy. Surgery team may choose wound infiltration with local anesthetics. As an IV agent, paracetamol 2 g/day may be chosen. Nonsteroidal anti-inflammatory agents should be avoided in urologic oncology patients because of possible nephrotoxicity. Morphine is a well-selected opioid which may be used as intermittent IV boluses (0.1 mg/kg) or patient controlled analgesie (PCA), however respiratory depression and nausea-vomiting should be taken into account. On the other hand, tramadol can be applied as an IV boluses of 1 mg/kg per 6 h. Its analgesic efficacy is weaker than morphine and may cause nausea-vomiting.

Epidural analgesia is considered as a gold standard for postoperative pain management, however newly defined ultrasound guided thoracic wall (paravertebral, erector spinae plane) or abdominal wall (transversus abdominis plane, rectus sheet, quadratus lumborum) blocks are preferred more for minimal invazive surgeries. Analgesic efficacy of these blocks is close to central block with a lower complication incidence [28–30].

References

1. Riad I, Abdelmalak B. Monitored anesthesia care and anesthesia outside the operating room. In: Longnecker DNN, Brown DL, Zapol WM, editors. Anesthesiology. The McGraw-Hill Company; 2012. p. 1260–74.
2. Sohn HM, Ryu JH. Monitored anesthesia care in and outside the operating room. Korean J Anesthesiol. 2016;69(4):319–26.
3. Vuyk JSE, Reekers M. Intravvenous anesthetics. In: Miller RDCH, Eriksson RI, editors. Miller's anesthesia. Philadelphia: Elsevier Saunders; 2015. p. 821–60.
4. Szumita PM, Baroletti SA, Anger KE, et al. Sedation and analgesia in the intensive care unit: evaluating the role of dexmedetomidine. Am J Health Syst Pharm. 2007;64(1):37–44.
5. Hawary A, Mukhtar K, Sinclair A, et al. Transurethral resection of the prostate syndrome: almost gone but not forgotten. J Endourol. 2009;23(12):2013–20.
6. Lai A, Davidson N, Galloway SW, et al. Perioperative management of patients on new oral anticoagulants. Br J Surg. 2014;101(7):742–9.
7. Rahman A, Latona J. New oral anticoagulants and perioperative management of anticoagulant/antiplatelet agents. Aust Fam Physician. 2014;43(12):861–6.
8. Tyritzis SI, Stravodimos KG, Vasileiou I, et al. Spinal versus general anaesthesia in postoperative pain management during transurethral procedures. ISRN Urol. 2011;2011:895874.
9. C M. (2013). Lower limb blocks. In: Mcleod GA, McCartney C, Wildsmith JAW, editors. Principles and practice of regional anaesthesia. Oxford textbooks in anaesthesia. p. 188–200.
10. Khorrami MH, Javid A, Saryazdi H, et al. Transvesical blockade of the obturator nerve to prevent adductor contraction in transurethral bladder surgery. J Endourol. 2010;24(10):1651–4.
11. Johnson GB, Portela D, Grasso M. Advanced ureteroscopy: wireless and sheathless. J Endourol. 2006;20(8):552–5.
12. Rozentsveig V, Neulander EZ, Roussabrov E, et al. Anesthetic considerations during percutaneous nephrolithotomy. J Clin Anesth. 2007;19(5):351–5.
13. Kuzgunbay B, Turunc T, Akin S, et al. Percutaneous nephrolithotomy under general versus combined spinal-epidural anesthesia. J Endourol. 2009;23(11):1835–8.
14. Trinh QD, Sammon J, Sun M, et al. Perioperative outcomes of robot-assisted radical prostatectomy compared with open radical prostatectomy: results from the nationwide inpatient sample. Eur Urol. 2012;61(4):679–85.

15. Hsu RL, Kaye AD, Urman RD. Anesthetic challenges in robotic-assisted urologic surgery. Rev Urol. 2013;15(4):178–84.
16. Kalmar AF, Foubert L, Hendrickx JF, et al. Influence of steep Trendelenburg position and CO(2) pneumoperitoneum on cardiovascular, cerebrovascular, and respiratory homeostasis during robotic prostatectomy. Br J Anaesth. 2010;104(4):433–9.
17. Aceto P, Beretta L, Cariello C, et al. Joint consensus on anesthesia in urologic and gynecologic robotic surgery: specific issues in management from a task force of the SIAARTI, SIGO, and SIU. Minerva Anestesiol. 2019;85(8):871–85.
18. Nasrallah G, Souki FG. Perianesthetic management of laparoscopic kidney surgery. Curr Urol Rep. 2018;19(1):1.
19. Park EY, Koo BN, Min KT, et al. The effect of pneumoperitoneum in the steep Trendelenburg position on cerebral oxygenation. Acta Anaesthesiol Scand. 2009;53(7):895–9.
20. Hong JY, Kim WO, Kil HK. Detection of subclinical CO2 embolism by transesophageal echocardiography during laparoscopic radical prostatectomy. Urology. 2010;75(3):581–4.
21. Choi EM, Na S, Choi SH, et al. Comparison of volume-controlled and pressure-controlled ventilation in steep Trendelenburg position for robot-assisted laparoscopic radical prostatectomy. J Clin Anesth. 2011;23(3):183–8.
22. Lestar M, Gunnarsson L, Lagerstrand L, et al. Hemodynamic perturbations during robot-assisted laparoscopic radical prostatectomy in 45 degrees Trendelenburg position. Anesth Analg. 2011;113(5):1069–75.
23. Kondo Y, Echigo N, Mihara T, et al. Intraocular pressure during robotic-assisted laparoscopic prostatectomy: a prospective observational study. Braz J Anesthesiol. 2021;71(6):618–22.
24. Herling SF, Dreijer B, Wrist Lam G, et al. Total intravenous anaesthesia versus inhalational anaesthesia for adults undergoing transabdominal robotic assisted laparoscopic surgery. Cochrane Database Syst Rev. 2017;4(4):CD011387.
25. Chin JH, Lee EH, Hwang GS, et al. Prediction of fluid responsiveness using dynamic preload indices in patients undergoing robot-assisted surgery with pneumoperitoneum in the Trendelenburg position. Anaesth Intensive Care. 2013;41(4):515–22.
26. Myles PS, Bellomo R, Corcoran T, et al. Restrictive versus liberal fluid therapy for major abdominal surgery. N Engl J Med. 2018;378(24):2263–74.
27. Cockcroft JO, Berry CB, McGrath JS, et al. Anesthesia for major urologic surgery. Anesthesiol Clin. 2015;33(1):165–72.
28. Gupta K, Mehta Y, Sarin Jolly A, et al. Anaesthesia for robotic gynaecological surgery. Anaesth Intensive Care. 2012;40(4):614–21.
29. Ardon A, Hernandez N. The use of peripheral nerve blockade in laparoscopic and robotic surgery: is there a benefit? Curr Pain Headache Rep. 2022;26(1):25–31.
30. Aniskevich S, Taner CB, Perry DK, et al. Ultrasound-guided transversus abdominis plane blocks for patients undergoing laparoscopic hand-assisted nephrectomy: a randomized, placebo-controlled trial. Local Reg Anesth. 2014;7:11–6.

Chapter 19
Endourological Management of Vesicoureteral Reflux

Aykut Akinci, Ezel Aydog, and Tarkan Soygur

Introduction

Vesicoureteral reflux is one of the most common urologic abnormalities in children with an average incidence rate of 1% of the general population. In children who present with urinary track infections, VUR is present in 30–50% of cases. The exact prevalence is not clear, since many asymptomatic cases may go undiagnosed. Prenatal hydronephrosis and VUR in siblings or parents raises the incidence rates to 16.2% and 27.4%, respectively [1].

Endoscopic subureteric injection of bulking agents is becoming a good alternative to conservative treatment and open surgery as biodegradable substances are getting more available worldwide. The procedure involves a standard cystoscope and injection of bulking material to the submucosal layer beneath the intramural part of the ureter. Improved backing of the intramural ureter, fixation of the uretero-vesical junction to the trigone and the narrowing of the ureteral orifice allows antegrade flow while preventing reflux.

A. Akinci
Department of Urology, Pamukkale University Faculty of Medicine, Denizli, Türkiye

E. Aydog
Department of Urology, Ankara University Faculty of Medicine, Ankara, Türkiye

T. Soygur (✉)
Department of Urology, Pediatric Urology, Ankara University Faculty of Medicine, Ankara, Türkiye

S. Tonyali et al. (eds.), *Current Endourology*,
https://doi.org/10.1007/978-3-032-00010-1_19

Bulking Agents

Polytetrafluoroethylene (PTFE, Teflon®) consisting of PTFE particles suspended in Glycerin carrier was the initially used bulking agent in 1981 and had some good results however it was never approved for usage on children due to concerns about particle migration [2, 3].

Silicone and bovine collagen were discontinued due to foreign body reactions [4].

Macroplastique, consists of a water-soluble polyvinylpyrrolidone gel, which is absorbed and eliminated by body, and a polydimethylsiloxane silicone elastomer implant material that remains in the body to provide a bulking effect. Macroplastique had some potentially oncogenic side effects [4].

Autologous chondrocytes were costly, required an additional harvesting procedure, and showed inconsistent cell growth, which affected success rates [5, 6].

Polyacrylamide hydrogel (PAHG) has been used to treat stress urinary incontinence (SUI) and has been shown to be safe [7, 8]. In a recent study by Cloutier et al. [9] PAHG in VUR was demonstrated to have a success rate comparable to Dx/HA, at a lower cost and without significant complications.

Deflux® (Dx/HA: Dextranomer/Hyaluronic Acid)

Deflux® was developed in 1995 [10]. It is supplied in 1 mL syringes of viscous gel, containing 50 mg dextranomer microspheres with an average size of 120 μm and 15 mg stabilized hyaluronic acid carrier.

After endoscopic injection, the dextranomer microspheres become encapsulated by the connective tissue. Deflux does not trigger any immunogenic reaction, carries no oncological risks and does not migrate from injection site [11–13]. Deflux® was approved [a] by the FDA for use on children in 2001. Initial clinical trials had good results for Deflux [14]; however, longer-term follow-up studies demonstrated high recurrence rates, as high as ~20% at 2 years post-injection [15].

In a meta-analysis [16] of 5527 patients, 8101 renal units, after one treatment resolution rates for reflux grades were: 78.5% for Grade I-II, 72% for Grade III, 68% for Grade IV and 51% for Grade V reflux. If the first injection failed, the success rate after a second injection was ~68%, and ~34% after a third one. The success rate in duplicated collecting systems was lower at 50% compared to 73% success rate of single system. In neuropathic bladders success rate was 62% compared to 74% success rate in normal bladders.

Dexell® is another Dx/HA copolymer with similar safety profile. It consists of cross-linked Dx particles with a size of 80–120 μm. A retrospective analysis of 240 patients (109 treated with Deflux; 131 with Dexell) found no significant differences in reflux resolution or postoperative UTI rates between the two agents [17].

Vantris® (PPC: Polyacrylate Polyalcohol Copolymer)

PPC is a synthetic, biocompatible, non-absorbable and distant-migration free bulking agent consisting of PPC particles in a 40% glycerol carrier gel. The average size of PPC particles are 300 μm, which is large enough to prevent distant migration.

In their retrospective study, Warchol et al. [18] compared 108 renal refluxing units (RRUs) receiving Dx/HA (Deflux) versus 109 RRUs receiving PPC (Vantris). Primary outcome was the resolution of VUR on MCUG at 3 months. In the Deflux group, reflux resolved in 63% of units after first injection and in 92.7% after two injections. In the Vantris group, the initial success after one injection was also 63%, but increased to 100% after a second injection. It should be noted that the Dx/HA group had fewer complex cases (duplex/bifid systems and persistent VUR after Deflux injection) compared to Vantris group; their ratios were 17.6% and 32.1%, respectively. The Dx/HA group also had less patients with grades IV and V reflux than the Vantris group; their numbers were 9 and 32, respectively. Both groups received 1 mL of the bulking agent; however, with different types of needles. A standard endoscopic needle was used for Deflux, versus a specialized bevel tip, concave-side-opening needle for Vantris (the latter replicates a "double-HIT" injection with a single puncture).

In another retrospective study by Kocaoglu [19], 24 RRU's in the Vantris group were compared to 64 RRUs in the Dx/HA group (Dexell) in children with Grade IV-V reflux. The initial success rate after one injection for Grade IV-V reflux was 53.9% with Dx/HA, compared to 80% with Vantris. Postoperatively, febrile UTIs occurred in 8 of 63 patients in the Dx/HA group versus 5 of 25 patients in the PPC group. Late ureterovesical junction obstruction developed in one patient of the PPC group, which was successfully treated with laser ablation in a secondary operation. Subgroup analysis revealed statistically significant superiority of Vantris in Grade IV reflux, however there was no difference in Grade V subgroup.

High grade reflux and ureteric dilation are risk factors for late obstruction, and studies so far have demonstrated a higher risk of late obstruction for polyacrylate-polyalcohol copolymer [20–22].

Current data suggest that PPC (Vantris) yields higher reflux resolution rates, however this comes with a higher risk of ureterovesical junction obstruction. High quality randomised controlled trials with long-term follow-up are needed before definitive recommendations can be made.

Technique

The standart endoscopic technique is the subureteric transurethral injection (STING). Under cystoscopy with a 0° or 30° lens, the bladder should be partially filled. Full bladder filling should be avoided. A rigid metal needle or a malleable needle (most commonly 3.7–4 Fr in size) is pierced through 6 o'clock position 2–3 mm below the ureteral orifice, into the submucosal layer. The needle is then advanced ~4–5 mm into the lamina propria of the submucosal portion of the ureter. For widely gaping orifices, the needle can be placed directly through the mucosa at the ureterovesical junction under hydrodistention. Note that the success rate of the classic STING technique is inferior to that of open surgical reimplantation.

It is important to observe the effect after injecting an initial 0.1–0.2 mL of bulking agent. A characteristic "volcanic" bulging should be observed, raising the ureteral meatus upward onto the dome of the mound. If this effect is not seen, the needle's direction and depth should be readjusted. The ideal final appearance is a crescent-shaped orifice at the dome.

Later, a variation of the classic STING technique in which material is implanted submucosally within the intramural ureter was reported, referred as hydrodistention implantation technique ("HIT"). This technique involves hydrodistension of the ureteral orifice to allow for injection of the bulking material through the ureteral lumen, instead of injecting in a subureteric position. Compared to standart STING, the "HIT" approach raises success rates above 90% with Deflux injection [23, 24]. A further refinement is the "double HIT" approach, which involves two intraluminal ureteric injections: one at 6 o'clock position in the mid-ureteral tunnel, and a second at the more distal part of the tunnel close to the ureteral orifice to allow for coaptation of the ureteral orifice [25]. In a study with a 1-year follow-up, the double-HIT technique achieved a 93% clinical and radiographic success rate, which challenged the necessity of any follow-up VCUG's in such cases[26].

During the endoscopic procedure, using hydrodistention of the ureteral orifice can give some insight into the degree of VUR before and after the injection [27].

Follow-Up

Due to the lack of high-quality studies, there is no clear evidence to guide an optimal follow-up regimen. Usually the patient is discharged on the same day of operation. After discharge, the patient remains on therapeutic dosage of antibiotics for 3 days. If indicated, antibiotic prophylaxis is often continued until the postoperative ultrasound and voiding cystourethrogram (VCUG) are performed at the 3-month follow-up. On follow-up ultrasound, a well-positioned mound is reassuring, although its presence does not reliably predict complete resolution of VUR. If the VCUG confirms reflux resolution antibiotic prophylaxis is discontinued and a follow-up ultrasound is done at 1 year. If reflux persists, a second endoscopic injection can be performed. After two failed endoscopic treatments, if any necessity for surgery occurs, the choice should be an open surgical reimplantation.

It is important to note that the injection site may appear calcified on computed tomography, and could be mistaken for ureteral stone [4].

The Role of Endoscopic Treatment in Overall Treatment of VUR

It should be kept in mind that approximately 80% %80 of Grade I-II VUR and 30–50% of Grade III-IV VUR will spontaneously resolve within 4–5 years of follow-up. However, in bilateral high-grade reflux, the spontaneous resolution rates are much lower [28]. Overall, success rates of VUR after a single injection have been reported as roughly 78–79% for Grade I-II, ~72% for Grade III, ~63% for Grade IV and ~51% for Grade V [28]. VUR itself does not cause renal injury in the absence of breaktrough febrile UTIs or lower urinary tract dysfunction. There is no evidence that small renal scars lead to hypertension, renal insufficiency, or problems during pregnancy. All treatment options should be discussed with parents. Surgical approaches should be suggested if parents prefer definitive treatment. Endoscopic treatment is preferred for lower grades of reflux (Grades I-II). If endoscopic treatment fails twice, any further surgical intervention should be an open reimplantation. Open surgery after an endoscopic treatment is only slightly harder than open surgery without prior endoscopic treatment [29].

A recent prospective randomized controlled trial [30] in 203 children between age of 1 to 12 with Grade III-IV reflux were compared in three treatment arms, consisting of: (1) endoscopic injection, (2) continuous antibiotic prophylaxis, (3) surveillance without prophylaxis. After 2 years, reflux resolution rates were; 71%, 39% and 47% for endoscopic surgery, antibiotic prophylaxis and surveillance without prophylaxis, respectively.

The validation of effectiveness of anti-reflux endoscopy compared to conservative treatment and open surgery is not yet clear due to lack of well structured randomized controlled trials with long-term follow-ups.

Complications

Endoscopic correction of reflux generally has good results in addition to its low risks. Bulking materials have some individal complication profiles. More generic complications, such as ureteric obstruction, are infrequent.

Tips and Tricks

- Before starting the procedure, always check all equipment-especially ensure that the injection needle is patent and not defective.
- Bladder overfilling should be avoided, as an overly distended bladder can make injection more difficult.

- Rapid administration of the bulking agent should be avoided. Inject slowly while observing the effect. The ureteral orifice should elevate, forming the characteristic 'volcanic' mound.
- In order to avoid unnecessary bleeding, the first entry point of the needle should be adjusted according to the visible vessels.

References

1. Radmayr C, Bogaert G, Dogan HS, Nijman JM, Rawashdeh YFH, Silay MS, Stein R, Tekgül S; members of the EAU Paediatric Urology Guidelines Panel. EAU Guidelines. Edn. presented at the EAU Annual Congress Milan 2021. ISBN 978-94-92671-13-4.
2. Puri P, et al. Multicenter survey of endoscopic treatment of vesicoureteral reflux using polytetrafluoroethylene. J Urol. 1998;160:1007–11.
3. Steyaert H, et al. Migration of PTFE paste particles to the kidney after treatment for vesicoureteric reflux. BJU Int. 2000;85:168–9.
4. Starmer B, McAndrew F, Corbett H. A review of novel STING bulking agents. J Pediatr Urol. 2019;15(5):484–90.
5. Atala A, Kim W, Paige KT, et al. Endoscopic treatment of vesicoureteral reflux with a chondrocyte-alginate suspension. J Urol. 1994;152:641–3; discussion 644. 10.
6. Kershen RT, Fefer SD, Atala A. Tissue-engineered therapies for the treatment of urinary incontinence and vesicoureteral reflux. World J Urol. 2000;18:51–5.
7. Lose G, Sorensen HC, Axelsen SM, Falconer C, Lobodasch K, Safwat T. An open multicenter study of polyacrylamide hydrogel (Bulkamid(R)) for female stress and mixed urinary 6 B. Starmer et al. + MODEL Please cite this article as: Starmer B et al., A review of novel STING bulking agents. J Pediatric Urol.
8. Toozs-Hobson P, Al-Singary W, Fynes M, Tegerstedt G, Lose G. Two-year follow-up of an open-label multicenter study of polyacrylamide hydrogel (Bulkamid) for female stress and stress-predominant mixed incontinence. Int Urogynecol J. 2012;23:1373–8.
9. Cloutier J, Blais AS, Moore K, Bolduc S. A prospective study using a new bulking agent for the treatment of vesicoureteral reflux: polyacrylamide hydrogel. J Urol. 2013;190:1034–7.
10. Stenberg A, Lackgren G. A new bioimplant for the endoscopic treatment of vesicoureteral reflux: experimental and shortterm clinical results. J Urol. 1995;154(2 Pt 2):800–3.
11. Stenberg A, Lackgren G. Treatment of vesicoureteral re ux in children using stabilized non-animal hyaluronic acid/– dextranomer gel (NASHA/DX): a long-term observational study. J Pediatr Urol. 2007;3(2):80–5.
12. Stenberg A, Larsson E, Lindholm A, Ronneus B, Stenberg A, Lackgren G. Injectable dextranomer-based implant: histopathology, volume changes and DNA-analysis. Scand J Urol Nephrol. 1999;33:35561.
13. Stenberg AM, Sundin A, Larsson BS, et al. Lack of distant migration after injection of a 125iodine labelled dextranomer based implant into the rabbit bladder. J Urol. 1997;158:1937–41.
14. Lightner DJ. Review of the available urethral bulking agents. Curr Opin Urol. 2002;12:333–8.
15. Brandstrom P, et al. The Swedish reflux trial in children: IV. Renal damage. J Urol. 2010;184:292.
16. Elder JS, et al. Endoscopic therapy for vesicoureteral reflux: a meta-analysis. I. Reflux resolution and urinary tract infection. J Urol. 2006;175:716.
17. Dogan HS, Altan M, Citamak B, Bozaci AC, Koni A, Tekgul S. Factors affecting the success of endoscopic treatment of vesicoureteral reflux and comparison of two dextranomer based bulking agents: does bulking substance matter? J Pediatr Urol. 2015;11(90):e1–5.

18. Warchol S, Krzemien G, Szmigielska A, Bombinski P, Toth K, Dudek-Warchol T. Comparison of results of endoscopic correction of vesicoureteral reflux in children using two bulking substances: dextranomer/hyaluronic acid copolymer (Deflux) vs. polyacrylate-polyalcohol copolymer (Vantris). J Pediatr Urol. 2016;12:256.
19. Kocaoglu C. Endoscopic treatment of Grades IV and V vesicoureteral reflux with two bulking substances: dextranomer hyaluronic acid copolymer vs. polyacrylate polyalcohol copolymer in children. J Pediatr Surg. 2016;51:1711–5.
20. Ben-Meir D, et al. Late-onset uretero-vesical junction obstruction following endoscopic injection of bulking material for the treatment of vesico-ureteral reflux. Urology. 2017;101:60–2.
21. Warchol S, et al. Endoscopic correction of vesicoureteral reflux in children using polyacrylate-polyalcohol copolymer (Vantris): 5-years of prospective follow-up. Centr Eur J Urol. 2017;70:314.
22. Okawada M, et al. Incidence of ureterovesical obstruction and Cohen antireflux surgery after Deflux(R) treatment for vesicoureteric reflux. J Pediatr Surg. 2018;53:310–2.
23. Routh JC, Inman BA, Reinberg Y. Dextranomer/hyaluronic acid for pediatric vesicoureteral reflux: systematic review. Pediatrics. 2010;125:1010–9.
24. Lee EK, Gatti JM, Demarco RT, Murphy JP. Long-term followup of dextranomer/hyaluronic acid injection for vesicoureteral reflux: late failure warrants continued follow-up. J Urol. 2009;181:1869–74.
25. Cerwinka W, Scherz H, Kirsch A. Dynamic hydrodistention classification of the ureter and the double HIT method to correct vesicoureteral reflux. Arch Esp Urol. 2008;61:882–7.
26. Kalisvaart JF, Scherz HC, Cuda S, Kaye JD, Kirsch AJ. Intermediate to long-term follow-up indicates low risk of recurrence after double HIT endoscopic treatment for primary vesico-ureteral reflux. J Pediatr Urol. 2012;8(4):359–65.
27. Kirsch, et al. Endoscopic Deflux injection for pediatric transplant reflux: a feasible alternative to open ureter-al reimplant. J Pediatr Urol. 2008;4:341–4.
28. Elder JS, et al. Pediatric vesicoureteral reflux guidelines panel summary report on the management of primary vesicoureteral reflux in children. J Urol. 1997;157:1846–51.
29. Canning DA. Deflux for vesicoureteral reflux: pro–the case for endoscopic correction. Urology. 2006;68:239–41.
30. Holmdahl G, et al. The Swedish reflux trial in children: II. Vesicoureteral reflux outcome. J Urol. 2010;184:280–5.

Chapter 20
Prone Percutaneous Nephrolithotomy

Panagiotis Kallidonis, Athanasios Vagionis, Theodoros Spinos, and Evangelos N. Liatsikos

Abbreviations

AoA	Angle of Approach
EAU	European Association of Urology
Ho:YAG	Holmium:Yttrium-Aluminum-Garnet
PCNL	Percutaneous nephrolithotomy
PCS	Pelvicalyceal system
SPECT-CT DMSA	Single-photon emission computed tomography/computed tomography scintigraphies with Dimercaptosuccinic acid
TFL	Thulium fiber lasers

Summary

Percutaneous nephrolithotomy is a complex endoscopic surgery that is performed to treat large renal stones. PCNL is comprised of several operative steps. Each step is susceptible to variations implying possible advantages and disadvantages. PCNL can be performed in two positions, prone and supine and each position has its advantages. The intraoperative puncture guidance can be performed using fluoroscopy, ultrasonography or the combination of the two imaging devices. The dilation of the track can be performed with telescopic/serial method with metal Alken or plastic Amplatz dilators and with balloon dilators. The size of the PCNL tract is the factor that characterizes the type of the surgery. Depending on the selected type of PCNL surgery, there are different options in the intracorporal lithotripsy devices

P. Kallidonis · A. Vagionis · T. Spinos · E. N. Liatsikos (✉)
Department of Urology, General University Hospital of Patras, Patras, Greece

S. Tonyali et al. (eds.), *Current Endourology*,
https://doi.org/10.1007/978-3-032-00010-1_20

that can be used. The success of a PCNL surgery is heavily based on a successful renal access avoiding injuries to the surrounding organs and respecting the structure of the kidney. Being familiar with renal anatomy and the neighboring organs positions is a necessity to proceed to the surgery. The complexity of PCNL represents a challenge during the learning curve of any endourologist. Tips and tricks are described in this chapter that could facilitate the safety and success outcomes of the procedure.

The Percutaneous Perspective in Urolithiasis

Indications and Contraindications

Percutaneous nephrolithotomy is a complex endoscopic surgery that is performed to treat large renal stones. According to the European Association of Urology (EAU) percutaneous nephrolithotomy (PCNL), PCNL has been established as the gold standard procedure for the treatment of renal calculi sized over 20 mm in maximal diameter. It can also be applied for lower pole stones sized 15–20 mm [1]. Other indications are the presence of renal fusion anomalies such as horseshoe kidneys [2], symptomatic lithiasis in calyceal diverticula [3] and large stone burden affecting the proximal ureter [4].

The absolute contraindications of PCNL include untreated urinary tract infections, potential malignant kidney tumors, tumor in the presumptive access tract area and pregnancy [1]. Relative contraindications include ongoing anticoagulant therapy and patient general health condition inappropriate for undergoing general anesthesia [5, 6].

Prone Percutaneous Nephrolithotomy

Description of the Surgery

PCNL is comprised of several operative steps. Each step is susceptible to variations implying possible advantages and disadvantages. Prior to the planned PCNL surgery, a computerized tomography for evaluation of the kidney anatomy along with surrounded organs is recommended. Moreover, a preoperative antibiotic regimen is administered for prophylaxis of infectious complications according to institutional regulations. Generally, a ureteral catheter can be placed in the pelvicalyceal system (PCS) to opacify the system and facilitate easier kidney puncture and PCNL tract establishment. Following the placement of ureteral catheter patients are set in prone position and a puncture targeting the PCS is performed in patient's flank area. The initial puncture technique and guidance defers among endourologists and can be performed using imaging devices such as radiography and ultrasonography with or without endoscopic control. The puncture is the initial step must be performed to create a percutaneous access tract (Fig. 20.1). After a successful puncture, a hydrophilic guidewire is passed in the pelvis and preferably down the ureter to secure the access to the renal system (Fig. 20.2). The hydrophilic guidewire should then be exchanged to a stiff guidewire enabling secure dilation of the PCNL tract. The dilations can be accomplished using different dilation techniques and instruments such as balloon, Amplatz or Metal dilators. After a successful dilation, an intracorporeal lithotripsy is performed by the introduction of a rigid or flexible nephroscope through the created working tract. The choice of the lithotripsy device, laser, pneumatic and/or ultrasonic energy devices, is based on the established tract size and urologists' preferences.

Since the introduction of PCNL in 1976 [7] many technical modifications in patient's position, intraoperative imaging approaches, puncture techniques, tract size, type of dilators and intracorporeal lithotripsy devices have been proposed [8].

PCNL can be performed in two positions, prone and supine and each position has its advantages. The prone PCNL is preferred to treat stones located in the upper pole, when the surgery is planned to be performed with multiple accesses and in bilateral procedures [5]. Main advantages of prone PCNL are the adequate

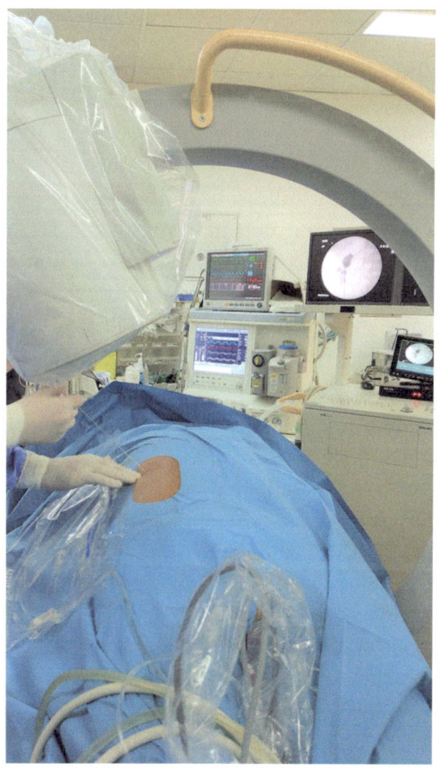

Fig. 20.1 Percutaneous puncture using "bullseye" technique

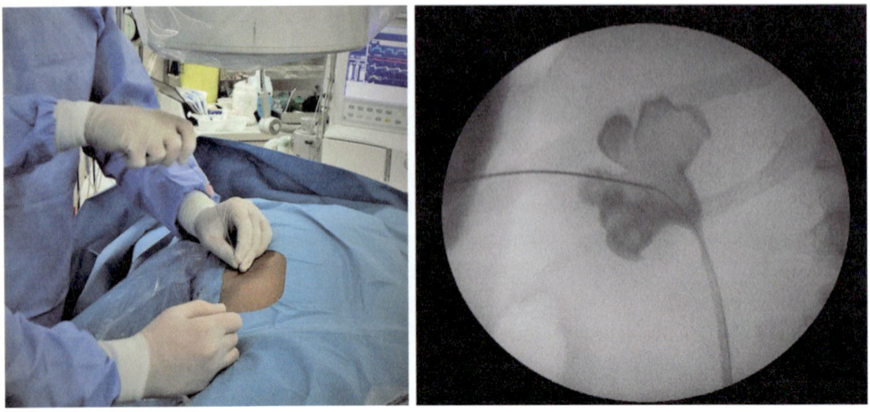

Fig. 20.2 Guidewire passing down to the ureter

puncturing space and wider space for instrument manipulation, the limited distance between skin and renal calyces and the possibility of bilateral simultaneous PCNL. Supine position offers better cardiovascular and airway management, it does not require repositioning of the patient and offers easier access to morbid obese patients and retrograde intrarenal surgery (RIRS) and PCNL combination can be performed easier in this position. Prone PCNL can also be combined with RIRS when the patient is in split-leg position. The two positions seem to offer similar efficacy and safety levels, as they result in similar rates in operative time, stone-free rate and hospital stay. The choice of position should be made according to the familiarity of each position to the surgeon and the other comorbidities of the patient [9].

As stated earlier the intraoperative puncture guidance can be performed using fluoroscopy, ultrasonography or the combination of the two imaging devices. Fluoroscopy excels in terms of image clarity offering the possibility of a more precise access to the pelvicalyceal system, which is depicted by retrograde contrast instillation. Ultrasonography provides information about the neighboring organs and can track real-time blood flow of the kidney using Doppler.

Currently, the fluoroscopy-guided puncture remains the preferred option for most of the urologists [10]. There are several techniques to choose the suitable puncturing spot and to navigate the needle inside the body. Two widely used fluoroscopy techniques are the eye of the needle or "bullseye" technique and the triangulation technique. The "bullseye" technique uses two planes in 0° and 30° towards the surgeon to set the direction of the needle while triangulation technique identifies the entering point by setting the c-arm to 0° and 30° towards the head of the patient and calculating the distance of the entering point from the projections on skin of the two planes [11].

Two common ultrasonography techniques are the longitudinal needle insertion, which allows the full visualization of the trajectory of the needle and the transverse needle insertion, which reduces the danger of rib shadowing and offers the possibility of a puncture in a greater distance from the ultrasound probe compared to the longitudinal access [12].

The dilation of the track can be performed with telescopic/serial method with metal Alken or plastic Amplatz dilators (Fig. 20.3). Balloon dilators are another option. Alken and Amplatz dilators seem to be equally effective [13], but the former dilators are significantly more cost-effective. The use of balloon dilators allows performing one-step dilation, offering reduced bleeding risk. However, is more expensive and can be less efficient than using dilators in patients with the history of prior renal surgery [14, 15]. Sequential use of dilators with increase in the diameter of the dilator is considered for tract dilation. One step dilation technique is a method that only one dilator or one balloon is used to dilate the percutaneous tract not its maximal diameter. Reducing the number of dilators that are used, the chance of traumatizing nearby vessels is minimized and the one step dilation technique is equally effective compared to other dilation methods [16].

The size of the PCNL tract is the factor that characterizes the type of the surgery. Since the introduction of PCNL in the 70's there have been many modifications in the procedure trying to reduce the size of the working tract to reduce the surgical trauma. Gradually many researchers proposed various miniaturized alternatives of PCNL and each one was named in a unique way so that it could be identified from the others. Many variants of PCNL shared similar tract sizes and this fact created a confusion even among endourologists. Schilling et al. [17] and Tepeler et al. [18] proposed categorizations of PCNL in order to resolve this confusion. According to Scilling et al. depending on the sheath outer diameter PCNL surgeries are divided in conventional PCNL (>22Fr), mini-PCNL (≤22Fr), minimally invasive PCNL (18Fr), ultra-mini PCNL (11-13Fr), mini-microPCNL (8Fr), super mini PCNL (7Fr) and micro-PCNL (<5Fr).

Depending on the selected type of PCNL surgery, there are different options in the intracorporal lithotripsy devices that can be used. In conventional PCNL lithotripters ballistic energy, ultrasound or the combination of the two ways of transmitting energy are used to disintegrate the stones. Newer models have also an integrated suction mechanism to remove the broken stone pieces [19] (Fig. 20.4). In

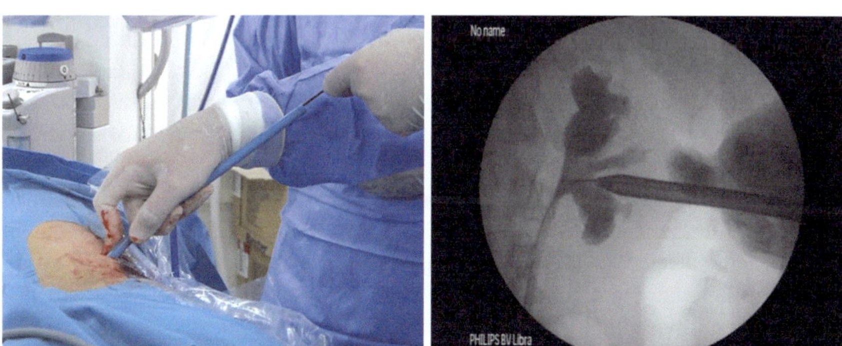

Fig. 20.3 Dilation using Amplatz dilators

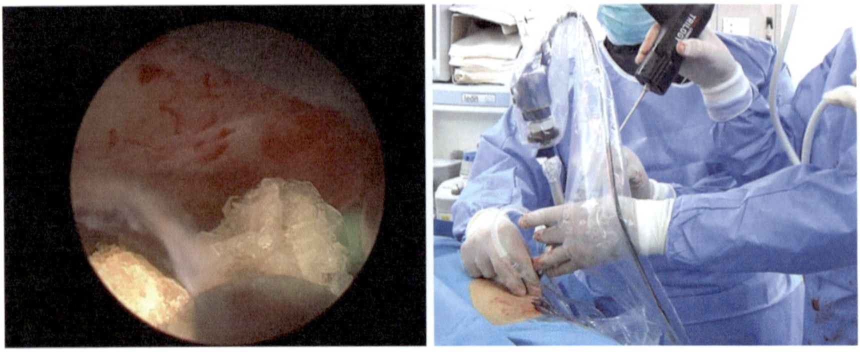

Fig. 20.4 Lithotripsy using ultrasonic and pneumatic lithotripter

mini-PCNL surgeries due to the narrow working channel of the nephroscope stone disintegration is mostly achieved with laser energy. There are different laser energy transmitting devices with different mechanisms and characteristics such as the Holmium:Yttrium-Aluminum-Garnet (Ho:YAG) and Thulium fiber lasers (TFL). Ho:YAG lasers offer the possibility of high-power lithotripsy, that can significantly reduce the operative time of the surgery compared to the low energy lasers [20]. Thulium technology is known in the endourological community for its use in prostate surgery but the recent introduction of TFL lithotripsy proposes that thulium laser lithotripsy has the potential to be significantly more efficient than Ho:YAG lithotripsy [21]. The generated fragments can be extracted with integrated suction of the lithotripter. Taking advantage of the active wash out, the vacuum cleaner effect that uses low pressure conditions to trap the fragments in a hydrodynamic pseydo-cavity and the purging effect the fragments can be extracted easier [22]. Other useful stone extracting devices include baskets and graspers. Stone extracting baskets differ in design and in the number of wires that create the basket.

Postoperative drainage is another point of debates. The use of a drainage at the end of PCNL is considered to provide important advantages such as renal drainage, bleeding tamponade and easy second-look nephroscopy. There are also different types of tubes that can be used at the end of the surgery for drainage of the pelvicalyceal system. A double-J stent and a nephrostomy tube have to be placed to drain the PCS, while in conventional PCNL a Malecot catherer can be placed as an alternative. However, many surgeons advocate that nephrostomy tubes increase postoperative morbidity and an external drainage is not essential. This type of surgery is called tubeless PCNL and relays an internal drainage such as a double-J stent for postoperative drainage. A totally tubeless PCNL is a surgery that no drainage tube is used for the collecting system postoperatively. Tubeless PCNL is superior in terms of patient length of stay and analgesic admission, but at the cost of losing access to the kidney that is crucial for second look and radiological assessments. Therefore it is advised to perform tubeless PCNL in uncomplicated cases only [23].

Anatomical Considerations

The success of a PCNL surgery is heavily based on a successful renal access avoiding injuries to the surrounding organs and respecting the structure of the kidney. Being familiar with renal anatomy and the neighboring organs positions is a necessity to proceed to the surgery. Kidneys lie between the two layers of Gerota's fascia in the retroperitoneal cavity. The upper poles are closer and more posterior to the skin compared to the lower poles and medial margins more anterior than the lateral margins. This fact gives to each kidney a definite inclination. Usually the left kidney can be located between the 11th and the 12th rib, while the right kidney lies 2 to 3 cm lower due to the existence of the liver in the right abdomen area. The pleura extends till the 12th rib and lungs till the 11th rib, it is possible to transverse the pleura while targeting an upper pole. Attempting to puncture over the 11th rib is not recommended. Furthermore, to avoid damaging the intercostal artery, it is recommended to target the middle of the intercostal space or just above the lower rib while puncturing over the 12th rib. Any injury of the intercostal artery could result in hemothorax [24, 25].

Familiarity with the vascular anatomy of the kidneys is important for performing PCNL Kidney blood supply is provided by the main renal artery. The renal artery is divided in two branches the anterior and the posterior. These branches are divided to interlobar arteries which follow parallel course to the calyceal infundibulum. While most renal tissue is supplied with a dense network of arteries, there is an avascular plane called the Brödel's bloodless line. This zone was used as an entry point to the kidney to treat staghorn stones in open anatrophic nephrolithotomies and it is still used as hallmark in nephrostomy insertion and in laparoscopic and robotic nephrolithotomies [26].

Because of the importance of minimizing the bleeding risk of PCNL, a number of experiments on fresh human cadaveric kidneys [27, 28] examined the probability of damaging arterial and venous vessels when puncturing different areas of the kidney [29–31]. The risk of arterial injury when puncturing a calyx in different renal poles was also assessed. It was found that puncturing the lower infundibulum was significantly safer in terms of bleeding complications compared to middle infundibulum, while puncturing the upper infundibulum has the highest probability for arterial and venous injury. The anterior pole had the densest vessel system and therefore it was the most dangerous for bleeding complications. In clinical practice, puncturing the upper calyces is a widely accepted way of entering the pelvicalyceal system that can be performed safely and effectively.

The tissue surrounding the infundibulum of the renal poles was divided in four quadrants and the probability of traumatizing the neighboring vessels was assessed. The anterior quadrant was found to be the most dangerous site, while the superior and the inferior quadrants were found to be the safest calyces.

Papillary Puncture for PCNL

Damaging major vessels can result in a number of severe complications such as hemorrhage and formation of pseudoaneurysms. Current literature suggests that the safest place to perform a renal puncture in a PCNL is the papilla of the calyx with an axis of the needle parallel to the infundibulum, while punctures that don't follow parallel direction and cross the infundibulum are dangerous to cause bleeding complications [28]. This "dogma" that was mainly structured based on results of bleeding complications in cadaveric kidneys had been keenly followed by the majority of the surgeons [32, 33]. The low rate of bleeding complications in clinical practice empowered even more this practice, which had not been questioned for years.

Non-papillary Puncture for PCNL

While in many aspects of the PCNL surgery such as patient position and tract dilation methods there was a continuous try to improve effectiveness of the surgery and to set the parameters of the surgery depending on the case, the viable positions of the PCS that can be targeted to gain access to the kidney and the possible complications have not been studied extensively. The studies accessing the risk of bleeding were performed in cadaveric kidneys and did not evaluate the risk after a dilation of the selected area to a tract up to 30Fr. Furthermore, the correlation of the neighboring organs with the kidney and how they affect the puncture has never been examined. The possibility of a more central puncture (non-papillary) has not been considered as in the common clinical practice the fornices of the calyces are the targeted area.

Performing non-papillary has been a common practice in our department for more than a decade. This approach offers important advantages compared to the traditional calyceal puncture such as improved instrument movement with wider angles and the direct insertion of a guidewire into the ureter. The safety of the non-papillary puncture was evident from the first cases and the evidence has been published in several published studies. Retrospective clinical studies examining safety and efficacy of non-papillary puncture in unselected cases in contemporary PCNL, in mini-PCNL and when treating staghorn stones have been performed [34–36]. To further investigate the efficacy and safety of non-papillary puncture, a prospective randomized trial comparing the operative time, hemoglobin drop and complication rate of papillary and non-papillary puncture was performed [37]. Again, there were no significant differences in terms of hemoglobin drop and complication rates. Moreover, we have conducted a prospective clinical study that examined not only the safety of puncture but also the safety of dilating the infundibulum of a middle renal calyx. Using the imaging tools of single-photon emission computed tomography/ computed tomography scintigraphies with Dimercaptosuccinic acid (SPECT-CT DMSA) and computed tomography perfusion we measured the angle of approach (AoA) in punctures in the infundibulum, the pelvis and the papilla comparing the vascularization of the renal areas that were affected during the dilation to create the percutaneous tract [38]. When comparing the AoA for the infundibulum and papilla punctures, no statistical significant differences were shown. Impressively all three different puncturing sites shared overlapping areas after the dilation. Evidence of the presented studies show that puncturing the infundibulum is a safe practice and this method could be advocated as an alternative to everyday clinical practice or in cases that the access of the papilla in not appropriate or impossible.

Tips and Tricks in Prone PCNL

The complexity of PCNL represents a challenge during the learning curve of any endourologist. Some specific tips and tricks could facilitate the safety and success outcomes of the procedure.

It is considered preferable to perform subcoastal punctures in order to avoid pleural complications.

Brodel's avascular line is the safest pathway to the PCS and therefore regardless of the puncture technique that is followed the puncture should have a direction of approximately 30° from the vertical axis targeting the posterolateral surface of the kidney.

Passing a guidewire in the ureter is essential for keeping the direction in the kidney and secures the access to the system.

A ureteral catheter is usually placed prior to PCNL procedure. The dilation by injecting contrast of the renal collecting system is crucial for a precise and safe puncture and a successful tract establishment. Ureteral catheters with an integrated balloon block the outflow of the contrast medium keeping the system inflated. When the classic ureteral catheters are used, it is required continuous flow of contrast during the puncture and at the time the tip of the dilator approaches the kidney. By injecting contrast only in the specified points of the procedure, the danger of contrast extravasation is reduced and visualization is preserved.

The success of tract dilation is affected by the adequacy of the skin incision. Friction between skin and dilators should be kept low because applying increased force to the dilator to overwhelm the friction could damage the collecting system or the nearby vessels. Especially when a balloon dilator is used, a small incision could restrict its expansion and attempting to extend the incision could injure the balloon or spill the contrast fluid.

It is recommended to create the PCNL tract over a stiff guidewire which is placed in the ureter. The guidewire leads the dilation forces with a direction aiming the ureter and prevents the system and the hilar structures from damage caused from the dilation. The advance of the dilator should follow the route of the guidewire without bending it. In cases where passing a guidewire to the ureter is impossible, the use of a stiff guidewire with a floppy J tip that can be coiled inside the system is recommended.

In case the access sheath remains inside the parenchyma due to insufficient dilation and shorter advancement of the dilators, the sheath should never be advanced without the direct vision such as a lithotripter probe. The alternative method is the reinsertion of the dilators.

Hypermobile kidneys can be quite tricky to perform a precise puncture. Selective apnea could be used in patients under general anesthesia to reduce the movement due to breathing.

Conclusion

Prone PCNL is a complex surgery that is used to treat large urinary calculi in the pelvicalyceal system. There many variations regarding every aspect of the surgery and depending on each case an individual way of treatment should be tailored. However, following general steps and knowing the alternatives that could be followed in each stage of the surgery can lead to great levels of efficacy and minimize the complications.

References

1. Türk C, Petřík A, Sarica K, Seitz C, Skolarikos A, Straub M, et al. EAU guidelines on interventional treatment for urolithiasis. Eur Urol. 2016;69(3):475–82. https://doi.org/10.1016/j.eururo.2015.07.041.
2. Purkait B, Sankhwar SN, Kumar M, Patodia M, Bansal A, Bhaskar V. Do outcomes of percutaneous nephrolithotomy in horseshoe kidney in children differ from adults? A single-center experience. J Endourol. 2016;30(5):497–503. https://doi.org/10.1089/end.2015.0794.
3. Srivastava A, Chipde SS, Mandhani A, Kapoor R, Ansari MS. Percutaneous management of renal caliceal diverticular stones: ten-year experience of a tertiary care center with different techniques to deal with diverticula after stone extraction. Indian J Urol. 2013;29(4):273–6. https://doi.org/10.4103/0970-1591.120091.
4. Goel R, Aron M, Kesarwani PK, Dogra PN, Hemal AK, Gupta NP. Percutaneous antegrade removal of impacted upper-ureteral calculi: still the treatment of choice in developing countries. J Endourol. 2005;19(1):54–7. https://doi.org/10.1089/end.2005.19.54.
5. Ecke TH, Barski D, Weingart G, Lange C, Hallmann S, Ruttloff J, et al. Presentation of a method at the exploration stage according to IDEAL: percutaneous nephrolithotomy (PCNL) under local infiltrative anesthesia is a feasible and effective method – retrospective analysis of 439 patients. Int J Med Sci. 2017;14(4):302–9. https://doi.org/10.7150/ijms.17963.
6. Solakhan M, Bulut E, Erturhan MS. Comparison of two different anesthesia methods in patients undergoing percutaneous nephrolithotomy. Urol J. 2019;16(3):246–50. https://doi.org/10.22037/uj.v0i0.4291.
7. Fernström I, Johansson B. Percutaneous pyelolithotomy. A new extraction technique. Scand J Urol Nephrol. 1976;10(3):257–9. https://doi.org/10.1080/21681805.1976.11882084.
8. Lahme S. Miniaturisation of PCNL. Urolithiasis. 2018;46(1):99–106. https://doi.org/10.1007/s00240-017-1029-3.

9. Falahatkar S, Mokhtari G, Teimoori M. An update on supine versus prone percutaneous nephrolithotomy: a meta-analysis. Urol J. 2016;13(5):2814–22.
10. Kamphuis GM, Baard J, Westendarp M, de la Rosette JJMCH. Lessons learned from the CROES percutaneous nephrolithotomy global study. World J Urol. 2015;33(2):223–33. https://doi.org/10.1007/s00345-014-1367-5.
11. Kyriazis I, Liatsikos E, Sopilidis O, Kallidonis P, Skolarikos A. European section of urotechnology educational video on fluoroscopic-guided puncture in percutaneous nephrolithotomy: all techniques step by step. BJU Int. 2017;120(5):739–41. https://doi.org/10.1111/bju.13894.
12. Chu C, Masic S, Usawachintachit M, Hu W, Yang W, Stoller M, et al. Ultrasound-guided renal access for percutaneous nephrolithotomy: a description of three novel ultrasound-guided needle techniques. J Endourol. 2016;30(2):153–8. https://doi.org/10.1089/end.2015.0185.
13. Ozok HU, Sagnak L, Senturk AB, Karakoyunlu N, Topaloglu H, Ersoy H. A comparison of metal telescopic dilators and Amplatz dilators for nephrostomy tract dilation in percutaneous nephrolithotomy. J Endourol. 2012;26(6):630–4. https://doi.org/10.1089/end.2011.0291.
14. Tomaszewski JJ, Smaldone MC, Schuster T, Jackman SV, Averch TD. Factors affecting blood loss during percutaneous nephrolithotomy using balloon dilation in a large contemporary series. J Endourol. 2010;24(2):207–11. https://doi.org/10.1089/end.2009.0402.
15. Aminsharifi A, Alavi M, Sadeghi G, Shakeri S, Afsar F. Renal parenchymal damage after percutaneous nephrolithotomy with one-stage tract dilation technique: a randomized clinical trial. J Endourol. 2011;25(6):927–31. https://doi.org/10.1089/end.2010.0638.
16. Wu Y, Xun Y, Lu Y, Hu H, Qin B, Wang S. Effectiveness and safety of four tract dilation methods of percutaneous nephrolithotomy: a meta-analysis. Exp Ther Med. 2020;19(4):2661–71. https://doi.org/10.3892/etm.2020.8486.
17. Schilling D, Hüsch T, Bader M, Herrmann TR, Nagele U, Training, et al. Nomenclature in PCNL or The Tower Of Babel: a proposal for a uniform terminology. World J Urol. 2015;33(11):1905–7. https://doi.org/10.1007/s00345-015-1506-7.
18. Tepeler A, Sarica K. Standard, mini, ultra-mini, and micro percutaneous nephrolithotomy: what is next? A novel labeling system for percutaneous nephrolithotomy according to the size of the access sheath used during procedure. Urolithiasis. 2013;41(4):367–8. https://doi.org/10.1007/s00240-013-0578-3.
19. Large T, Nottingham C, Brinkman E, Agarwal D, Ferrero A, Sourial M, et al. Multi-institutional prospective randomized control trial of novel intracorporeal lithotripters: ShockPulse-SE vs Trilogy Trial. J Endourol. 2021; https://doi.org/10.1089/end.2020.1097.
20. Chen S, Zhu L, Yang S, Wu W, Liao L, Tan J. High- vs low-power holmium laser lithotripsy: a prospective, randomized study in patients undergoing multitract minipercutaneous nephrolithotomy. Urology. 2012;79(2):293–7. https://doi.org/10.1016/j.urology.2011.08.036.
21. Traxer O, Keller EX. Thulium fiber laser: the new player for kidney stone treatment? A comparison with Holmium:YAG laser. World J Urol. 2020;38(8):1883–94. https://doi.org/10.1007/s00345-019-02654-5.
22. Nagele U, Nicklas A. Vacuum cleaner effect, purging effect, active and passive wash out: a new terminology in hydrodynamic stone retrival is arising – Does it affect our endourologic routine? World J Urol. 2016;34(1):143–4. https://doi.org/10.1007/s00345-015-1575-7.
23. Tirtayasa PMW, Yuri P, Birowo P, Rasyid N. Safety of tubeless or totally tubeless drainage and nephrostomy tube as a drainage following percutaneous nephrolithotomy: a comprehensive review. Asian J Surg. 2017;40(6):419–23. https://doi.org/10.1016/j.asjsur.2016.03.003.
24. Netto NR Jr, Ikonomidis J, Ikari O, Claro JA. Comparative study of percutaneous access for staghorn calculi. Urology. 2005;65(4):659–62; discussion 662-653,. https://doi.org/10.1016/j.urology.2004.10.081.
25. Aron M, Goel R, Kesarwani PK, Seth A, Gupta NP. Upper pole access for complex lower pole renal calculi. BJU Int. 2004;94(6):849–52; ; discussion 852. https://doi.org/10.1111/j.1464-410X.2004.05045.x.
26. Macchi V, Picardi E, Inferrera A, Porzionato A, Crestani A, Novara G, et al. Anatomic and radiologic study of renal avascular plane (Brödel's line) and its potential relevance on

percutaneous and surgical approaches to the kidney. J Endourol. 2018;32(2):154–9. https://doi.org/10.1089/end.2017.0689.
27. Sampaio FJ. Renal anatomy. Endourologic considerations. Urol Clin North Am. 2000;27(4):585–607., vii. https://doi.org/10.1016/s0094-0143(05)70109-9.
28. Sampaio FJ, Zanier JF, Aragão AH, Favorito LA. Intrarenal access: 3-dimensional anatomical study. J Urol. 1992;148(6):1769–73. https://doi.org/10.1016/s0022-5347(17)37024-6.
29. Sampaio FJ, Aragao AH. Anatomical relationship between the intrarenal arteries and the kidney collecting system. J Urol. 1990;143(4):679–81. https://doi.org/10.1016/s0022-5347(17)40056-5.
30. Sampaio FJ. Renal collecting system anatomy: its possible role in the effectiveness of renal stone treatment. Curr Opin Urol. 2001;11(4):359–66. https://doi.org/10.1097/00042307-200107000-00004.
31. Sampaio FJ, Passos MA. Renal arteries: anatomic study for surgical and radiological practice. Surg Radiol Anat. 1992;14(2):113–7. https://doi.org/10.1007/bf01794885.
32. Pearle MS. Puncture for percutaneous surgery: is the papillary puncture a dogma? No! Curr Opin Urol. 2019;29(4):472–3. https://doi.org/10.1097/mou.0000000000000627.
33. Campobasso D, Ferretti S, Frattini A. Papillary puncture: still a good practice. World J Urol. 2019;37(3):573–4. https://doi.org/10.1007/s00345-018-2527-9.
34. Kyriazis I, Kallidonis P, Vasilas M, Panagopoulos V, Kamal W, Liatsikos E. Challenging the wisdom of puncture at the calyceal fornix in percutaneous nephrolithotripsy: feasibility and safety study with 137 patients operated via a non-calyceal percutaneous track. World J Urol. 2017;35(5):795–801. https://doi.org/10.1007/s00345-016-1919-y.
35. Kallidonis P, Vagionis A, Lattarulo M, Adamou C, Tsaturyan A, Liourdi D, et al. Non-papillary percutaneous nephrolithotomy for treatment of staghorn stones. Minerva Urol Nefrol. 2020; https://doi.org/10.23736/S0393-2249.20.04124-7.
36. Kallidonis P, Vagionis A, Vrettos T, Adamou K, Pagonis K, Ntasiotis P, et al. Non papillary mini-percutaneous nephrolithotomy: early experience. World J Urol. 2021;39(4):1241–6. https://doi.org/10.1007/s00345-020-03267-z.
37. Kallidonis P, Kyriazis I, Kotsiris D, Koutava A, Kamal W, Liatsikos E. Papillary vs nonpapillary puncture in percutaneous nephrolithotomy: a prospective randomized trial. J Endourol. 2017;31(S1):S4–9. https://doi.org/10.1089/end.2016.0571.
38. Kallidonis P, Kalogeropoulou C, Kyriazis I, Apostolopoulos D, Kitrou P, Kotsiris D, et al. Percutaneous nephrolithotomy puncture and tract dilation: evidence on the safety of approaches to the infundibulum of the middle renal calyx. Urology. 2017;107:43–8. https://doi.org/10.1016/j.urology.2017.05.038.

Chapter 21
Laparoscopy and Robotics in Pelvic Reconstructive Surgery

Mija Blaganje and Emmanuel Chartier-Kastler

Introduction

As mean life expectancy is extending, needs for surgical management of pelvic organ prolapse and urinary incontinence increase. Along with them, in the light of previous interventions and various surgical approaches and materials used, exists an increasing demand for tape and mesh revision surgery, but also a relatively constant need of fistula repair.

There are different techniques of pelvic reconstructive surgery for pelvic organ prolapse (POP), urinary incontinence (UI), fistula repair and mesh revision surgeries, combining vaginal, abdominal and laparoscopic approaches.

Laparoscopic approach has many advantages over open abdominal approach, including better anatomic visibility as a result of magnification, insufflation, and improved hemostasis. Other advantages include shorter hospitalization, decreased postoperative pain, and mostly better cosmetic result due to smaller incisions. Rather than using a large incision, laparoscopy involves using several small incisions to perform a surgical procedure. Robotic surgery is a laparoscopic procedure, with an added layer of technology. Urologists have always been leaders in advancing surgical technology and were the first to utilize modern robotic surgery which is now used for all intra-abdominal, retroperitoneal, and pelvic procedures. More than 20 years after the first urological robotic procedure, it has become an established part of the urologist's armamentarium. For some procedures it has become accepted

M. Blaganje
Department of Gynecology, Division of Gynecology and Obstetrics, University Medical Centre Ljubljana, Ljubljana, Slovenia

Department of Gynecology, Medical Faculty, University of Ljubljana, Ljubljana, Slovenia

E. Chartier-Kastler (✉)
Department of Urology, AP-HP Pitie-Salpetriere, Sorbonne University, Paris, France
e-mail: emmanuel.chartier-kastler@aphp.fr

S. Tonyali et al. (eds.), *Current Endourology*,
https://doi.org/10.1007/978-3-032-00010-1_21

practice and this has allowed it to be explored in the entire spectrum of complex reconstructive procedures. Modern robotic surgery is relatively new to pelvic reconstructive surgery, where the major benefit in comparison to conventional laparoscopic surgery includes improved dexterity with increased degrees of freedom of movement, 3-dimensional image providing depth perception similar to that of open surgery, enhanced magnification, sitting position with increased surgeon's comfort and decreased surgeon hand fatigue. Procedures that involve high precision and technical skill such as suturing appear to be the first areas of application of this technology. The benefit of robotic surgery is achieving clear tissue plains and hemostasis in the pelvis and retropubic space with the added ergonomic advantages over the conventional laparoscopic approach. However, use of an additional trocar, larger trocar port incisions and their higher placement in the upper abdomen may esthetically be less acceptable for some patients weighing robot against conventional laparoscopy. Although seen as an evolution of laparoscopy, the novice to the robotic system has to learn to control the console, perform procedures without haptic feedback and use instruments with greater degrees of freedom.

Surgery for Pelvic Organ Prolapse

In 1957, the sacrum was first used as the site of attachment of the prolapsed uterus, thus re-establishing the anatomically natural axis of the vagina [1]. A year later, an implant was first used vaginal vault prolapse [2]. Since then, the field of POP surgery has changed significantly, and for many, sacrocolpopexy has become the surgical method of choice for the treatment of vaginal vault prolapse with a success rate up to 98% [3, 4]. The recurrence of prolapse is several times less likely and dyspareunia up to 10 times less likely with laparoscopic sacrocolpopexy (LSC) compared to vaginal surgery [4, 5]. For vaginal sacrospinous ligament fixation and sacrouterine ligament plication failure rates reported 5 years after surgery were 70.3% and 61.5% [6]. Sacrocolpopexy was first performed laparoscopically in 1994 in the USA. With laparoscopic performance, they achieved efficacy comparable to the open abdominal approach in a much less invasive way, and reported 100% treatment success in a series of 15 patients. LSC is effective as the first choice treatment and offers better preservation of sexual function compared to transvaginal synthetic mesh, now-a-days banned in several countries around the world, and fewer mesh-related complications [7]. The laparoscopic approach allows better visibility and display of some target organs, especially the posterior wall of the vagina, faster recovery, less bleeding and shorter hospital stay. Robotic assistance seems to contribute some advantages associated with significantly lower blood loss and lower conversion rate, but longer operative time compared to conventional laparoscopic surgery. Both approaches appear to promote equivalent clinical outcomes [8].

The following are the most important laparoscopic approaches and techniques represented in the scientific literature of the last 10 years, with an emphasis on the oldest laparoscopic surgical technique—LSC.

Laparoscopic Sacrocolpopexy

Laparoscopic sacrocolpopexy is the surgical technique of choice for the treatment of vaginal vault prolapse with strong recommendation according to the literature evidence [3]. Although the basic principle of LSC is the attachment of the vaginal vault—with more or less extensive dissection of the vesico-vaginal and recto-vaginal space—to the anterior longitudinal ligament at the level of the sacral promontory with a mesh implant, various technical variants have evolved over time. In addition to apical vault prolapse, any associated cystocele, rectocele, or rectal prolapse can be treated concomitantly with LSC. From a review of 953 articles of the last 10 years, we list the most important findings [9]. At present, it is not possible to recommend a specific variant of any existing surgical technique versions. Deeper dissection of the vesico-vaginal space provides fewer recurrences of anterior vaginal wall prolapse, but may cause more *de novo* dysuria. Currently, the use of polypropylene mesh type 1 is recommended, which can be sutured to the vagina with a knitted or monofilament thread, by stringing single or running sutures, which can be resorbable or non-resorbable. Either non-absorbable titanium screws (tackers) or a non-absorbable suture can be used to attach the mesh to the promontory. At the same time, if necessary, a subtotal or total hysterectomy can be performed. However, when uterus preservation is desired, an alternative laparoscopic sacro-hystero-colpopexy can be performed (Fig. 21.1). To date, there is insufficient evidence to advise on the use of different shapes of meshes, the exact location of their attachment to the promontory, the tension of the laid mesh, or peritonisation. The main limitation of LSC is the longer duration of surgery and the longer learning curve. The operation appears to be completely mastered after its 60 executions [10]. Various curricula provide for a surgeon to first assist with 20 surgeries and then to be guided by the mentor for further 30 surgeries, this reducing the time required to perform the surgery to the acceptable time of 90 minutes after 10 to 30 performed procedures [11, 12]. Average operative time for robotic sacrocolpopexy is 226 minutes [8] and operation is usually mastered after 20 performed cases.

Alternatives to Laparoscopic Sacrocolpopexy Including Mesh

Although very rare, at the time of surgery we may come across circumstances when attachment to the promontory is either not possible or not safe enough to perform. These could be related to the anatomy of the structures surrounding the promontory (Fig. 21.2), extensive obliterating adhesions of this part of the abdomen following previous surgery or extensive intraoperative complications. Although presented as independent surgical techniques, some among the following could be used as an alternative, not converting from the laparoscopic approach.

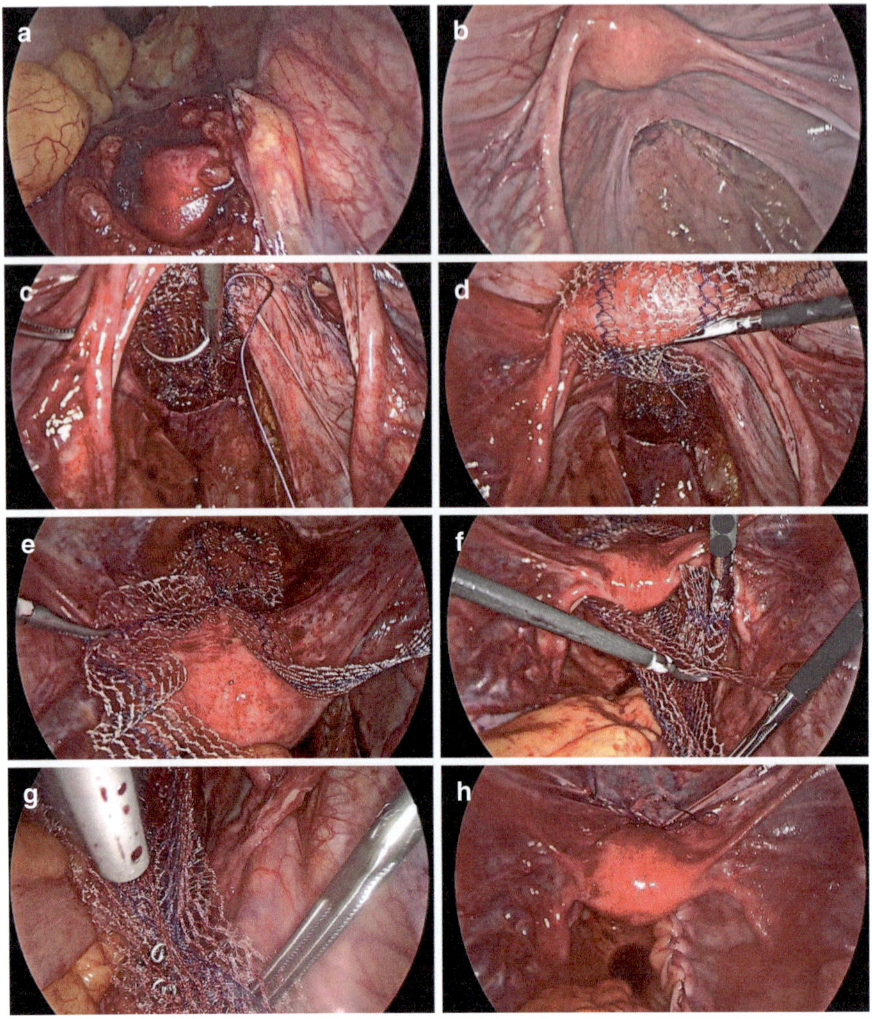

Fig. 21.1 Laparoscopic sacral hystero-colpopexy. Performed by anterior and posterior mesh for combined apical, anterior and posterior prolapse. Conventional laparoscopy. (**a**) Disection of the promontory; (**b**) Disection of the peritoneum between the promontory and the Douglas space; (**c**) Posterior mesh attachment along the posterior vaginal wall; (**d**) View of the pelvis after posterior mesh attachment; (**e**) View of the pelvis after anterior mesh attachment along the anterior vaginal wall and before passing the two split ends through the broad ligament bilaterally; (**f**) Adjustment of the mesh ends and positioning of the uterus and vaginal walls; (**g**) Fixing the mesh ends to the promontory by titanium tackers; (**h**) View of the pelvis after peritonisation

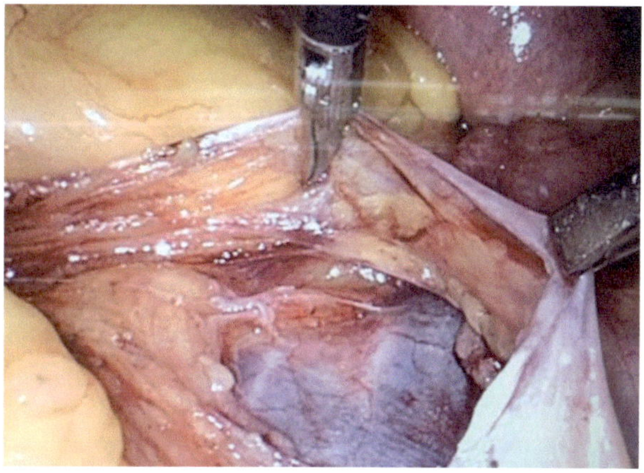

Fig. 21.2 Aberant iliac vain bifurcation anatomy over the promontory

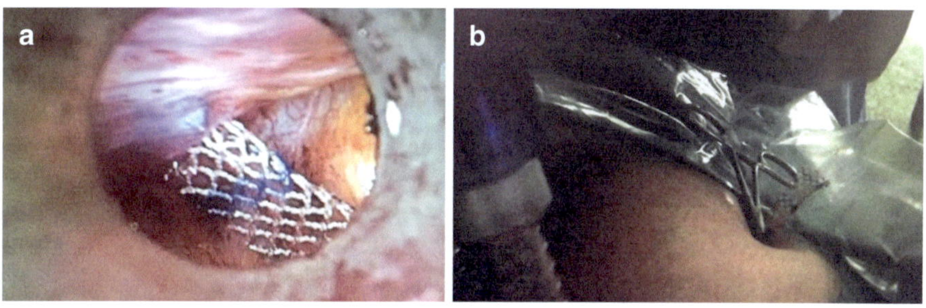

Fig. 21.3 Laparoscopic lateral abdominal suspension. (**a**) View of a mesh end entering the retroperitoneal space at the site of a round ligament; (**b**) the mesh is lead to the surface through the abdominal wall, where it is cut

Laparoscopic Lateral Abdominal Suspension

This technique for the treatment of POP was first reported by Dubuisson [13]. Instead of attaching the free arms of the mesh to the sacral promontory, the mesh is bilaterally inserted under the peritoneum, entering the retroperitoneal space at the site of round ligaments and then sled under the peritoneum all the way to the point 5 cm above the anterior superior iliac spine. At this point, the mesh is lead through the abdominal wall to the surface, where it is cut (Fig. 21.3). The retroperitoneal space and the layers of the abdominal wall that the mesh passes retain its position and thus maintain a new anatomical position of the attached organs. According to the original version, the mesh is fastened to the vagina with resorbable nylon screws instead of sutures, which saves suturing time to inexperienced, with the disadvantage of long resorption time of sharp screws in an otherwise physiologically sensitive place of the vagina. Of course, the surgery is also feasible with attachment of the mesh with classic suturing. With the technique of lateral abdominal suspension, important retroperitoneal structures such as vessels and nerves are avoided and thus the risk of intraoperative lesion that exists with LSC. A recent report suggests that the laparoscopic lateral abdominal suspension technique is safe and effective for the treatment of prolapse [14].

Laparoscopic Pectopexy

Laparoscopic pectopexy is another alternative to LSC. While the principle of attaching the mesh to the vagina or uterus is the same as for LSC, the free arms of the mesh are attached with a nonresorbable suture to the pectineal ligament of the pubis (Fig. 21.4), both anterior to the junction of the external iliac vein crossing instead of to the promontory. The arms of the mesh thus run approximately parallel to the round ligaments. Compared to LSC, pectopexy has been shown to be equally effective in the medium term, with significantly less constipation which may occur in LSC due to hypogastric nerve plexus injury [15]. Nevertheless, due to currently small volume of published data on laparoscopic pectopexy, the use of this technique is currently recommended in research settings, according to the recommendations of the British National Institute for Health and Care Excellence (NICE) [16].

Alternatives to Laparoscopic Sacrocolpopexy Without Mesh

Laparoscopic Correction of Paravaginal Defect

Laparoscopic correction of paravaginal defect by colposuspension on Cooper's ligament is founded on the principle of Burch colposuspension surgery, a surgical technique for stress urinary incontinence treatment, in which the lateral parts of the anterior vaginal wall are fixed on both sides to the Cooper's ligament of the pubis at the level of the bladder neck. The technique used to treat prolapse can successfully correct a paravaginal defect, caused by an interrupted or weakened connective tissue attachment of the pubocervical fascia in the direction of the lateral pelvic wall and its arcus tendineus fasciae pelvis. By dissecting the retroperitoneal space along

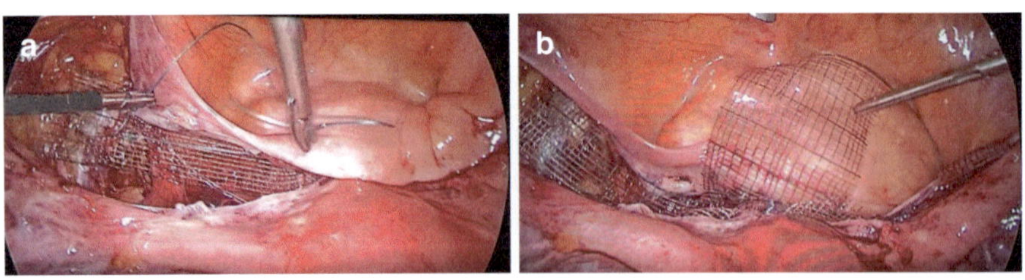

Fig. 21.4 Laparoscopic pectopexy. A uterus preserving procedure by conventional laparoscopy. (**a**) Mesh attachment to the left pectineal ligamnet; (**b**) free mesh attached to the uterine isthmus intended for anterior vaginal wall placement. Vesico-vaginal space has been disected, but not exposed on the image

the pubic bone and lateral pelvic wall, the entire length of the vagina on both sides is exposed and then suspended onto the Cooper's ligament with running or individual sutures, from the level of the bladder neck to the height of the fornix, without the use of mesh (Fig. 21.5). In this way, anterior vaginal wall prolapse, apical vaginal or uterine prolapse can successfully be corrected at the same time, but the technique has not been compared to LSC [17, 18]. The laparoscopic paravaginal repair with reported success rates of 60% to 89% could be considered as a concomitant treatment of anterior vaginal wall prolapse caused by lateral defects, including at time of laparoscopic/robotic sacralcolpopexy.

Laparoscopic Plication of Sacrouterine Ligaments

Laparoscopic plication of sacrouterine ligaments is described either as a preventive measure or as a method of treating prolapse either with uterus in place or after hysterectomy. So far, it has not been compared to LSC. It could represent a surgical alternative for apical prolapse or anterior vaginal wall prolapse treatment in well-selected patients. According to some data, 19% of patients have recurrences of prolapse in 2 years [19, 20].

Laparoscopic Colporraphy

Laparoscopic colporrhaphy is described as an associated intervention to other laparoscopic corrections of POP [21] and not as a stand-alone technique, as it would be more difficult to justify as such, compared to simpler and less invasive vaginal colporrhaphy. Laparoscopically it is applied to reduce the volume of anterior or posterior vaginal wall prolapse, observed concomitantly with apical prolapse. After dissection of the rectovaginal space and vesicovaginal space, exposing the surface of the vaginal wall, colporraphy is performed with several longitudinally placed running sutures, thus achieving plication in the cranio-caudal direction. In addition to reducing the volume of the prolapse, a greater thickness of the naturally thinned tissue of the vagina before suturing of the mesh is achieved in this manner [22].

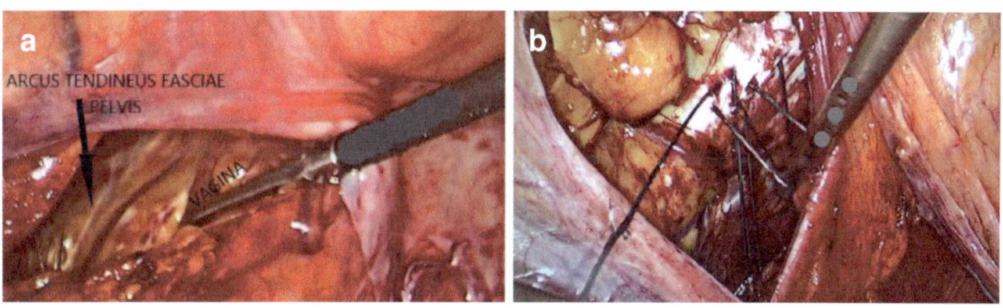

Fig. 21.5 Paravaginal defect correction. Conventional laparoscopy. (**a**) Exposed left pelvic side wall, vagina is identified; (**b**) Vagina is suspended onto the Cooper's ligament with running sutures from the level of the bladder neck to the height of the left fornix

Continence Surgery

Burch Urethropexy

The Burch c has an over 50-year history demonstrating good long-term outcomes with few complications. Laparoscopic and robotic approaches appear to have equal efficacy to the open procedure. Although the application of the Burch urethropexy has faded with the shift toward less invasive suburethral tape surgery due to surgical practicality of the latter, it continues to have a role in the treatment of stress urinary incontinence and is again regaining popularity in parts of the world with vaginal mesh ban. A Burch urethropexy should be considered when vaginal access is limited, when concurrent intra-abdominal surgery is planned, and when mesh is contraindicated, not wished for or not available.

A systematic review of 53 trials had reported success rates of 85–90% one year postoperatively and 70% five years postoperatively [23]. Later, minimally invasive techniques for Burch described the advantages over open surgeries, such as shorter length of hospital stays, faster recovery, and faster return to activity. A Cochrane review of laparoscopic Burch included 22 randomised controlled trials [24]. Cure rates and safety of laparoscopic and open Burch colposuspension were similar, but this review revealed that laparoscopy was associated with a shorter length of hospital stays, lower morbidity, significantly fewer postoperative complications, lower estimated blood losses, shorter duration of catheterisation and significantly less pain. A robotic-assisted Burch urethropexy was first reported with two cases performed in 145 minutes in 2007 by Khan et al. [25]. Robotic assistance provided the advantages of increased magnification, visualisation and surgeon comfort over traditional laparoscopy. Results of a large case series suggest that robotic-assisted Burch urethropexy is a safe and effective procedure with low complication rates. An 85% cure of symptoms reported on a short term with mean operative time 143 (±58) min and minimal blood loss is comparable to laparoscopic Burch urethropexy [26].

Due to these less invasive laparoscopic approaches the Burch procedure continues to have a place in the operative armamentarium.

Artificial Urinary Sphincter Placement

The management of women patients with intrinsic sphincter deficiency (ISD)-related SUI is less clear than of those with urethral hypermobility in whom suburethral tape placement is recognized as the gold standard surgical treatment. As supported by the American Urological Association (AUA) guidelines in some parts of the World and the USA retropubic tapes, autologous fascia slings, and bulking agents are favored in these patients. Additionally, the European Association of Urology (EAU) guidelines emphasize the possible role of external compression device, such as the Adjustable Continence Therapy (ACT®) balloons or the artificial urinary sphincter (AUS) AMS 800™, providing the patient would be informed of the high risk of complications, mechanical failure or need for explantation [27]. However, in some countries, especially in France, AUS AMS 800™ is considered the standard of care in female patients with SUI due to ISD [28].

In theory there may be several advantages of using AUS in women with failed previous anti-incontinence surgery, with possibly lower risk of urinary retention and self-catheterization than with "obstructive" therapeutic options such as fascia sling or adjustable continence therapy [29].

The difficulty of AUS implantation in women represents the dissection of the bladder neck, because there is no natural plane between the urethra and vagina and the bladder neck lies deeply in the pelvis. Laparoscopic and robotic approaches may offer an advantage over open techniques due to easier access and better visualization. Laparoscopic and robotic series reported so far were limited by their relatively small sample size and short follow-up. The surgical approach may have a significant influence on outcomes, as observed by the promising results of most laparoscopic and robotic series [30–33] reporting outcomes similar to large open series. A systematic review on the subject states that according to the existing literature, AUS AMS-800™ may provide excellent functional outcomes in female patients with SUI due to ISD with 61.1–100% being fully continent post-operatively, paralleling results of AUS implantation in male patients. However, this comes in hand with relatively high morbidity with reported erosion rates of up to 22.2% and explantation rates up to 45.3% [29].

Fistula Repair

Vesico-Vaginal Fistula

The most common cause of vesicovaginal fistula (VVF) in the developed countries is hysterectomy. Although the vaginal approach is the most common for repair of VVF, the laparoscopic approach with or without robot-assistance can be applied in patients for whom the vaginal approach is not possible. It successfully replaces an open abdominal approach when the defect is large, multiple, involves other pelvic structures including the ureters and when there is poor mobility of the vaginal wall, making adequate visualization from a vaginal approach difficult. Criteria for a good surgical repair include: good visualization, good dissection, good approximation of the margins, tension-free watertight closure, use of a well vascularized tissue flaps and adequate post-operative urinary drainage [34]. The surgical approach can be performed either by extravesical technique or accompanied by intentional cystotomy—transvesical technique. Pollack stent can be inserted through the fistula by cystoscopy, allowing better visualization of the fistula at the time of sharp laparoscopic dissection. Stenting of the ureters is performed occasionally or systematically. Indigo carmine or methylene blue instillation into the bladder is sometimes used to better visualize the fistula. Bladder can be closed by single or double layer suture and vaginal defect closed in different ways, with or without interposition flap (fatty tissue, peritoneum or fibrin glue). A systematic review of literature [35, 36] showed that the general success of laparoscopic repair is approximately 90% and conclusion on the best technique couldn't be drawn. There was no difference in success rates with different number of layers in the fistula closure or with use of interposition flaps, but there was a small increase in success in the cases that documented intraoperative bladder filling to test the integrity of the bladder closure.

Advances in robotic repair have been adopted since 2005 and current data underline the successful robotic repair of supratrigonal nonobstetric VVF. When considering robotic repair, it is essential to establish the size, number, location, and etiology of the VVF. Robotic assistance facilitates dissection of the vesicovaginal space and a tension-free closure of the bladder with low morbidity for the patient being operated in the deep pelvis with delicate anatomical structures. Robotic repair of a VVF can be applied safely with an excellent success rate and very low morbidity. Robotic-assisted VVF repair is now well established in the literature, with a comprehensive review of 19 studies [36] demonstrating nearly a 100% resolution rate especially with more recent publications. Delineation of the ideal flap for interposition, as well as the timing of robotic-assisted fistula repair, is still needed. Recommended in a consensus report by the European Association of Urology Robotic Section Scientific Working Group for reconstructive urology the robotic repair of a VVF can be applied safely with an excellent success rate and very low morbidity [37].

Uretero-Vaginal Fistula

Uretero-vaginal fistula commonly occurs due to an iatrogenic ureteral injury in the process of gynaecological surgeries with a reported incidence of up to 5% [38]. When initial management with ureteral stenting fails, ureteroneocystostomy is prefered over the end-to-end ureteral anastomosis. Although not commonly performed, ureteral reconstruction, reimplantation and ureterolysis have traditionally involved a laparotomy, with its associated morbidity, as a gold standard. Although technically demanding, with increasing experience in laparoscopic procedures, laparoscopic reimplantation has become a feasible option for management of such injuries either by conventional laparoscopic or robotic-assisted ureteroneocystostomy with a success rate compared to that of open surgery but with less morbidity and quick convalescence [39–41]. Extensive ureteral mobilization can be replaced by mobilizing the bladder and doing the psoas hitch and when necessary additional Boari flap. First described in 1994 and mostly used in reflux patients [42, 43], laparoscopic extravesical Lich–Gregoir ureteroneocystostomy and psoas hitch for posthysterectomy ureterovaginal fistula was shown to have a success rate of 90–100% [44].

The ergonomics, dexterity and minimally invasive nature of the robotic system offer itself well to these precise procedures. The first robotic ureteral ureteroneocystostomy was reported in 2004 [45] and the first robotic ureterolysis with omental wrap in 2006 [46]. Robotic ureteroneocystostomy provides similar outcomes when compared with an open approach in well-selected patients when assessing for recurrent ureteral obstruction or adverse events. Robotic surgery is associated with lower postoperative narcotic pain prescriptions at discharge, lower PCA usage, and shorter LOS, which are important benefits when compared with open surgery [47].

Tape and Mesh Revision Surgery

Synthetic suburethral tapes are the most commonly used surgical procedures performed in Europe for the treatment of SUI and synthetic mesh placed abdominally or vaginally, has widely been used for POP surgical treatment. At the time of reclassification of transvaginal surgical mesh for pelvic organ prolapse treatment from class II to class III medical device by the Food and Drug Administration (FDA), the serious risk of complications that may be associated with transvaginal surgical mesh was emphasized and transvaginal mesh placement surgery discontinued in several countries.

The use of synthetic material has generated new type of complications including erosion and extrusion of the material, material contraction, pelvic pain and dispareunia [48], which are being underreported, especially in countries without existent national registries and for which surgical management can be complex and challenging. Complications of erosion, extrusion and contraction usually present 12 months and later following initial surgery and often require more than one surgical procedure, where the first revision surgery tends not to be over extensive (i.e. local or partial excision of the tape or mesh), to reduce the rates and severity of possible complications and a subsequent revision surgery, when needed, tends to be more radical [49].

The complications of transobturator and single incision tapes and mesh surgery inserted by a vaginal approach are normally managed by a vaginal approach. Revision surgery may involve tape loosening and tape section in patients with urinary obstruction, and the partial or entire removal in patients with storage symptoms, mixed urinary symptoms, bladder and urethral erosions, vaginal extrusion, chronic pelvic pain symptoms and dyspareunia. Mesh inserted laparoscopically and retropubic tapes are removed from the abdominal approach, preferably laparoscopically. A combination surgery is sometimes needed, depending on accessibility of the mesh through different approaches (Fig. 21.6). The difficulty in mesh and tape removal is represented in the identification of the mesh integrated into the native tissue, the loss of natural planes, the dissection of the scar tissue adjacent to the mesh and preservation of the intactness of the adjacent organs, detection of potential intraoperative lesions and perforations, followed by surgical reparation with

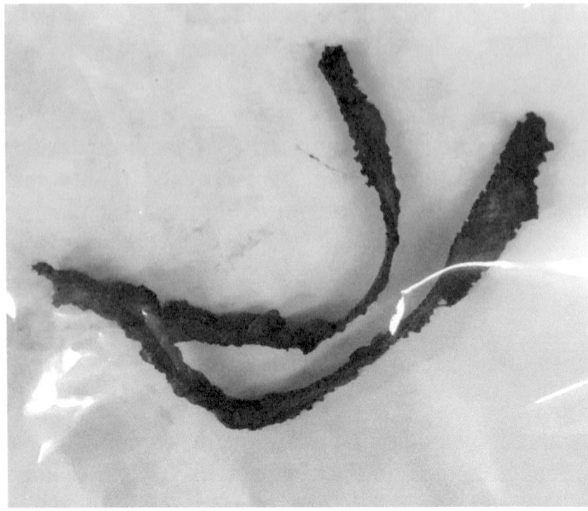

Fig. 21.6 Retropubic suburethral tape after complete removal with a combined surgical approach. Suburethral part of the tape was dissected through a vaginal approach, while the upper part was dissected by laparoscopy

suturing when needed, all performed deep in the pelvis. Laparoscopic (and robot-assisted) approaches may offer an advantage over open techniques due to better visualization, higher precision and improved dexterity in difficultly accessible areas of the pelvis.

Tips and Tricks

1. When performing laparoscopy deep in the pelvis I place a suture through the sigmoid epiploicae and place it to traction through the abdominal wall, lateral and cranially to the left lower quadrant port to retract the rectosigmoid to the left of the promontory and out from the pelvis, which enables me better visibility and more maneuver space.
2. When dissecting the peritoneum above the promontory, I lift and tighten the peritoneum to avoid vessel injury.
3. I stay to the right of the promontory to prevent hypogastric nerve plexus injury.
4. For fixing the sutures onto the Cooper's or Pectineal ligament, the backhand position of the needle in the needle holder assures better maneuverability.

Literature

1. Arthure HG, Savage D. Uterine prolapse and prolapse of the vaginal vault treated by sacral hysteropexy. J Obstet Gynaecol Br Em. 1957;64:355–60.
2. Ameline A, Huguier J. Posterior suspension to the lumbo-sacral disk; abdominal method of replacement of the utero-sacral ligaments. Gynecol Obstet. 1957;56:94–8.
3. Maher C, Feiner B, Baessler K, et al. Surgery for women with apical vaginal prolapse. Cochrane Database Syst Rev. 2016;10:CD012376.

4. Haya N, Maher M, Ballard E. Surgical management of recurrent upper vaginal prolapse following sacral colpopexy. Int Urogynecol J. 2015;26:1243–5.
5. Nezhat CH, Nezhat F, Nezhat C. Laparoscopic sacral colpopexy for vaginal vault prolapse. Obstet Gynecol. 1994;84:885–8.
6. Jelovsek JE, Barber MD, Brubaker L, et al. Pelvic Floor Disorders Network. Effect of uterosacral ligament suspension vs sacrospinous ligament fixation with or without perioperative behavioral therapy for pelvic organ vaginal prolapse on surgical outcomes and prolapse symptoms at 5 years in the OPTIMAL randomized clinical trial. JAMA. 2018;319:1554–65.
7. Lucot JP, Cosson M, Bader G, et al. Safety of vaginal mesh surgery versus laparoscopic mesh sacropexy for cystocele repair: results of the prosthetic pelvic floor repair randomized controlled trial. Eur Urol. 2018;74:167–76.
8. Yang J, He Y, Zhang X, et al. Robotic and laparoscopic sacrocolpopexy for pelvic organ prolapse: a systematic review and meta-analysis. Ann Transl Med. 2021;9(6):449.
9. Gluck O, Blaganje M, Veit-Rubin N, et al. Laparoscopic sacrocolpopexy: a comprehensive literature review on current practice. Eur J Obstet Gynecol Reprod Biol. 2019;245:94–101.
10. Brubaker L, Nygaard I, Richter HE, et al. Two-year outcomes after sacrocolpopexy with and without burch to prevent stress urinary incontinence. Obstet Gynecol. 2016;112:49–55.
11. Costantini E, Mearini L, Lazzeri M, et al. Laparoscopic versus abdominal sacrocolpopexy: a randomized, controlled trial. J Urol. 2016;196:159–65.
12. Coolen A-LWM, van IJsselmuiden MN, van Oudheusden AMJ, et al. Laparoscopic sacrocolpopexy versus vaginal sacrospinous fixation for vaginal vault prolapse, a randomized controlled trial: SALTO-2 trial, study protocol. BMC Womens Health. 2017;17:52.
13. Dubuisson JB, Jacob S, Chapron C, et al. Laparoscopic treatment of genital prolapse: lateral utero-vaginal suspension with 2 meshes. Results of a series of 47 patients. Gynecol Obstet Fertil. 2002;30:114–20.
14. Veit-Rubin N, Dubuisson J-B, Gayet-Ageron A, et al. Patient satisfaction after laparoscopic lateral suspension with mesh for pelvic organ prolapse: outcome report of a continuous series of 417 patients. Int Urogynecol J. 2017;28:1685–93.
15. Noé K-G, Schiermeier S, Alkatout I, et al. Laparoscopic pectopexy: a prospective, randomized, comparative clinical trial of standard laparoscopic sacral colpocervicopexy with the new laparoscopic pectopexy-postoperative results and intermediate-term follow-up in a pilot study. J Endourol. 2015;29:210–5.
16. Laparoscopic mesh pectopexy for apical prolapse of the uterus or vagina (IPG608). Available via NICE. https://www.nice.org.uk/guidance/IPG608/chapter/1-recommendations of subordinate document. Accessed 25 Jan 2024.
17. Chinthakanan O, Miklos JR, Moore RD. Laparoscopic paravaginal defect repair: surgical technique and a literature review. Surg Technol Int. 2015;27:173–83.
18. Yoon WS, Lee HN, Lee YS, et al. Laparoscopic colposuspension to the Cooper's ligament after hysterectomy for uterovaginal prolapse. J Obstet Gynaecol Res. 2013;39:714–9.
19. Nishimura K, Yoshimura K, Hoshino K, et al. Laparoscopic uterosacral ligament colpopexy for apical support in addition to hysterectomy for pelvic organ prolapse. J Obstet Gynaecol Res. 2019;45:1522–9.
20. Serati M, Laganà AS, Casarin J, et al. Laparoscopic duplication of the uterosacral ligaments following hysterectomy for stage III-IV apical pelvic organ prolapse. Updat Surg. 2019;72(1):199–204.
21. Noé GK, Schiermeier S, Papathemelis T, et al. Prospective International Multicenter Pelvic Floor Study: short-term follow-up and clinical findings for combined pectopexy and native tissue repair. J Clin Med. 2021;10(2):217.
22. Noé GK, Alkatout I, Schiermeier S, et al. Laparoscopic anterior and posterior native tissue repair: a new pelvic floor approach. Minim Invasive Ther Allied Technol. 2019;28:241–6.
23. Lapitan MC, Cody JD. Open retropubic colposuspension for urinary incontinence in women. Cochrane Database Syst Rev. 2012;13(6):CD002912. Update in: Cochrane Database Syst Rev (2016) 2:CD002912

24. Dean N, Ellis G, Herbison GP, Wilson D, et al. Laparoscopic colposuspension for urinary incontinence in women. Cochrane Database Syst Rev. 2017;7(7):CD002239. Update in: Cochrane Database Syst Rev (2019) 10;12:CD002239
25. Khan MS, Challacombe B, Rose K, et al. Robotic colposuspension: two case reports. J Endourol. 2007;21(9):1077–9.
26. Lee TG, Unlu BS, Petruzzi VA, et al. Safety and efficacy of robotic-assisted Burch for pure stress urinary incontinence: a large case series. J Obstet Gynaecol. 2021;41(5):803–6.
27. Burkhard F, Bosch J, Cruz F, et al. EAU guidelines on urinary incontinence in adults. 2018. Available via EAU. http://uroweb.org/guideline/urinaryincontinence of subordinate document. Accessed 25 Jan 2024.
28. Cour F, Le Normand L, Lapray JF, et al. Intrinsic sphincter deficiency and female urinary incontinence. Prog Urol. 2015;25:437–54.
29. Peyronnet B, O'Connor E, Khavari R, Capon G, et al. AMS-800 Artificial urinary sphincter in female patients with stress urinary incontinence: a systematic review. Neurourol Urodyn. 2019;38(Suppl 4):S28–41.
30. Peyronnet B, Vincendeau S, Tondut L, et al. Artificial urinary sphincter implantation in women with stress urinary incontinence: preliminary comparison of robotassisted and open approaches. Int Urogynecol J. 2016;27:475–81.
31. Rouprêt M, Misraï V, Vaessen C, et al. Laparoscopic approach for artificial urinary sphincter implantation in women with intrinsic sphincter deficiency incontinence: a single-centre preliminary experience. Eur Urol. 2010;57:499–504.
32. Ferreira C, Brychaert PE, Menard J, et al. Laparoscopic implantation of artificial urinary sphincter in women with intrinsic sphincter deficiency: mid-term outcomes. Int J Urol. 2017;24:308–13.
33. Fournier G, Callerot P, Thoulouzan M. Robotic-assisted laparoscopic implantation of artificial urinary sphincter in women with intrinsic sphincter deficiency incontinence: initial results. Urology. 2014;84:1094–8.
34. Couvelaire R. Reflections on a personal statistics of 136 vesicovaginal fistulas. J Urol Medicale Chir. 1953;59(3–4):150.
35. Miklos JR, Moore RD, Chinthakanan O. Laparoscopic and robotic-assisted vesicovaginal fistula repair: a systematic review of the literature. J Minim Invasive Gynecol. 2015;22(5):727–36.
36. Bodner-Adler B, Hanzal E, Pablik E, et al. Management of vesicovaginal fistulas (VVFs) in women following benign gynaecologic surgery: a systematic review and meta-analysis. PLoS One. 2017;12(2):e0171554.
37. Randazzo M, Lengauer L, Rochat CH, et al. Best practices in robotic-assisted repair of vesicovaginal fistula: a consensus report from the European Association of Urology Robotic Urology Section Scientific Working Group for Reconstructive Urology. Eur Urol. 2020;78(3):432–42.
38. Moawad G, von Walter GA. Management of urinary tract injuries in minimally invasive gynecologic surgery. Postgrad Obstet Gynecol. 2013;33:1–7.
39. Yang C, Jones L, Rivera ME, et al. Robotic-assisted ureteral reimplantation with Boari flap and psoas hitch: a single-institution experience. J Laparoendosc Adv Surg Tech A. 2011;21:829–33.
40. Kozinn SI, Canes D, Sorcini A, et al. Robotic versus open distal ureteral reconstruction and reimplantation for benign stricture disease. J Endourol. 2012;26:147–51.
41. Callewaert PR, Biallosterski BT, Rahnama'i MS, et al. Robotic extravesical anti-reflux operations in complex cases: technical considerations and preliminary results. Urol Int. 2012;88:6–11.
42. Ehrlich RM, Gershman A, Fuchs G. Laparoscopic vesicoureteroplasty in children: initial case reports. Urology. 1994;43:255–61.
43. Reddy PK, Evans RM. Laparoscopic ureteroneocystostomy. J Urol. 1994;152:2057–9.
44. Modi P, Gupta R, Rizvi SJ. Laparoscopic ureteroneocystostomy and psoas hitch for posthysterectomy ureterovaginal fistula. J Urol. 2008;180:615–7.
45. Dinlenc CZ, Gerber E, Wagner JR. Ureteral reimplantation during robot assisted laparoscopic radical prostatectomy. J Urol. 2004;172(3):905.

46. Mufarrij PW, Lipkin ME, Stifelman MD. Robot-assisted ureterolysis, retroperitoneal biopsy, and omental wrap: pilot series for the treatment of idiopathic retroperitoneal fibrosis. J Endourol. 2008;22(8):1669–75.
47. Skupin PA, Stoffel JT, Malaeb BS, et al. Robotic versus open ureteroneocystostomy: is there a robotic benefit? J Endourol. 2020;34(10):1028–32.
48. Lee D, Zimmern PE. Management of complications of mesh surgery. Curr Opin Urol. 2015;25(4):284–91.
49. Ismail S, Chartier-Kastler E, Reus C, et al. Functional outcomes of synthetic tape and mesh revision surgeries: a monocentric experience. Int Urogynecol J. 2019;30(5):805–13.

Chapter 22
Robot-Assisted Laparoscopic Partial Nephrectomy

Nicolas A. Soputro, Aaron Kaviani, Mahmoud Abou Zeinab, and Jihad Kaouk

Introduction

For many years, partial nephrectomy has been considered the gold standard for the management of suspicious small renal masses. The goals of nephron-sparing surgeries included the maximal preservation of normal renal parenchyma and the absence of perioperative complications whilst ensuring a negative surgical margin and satisfactory oncological outcomes. In recent decades, several minimally invasive surgical techniques for partial nephrectomy have been introduced, with both laparoscopic and robotic partial nephrectomy demonstrated to confer comparable oncological and functional outcomes but with significant improvements in perioperative outcomes and patient comfort. Of note, the enhanced intraoperative visions, ergonomics, and maneuverability offered by the robotic surgical platform allowed for marked reductions in operative time, intraoperative blood loss, as well as perioperative morbidity and mortality. Further technological and technical advancements in robotic partial nephrectomy have also provided the opportunity to expand the clinical indications for the procedure, including in patients with higher body mass index, previous abdominal surgery, and with higher complexity tumors [1, 2].

With the continuing evolution of robotic surgical techniques, significant emphasis has been placed towards further improvement in long-term renal functional outcomes following partial nephrectomy. While the volume of excision remains highly dependent on the size, location, and complexity of the tumor, different intraoperative considerations have been proposed to promote better preservation of vascularized, functional renal parenchyma. These included previously described attempts to minimize or eliminate ischemia, performing tumor enucleation or resection with thin parenchymal margins, as well as meticulous suturing techniques to ensure

N. A. Soputro · A. Kaviani · M. A. Zeinab · J. Kaouk (✉)
Glickman Urological & Kidney Institute, Cleveland Clinic, Cleveland, OH, USA
e-mail: kaoukj@ccf.org

S. Tonyali et al. (eds.), *Current Endourology*,
https://doi.org/10.1007/978-3-032-00010-1_22

hemostasis and quality renorrhaphy. Despite the theoretical benefits of the different approaches, further clinical studies remain necessary to ensure their respective clinical utility without additional impacts on surgical complexity and perioperative morbidity [3–6].

In addition to the aforementioned technical modifications, the recent introduction of the purpose-built Single Port (SP) surgical platform (Intuitive Surgical, Sunnyvale, CA, USA) has also altered the contemporary landscape of minimally invasive surgical practices for partial nephrectomy. Compared to the traditional multi-port robotic surgical platform, the SP offered several unique features, such as a narrow profile and double-jointed instruments, which improved the ergonomics and maneuverability, especially when performing procedures in smaller surgical working spaces. These provided the opportunity for surgeons to regionalize surgical approaches to the anatomy of interest and to implement novel surgical access, as evident by the advent of Low Anterior Access (LAA) for various retroperitoneal upper tract procedures, with demonstrable benefits in enhancing perioperative outcomes and patient comfort [7–10].

This chapter sought to describe the various technical nuances and innovations pertaining to the expanding minimally invasive surgical repertoire for partial nephrectomy, focusing on their correlation with the primary objectives of the procedure in improving patient comfort as well as the long-term functional and oncological outcomes.

Preoperative Evaluation

Preoperative evaluation prior to partial nephrectomy typically involves a detailed clinical history and physical examination, along with baseline laboratory values including baseline creatinine and estimated glomerular filtration rate (GFR). For solid or complex cystic renal mass, the current guideline from the American Urological Association (AUA) recommends the utility of high-quality, multiphase, cross-sectional imaging through Computed Tomography (CT) or Magnetic Resonance Imaging (MRI) to better characterize and clinically stage the respective lesion. The characterization of the renal mass should include comprehensive assessments of tumor complexity, location of the tumor with respect to the renal poles and hilum, the exophytic or endophytic nature of the lesion, level of invasiveness, degree of contrast enhancements, as well as the presence of fat.

In addition, the AUA guidelines also recommends preoperative assessment for possible metastasis, especially in the thoracic region. In most cases, renal mass biopsy is often not required and should be cautioned, particularly when it does not contribute to any changes in the management plans. When renal mass biopsy is considered, core biopsy is usually preferred in lieu of fine needle aspirate. Genetic counselling is also not routinely performed but can be opted in younger patients with known renal malignancy, multifocal or bilateral disease, those with first or second degree relative with renal malignancy, or in patients with known familial renal neoplastic syndrome. The latter may include but is not limited to tuberous sclerosis, Birt-Hogg-Dube, or Von-Hippel-Lindau syndrome.

Surgical Techniques

Transperitoneal Multi-Port Robotic Partial Nephrectomy

Multi-Port Robotic Partial Nephrectomy (MP-RAPN) is commonly performed using the DaVinci Xi robotic surgical platform (Intuitive Surgical, Sunnyvale, CA, USA) via a Transperitoneal technique. Following the induction of general anesthesia, the patient is positioned in a 60° lateral decubitus position with the operating table mildly flexed at the level of the umbilicus. A slight Trendelenburg position can also be applied to assist in bowel manipulation. Appropriate padding with pillows and foam pads should be applied to the respective pressure points, following which the patient is secured to the operating table and a Foley catheter is inserted.

Pneumoperitoneum can be achieved following a careful insertion of a Veress needle at the lateral border of the rectus muscle at the level of the 12th rib. After the peritoneum is insufflated to 15 mmHg, the Veress needle is replaced with a 12 mm robotic port for the 30° endoscope. Following a careful inspection of the peritoneal cavity to ensure the absence of injury during the initial access and insufflation, three 8 mm robotic ports can be inserted under vision—the first at approximately 3 cm below the costal margin along the pararectal line, the second about two fingers breadth cephalad to the anterior superior iliac spine, and another in the lower quadrant of the abdomen along the pararectal line. A laparoscopic assistant port for insufflation is subsequently inserted more medially between the camera and the lower pararectal robotic ports, aiming to create an equilateral triangle among the three ports. For right-sided procedure, an additional 5 mm assistant port can be placed in the subxiphoid area to accommodate a locking Allis clamp for liver retraction. Depending on the clinical scenarios, each port position can be configured at the surgeon's discretion (Fig. 22.1).

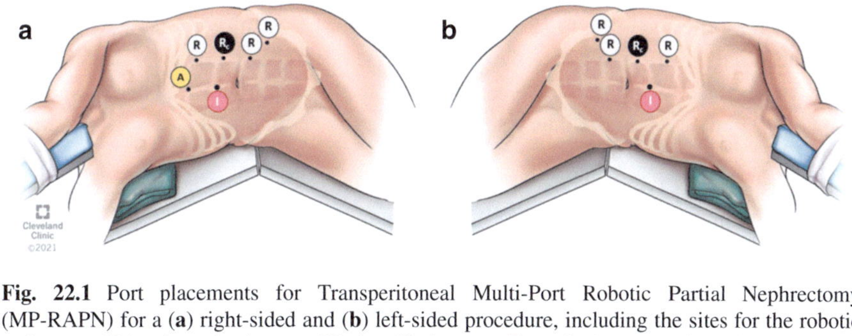

Fig. 22.1 Port placements for Transperitoneal Multi-Port Robotic Partial Nephrectomy (MP-RAPN) for a (**a**) right-sided and (**b**) left-sided procedure, including the sites for the robotic endoscope ($\mathbf{R_c}$), other robotic ports (**R**), insufflation port (**I**), and a laparoscopic assistant port (**A**)

Following port placement, the patient cart of the robotic platform can be approached from the posterior aspect over the patient's shoulder making an obtuse angle relative to the axis of the operating table. The camera is subsequently aligned towards the kidney of interest and the robotic instruments are introduced to the peritoneal cavity under vision. Using the ProGrasp forceps on the left and a monopolar curved scissor on the surgeon's right hand, the peritoneum is first incised along the white line of Toldt and the bowel is mobilized medially to develop a plane anterior to the Gerota's fascia and posterior to the mesocolon.

Once the retroperitoneum is entered, dissections can be continued towards the renal hilum by first identifying the psoas major muscle and the gonadal vein as important landmarks. On the right side, the gonadal vein is usually kept medially towards the inferior vena cava, whilst on the left, the gonadal vein can be lifted along with the left ureter for adequate exposure of the left renal hilum. Using the preoperative images as a guide, meticulous dissections can then be performed on the renal hilum to better appreciate the renal artery and vein in preparation for vascular control, especially to properly identify any evidence of early arterial branching. In most cases, surgeons can opt only for arterial control and not to pursue any venous clamping. This is given the risk of venous congestion associated with venous occlusion that can increase the risk of bleeding during the subsequent dissection steps.

After adequate exposure of the hilar landmarks is achieved, the Gerota's fascia can be opened down to the renal capsule. Following this, the dissections can continue along the renal capsule with minimal fat excision until the tumor or the surface overlying the tumor is exposed. Intraoperative ultrasound can then be performed using a laparoscopic ultrasound probe or a drop-in robotic ultrasound probe (ProART Robotic Drop-In Transducer 8826, BK Medical, Peabody, MA, USA). The latter was purpose-built for a robotic surgical platform and can be maneuvered independently by the surgeon intracorporeally (Fig. 22.2a). The live intraoperative images from the ultrasound probe can be visualized as a picture-in-picture display in the surgeon console as facilitated by the built-in TilePro function of the DaVinci robotic system (Intuitive Surgical, Sunnyvale, CA, USA). Once the borders of the tumors are visualized, the surrounding renal capsule is circumferentially scored with electrocautery to delineate the resection boundaries.

Prior to tumor excision, robotic bulldog clamp(s) (Scanlan International, St. Paul, MN, USA) can be applied using the ProGrasp forceps to clamp renal artery ± vein, marking the beginning of ischemia time. Should the surgeon decide to clamp both the renal artery and vein, the renal artery is typically clamped first. Under warm ischemia, the tumor is excised using a combination of cold scissors and electrocautery, ensuring adequate surgical margin and hemostasis throughout (Fig. 22.2b).

Renorrhaphy is typically performed in two layers. The deep layer can be closed using a running 3–0 V-loc suture (Medtronic, Minneapolis, MN, USA) that is secured with a Hem-o-lok clip (Teleflex Medical, Research Triangle Park, NC, USA) in a sliding clip fashion. Each suture point is placed to facilitate the closure of intrarenal vessels and/or any entry into the collecting system (Fig. 22.2c). Throughout our experience, early unclamping is routinely preferred prior to

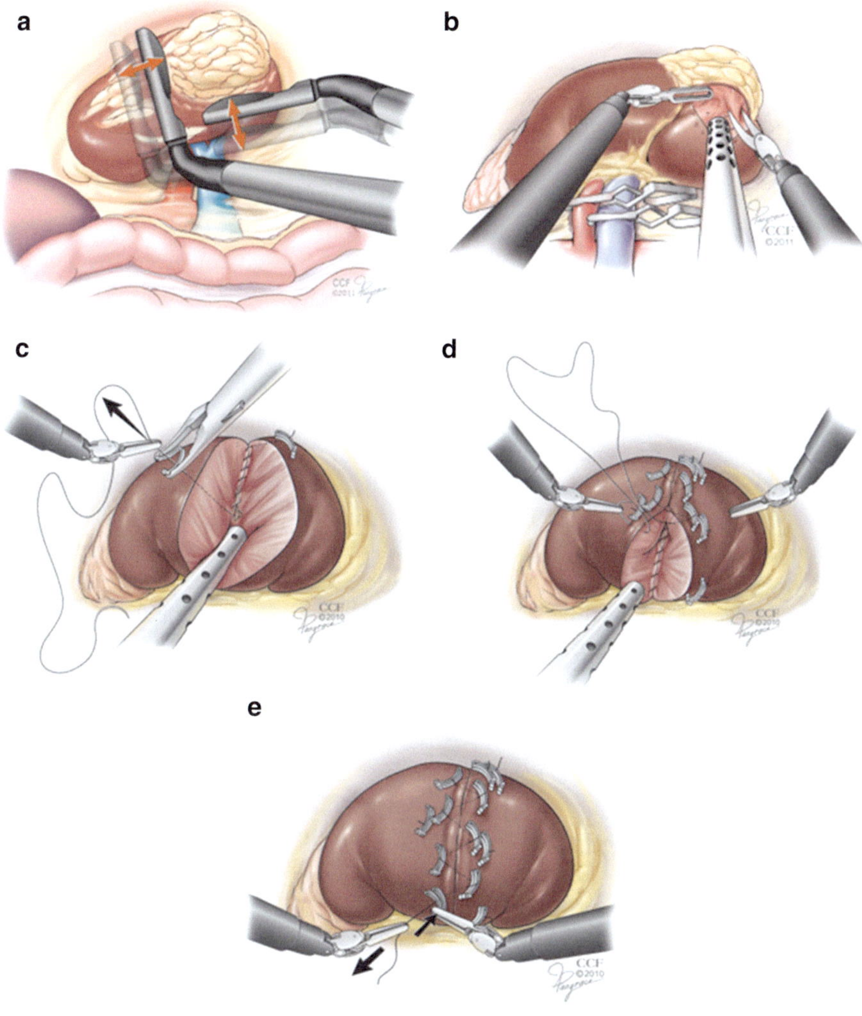

Fig. 22.2 Illustrations of several surgical steps during Transperitoneal Multi-Port Robotic Partial Nephrectomy (MP-RAPN) including (**a**) intraoperative ultrasound for tumor identification, (**b**) tumor excision under warm ischemia with both renal artery and vein clamped, (**c**) deep-layer renorrhaphy, (**d**) outer layer renorrhaphy, and (**e**) the completion of renorrhaphy. (*Retroperitoneal Multi-Port Robotic Partial Nephrectomy)*

capsular renorrhaphy, defined as the release of vascular clamp prior to the completion of renorrhaphy. In addition to reducing the total ischemia time, early unclamping can provide additional benefits in allowing any remaining sources of bleeding to be identified and addressed before the subsequent closure. Outer layer renorrhaphy is performed using 0-Vicryl suture on a CT-1 needle (Ethicon Inc., Sommerville, NJ, USA) to reapproximate the renal capsule. The suture points should be placed at a safe distance from the resection edge to reduce the risk of capsular tear (Fig. 22.2d).

A sliding Hem-o-lok clip can be placed after each suture needle passage. Depending on the depth of the excision and tumor location, an extra layer of renorrhaphy can be performed at the discretion of the surgeon. In recent years, hemostatic agents, such as Surgicel (Ethicon Inc., Sommerville, NJ, USA), are not routinely indicated but can be used depending on the different clinical scenarios and/or surgeon preference.

Following the completion of renorrhaphy, the Gerota's fascia can be closed with Hem-o-lok clips. An EndoCatch Specimen Retraction Pouch (Medtronic, Minneapolis, MN, USA) can then be introduced for the subsequent removal of the specimen. Prior to the port removals and wound closure, a Jackson-Pratt drain can be placed through the most caudal port site [2].

Postoperatively, patients are normally commenced on a clear diet that can be advanced as tolerated. The Foley catheter and optional Jackson-Pratt drain are commonly removed on postoperative day 1. Drain fluid Creatinine analysis can be used to evaluate for the presence of urine leak prior to drain removal if suspected. To reduce the risk of thromboembolic events, early mobilization is often encouraged. The use of pharmacological or mechanical thromboprophylaxis remains at the discretion of the surgical team, weighing the risks and benefits depending on the specific clinical scenarios.

While patients are routinely admitted as inpatients following RAPN, a recent large cohort study involving 5353 patients highlighted a significantly reduced length of stay (LOS) following RAPN, as compared to the laparoscopic (LPN) approach (mean, RAPN 2.25 vs. LPN 2.58 days, $p < 0.001$) [11]. Throughout the years, several studies have highlighted the favorable perioperative, oncological, and functional outcomes following RAPN. Previous multi-institutional studies have highlighted the relatively low risks of major postoperative complications of up to 5.4% which remains comparatively lower than LPN (9.4%) and open partial nephrectomy (11.5%) [12–14]. In terms of oncological outcomes, the 5-year and 7-year cumulative incidence of Renal Cell Carcinoma (RCC)-related deaths following RAPN were estimated to be 1.8%, while the 5-year and 7-year cumulative incidence of local recurrence was 3.6% and 4.2%, respectively. The cumulative incidence for metastatic disease was reported at 3.2% at 5 years and 4.6% at 7 years [1]. With regards to functional outcomes, approximately 6% were previously noted to experience clinically significant CKD upstaging at 5 years, which was defined as any progression from CKD Stages of 1–2 (GFR ≥60 mL/min/1.73 m^2) to 3a (GFR 45–59 mL/min/1.73 m^2) or above, Stage 3a to 3b (GFR 30–44 mL/min/1.73 m^2) or above, Stage 3b to 4 (GFR 15–29 mL/min/1.73 m^2) or above, or from Stage 4 to 5 (GFR <15 mL/min/1.73 m^2) [1, 14].

In addition to the Transperitoneal approach, MP-RAPN can also be performed using a Retroperitoneal technique. In this approach, the patient is positioned in a full 90° lateral flank position with the operating table adequately flexed to open the space between the 12th rib and the iliac crest. A small incision is then made at the mid-axillary line above the iliac crest to enter the lumbodorsal fascia. A blunt dissection using the surgeon's finger is then used to gently sweep the peritoneum and to open the space for the insertion of the retroperitoneal Spacemaker™ Dissection

Balloon (Medtronic, Minneapolis, MN, USA). To ensure adequate exposure for the partial nephrectomy, the balloon should be inserted under vision and oriented along the psoas major muscle towards the kidney.

Following the creation of the retroperitoneal space, the 30° endoscopic camera can be inserted through the 12 mm robotic port placed in the mid-axillary line just above the iliac crest. The transversus abdominis muscle should be clearly visualized superiorly while the psoas major muscle with or without the ureter should be identifiable inferiorly. The remaining robotic ports is then inserted under vision, with one inserted along the posterior axillary line, another inserted along the anterior axillary line, and the fourth port placed about 6 cm medial to the previous port. The different ports typically adopt a slight arch-like configuration at approximately 6 cm distance between each other. An assistant port can also be inserted about 8 cm caudal to the fourth port.

The Retroperitoneal approach often involves the mobilization of the paranephric fat outside of the Gerota's fascia. The Gerota's fascia can then be approached posteriorly and incised just above the psoas major muscle to gain exposure of the kidney. The remaining dissection steps, including exposure of the renal hilum, intraoperative ultrasound, tumor excision, renorrhaphy, and specimen extraction remain similar to the previously described Transperitoneal MP-RAPN.

Compared to the Transperitoneal technique, Retroperitoneal MP-RAPN offers more direct access and exposure to the renal hilum. The complete preservation of the peritoneum and intraperitoneal organs has also been beneficial in providing surgical options in patients with previous abdominal surgery, improving postoperative recovery, and reducing perioperative morbidity, particularly the risk of postoperative ileus.

Retroperitoneal Single-Port Robotic Partial Nephrectomy via a Low Anterior Access

The purpose-built SP robotic platform consists of three main components, including the patient cart, the vision cart, and the surgeon console. While the vision cart and surgeon console bear resemblance to other DaVinci robotic surgical platforms, the SP patient cart is distinctively unique as it possesses a single arm with four instrument drives that can simultaneously accommodate a double-jointed 8 mm endoscopic camera and three other 6 mm robotic instruments. Both the endoscopic camera and robotic instruments can facilitate seven degrees of freedom, which allows for 360° anatomic access from a single pivot point.

The current armamentarium of the SP instruments includes the Maryland bipolar forceps, Cadiere forceps, monopolar hook and scissor, round tooth retractor, needle driver, and Hem-o-lok Weck clip applier. Extracorporeally, the instruments are arranged in a 12, 3, 6, and 9 o'clock configurations. They are then introduced through a 25 mm multichannel cannula of the purpose-built SP Access Kit (Intuitive

Surgical, Sunnyvale, CA, USA). As initially conceptualized by the Cleveland Clinic group, the unique bubble chamber design of the SP port facilitates the 'Floating Docking Technique', which significantly improves the flexibility and range of the instruments by up to 390° and addresses the required 10 cm minimum working distance for the SP instruments [9]. In addition, the SP Access Kit also houses a 12 mm assistant port adjacent to the multichannel cannula and a separate 8 mm assistant port on the side of the bubble chamber. The former is typically used for the Remotely Operated Suction Irrigation (ROSI) system (Vascular Technology Inc., Nashua, NH, USA), whereas the latter accommodates an insufflation trocar. The two assistant ports can also be used for various laparoscopic instruments, including a vascular stapler.

Of note, the first human clinical trial of the SP platform was performed by Kaouk et al. in 2010 using the DaVinci SP999 (Intuitive Surgical, Sunnyvale, CA, USA). The trial included four cases of RAPN that were successfully completed via a Transperitoneal approach without any conversion, additional port, or perioperative complications [8]. Following Food & Drug Administration (FDA) approval in 2018, the technique has been replicated across various institutions throughout the United States, maintaining favorable perioperative outcomes with a minimal morbidity profile [7].

Similar to its MP counterpart, SP-RAPN can be completed either via Transperitoneal or Retroperitoneal approaches with a recent publication from the Single Port Advanced Research Consortium (SPARC) highlighting comparable clinical outcomes between the two approaches. The unique features of the SP platform, however, provided the opportunity to regionalize our surgical approach and to develop alternate surgical access as evident through the advent of a LAA that was first implemented by the Cleveland Clinic group for a retroperitoneal dismembered pyeloplasty [15]. While several names have been introduced in the literature to describe the same approach (e.g. Mini-Pfannenstiel and Superior Anterior Retroperitoneal Access/SARA) [16, 17], the recent consensus from the SPARC collaborative group has decided to continue with LAA to describe the technique moving forward.

Regardless of the procedure types, LAA can be consistently used with the patient first positioned in a lateral decubitus position and with a 3-4 cm incision made at approximately two fingers breadth above the superior pubic ramus. After separating the external oblique fascia, blunt dissection is performed using the surgeon's finger to open the retroperitoneal space in preparation for the insertion of the SP Access Kit. The patient cart can then be approached from the patient's posterior aspect and the single robotic arm is positioned and docked at an acute angle towards the ipsilateral kidney (Fig. 22.3). The endoscope can be positioned at either 12 or 6 o'clock, while the Cadiere forceps and monopolar curved scissors are usually placed on the left and right, respectively. As the robotic instruments are introduced, the psoas major muscle can be visualized and forms an important landmark. Dissections are then pursued to first identify the ureter and to follow its course proximally towards the renal hilum. Once the hilar structures are isolated, the remaining dissection steps are identical to the previously described techniques for MP-RAPN [18].

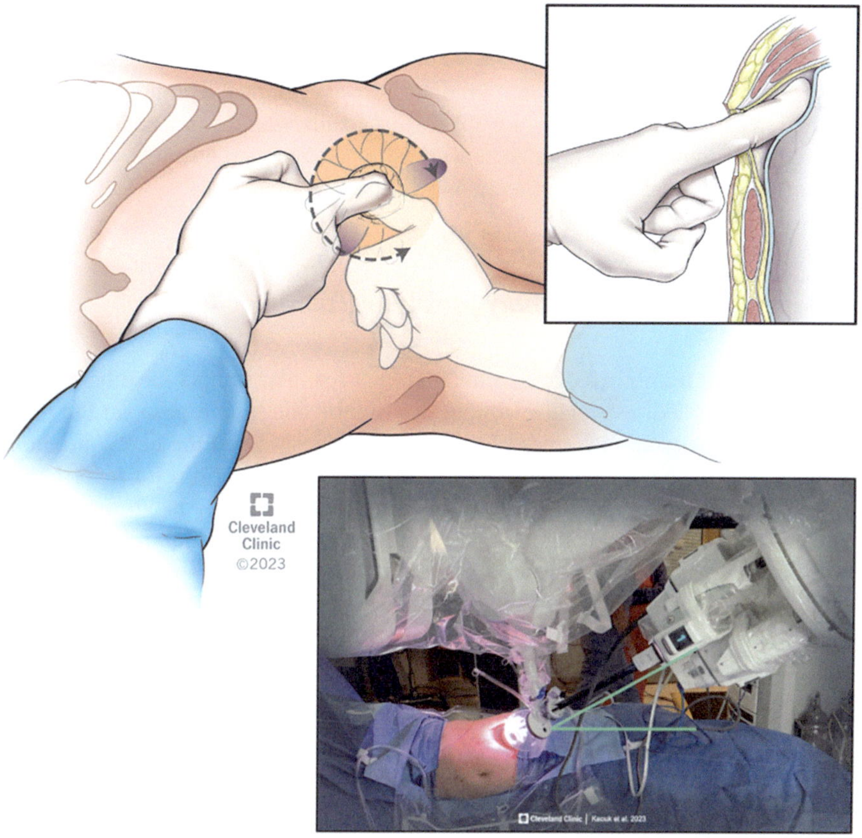

Fig. 22.3 **(Main & In-Picture Top)** Blunt finger dissection to develop the extraperitoneal during Low Anterior Access (LAA) Single Port (SP) RAPN. **(In-Picture Bottom)** SP robot docking at an acute angle aiming towards the kidney using the 'floating docking technique', as facilitated by the purpose-built SP Access Kit

A recently published initial experience highlighted the feasibility of performing the technique for various tumor locations. The efficacy of partial nephrectomy as often described in terms of the trifecta of negative surgical margin, warm ischemia time of within 25 minutes, and the absence of major postoperative complications of Clavien-Dindo grades 3a and above, was achieved in 94%. Importantly, the technique has facilitated further enhancements in postoperative outcomes and patient comfort, with 83% being discharged on the same day without any opioid analgesia. Furthermore, the complete preservation of the peritoneum and accessory respiratory muscles has also allowed for significant reductions in the risk of postoperative ileus and respiratory complications, respectively [10, 17, 19].

Special Scenarios

The continuing advancements in minimally invasive surgical techniques have also resulted in expanded indications for RAPN, especially with the procedure able to be pursued for complex hilar tumors, as well as in patients with a solitary kidney [20, 21] or previous renal transplant recipients [22].

Robotic Partial Nephrectomy for Hilar Tumors

The safety and feasibility of performing RAPN for hilar tumors have been previously demonstrated, especially without any significant compromise on the oncological and functional outcomes [23, 24]. Nevertheless, given the likely proximity of the tumor to the renal vessels and limited parenchymal margins for renorrhaphy, it is important to consider several technical nuances that may need to be implemented with one example being the V-Hilar Suture (VHS) technique. The technical modification with VHS includes the reapproximation of the deep layer starting close to the renal hilum towards the lateral edges of the resection bed to make up a V-like configuration diverging from the renal hilum (Fig. 22.4) [25].

Redo Robotic Partial Nephrectomy

As highlighted in the previous section, local tumor recurrence remains one of the most important risks to consider following RAPN. While salvage or redo partial nephrectomy can be performed robotically, there are important challenges that need to be considered both in the preoperative and intraoperative settings.

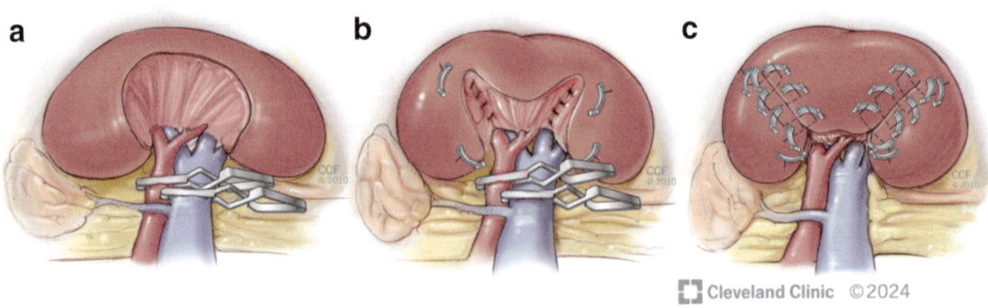

Fig. 22.4 V-Hilar Suture (VHS) technique for partial nephrectomy for hilar tumors, starting with (**a**) an exposed resection bed, (**b**) deep layer renorrhaphy, and (**c**) outer layer renorrhaphy following a V-shape configuration from the renal hilum

Firstly, preoperative radiologic characterization of the renal mass using CT or MRI modalities may be limited by the reduced volume of normal renal parenchyma and the presence of radiopaque surgical clips from the previous procedure [26].

Intraoperatively, the presence of adhesions from the prior procedure and fibrosis secondary to the peripheral tissue reaction surrounding the tumor can impose additional challenges during the establishment of pneumoperitoneum and hilar dissection. The presence of fibrotic tissues may also add to the complexity during the opening of Gerota's fascia and intraoperative tumor identification and its subsequent resection. To assist in reopening the Gerota's fascia during redo RAPN, our conventional technique for primary RAPN routinely involves a single, minimal incision to bivalve the Gerota's fascia that was later closed with medium Hem-o-lok clips. To improve the precision during the identification of the tumor and its margins, the use of intraoperative ultrasound with or without Doppler imaging is highly recommended. Depending on the tumor complexity and available resources, additional intraoperative navigation tools, such as Indocyanine Green (ICG) may be employed to better distinguish the renal tumor from normal renal tissues. Following tumor excision, renorrhaphy can also be complicated depending on the tumor location and their proximity to the renal hilum.

Previous multi-institutional studies have reported the feasibility and safety of performing redo RAPN with minimal risk of intraoperative complication and conversion to other surgical approaches, including radical nephrectomy. Of note, many of the procedures of up to 25.7% were completed off-clamp. Major postoperative complications were identified in up to 7% of cases, which more commonly involved postoperative bleeding. In terms of oncological outcomes, positive surgical margins were identified in up to 11.5% with limited information on disease progression given the limited duration of follow-up [27, 28].

Robotic Partial Nephrectomy in a Renal Allograft

It was previously estimated that kidney transplant recipients were at 5–10 times increased risk of developing RCC. Nevertheless, RCC commonly occurs in the native kidney and the risk of RCC in the allograft remained low between 0.02% and 0.4%. While most cases are usually managed with radical nephrectomy, nephron-sparing surgery warrants an important consideration, particularly to not render the patient anephric and becoming dialysis-dependent. The technique for RAPN in a renal allograft has been previously described, with several technical modifications, especially when compared to the traditional Transperitoneal MP-RAPN.

With the patient positioned in a lateral decubitus position with the operating table slightly flexed, the ports are arranged to ensure adequate access towards the transplanted kidney in the iliac fossa. In terms of the robotic ports, the endoscope port is first placed in the supraumbilical area. The left robotic arm is then inserted along the pararectal line at approximately 3 cm below the costal margin. The right robotic arm can be kept midline in the suprapubic area, while the fourth robotic arm is placed at the level of the 12th rib in the upper quadrant ipsilateral to the allograft. An assistant port can subsequently be placed along the pararectal line on the contralateral side between the ports for the camera and the right robotic arm [22]. Surgical techniques are otherwise similar to the previously described steps for MP-RAPN. The decision to perform an intraoperative frozen section should be at the discretion of the surgical team and remains dependent on the preoperative evaluation.

The outcomes of partial nephrectomy in a renal allograft have been previously reported, with cancer recurrence identified in 3.6% after 3 years, which was comparable to the prevalence in the non-transplant population [29].

Other Technical Modifications and Intraoperative Considerations

While maturing RAPN experience has provided continuing assurance towards satisfactory cancer control and further enhancements in perioperative outcomes, there remains an ongoing discussion surrounding different modifiable intraoperative factors that can improve the long-term functional outcomes following RAPN. Examples of the different factors can include the preferred surgical approach (such as Transperitoneal versus Retroperitoneal), as well as the techniques for vascular control, tumor extirpation, and renorrhaphy.

Firstly, when comparing Transperitoneal versus Retroperitoneal RAPN, previous studies have identified comparable long-term functional outcomes between the two approaches [30, 31]. In terms of vascular control, although off-clamp partial nephrectomy theoretically eliminates the risk of ischemic renal injury, the technique did not contribute to significant improvements in functional preservation. Rather, it may be associated with increased risks of complications, including intraoperative bleeding requiring transfusion and conversion to radical nephrectomy [3, 32, 33]. In cases with higher degrees of complexity, an alternative cold ischemia technique has been previously introduced, which included the use of ice slush to cool the kidney to temperatures of 10–20 °C (Fig. 22.5). While renal hypothermia facilitated by cold ischemia allows for a longer ischemia time, the technique may not translate to detrimental improvements in postoperative renal function, especially when compared to the conventional warm ischemia technique [4, 34].

In recent years, several studies have introduced the possibility of performing tumor enucleation in place of standard partial nephrectomy based on the understanding towards the presence of a distinct layer of pseudocapsule around the renal mass that can serve as a dissection plane. While the technique may allow for better preservation of normal renal parenchyma and thus postoperative renal function, there is a paucity of evidence on the oncological outcomes and concerns surrounding the reproducibility of the technique [35, 36]. Of note, there may be some heterogeneity in the existence and thickness of the pseudocapsule [37]. Furthermore, there remains an ongoing question surrounding tumor invasion of the pseudocapsule, especially in deeper, more endophytic tumors that will undoubtedly compromise the oncological outcomes [6, 36].

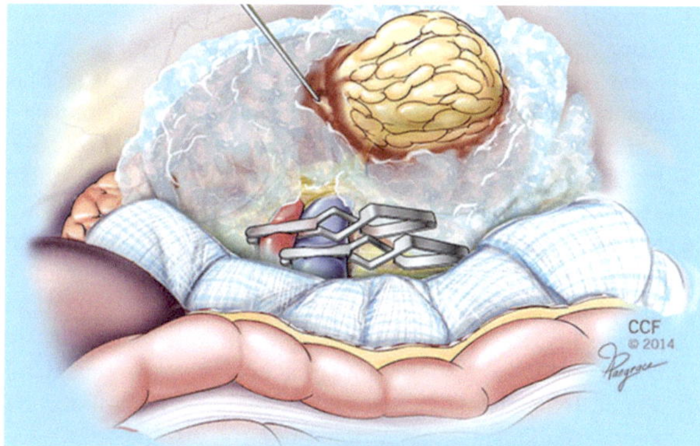

Fig. 22.5 Cold ischemia during Transperitoneal MP-RAPN following the introduction of ice slush

With renorrhaphy often considered an important yet time-consuming step of RAPN, several groups have considered adopting 'sutureless renorrhaphy' as part of their routine RAPN practice. This technical modification relies on the utility of either hemostatic agents, electrocautery, or both to ensure adequate hemostasis and the absence of urine leak following the tumor resection. Nevertheless, the current levels of evidence to support this technique remain limited with most of the studies being retrospective, single-institutional analyses over a relatively short duration of follow-up [5].

Conclusion

Herein, we present the standardized approaches to performing RAPN using the standard MP robotic platform and the more recently introduced purpose-built SP robotic system. With the continuing surgical technological and technical advancements, recent years have witnessed an expansion in the clinical indications of RAPN, allowing the procedure to be performed in tumors of higher complexity, patients with higher BMI and hostile abdomen, as well as those with solitary and kidney and previous renal transplant recipients. While certain technical modifications can be implemented, there remains an ongoing need for further research to better guide the different intraoperative factors that can translate into additional improvements in the perioperative, oncological, and functional outcomes for RAPN.

References

1. Bertolo R, Garisto J, Dagenais J, et al. Transperitoneal robot-assisted partial nephrectomy with minimum follow-up of 5 years: oncological and functional outcomes from a single institution. Eur Urol Oncol. 2019;2:207–13.
2. Kaouk JH, Khalifeh A, Hillyer S, et al. Robot-assisted laparoscopic partial nephrectomy: step-by-step contemporary technique and surgical outcomes at a single high-volume institution. Eur Urol. 2012;62:553–61.

3. Antonelli A, Veccia A, Francavilla S, et al. On-clamp versus off-clamp robotic partial nephrectomy: a systematic review and meta-analysis. Urol J. 2019;86:52–62.
4. Lane BR, Russo P, Uzzo RG, et al. Comparison of cold and warm ischemia during partial nephrectomy in 660 solitary kidneys reveals predominant role of nonmodifiable factors in determining ultimate renal function. J Urol. 2011;185:421–7.
5. Liu P, Li Y, Shi B, et al. The outcome of sutureless in partial nephrectomy: a systematic review and meta-analysis. Biomed Res Int. 2022;2022:5260131.
6. Minervini A, Campi R, Di Maida F, et al. Tumor–parenchyma interface and long-term oncologic outcomes after robotic tumor enucleation for sporadic renal cell carcinoma. Presented at the Urologic Oncology: Seminars and Original Investigations; 2018.
7. Kaouk J, Garisto J, Eltemamy M, et al. Pure single-site robot-assisted partial nephrectomy using the SP surgical system: initial clinical experience. Urology. 2019;124:282–5.
8. Kaouk JH, Haber G-P, Autorino R, et al. A novel robotic system for single-port urologic surgery: first clinical investigation. Eur Urol. 2014;66:1033–43.
9. Lenfant L, Kim S, Aminsharifi A, et al. Floating docking technique: a simple modification to improve the working space of the instruments during single-port robotic surgery. World J Urol. 2021;39:1299–305.
10. Okhawere KE, Beksac AT, Wilson MP, et al. A propensity-matched comparison of the perioperative outcomes between single-port and multi-port robotic assisted partial nephrectomy: a report from the single port advanced research consortium (SPARC). J Endourol. 2022;36:1526–31.
11. Okhawere KE, Milky G, Razdan S, et al. One-year healthcare costs after robotic-assisted and laparoscopic partial and radical nephrectomy: a cohort study. BMC Health Serv Res. 2023;23:1099.
12. Spana G, Haber G-P, Dulabon LM, et al. Complications after robotic partial nephrectomy at centers of excellence: multi-institutional analysis of 450 cases. J Urol. 2011;186:417–22.
13. Bic A, Mazeaud C, Salleron J, et al. Complications after partial nephrectomy: robotics overcomes open surgery and laparoscopy: the PMSI French national database. BMC Urol. 2023;23:146.
14. Margue G, Ingels A, Bensalah K, et al. Late complications and 5 years outcomes of robotic partial nephrectomy in France: prospective assessment in the French Kidney Cancer Research Network (UroCCR 10). World J Urol. 2023;41:2281–8.
15. Lenfant L, Wilson CA, Sawczyn G, et al. Single-port robot-assisted dismembered pyeloplasty with mini-pfannenstiel or peri-umbilical access: initial experience in a single center. Urology. 2020;143:147–52.
16. Beksac AT, Wilson CA, Lenfant L, et al. Single-port mini-pfannenstiel robotic pyeloplasty: establishing a non-narcotic pathway along with a same-day discharge protocol. Urology. 2022;160:130–5.
17. Pellegrino AA, Chen G, Morgantini L, et al. Simplifying retroperitoneal robotic single-port surgery: novel supine anterior retroperitoneal access. Eur Urol. 2023;84:223–8.
18. Soputro N, Ferguson E, Ramos-Carpinteyro R, et al. Low anterior access for retroperitoneal single-port robotic partial nephrectomy. Eur Urol Open Sci. 2023;55:S219.
19. Rich JM, Okhawere KE, Nguyen C, et al. Transperitoneal versus retroperitoneal single-port robotic-assisted partial nephrectomy: an analysis from the Single Port Advanced Research Consortium. Eur Urol Focus. 2023;9:1059–64.
20. Hillyer SP, Bhayani SB, Allaf ME, et al. Robotic partial nephrectomy for solitary kidney: a multi-institutional analysis. Urology. 2013;81:93–7.
21. Kaouk JH, Malkoç E. Is robotic partial nephrectomy convenient for solitary kidney? Turk J Urol. 2016;42:127–9.
22. Kaouk J, Spana G, Hillyer S, et al. Robotic-assisted laparoscopic partial nephrectomy for a 7-cm mass in a renal allograft. Am J Transplant. 2011;11:2242–6.
23. Eyraud R, Long J-A, Snow-Lisy D, et al. Robot-assisted partial nephrectomy for hilar tumors: perioperative outcomes. Urology. 2013;81:1246–52.

24. Dulabon LM, Kaouk JH, Haber G-P, et al. Multi-institutional analysis of robotic partial nephrectomy for hilar versus nonhilar lesions in 446 consecutive cases. Eur Urol. 2011;59:325–30.
25. Khalifeh A, Autorino R, Hillyer SP, et al. V-hilar suture renorrhaphy during robotic partial nephrectomy for renal hilar tumors: preliminary outcomes of a novel surgical technique. Urology. 2012;80:466–73.
26. Matsushita K, Matsubara S, Tsumura K, et al. Computed tomography appearance of Hem-o-lok clips in patients who have undergone laparoscopic nephrectomy or nephroureterectomy. JSLS. 2011;15:517–9.
27. Beksac AT, Carbonara U, Abou Zeinab M, et al. Redo robotic partial nephrectomy for recurrent renal tumors: a multi-institutional analysis. J Endourol. 2022;36:1296–301.
28. Di Maida F, Grosso AA, Campi R, et al. Redo partial nephrectomy for local recurrence after previous nephron-sparing surgery. Surgical insights and oncologic results from a high-volume robotic center. Eur Urol Open Sci. 2023;57:84.
29. Griffith J, Amin K, Waingankar N, et al. Solid renal masses in transplanted allograft kidneys: a closer look at the epidemiology and management. Am J Transplant. 2017;17:2775–81.
30. Paulucci DJ, Beksac AT, Porter J, et al. A multi-institutional propensity score matched comparison of transperitoneal and retroperitoneal partial nephrectomy for cT1 posterior tumors. J Laparoendosc Adv Surg Tech A. 2019;29:29–34.
31. Porpiglia F, Mari A, Amparore D, et al. Transperitoneal vs retroperitoneal minimally invasive partial nephrectomy: comparison of perioperative outcomes and functional follow-up in a large multi-institutional cohort (The RECORD 2 Project). Surg Endosc. 2021;35:4295–304.
32. Bertolo R, Simone G, Garisto J, et al. Off-clamp vs on-clamp robotic partial nephrectomy: perioperative, functional and oncological outcomes from a propensity-score matching between two high-volume centers. Eur J Surg Oncol. 2019;45:1232–7.
33. Sharma G, Shah M, Ahluwalia P, et al. Off-clamp versus on-clamp robot-assisted partial nephrectomy: a propensity-matched analysis. Eur Urol Oncol. 2023;83:S1470–1.
34. Funahashi Y, Yoshino Y, Sassa N, et al. Comparison of warm and cold ischemia on renal function after partial nephrectomy. Urology. 2014;84:1408–13.
35. Culpan M, Atis G, Sanli O, et al. Comparison of tumor enucleation and standard partial nephrectomy according to trifecta outcomes: a multicenter study by the Turkish Academy of Urology, Uro-Oncology Working Group. J Investig Surg. 2022;35:1112–8.
36. Minervini A, Campi R, Sessa F, et al. Positive surgical margins and local recurrence after simple enucleation and standard partial nephrectomy for malignant renal tumors: systematic review of the literature and meta-analysis of prevalence. Minerva Urol Nefrol. 2017;69(6):523–38.
37. Tsivian M, Packiam VT, Thompson RH. Tumor enucleation is appropriate during partial nephrectomy: against. Eur Urol Focus. 2019;5:925–6.

Chapter 23
Retrograde Intrarenal Surgery

Mrigyanka Sinha, Amelia Pietropaolo, and Bhaskar K. Somani

History

The origin of modern day ureteroscopes (URS) dates back to 1912 when Hugh Hampton Young serendipitously introduced a paediatric cystoscope into a dilated ureter that was being treated for congenital posterior urethral valve. This event led to further research into endoscopic management of urological pathologies leading to the development of the equipment we use today.

Karl Storz in 1980 introduced the first ureteroscope [1]; a 12 Fr, 50 cm long rigid ureteroscope with dual working channels. This was however rather cumbersome to use due to the nature of the initial design. Around the same time Olympus modified a paediatric bronchoscope into a deflectable flexible ureteroscope to help improve access. The rigid ureteroscopes were improved by replacing the rod-lens imaging to fibre-optic imaging allowing miniaturisation of the outer diameter.

In 1964 Marshall et al. [2] reported the first use of ureteroscope to visualise an impacted ureteral calculus. Later the flexible ureteroscope was enhanced by addition of a working channel, deflection of active tip and alteration of stiffness of endoscopic shaft [3]. By 2001 smaller scopes were introduced with a diameter of 8Fr and a standard 3.6 Fr working channel (3Fr = 1 mm). This in turn helped improve ureteroscopy and decrease ureteric trauma and failed procedure due to large instruments. In 2014 digital imaging was introduced in addition to the pre-existing fiberoptic imaging, thus improving the image quality. This digital image flexible

M. Sinha
Clinical Fellow, University Hospital Southampton, Southampton, UK

A. Pietropaolo
University Hospital Southampton, Southampton, UK

B. K. Somani (✉)
University Hospital Southampton NHS Trust, Southampton, UK
e-mail: b.k.somani@soton.ac.uk

S. Tonyali et al. (eds.), *Current Endourology*,
https://doi.org/10.1007/978-3-032-00010-1_23

URS has an chip at the tip which allows for the progression of procedure without camera head and light cord, making the procedure ergonomically better for the surgeon.

URS is most commonly used for renal tract stone management. The lifetime prevalence of renal tract calculi is at 14% and expected to increase with lifestyle changes, due to metabolic syndrome and climate change leading to warmer temperature. The prevalence varies from 1% to 20% across the globe with some areas reporting >37% in last two decades [4]. First time stone formers had recurrence of 26% in 5 years with some patients having recurrences which were more common. URS offers an optimal surgical intervention for stone treatment with success comparable to PCNL (percutaneous nephrolithotomy) but with a lower risk of high grade complications, and with reported success superior to ESWL (extra-corporeal Shock wave lithotripsy) [5].

Bhanot et al. [6] found that semi-rigid URS offers 80% overall stone clearance and is particularly useful for distal ureteric calculus. Following this section are details of indications, guidelines and further details of ureteroscopy, which are as described ahead in this chapter.

Indications

Rigid and flexible URS are routinely used for diagnostic and therapeutic purposes for renal and ureteric pathologies on a routine basis. This can be done via an antegrade or a retrograde approach. In retrograde approach, the access is per-urethra, usually after a routine cystoscopy and in antegrade it is via a percutaneous approach usually from the kidney. A description of indications, contraindications and complications is presented in Table 23.1.

Recent research [7] shows that 75% of stones <5 mm and 62% of stones ≥5 mm can pass spontaneously averaging on 17 days (range: 6–29 days). This was found to be in 49% of upper ureteral stones, 58% of mid ureteric stones and as high as 68% in distal ureteric stones.

Indications for active ureteral stone removal according to European Association of Urologists (EAU) guidelines [7] are as follows:

- Stones with low likelihood of spontaneous passage
- Persistent pain despite adequate analgesia
- Persistent obstruction
- Renal insufficiency (renal failure, bilateral obstruction, or single kidney)

Indications for active renal stone removal according to EAU guidelines [7] are as follows:

- Stone growth
- Stones in high-risk patients for stone formation
- Obstruction due to stones
- Symptomatic stones—pain, haematuria, infection

Table 23.1 Showing indications and contra-indications of URS (ESWL and PCNL which are alternatives for URS)

Procedure	Indication	Relative and Absolute Contra-indications	Most common complications (incidence)
Ureteroscopy (URS)	Retrograde: Ureteric calculus<2 cm Multiple small ureteric calculi Renal calculus <2 cm Ureteric transitional cell carcinoma (TCC)- diagnostic, biopsy and laser ablation Diagnosis and management of ureteric strictures Management of calculi in solitary kidneys and horse-shoe kidneys Renal diverticulum management Pre or intra renal transplant for donor renal stone disease Stone disease treatment in morbid obesity and those with bleeding diathesis	Active and untreated urinary tract infections/ active urosepsis Anticoagulation (must be discontinued/ bridged) Anaesthesia related contra-indications or unsuitability There are no specific absolute contra-indications for performing URS	Overall complication rate: (9–25%) Infection (0.2–15%) Urosepsis (0.1–4.3%) Perirenal abscess (0.06%) Urinary clot retention (1.6%) Subcapsular, peri-renal and retroperitoneal haematoma (upto 2.2%) Failure to access ureter (1–37%) Ureteral wall injury (0.13–46.5%) Extra-renal stone migration (0.15%) Ureteral avulsion and strictures (<1%)
	Antegrade: Large calculi in upper renal tract >2 cm Impacted proximal ureteric calculus Unable to access ureter or upper renal tract via retrograde approach		

(continued)

Table 23.1 (continued)

Procedure	Indication	Relative and Absolute Contra-indications	Most common complications (incidence)
Extracorporeal Shock Wave Lithotripsy (ESWL)	Ureteric calculus <20 mm Renal calculi <20 mm Stone to skin ratio of <10–12 cm Hardness of stone 800-1000HU	Pregnancy Bleeding disorders (compensation required if treatment contemplated) Active UTIs Severe skeletal malformations Severe obesity Close vicinity arterial aneurysm	Steinstrasse (4–7%) Regrowth of residual stone fragment (21–59%) Renal colic (2–4%) Bacteriuria in non-infection stones (7.7–23%) Sepsis (1–2.7%) Renal haematoma-symptomatic (<1%) Renal haematoma—asymptomatic (4–19%) Morbid cardiac events (case report) Bowel perforation (case report) Liver and splenic haematoma (case report)
Percutaneous Nephrolithotomy (PCNL)	Large calculi (>15 mm)	Untreated UTI Tumour in the access tract for surgery Potential diagnosis of renal malignancy Pregnancy Anti-coagulants (must be discontinued/ bridged)	Fever (10.8%) Sepsis (0.5%) Blood loss requiring transfusion (7%) Haemorrhage requiring embolization (0.4%5) Thoracic complications (1.5%) Organ injury (0.4%) Urinoma formation (0.2%) Death (0.05%)

- Stones >15 mm
- Stones ≤15 mm if unsuitable for observation
- Patient preference or social situation
- Comorbidity

According to EAU guidelines [7], Holmium: yttrium-aluminium-garnet (Ho:YAG) is the current optimum standard for URS and flexible nephroscopy for laser treatment of stone. Thulium fiber laser (TFL) is a promising alternative; but there is a dearth of clinical data for it currently.

While URS offers a great management option for stone disease, treatment should not be employed in an acutely infected system. The high intra-renal pressure induced during introduction of scope into kidney can worsen any underlying infection. Also, the stone which would potentially be the source of sepsis should first be treated with appropriate antibiotics and contained before this source is disseminated via laser treatment. If there is obstructed infected system, this should be drained via a percutaneous nephrostomy (PCN) or ureteric stent first with definitive treatment planned for later. Apart from this, there appear to be no absolute contra-indications to URS. It is the preferred modality in obese patients as well.

Procedure

This is reflective of best clinical practice or standard technique, but different surgical approaches can be tried based on the expertise and experience of the team. The procedure should be carried out depending on the clinical situation/presentation and patient preference after counselling for available options (Figs. 23.1 and 23.2).

Initially the bladder is accessed using a rigid cystoscope. A cystoscopic assessment can be initially performed and the ureter on the side of the pathology is then identified, with a 'safety' guidewire introduced, and position of the same confirmed

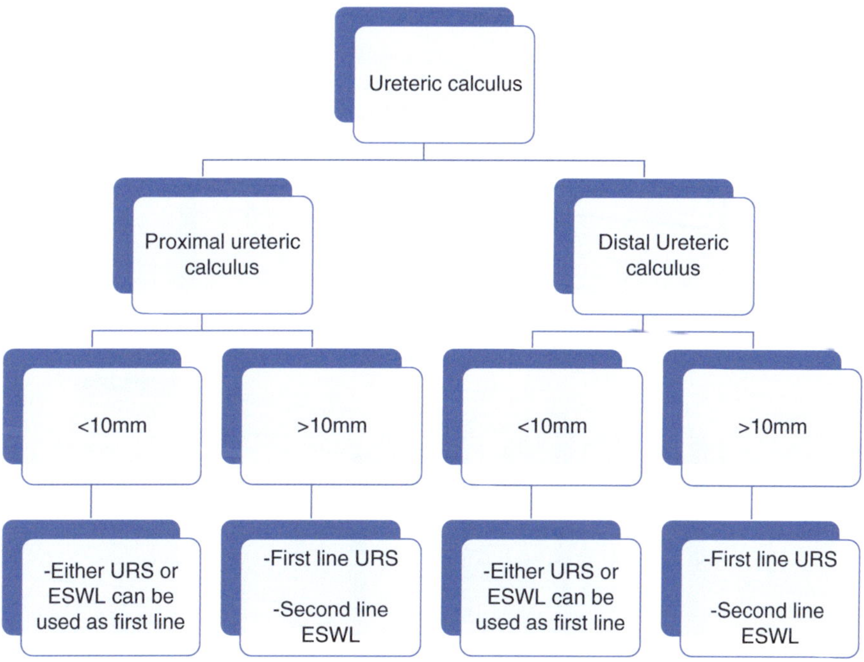

Fig. 23.1 Flowchart for ureteric calculus management as per EAU guidelines [7]

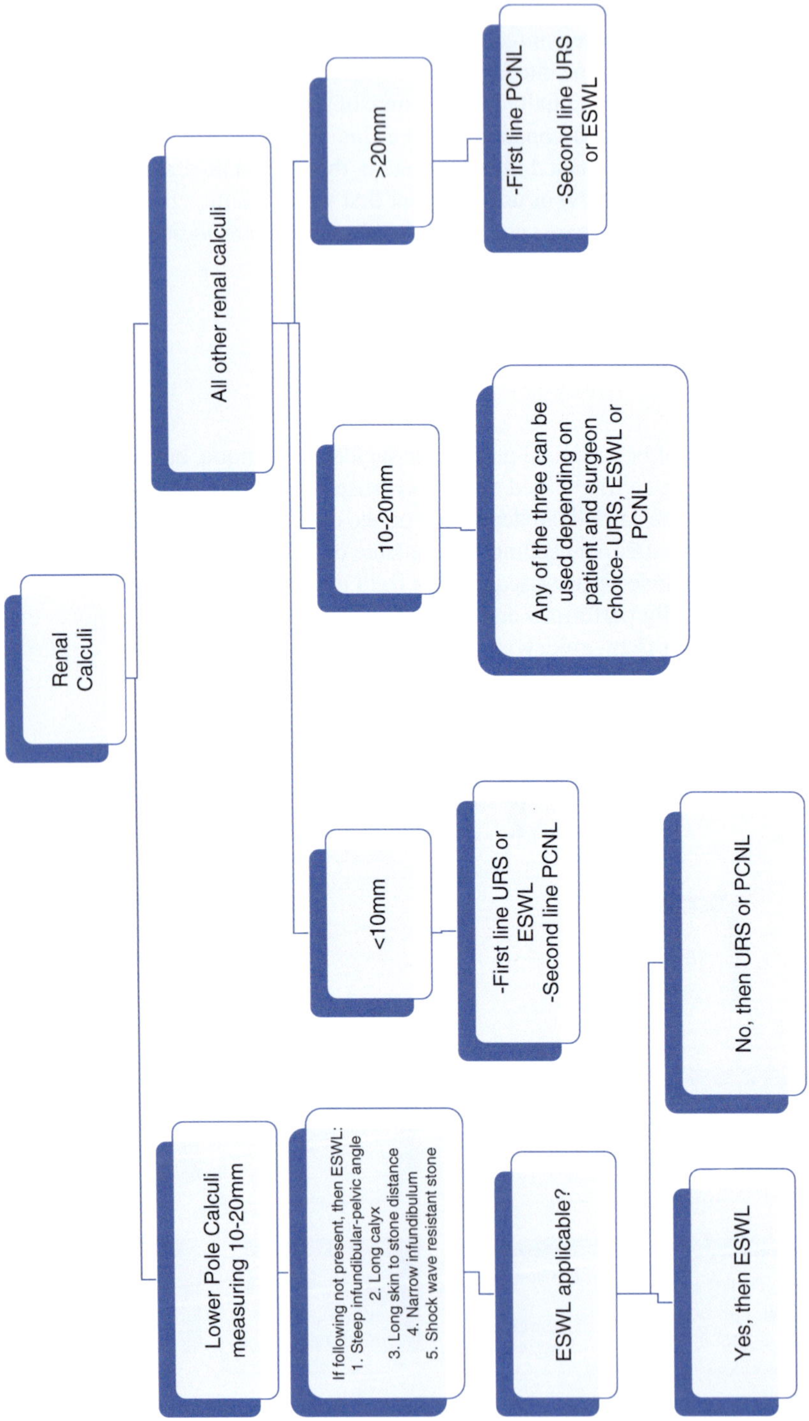

Fig. 23.2 Flowchart for renal calculus management as per EAU guidelines [7]

in the kidney via on-table imaging. This can be further confirmed by performing a retrograde pyelogram which also gives the added advantage of visualising ureteric anatomy or kinking. A soft tip guidewire can be used to avoid injury to ureteric mucosa or to get is past an impacted ureteric stone.

The cystoscope can now be withdrawn keeping the 'safety' guidewire in position. A semi-rigid URS is then introduced atop a 'working' guidewire. This helps in defining intramural anatomy and is often helpful in difficult ureters with kinking. It is also useful in causing passive dilatation of a relatively narrow ureter. It is introduced up to or just below the pelvi-ureteric junction (PUJ) and the position confirmed endoscopically or via imaging. However, if the ureter is found to be particularly narrow it is advisable to insert a JJ ureteric stent and bring the patient back for elective ureteroscopy after 10–14 days to avoid ureteral injury. The alternate is to try and access the ureter via a flexible ureteroscope which might allow negotiating through this narrow area. Excessive force should not be applied as it leads to ureteral injury and if the ureter does not allow a safe access, placing a ureteric stent and performing a delayed ureteroscopy should be the preferred option. Balloon or sequential dilatation in this scenario should also be avoided in a virgin ureter.

Many experience surgeons may choose to proceed with flexible ureteroscopy as the initial instrument of choice after cystoscopy. If multiple entries are anticipated then it is often safe to use a ureteric access sheath (UAS) to avoid ureteric trauma, improve outflow and vision with a reduced intrarenal pressure. All renal calyces are then walked using the flexible URS and the pathology can be dealt with accordingly.

A post-op stent is not mandatory but is recommended [7] in case of ureteric trauma, stone debris, risk of infection, solitary kidney and in pregnancy. The stent duration is decided by the surgeon and often varies between 1 and 2 weeks. If a shorter duration of 24–48 hours is desired, then a stent on string or ureteric catheter can be inserted which can be removed by patients as well. The bladder is then emptied at the conclusion of the procedure. In some instances, an overnight urethral catheter might be placed post-URS depending on the surgeon practice.

Flexible Ureteroscopes

Flexible ureteroscopes are indispensable surgical working tools for renal stone treatment and endoscopic management of upper tract urothelial cancers. Together with the irrigation systems and disposable equipment, they represent the surgical armamentarium necessary to carry out flexible ureteroscopy (fURS) and retrograde intrarenal surgery (RIRS) of different complexities. With technological advancements that have characterised over the last few years, they have gradually been optimised with the introduction of the digital chip-on-the-tip technology [8]. This allows a much better image resolution, improved diagnostics, and reduction in the weight of the scopes [9].

Newer scopes, despite being more expensive, are characterised by longer durability and increased stone free rate thanks to their better vision [10]. Flexible ureteroscopes are durable, but can sometimes be damaged during surgical use, transport, sterilisation and handling [11]. It has been shown how high-volume stone centers are burdened by less ureteroscopes breakages compared to non-specialised endourological centers, however the participation of trainees during the procedure can also increase the risk of damages [12]. Reusable flexible ureteroscopes can lead to significant cost of repair when damaged. Unfortunately, maintenance cost [13] and repair of damages are sometimes very prohibitive for hospitals and if multiples scopes undergo repair simultaneously, the efficiency of the whole department can be affected. Disposable or single use ureteroscopes were more recently introduced to overcome this issue. The main advantage of these new generation devices are the reduced risk of cross-contamination as they do not go through reprocessing steps, and they are not burdened by repair costs. However, the cost of procuring it is still high to completely migrate to the new disposable devices [14]. A more rational and hybrid system has been introduced by most hospitals in order to decide which scope to use according to the case mix [15]. This has shown how disposable scopes can be purchased and used in complex endourological procedures where reusable scopes have a high risk of scope damage or sepsis. Ergonomics of flexible scope is also important. Complex series of movements involving several muscles are recruited for the fine movements necessary for the handling and manoeuvring of a flexible ureteroscope. Laboratory studies [16] have shown how both the single use and reusable digital ureteroscopes have better ergonomics than the reusable fiber-optic ureteroscopes. Many new single use ureteroscopes have been recently introduced in the international market, their characteristics have been compared in vitro and in vivo studies and each of them can offer similar features in term of availability, ergonomics, ease of use and cost [17]. The future for these devices is bright and set to achieve more affordable prices associated with highly valuable technological advancements [18]. Future generation of scopes plan to incorporate pressure and temperature sensors, artificial intelligence and suction irrigation to improve patient outcomes and surgeon comfort.

Consumables

Guidewires, baskets and access sheaths are the necessary endourological equipment that are used daily in clinical practice.

Guide wires are usually chosen according to the surgeons' preference, a wide choice is available on the market, and we can distinguish two different classes according to the coatings. All guide wires are in fact made of stainless steel or nitinol material. The coating plays a difference in their hydrophilic property and stiffness. The Polytetrafluoroethylene (PTFE) coating is characterized by stiffness and PTFE coated guidewires are excellent as working tools to insert access sheaths and ureteroscopes. However, being stiff, they have a higher risk of perforation hazard.

The wires coated with hydrophilic polymers can easily overcome narrowing and obstruction due to their hydrophilic properties, but are less stiff and not appropriate as working guide wires. Some hybrid guidewires are also available in the market that combines the stiffness of the PTFE core with a hydrophilic soft tip, ideal for initial ureteric access [19].

Several retrieval devices are available on the market for a huge variety of circumstances. Most of them are Nitinol baskets and the choice of use also depends on the case mix, surgeon preference, price, usability and availability. The most commonly used is the tipless retrieval device that allows it to be positioned closed to the ureteric mucosa in order to trap the stones. Newer models can be used together with the laser fibres to trap the stone while lasering. Advanced single use ureteroscopes allow the surgeon to manipulate the basket independently using the Empower device attached to the handle of the ureteroscope [20].

Ureteral access sheaths (UAS) are useful aids in flexible ureterorenoscopy. The physical properties of UAS vary by their model and manufacturer [21] but in general they are radiopaque hollow sheaths inserted under fluoroscopic guidance on a guide wire, through the ureter up to or just below the PUJ. Their diameter can be selected according to the ureteric compliance assessed intraoperatively and the length is dependent on the patient's gender and height. The effect of using a UAS is seen in reducing operative time, allowing multiple passes of instruments, protecting the ureteroscope and reducing intrarenal pressure [22]. Use of modified access sheath that is able to develop negative pressure during fURS has been recently demonstrated [23]. These studies have found how the new suctioning UAS may improve the vision by reducing the amount of stone dust [24, 25]. However, higher levels of evidence via clinical trials are necessary to corroborate those findings.

Irrigation devices are essential to guarantee a good vision during flexible ureterorenoscopy and several irrigation methods have been introduced over the years. These vary from gravity pressure to manual or pedal pump irrigation devices, to controlled irrigation pressure devices. Their efficacy has been compared in vitro [26] and future developments are expected to involve artificial intelligence for intrarenal temperature and pressure control [27].

Ureteroscopy in Special Scenarios

Large Stones (>2 cm)

Over the years, with the advent of the UAS and higher power lasers, the boundaries and indications for fURS have been extended to treat larger stones. Excellent results have been demonstrated in several recent studies. A recent systematic review and meta-analysis by Geraghty et al. [28] included 12 articles with a total number of 651 patients. The stone free rate (SFR) described was 91% for a mean stone size of 2.6 cm and it took an average of 1.5 procedures per patient to achieve this. More recently, Pietropaolo et al. [29] analysed a prospective cohort of 50 patients with stones larger than 15 mm. They underwent fURS with high power 100w laser using pop-dusting technique with setting of 0.3–0.6 J and a frequency of 20–50 Hz and a long-pulse setting. The SFR in this case was 93% after the first procedure rising to 98% after the second procedure (needed in 3 patients) and the operative time was reduced to 51 minutes. Alsmadi et al. [23] have added to the technique a suctioning UAS to treat a cohort of 103 patients with stone size of 12–14 mm. In the group where the special device was used, the SFR rated reached 93%. Another study by the Chinese team of Huang et al. [30] analysed 251 patients with mean stone size of 2.7 cm and mean number of procedures at 1.4 (range: 1–5). The initial and final SFR was 61.9% and 89.5% respectively, showing fURS as a valid option for large stones.

Paediatric Patients

Treatment of urinary stones in children is usually performed in specialised centres with high experience and case volume. Ureteroscopy is now more commonly used for the treatment of renal and ureteric stones in paediatric patients. A recent systematic review by Whatley et al. [31] looked at 11 studies on outcomes of fURS in paediatric patients. This described 431 patients with mean stone size of 13 mm finding an overall SFR of 87%. Considering that shockwave lithotripsy (SWL) often requires multiple sessions and general anaesthesia in paediatric patients, fURS affirm its role as a more effective and minimally invasive option [32]. This is even more true when using high power laser. Reeves et al. [33] showed a good SFR and low complication rate when using 100 W with pop dusting technique in patients with mean age of 6.5 year old. A bigger patient cohort of 57 patients between 2 high volume European stone centre was analysed by Mosquera et al. [34] The patients with a mean age of 10.1 years and stone size of 9.5 mm reached initial and final SFR of 82.4% and 98.2% respectively with a minor complication rate of 7%. Another review by Ishii et al. [35] included 14 articles with 1664 patients (mean age of 7.8 years). The SFR was 86.3%, and the complication rate was 10.6%. demonstrating again the effectiveness and safety of URS in the paediatric population.

Elderly Patients

In view of its minimally invasive nature, URS is also widely used as stone treatment technique in old and frail patients. Prattley et al.'s article [36] included a review of six articles where 560 patients over 70 years (range: 70–91 years) underwent URS. The final SFR ranged from 66% to 97%, with overall complication rate of 9%, with a very low rate of major complications and no deaths reported in this review.

Stones in Pregnancy

In pregnancy, stone treatment should be deferred if no urgent criteria for stone removal exist. Ishii et al. [37] performed a systematic review including 21 articles (271 procedures), with patients between the second or third trimester of pregnancy. The SFR was 85% and the complication rate (11.4%) were mostly non-obstetric complications. This helped to understand that URS in pregnancy is a safe and effective procedure. A similar review by Semins et al. [38] showed that the complication rate of URS during pregnancy was comparable to the general population. However, Johnson et al. [39] showed a concerning 4% rate of obstetric complications, reiterating the importance of the case selection in this specific cohort of patients.

Stones in Obese Patients

Obese and morbidly obese patients have a higher risk of stone formation and therefore often require treatment. To reduce the anaesthetic risk and choose a lesser invasive option, URS is the favourite option in this group of patients. Ishii et al. [40] described in their systematic review 835 patients with mean BMI of 40.5 kg/m^2. The overall SFR was 82.5% and the complication rate was 9.3%, which was similar when compared to the general population.

Stones in Patients with a Solitary Kidney

Treating stones in a solitary kidney is often indicated to prevent obstruction, anuria and renal failure. However, preserving the single kidney is paramount and ureteroscopy seems to be the safest stone treatment method to preserve the renal functionality. Pietropaolo et al. [41] performed a systematic review with 696 patients with single functioning kidney. The SFR of 85.2% was achieved with an average of 1.2 procedures per patient. This patient cohort showed a complication rate of 16.4%, however most of these were minor complications. Together with URS, SWL has also been found to be effective and relatively free from complications [42], however burdened by the need of repeat sessions and risk of steinstrasse and consequent anuria, URS in preferred in this patient cohort.

Stones in Bleeding Diathesis and Anticoagulated Patients

Among the other surgical procedure for renal stones treatment, ureteroscopy has the lowest risk of bleeding. Sharaf et al. [43] in their systematic review about patients undergoing URS with bleeding diathesis, identified a complication rate of just 6%.

Only 5% of these were major complications, two anti-coagulated patients with haematomas requiring embolisation and one ureteric perforation. An American paper [44] on 4799 URS performed across 31 practices, showed that URS on anticoagulants is safe, however antiplatelets therapy increases the risk of hospitalization.

A patient-centred approach should therefore be taken with regards to continuing these agents, only if really necessary, or correcting bleeding diatheses prior to URS.

Bilateral URS in Stone Disease

In patients with bilateral urolithiasis, simultaneous ureteroscopic procedures is a possible option. Geraghty et al. [45] analysed in a systematic review a total of 491 patients who underwent bilateral URS. The SFR was 92% and the complication rate of 25.6%. Several authors have described the procedure as effective, representing a safe viable standard of care in high volume centres with experienced surgeons [46–48]. Fiscus et al. [49] compared patients undergoing single session bilateral and staged bilateral URS and found that the former has an overall shorter operative time and similar SFR compared to planned staged URS.

Anatomical Abnormalities and Anomalous Kidneys

Ingimarsson et al. [50] have described in their systematic review several abnormal cases that can make ureteroscopy very difficult. These are mainly secondary to patients' anatomic and physiological characteristics such as altered urinary tract anatomy, congenital anomalies and spinal deformities. Anomalous kidneys can be abnormal ascent, fusion or rotation and they are normally originated in embryological age. In these cases, the access to the stone can be more challenging and Lavan et al. [51] performed a systematic review showing that URS in expert hands can be decisive. The initial and final SFR after the procedure was 76.6% and 82.3% respectively. Incidence of 17.2% complications was reported of which 2.4% were Clavien–Dindo ≥III complications and the authors have concluded that despite the technical difficulties, URS can be safe and effective in anomalous kidneys [52].

Chronic Kidney Disease

Until few years ago, there was uncertainty towards the possibility of long-term renal damage following URS mainly in patients with previous chronic kidney disease (CKD). Reeves et al. [53] performed a prospective data collection to analyse the post operative renal function after fURS. In 227 patients, after mean follow-up of 112 weeks, a significant improvement of the estimated glomerular filtration rate (eGFR) from baseline was observed. The results were corroborated by a systematic review [54] which confirmed how endourological interventions (PCNL and fURS) do not cause a deterioration of long-term renal function but tends to improve it.

Transplant Kidneys

In cases of patients who need renal transplant for end stage renal failure, donor renal stones may need treatment either pretransplant or posttransplant to maintain the allograft function. A recent systematic review [55] analysed URS outcomes before and after transplant. In the post transplant cohort, the procedure can be more challenging, and the consequent complications were 12.4%. However, several advancements in endourological technique have made URS for donor and post-transplant urolithiasis a safe and effective procedure.

Diagnostic Ureteroscopy for UTUC

Upper-tract urothelial carcinoma (UTUC) is a relatively uncommon disease. This has common risk factors to bladder cancer but different biological and clinical characteristics [56].

According to focality, number and size and histological grade, UTUC be differentiated into high and low risk (Fig. 23.3).

According to the EAU guidelines [57], endoscopic ablation of UTUC should be considered in patients with clinically low-risk cancer (Fig. 23.4). A fURS is useful in

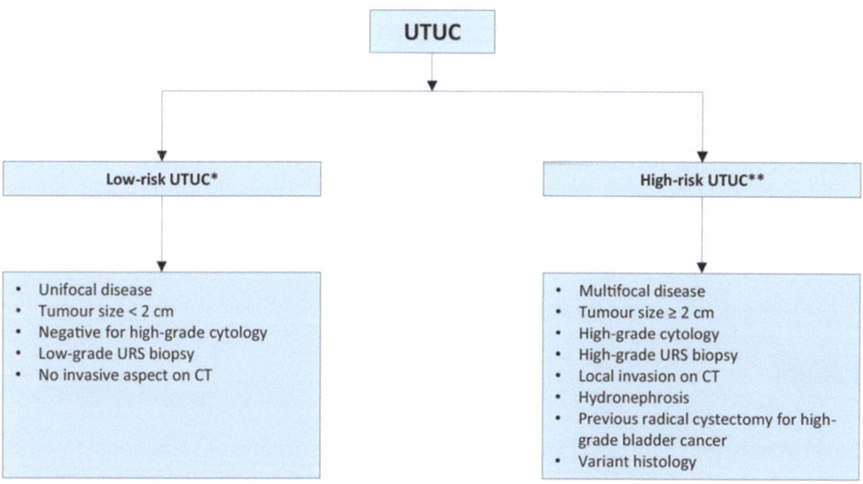

Fig. 23.3 Risk stratification of non-metastatic UTUC (as per EAU guidelines [57])

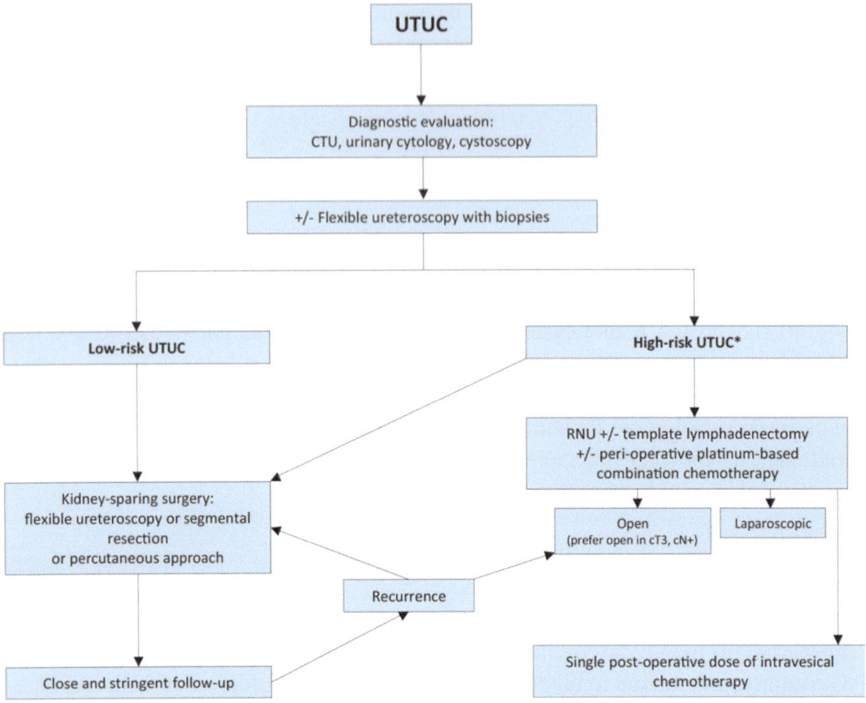

Fig. 23.4 Proposed flowchart for the management of UTUC (as per EAU guidelines [57])

the management of pelvicalyceal tumours and a recent systematic review [58] showed that in low-grade disease, similar survival was observed between nephroureterectomy and ureteroscopic ablation [59]. However, patient selection is paramount in these cases. Technological advancements have improved the image quality during ureteroscopy. Keller et al. [60] have analysed different types of flexible digital ureteroscopes to identify the key features to guarantee a better vision. Most new generation videoscopes are also supplied with Image enhancement technologies such as narrow-band imaging (NBI), photodynamic diagnosis (PDD) and Image 1-S (formerly SPIES). The best quality is reached by Image 1-S technology "Clara + Chroma" mode. NBI technology [61] provides increased quality of UTUC specially to differentiate the border between tumour and normal tissue with its ability to highlight the vascular architecture. All these new tools improve the detection and diagnosis of UTUC.

Lasers

Laser stands for Light amplification by stimulated emission of radiations, in other words, a device capable of converting light or electrical energy into a focused, high energy beam [62]. The application of lasers in endourology has broadened in the past three decades. Pulsed lasers such as the holmium:yttrium–aluminum–garnet (Ho:YAG) are able to deliver their energy in pulses that are very efficient at stone lithotripsy [63]. The surgeon can manipulate the energy and the pulse frequency parameters to change the effect of the laser on the stone. Several types of lithotripsies can in fact be performed adjusting the laser setting [64], such as fragmentation, pop corning, dusting and pop dusting [65]. The response of the stone to the laser depends also on the stone composition and hardness. The dual-phase MOSES 'pulse modulation' technology has been introduced in high-power laser machines with the benefit to decrease the retropulsion, increase the stability during laser lithotripsy with improved efficiency. Ho:YAG laser has been the gold standard for laser lithotripsy for 20 years, and more recently we have the new thulium fiber laser (TFL) lithotripter [66]. This offers pulse frequencies up to 2200 Hz and a total power level up to 55 W. The stone ablation is four-times that of the Ho:YAG laser with clear reduction of operating time and formation of finer stone dust. Not many randomised controlled trials exist on the matter yet, but it is already evident that it has become an attractive alternative to conventional laser techniques, and it is here to stay [67].

Complications

Being a minimally invasive endoscopic procedure, ureteroscopy can be burdened by different grades of complications [68]. Haematuria and pain are expected and common after the procedure, but more life-threatening complications have been documented in rare cases [69].

Ureteric Perforation / Avulsion

One of the most dreaded intraoperative complications after URS can be ureteric injury. This can present in different stages of severity (type 0–3) according to the involvement of the superficial mucosa, or the underlining tissues including the extramucosal fat [70]. Early diagnosis of it is paramount to prevent the potentially fatal consequences such as retroperitoneal urine leak and urinoma. Ureteric avulsion is a rare complication and caused by disinsertion of the ureter from its distal attachment to the bladder [71]. This is a serious complication that requires immediate major surgical repair with devastating long-term sequalae. This is precisely why a ureteric stent should be placed in the first instance when the ureter is narrow and does not allow primary ureteroscopy, for passive dilatation of the ureter which allows delayed ureteroscopy, minimising the risk of ureteric damage.

Urosepsis

This is one of the most life-threatening complications for fURS and can be facilitated by the use of high-pressure irrigation and infective nature of the stones. This can often cause urinary tract infections (UTIs), and, in rare cases can lead to severe systemic infection and sepsis. Post-ureteroscopic infectious complications and urosepsis are uncommon but serious life-threatening complications, a source of morbidity and potential mortality. The rate of urospesis after URS for stone disease varies between 2.2% and 20% in some studies [72]. According to a recent systematic review [73], predisposing factors for post URS sepsis includes female gender, large stone burden and long operative time. These can be associated with patient factors such as multiple comorbidities, history of recurrent UTIs or positive urine culture, immunocompromission, pre-operative stent dwell time [74], previous indwelling catheter or neurogenic bladder. Pietropaolo et al. [75] used a machine learning model to create a predictive tool for post-operative urosepsis, able to select high risk patients, and to be able to adjust preventative measures and improve pre-operative counselling.

Training

European Association of Urology (EAU) Section of Uro-Technology (ESUT) and Urolithiasis (EULIS) have been long involved in training modules and courses. Over the years, they have established a standardized training program in endoscopic stone treatment, laparoscopic surgery, and transurethral procedures on hands-on-training (HOT) models [76]. The endoscopic stone treatment step 1 (EST S1) [77] was indeed validated, and it is now a standardised training protocol used in 25 countries. This evaluates trainee's ability to perform a full dry lab procedure, from the simple cystoscopy to a flexible ureteroscopy. More complex tasks have been added to the endoscopic stone treatment step 2/A [78] to allow the trainee to become sufficient in laser lithotropsy.

Tips and Tricks

Videos and webinars gained renewed interest to learn tip and tricks from expert. The current Covid pandemic has reaffirmed their utility in absence of other face to face tools such as hand on training. Tip and tricks papers have also been published with step-by step approach to endourological procedure such as rigid and flexible ureteroscopy with specific attention drawn to difficult or challenging parts of it. Whitehurst et al. [79] and PETRA group [80] have in fact focussed on the use of pictorial advice about how to overcome common difficulties in the URS procedures.

Similarly, a pool of experienced endourological surgeons have created an "expert consensus view" in 2 parts [81, 82] for basic and advanced ureterorenoscopy. Traxer et al. [83] in their recent review described the surgical technique for fURS as well as tips and tricks for the treatment of intrarenal stones.

Summary

In this chapter we have shown the current literature pertaining to the use of RIRS in a variety of complex patients and stone disease with efficacy and complications in these sceneries. RIRS seems to be a safe and efficient method for treatment of these patients and will have expanding role in future through use of modern technology such as use of artificial intelligence, intrarenal pressure and temperature monitoring.

References

1. Wason SE, Monfared S, Lonson A, et al. Ureteroscopy. In: StatPearls [Internet]. Treasure Island (FL): StatPearls Publishing; 2021.
2. Marshall, et al. Fiber optics in urology. J Urol. 1964;91:110–4. https://doi.org/10.1016/s0022-5347(17)64066-7.
3. Grasso M, Alexander BS, Pyo P, et al. Ureteroscopy. Medscape. 2018.
4. Trinchieri A, et al. Epidemiology of urolithiasis: an update. Clin Cases Miner Bone Metab. 2008;5(2):101–6.
5. Prattley S, Voss J, Cheung S, et al. Ureteroscopy and stone treatment in the elderly (≥70 years): prospective outcomes over 5- years with a review of literature. Int Braz J Urol. 2018;44(4):750–7. https://doi.org/10.1590/S1677-5538.IBJU.2017.0516.
6. Bhanot R, Jones P, Somani BK. Minimally invasive surgery for the treatment of ureteric stones- state-of-the-art review. Res Rep Urol. 2021;(13):227–36. https://doi.org/10.2147/RRU.S311010. eCollection 2021.
7. Türk C, Neisius A, Petřík A, et al. EAU guidelines on urolithiasis. Eur Urol. 2016;69(3):468–74. https://doi.org/10.1016/j.eururo.2015.07.040. Epub 2015 Aug 28
8. Bach C, Nesar S, Kumar P, et al. The new digital flexible ureteroscopes: 'size does matter' – increased ureteric access sheath use! Urol Int. 2012;89(4):408–11.
9. Şener TE, Pietropaolo A, Talso M. An overview of the advantages of digital flexible ureteroscopes. A review by young academic urologists endourology and urolithiasis Working Party of the European Association of Urology. J Urol Surg. 2020;7(2):76–8.
10. Talso M, Proietti S, Emiliani E. Comparison of flexible ureterorenoscope quality of vision: an in vitro study. J Endourol. 2018;32(6):523–8.
11. Banerjee I, Katz JE, Bhattu AS, et al. Durability of digital flexible ureteroscope in university hospital and ambulatory surgical center: is it time to rethink? J Endourol. 2021;35(3):289–95.
12. Ozimek T, Cordes J, Wiessmeyer JR, et al. Steep infundibulopelvic angle as a new risk factor for flexible ureteroscope damage and complicated postoperative course. J Endourol. 2018;32(7):597–602.
13. Mager R, Kurosch M, Höfner T, et al. Clinical outcomes and costs of reusable and single-use flexible ureterorenoscopes: a prospective cohort study. Urolithiasis. 2018;46(6):587–93.

14. Ventimiglia E, Godínez AJ, Traxer O, et al. Cost comparison of single-use versus reusable flexible ureteroscope: a systematic review. Turk J Urol. 2020;46(Supp. 1):S40–5.
15. Ventimiglia E, Smyth N, Doizi S, et al. Can the introduction of single-use flexible ureteroscopes increase the longevity of reusable flexible ureteroscopes at a high volume centre? World J Urol. 2021;40:251–6.
16. Ludwig WW, Lee G, Ziemba JB, et al. Evaluating the ergonomics of flexible ureteroscopy. J Endourol. 2017;31(10):1062–6.
17. Bahaee J, Plott J, Ghani KR. Single-use flexible ureteroscopes: how to choose and what is around the corner? Curr Opin Urol. 2021;31(2):87–94.
18. Somani BK, Talso M, Bres-Niewada E. Current role of single-use flexible ureteroscopes in the management of upper tract stone disease. Cent Eur J Urol. 2019;72(2):183–4.
19. Clayman M, Uribe CA, Eichel L. Comparison of guide wires in urology. Which, when and why? J Urol. 2004;171(6 Pt 1):2146–50.
20. Ventimiglia E, Sindhubodee S, Besombes T, et al. Operator-assisted vs self-achieved basketing during ureteroscopy: results from an in vitro preference study. World J Urol. 2021;39(6):2169–75.
21. Patel N, Monga M. Ureteral access sheaths: a comprehensive comparison of physical and mechanical properties. Int Braz J Urol. 2018;44(3):524–35.
22. Lima A, Reeves T, Geraghty R. Impact of ureteral access sheath on renal stone treatment: prospective comparative non randomised outcomes over a 7 year period. World J Urol. 2020;38:1329–33.
23. Alsmadi KJ, Li X, Zeng G. Use of a modified ureteral access sheath in semi-rigid ureteroscopy to treat large upper ureteral stones is associated with high stone free rates. Asian J Urol. 2019;6(3):217–21.
24. Huang J, Xie D, Xiong R. The application of suctioning flexible ureteroscopy with intelligent pressure control in treating upper urinary tract calculi on patients with a solitary kidney. Urology. 2018;111:44–7.
25. Zhu Z, Cui Y, Zeng F. Comparison of suctioning and traditional ureteral access sheath during flexible ureteroscopy in the treatment of renal stones. World J Urol. 2019;37(5):921–9.
26. Proietti S, Dragos L, Somani BK, et al. In vitro comparison of maximum pressure developed by irrigation systems in a Kidney Model. J Endourol. 2017;31(5):522–7.
27. Doizi S, Letendre J, Cloutier J. Continuous monitoring of intrapelvic pressure during flexible ureteroscopy using a sensor wire: a pilot study. World J Urol. 2021;39(2):555–61.
28. Geraghty R, Abourmarzouk O, Rai B, et al. Evidence for ureterorenoscopy and laser fragmentation (URSL) for large renal stones in the modern era. Curr Urol Rep. 2015;16(8):54.
29. Pietropaolo A, Jones P, Whitehurst L, et al. Role of 'dusting and pop-dusting' using a high-powered (100 W) laser machine in the treatment of large stones ($\geq$ 15 mm): prospective outcomes over 16 months. Urolithiasis. 2019;47(4):391–4.
30. Huang JS, Xie S, Huang X-J, et al. Flexible ureteroscopy and laser lithotripsy for renal stones 2 cm or greater. Medicine (Baltimore). 2020;99(43):e22704.
31. Whatley A, Jones P, Aboumarzouk O, et al. Safety and efficacy of ureteroscopy and stone fragmentation for pediatric renal stones: a systematic review. Transl Androl Urol. 2019;8(Suppl 4):S442–7.
32. Bowen DK, Song L, Faerber J, et al. Retreatment after ureteroscopy and shockwave lithotripsy: a population-based comparative effectiveness study. J Urol. 2020;203(6):1156–62.
33. Reeves T, Griffin S, Pietropaolo A, et al. Feasibility of dusting and pop-dusting using high-power (100W) Holmium YAG (Ho:YAG) laser in treatment of paediatric stones: results of first worldwide clincial study. Cent Eur J Urol. 2019;72(4):398–401.
34. Mosquera L, Pietropaolo A, Madarriaga YQ, et al. Is flexible ureteroscopy and laser lithotripsy the new gold standard for pediatric lower pole stones? outcomes from two large European tertiary pediatric endourology centers. J Endourol. 2021;35(10):1479–82.
35. Ishii H, Griffin S, Somani BK. Ureteroscopy for stone disease in the paediatric population: a systematic review. BJU Int. 2015;115(6):867–73.

36. Prattley S, Voss J, Cheung S, et al. Ureteroscopy and stone treatment in the elderly (≥70 years): prospective outcomes over 5-years with a review of literature. Int Braz J Urol. 2018;44(4):750–7.
37. Ishii H, Abourmarzouk O, Somani BK. Current status of ureteroscopy for stone disease in pregnancy. Urolithiasis. 2014;42(1):1–7.
38. Semins MJ, Trock BJ, Matlaga BR. The safety of ureteroscopy during pregnancy: a systematic review and meta-analysis. J Urol. 2009;181(1):139–43.
39. Johnson EB, Krambeck AE, White WM, et al. Obstetric complications of ureteroscopy during pregnancy. J Urol. 2012;188(1):151–4.
40. Ishii H, Couzins M, Abourmarzouk O, et al. Outcomes of systematic review of ureteroscopy for stone disease in the obese and morbidly obese population. J Endourol. 2016;30(2):135–45.
41. Pietropaolo A, Jones P, Whitehurst L, et al. Efficacy and safety of ureteroscopy for stone disease in a solitary kidney: findings from a systematic review. Urology. 2018;119:17–22.
42. Yuruk E, Binbay M, Ozgor F, et al. Comparison of shockwave lithotripsy and flexible ureteroscopy for the treatment of kidney stones in patients with a solitary kidney. J Endourol. 2015;29(4):463–7.
43. Sharaf A, Amer T, Somani BK, Abourmarzouk O. Ureteroscopy in patients with bleeding diatheses, anticoagulated, and on anti-platelet agents: a systematic review and meta-analysis of the literature. J Endourol. 2017;12:1217–25.
44. Westerman ME, Scales JA, Sharma V, et al. The effect of anticoagulation on bleeding-related complications following ureteroscopy. Urology. 2017;100:45–52.
45. Geraghty R, Rai B, Jones P, Somani BK. Bilateral simultaneous ureteroscopic (BS-URS) approach in the management of bilateral urolithiasis is a safe and effective strategy in the contemporary era-evidence from a systematic review. Curr Urol Rep. 2017;18(2):11.
46. Ingimarsson JP, Rivera M, Knoedler JJ, et al. Same-session bilateral ureteroscopy: safety and outcomes. Urology. 2017;108:29–33.
47. Ge H, Zheng X, Na Y, et al. Bilateral same-session ureteroscopy for treatment of ureteral calculi: a systematic review and meta-analysis. J Endourol. 2016;30(11):1169–79.
48. Rai BP, Ishii H, Jones P, et al. Bilateral simultaneous ureteroscopy for bilateral stone disease: a systematic review. Can J Urol. 2016;23(2):8220–6.
49. Fiscus G, Marien T, Tangpaitoon T, et al. Single session bilateral vs staged bilateral ureteroscopy for nephrolithiasis: an assessment of safety and efficacy. Urology. 2019;123:64–9.
50. Ingimarsson JP, Krambeck AE. Special situations in ureteroscopy. Minerva Urol Nefrol. 2016;68(6):547–59.
51. Lavan L, Herrmann T, Netsch C, et al. Outcomes of ureteroscopy for stone disease in anomalous kidneys: a systematic review. World J Urol. 2020;38(5):1135–46.
52. Astolfi RH, Freschi G, Berti FF, et al. Flexible ureterorenoscopy in position or fusion anomaly: is it feasible? Rev Assoc Med Bras (1992). 2017;63(8):685–8.
53. Reeves T, Pietropaolo A, Somani BK, et al. Ureteroscopy and laser stone fragmentation is safe and tends to improve renal function in patients with chronic kidney disease: prospective outcomes with a minimum follow-up of 6 months. J Endourol. 2020;34(4):423–8.
54. Reeves T, Pietropaolo A, Gadzhiev N, et al. Role of endourological procedures (PCNL and URS) on renal function: a systematic review. Curr Urol Rep. 2020;21(5):21.
55. Reeves T, Agarwal V, Somani BK, et al. Donor and post-transplant ureteroscopy for stone disease in patients with renal transplant: evidence from a systematic review. Curr Opin Urol. 2019;29(5):548–55.
56. Soria F, Shariat SF, Lerner SP, et al. Epidemiology, diagnosis, preoperative evaluation and prognostic assessment of upper-tract urothelial carcinoma (UTUC). World J Urol. 2017;35(3):379–87.
57. Rouprêt M, Babjuk M, Burger M, et al. European Association of Urology Guidelines on Upper Urinary Tract Urothelial Carcinoma. Eur Assoc Urol. 2021;79:62–79.
58. Ng Chieng Hin J, Hettiarachchilage D, Gravestock. Role of ureteroscopy in treatment of upper tract urothelial carcinoma. Curr Urol Rep. 2021;22(10):49.

59. Seisen T, Peyronnet B, Dominguez-Escrig JL, et al. Oncologic outcomes of kidney-sparing surgery versus radical nephroureterectomy for upper tract urothelial carcinoma: a systematic review by the EAU non-muscle invasive bladder cancer guidelines panel. Eur Urol. 2016;70(6):1052–68.
60. Keller EX, Doizi S, Villa L, Traxer O. Which flexible ureteroscope is the best for upper tract urothelial carcinoma treatment? World J Urol. 2019;37(11):2325–33.
61. Hao YC, Xiao CL, Liu K, et al. Application of narrow-band imaging flexible ureteroscopy in the diagnosis, treatment and follow-up of upper tract urothelial carcinomas. Zhonghua Wai Ke Za Zhi. 2018;56(3):222–6.
62. Brewin AE, Somani BK. What is new in lasers for endourology: looking into the future. Urol News. 2021;25(2).
63. Kronenberg P, Somani BK. Advances in lasers for the treatment of stones—a systematic review. Curr Urol Rep. 2018;19(6):45.
64. Aldoukhi AH, Black KM, Ghani KR. Emerging laser techniques for the management of stones. Urol Clin North Am. 2019;46(2):193–205.
65. Pietropaolo A, Schembri M, Somani BK. Dusting and pop-dusting for kidney stone disease: video and outcomes. Turk J Urol. 2020;46(4):326–7.
66. Kronenberg P, Traxer O. The laser of the future: reality and expectations about the new thulium fiber laser-a systematic review. Transl Androl Urol. 2019;8(Suppl 4):S398–417.
67. Schembri M, Sahu J, Aboumarzouk O, et al. Thulium fiber laser: the new kid on the block. Turk J Urol. 2020;46(Supp. 1):S1–S10.
68. De Coninck V, Keller EX, Somani B, et al. Complications of ureteroscopy: a complete overview. World J Urol. 2020;38(9):2147–66.
69. Cindolo L, Castellan P, Primiceri G, et al. Life-threatening complications after ureteroscopy for urinary stones: survey and systematic literature. Minerva Urol Nefrol. 2017;69(5):421–31.
70. Traxer O, Thomas A. Prospective evaluation and classification of ureteral wall injuries resulting from insertion of a ureteral access sheath during retrograde intrarenal surgery. J Urol. 2013;189(2):580–4.
71. Denis D, Moreno S, Velasco A, et al. Ureteral avulsion during retrograde intrarenal surgery: when the unexpected happens. J Endourol Case Rep. 2020;6(3):177–9.
72. Bonkat G, Cai T, Veeratterapillay R, et al. Management of urosepsis in 2018. Eur Urol Focus. 2019;5:5–9.
73. Chugh S, Pietropaolo A, Montanari E, et al. Predictors of urinary infections and urosepsis after ureteroscopy for stone disease: a systematic review from EAU Section of Urolithiasis (EULIS). Curr Urol Rep. 2020;21(4):16.
74. Nevo A, Mano R, Baniel J, et al. Ureteric stent dwelling time: a risk factor for post-ureteroscopy sepsis. BJU Int. 2017;120(1):117–22.
75. Pietropaolo A, Geraghty RM, Veeratterapillay R, et al. A machine learning predictive model for post-ureteroscopy urosepsis needing intensive care unit admission: a case–control YAU endourology study from Nine European Centres. J Clin Med. 2021;10(17):3888.
76. Somani BK, Brouwers T, Veneziano D, et al. Standardization in Surgical Education (SISE): development and implementation of an innovative training program for urologic surgery residents and trainers by the European School of Urology in Collaboration with the ESUT and EULIS Sections of the EAU. Eur Urol. 2021;79(3):433–4.
77. Veneziano D, Ploumidis A, Proietti S, et al. Validation of the endoscopic stone treatment step 1 (EST-s1): a novel EAU training and assessment tool for basic endoscopic stone treatment skills-a collaborative work by ESU. ESUT and EULIS World J Urol. 2020;38(1):193–205.
78. Veneziano D, Ploumidis A, Cleynenbreugel BV, et al. Development methodology of the novel endoscopic stone treatment step 2/A training/assessment curriculum and a roadmap on developing hands-on training curriculums in future: an International Collaborative Work by European Association of Urology Sections. J Endourol. 2021;35(9):1419–26.

79. Whitehurst LA, Somani BK. Semi-rigid ureteroscopy: indications, tips, and tricks. Urolithiasis. 2018;46(1):39–45.
80. Somani BK, Ploumidis A, Pappas A, et al. Pictorial review of tips and tricks for ureteroscopy and stone treatment: an essential guide for urologists from PETRA research consortium. Transl Androl Urol. 2019;8(Suppl 4):S371–80.
81. Rukin NJ, Somani BK, Patterson J, et al. Tips and tricks of ureteroscopy: consensus statement part I. Basic ureteroscopy. Cent Eur J Urol. 2015;68(4):439–46.
82. Rukin NJ, Somani BK, Patterson J, et al. Tips and tricks of ureteroscopy: consensus statement. Part II. Advanced ureteroscopy. Cent Eur J Urol. 2016;69(1):98–104.
83. Doizi S, Traxer O. Flexible ureteroscopy: technique, tips and tricks. Urolithiasis. 2018;46(1):47–58.

Chapter 24
Robot Assisted Laparoscopic Upper Urinary Tract Reconstruction

Maria C. Velasquez, Nicholas A. Smith, and Leslie A. Deane

Introduction

Imaging

CT Urogram and 3D Reconstruction

Given the widespread use of computed tomography (CT) in different settings, the diagnosis of ureteral abnormalities has also increased over the last decades. However, plain imaging is insufficient for the proper diagnosis and detailed evaluation necessary for the assessment of ureteral pathologies. CT urography (Fig. 24.1), which has largely replaced intravenous urography, has therefore emerged as the primary imaging modality for evaluation of the urinary tract, allowing detailed assessment of the ureters, as well as direct visualization of adjacent structures and complete evaluation of the abdomen and pelvis [1]. CT urography is defined as CT examination of the urinary tract that includes a non-enhanced phase, which allows

M. C. Velasquez
Department of Urology, University of California San Francisco, San Francisco, CA, USA
e-mail: maria.velasquezescobar@ucsf.edu

N. A. Smith
Department of Urology, Columbia University, Mount Sinai Medical Center, Miami Beach, Miami, FL, USA
e-mail: nicholas.smith@msmc.com

L. A. Deane (✉)
Division of Urology, Department of Surgery, Howard University College of Medicine, Washington, DC, USA
e-mail: leslie.deane@howard.edu

S. Tonyali et al. (eds.), *Current Endourology*,
https://doi.org/10.1007/978-3-032-00010-1_24

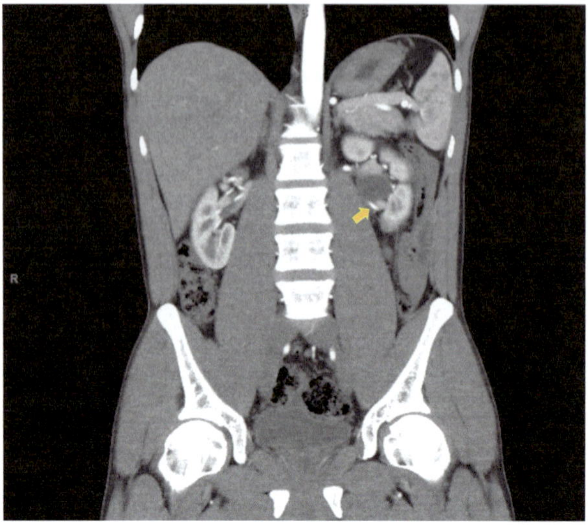

Fig. 24.1 Contrast-enhanced computed tomography scan reveals apparent left ureteropelvic junction obstruction in this patient with left flank pain. A crossing lower pole artery is visible on this coronal section (yellow arrow)

detection of stones and evaluation of masses for fat or calcium, a contrast-enhanced phase (by using intravenous contrast material that contains 30–42 g of iodine) designed for the characterization of masses, providing a baseline attenuation value to calculate enhancement of urinary tract lesions, and finally an excretory phase (performed 7 min after the injection of the contrast media) which evaluates the urothelium for potential luminal filling defects within the ureters and bladder. However, this final phase is subject to intermittent peristaltic contractions of the ureter, rendering the distal ureter the most difficult area to distended and opacify. Therefore, some ancillary maneuvers have been implemented with mixed results and acceptance, including preemptive intravenous saline hydration forced diuresis, the use of abdominal compression devices, prone patient positioning and low dose furosemide injection. Nevertheless the advantages of such techniques have been inconsistent and with the potential for side effects from furosemide administration, these techniques are not routinely used or recommended [2]. Furthermore, CT urography with 3D reconstruction, provides detailed anatomical information and a more accurate diagnostic approach for surgical planning, facilitating the precise location for endopyelotomy incision, safely avoiding crossing vessels in patients with ureteropelvic obstruction and lowering the risk of significant hemorrhage. Most recent technology is directed towards 3D printed organ modeling, using a novel technique that combines 3D wax printer and polymer molding. A recent study [3], in which 3D CT data sets of human cadaveric kidneys were used, demonstrated that the anatomical details of the models, including the pyelocaliceal system, were validated in detail by CT scan, ultrasound and endoscopy, proving to be a cost-effective method to obtain a reproducible model suitable for surgical simulation and training.

Mercaptoacetyltriglycine-3 (MAG-3) Diuretic Renal Scan

Commonly used for routine dynamic renal imaging, it is the radioisotope of choice in patients suspected of having ureteral obstruction. In this imaging technique, the radioisotope is injected into the circulatory system and then filtered by the kidneys, allowing dynamic images that assess function. The collecting system can be challenged, by administering a diuretic (usually furosemide) 15 min before, at the same time, or 15 min after the tracer is administered. Parameters evaluated include measurement of renal blood flow, absolute tracer clearance rates, differential renal function and response to the diuretic challenge. One of the most common indications for a MAG 3 diuretic renal scan is suspected outflow tract obstruction and renal functional evaluation. Furthermore, this can only be assessed if the disease in question is unilateral, allowing for the differential renal function to be compared with the healthy contralateral kidney. Differential function is evidently less useful in bilateral renal disease, a scenario in which measurement of GFR with Cr-51-EDTA is indicated to evaluate renal impairment [4]. Results, however, are highly subjective and dependent on the reader's experience. Moreover, there are several well-known pitfalls to this imaging modality, which can affect the quality of renal imaging, including motion artifact, dehydration and impaired renal function, as the success of the diuretic challenge depends on renal response to the medication. Obstruction cannot be adequately evaluated if there is an impaired drainage response to a diuretic challenge [5].

MRI Urography

Used to meticulously evaluate the renal parenchyma, the pelvicalyceal system and ureters, with the advantage of no radiation exposure or iodinated contrast administration, unlike CT urography. Therefore, is the preferred image modality in patients with impaired renal function or iodine allergy. Nevertheless, MR urography is limited by decrease spatial resolution, longer examination times, significantly higher cost and inability to appropriately assess for calculi and calcifications. MRI urography consists of static fluid urography with T2-weighted sequences; which is independent of the renal excretory function and is useful to differentiate between obstructed and non-obstructed ureters, and excretory urography with T1-weighted sequences after IV contrast administration (gadolinium based agents are most commonly used), used to evaluate the anatomy and function of the renal system with the corticomedullary, nephrographic and excretory phases [6].

Antegrade and Retrograde Pyelogram

Antegrade and retrograde pyelography are commonly used to further evaluate patients with incompletely opacified segments on CT urography and to further characterize ureteric lesions (Fig. 24.2). It consists of injecting water-soluble contrast,

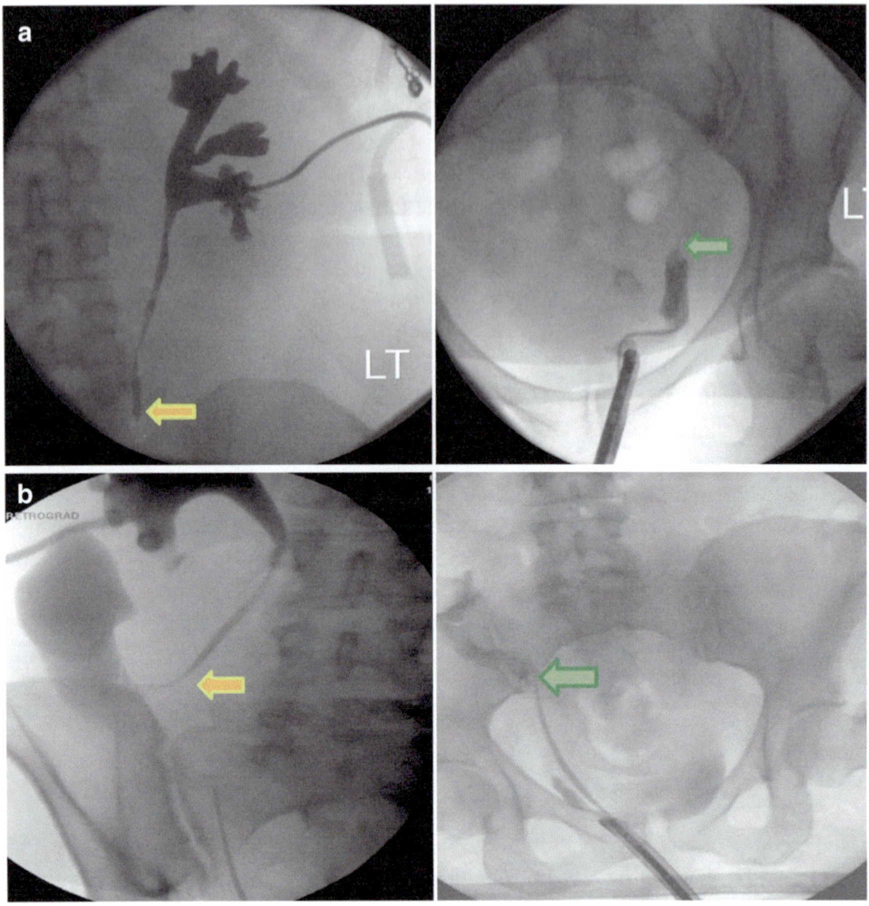

Fig. 24.2 Antegrade and retrograde pyelograms. (**a**) Left ureter: Long mid-distal stricture secondary to pelvic radiation in a patient with history of uterine cancer. Note significant narrowing of the proximal and mid ureter with an abrupt termination (yellow arrow). Distally there is abrupt termination of the ureter below the pelvic brim (green arrow). (**b**) Right ureter: Patient with a ureteral injury. The yellow arrow demonstrates the proximal end of the ureteral defect. Distally there is abrupt termination of the ureter at the pelvic brim level (green arrow), for this patient a ureteral re-implant with Boari flap was performed

typically diluted to 50% using sterile saline, in an antegrade (depending on the prior existence of a nephrostomy tube) or retrograde fashion into the ureter and collecting system under fluoroscopic guidance, allowing better anatomical characterization of the ureter for surgical planning. For example, antegrade/retrograde pyelography plays an important role in the diagnosis and management of ureteropelvic junction obstruction, as it not only confirms the diagnosis, but also determines the exact location and extent of the obstruction [7], thereby dictating if an endoscopic intervention such as endopyelotomy is suitable, versus a more complex reconstructive procedure such as pyeloplasty. Retrograde pyelogram should also be performed during ureteral stent placement, while attempting to temporarily relieve the ureteral obstruction, with the aim of confirming adequate stent position. Overall, antegrade/retrograde pyelogram is a safe procedure, although one must remain cognizant of the risk of complicated urinary tract infection (UTI) and institute appropriate antimicrobial prophylaxis [8].

Diagnostic Ureteroscopy

Diagnostic ureteroscopy can be performed to better assess ureteral strictures in patients in which imaging modalities such as CT urogram or MR urography were insufficient to provide details needed for surgical planning. Moreover, it is a useful tool when diagnostic uncertainty exists, allowing direct visualization of the stricture and ruling out differential pathologies such as malignancy, providing tissue diagnosis if warranted [9, 10]. The choice of semirigid or flexible ureteroscopy is based on the location of the pathology being evaluated, with distal lesions being more amenable to the former and more proximal lesions, the latter. It is important that all pre-operative images are available and displayed in the operative suite and that a urinalysis is done to exclude infection. Overall, diagnostic ureteroscopy is an established minimally invasive procedure that is very well tolerated. Nonetheless, significant complications may arise in the perioperative and/or postoperative period. Ureteral stent discomfort (if it is decided that patient will benefit from stent placement after the intervention), ureteral wall injury and infection are the most commonly reported complications. Therefore, patients should always be counseled appropriately regarding these risks [11].

Anatomy

Embryologically, the ureter originates from the ureteric bud, which is a protrusion of the mesonephric duct. In adulthood it measures 25–30 cm long, with a diameter of 1.5–6 mm. The ureters begin at the ureteropelvic junction, posterior to the renal vein and artery at the hilum, and then travel inferiorly along the psoas muscle and enter the bladder posteriorly on the trigone. Anatomically, the ureter can be divided into abdominal, pelvic and intramural segments. There are important differences in blood supply to these 3 anatomic regions. Clinically, however, when determining an approach to stricture repair, the ureter is divided into proximal, mid and distal, with the proximal including from the ureteropelvic junction to the upper border of the sacroiliac joint, the mid from this latter point to the lower border of the sacroiliac joint and the distal then continuing to the ureteric orifice. Additionally, there are 3 specific areas of normal anatomical narrowing along the ureter, located at the levels of the ureteropelvic junction, the crossing of the iliac vessels and ureterovesical junction. These areas can be inadvertently labeled as strictures on images in the pre-operative setting [12].

Abdominal Segment

This segment extends from the renal pelvis to the pelvic brim. The right ureter begins behind the descending part of the duodenum. Just below their origin, the ureters are crossed by gonadal (testicular or ovarian) vessels. On the left side, the sigmoid arteries and veins run in front of the ureter and reach the sigmoid colon. The genitofemoral nerve is located behind the ureter and runs along the anterior surface of the psoas major. At the area of the sacroiliac joints, the ureters cross the pelvic brim, as well as the bifurcation of the common iliac arteries and enter the pelvis. The upper ureter is supplied by branches arising medially from the renal artery and occasionally the abdominal aorta, gonadal artery and common iliac arteries. Two of the most common areas of ureteric injury are near the pelvic brim, given the proximity of the infundibulopelvic ligament and further distally, the crossing of the uterine artery in surgical interventions such as hysterectomy [14, 15].

Pelvic Segment

This segment accounts for roughly half of the total length, measuring approximately 15 cm. It starts at the pelvic inlet and then crosses near the bifurcation of the common iliac vessels. Once within the pelvic cavity, the ureters travel along the lateral pelvic wall along the internal iliac artery distally crossing the obturator artery, vein and nerve. At this point, the vas deferens loops medially over the ureter. In females the ovarian and the uterine artery run anteriorly. Subsequently, the ureters proceed to the bladder along the inferior vesical vessels and the inferior hypogastric plexus. This ureteral segment is supplied by the superior and inferior vesical arteries. In the male the artery to the vas deferens and in the female, the uterine artery also supplies this portion of the pelvic segment of the ureter. The anatomical course of this ureteral segment is of surgical importance, as they travel in close proximity to the ovarian and uterine vessels, therefore putting them at risk of injury during gynecological interventions. Additionally, when performing vaginal surgery, there is an increased risk of injury to the ureter [13, 14].

Intramural Segment

The intramural segment of the ureter involves the ureter which runs obliquely through the bladder wall, from its point of entry in the lateral wall to the orifice located on the trigone. This segment is slightly narrower in caliber than the extravesical ureter, and only measures 1.2–2.5 cm in the adult. Near the bladder, the terminal ureter is enveloped by the muscular layer of Waldeyer, which fuses with detrusor muscle fibers creating a ureterovesical valve and preventing reflux [13, 15].

Renal Pelvis and UPJ Reconstruction

Surgical Principles

Pre-operative Planning

In patients with a diagnosis of UPJ obstruction, nephrostomy tube (NT) placement is recommended for urinary diversion and preservation of renal function in those who are symptomatic, as long term ureteral stents may induce ureteral edema and periureteral fibrosis resulting in untoward challenges during surgery [16]. As previously mentioned, nephrostomy placement may be helpful in confirming the diagnosis of obstruction via antegrade nephrostogram, before or during the definitive surgical procedure. It should be noted that in patients with a relatively noncompliant collecting system or when there is poor underlying renal function and reduced urine production, UPJ obstruction might not be associated with hydronephrosis, in which case percutaneous access can be challenging [17]. On the other hand, in hydronephrotic kidneys, renal stones can develop due to urinary stasis. This also needs to be carefully assessed before planning a surgical intervention. In patients who were previously managed with indwelling ureteral stents, ureteral rest for 2–4 weeks is recommended, as recent studies have shown that implementing ureteral rest prior to ureteral reconstruction of proximal and middle ureteral strictures, allows stricture maturation and is associated with higher surgical success rates and lower blood loss [16]. If a renal scan has not been performed, it should be done after a period of drainage and ureteral rest to determine the function of the affected kidney as overall, simple nephrectomy may be indicated when split renal function is less than 20% in the setting of recurrent infections, although many surgeons take the full clinical picture into consideration rather than a single split function number [18]. Once all the required imaging studies have been done, patients should be counseled on the findings before definitive repair. It is recommended to obtain routine laboratory studies, including complete blood count, basic metabolic panel and urine culture prior to surgery, as patients with nephrostomy tubes and/or indwelling ureteral stents are at higher risk for bacterial or fungal colonization, which can be associated with surgical site infections and post-operative complications resulting in increased post-operative length of stay, if not appropriately addressed before surgery. In asymptomatic patients, if the bacteria isolated in the pre-operative urine culture is resistant to oral antimicrobials, the patient should be admitted to the hospital to commence culture directed intravenous antibiotics 24 h before surgical intervention. Otherwise, if the bacteria are susceptible to oral antimicrobials, patients should start an oral regimen at least 24 h before the intervention. Additionally, if the pre-operative urine culture is negative, antimicrobial surgical prophylaxis is recommended as per local guidelines [8]. Routine bowel preparation is not recommended.

Positioning and Port Placement

Patients are placed in a modified flank position with the ipsilateral arm placed along the side, padded and secured. All pressure points are adequately padded, and gel rolls are placed under the patient's shoulder and hip to prevent nerve compression injuries. A pillow is placed between the patient's knees, and the patient is then safety secured to the bed using tape or straps over the patient's arms, hips and legs. Then the surgical bed is mildly flexed if at all, with the aim of bridging the surgical area and to increase the space between the iliac crest and the inferior costal margin. Of note, genitalia and nephrostomy tubes should be adequately prepped and are included in the sterile field. A Foley catheter is inserted within the sterile field.

Pneumoperitoneum is most frequently achieved using the Veress needle technique, in which the needle is usually placed two finger breadths below the costal margin and in the midclavicular line. Adequate placement of the needle in the peritoneum is confirmed by the aspiration and saline drop test, with maintenance of a low-pressure pneumoperitoneum (<10 mm Hg) with slow insufflation of carbon dioxide and symmetrical distention of the abdomen. Once a satisfactory pneumoperitoneum has been achieved, robotic ports can be placed under direct vision (Fig. 24.3). If using the Xi DaVinci robotic system, 4 trocars are placed in a straight-line configuration along the para-rectus midclavicular line, starting 2 finger breadths below the costal margin and 2 finger breadths above the iliac crest. There should be approximately 8 cm between each trocar, with the second port (from superior to inferior) being placed over the renal hilum. Additionally, a 5 mm or 12-mm assistant port is placed for the assistant surgeon, to allow for passage and retrieval of needles, aid in retraction and suctioning. Port placement may be modified as needed based on the patient's body habitus, prior surgical incisions and/or the presence of

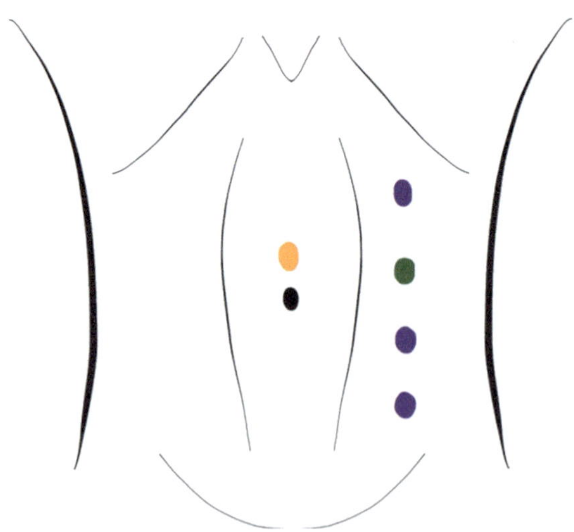

Fig. 24.3 Port placement for UPJ, proximal and mid ureteral strictures
●12 mm Assistant port
●8 mm Camera port
●8 mm Robotic port

adhesions [19–21]. It is the preference of the authors to enter the abdomen with a 5 mm visual port and zero-degree lens and then observe the insertion of each subsequent port, followed finally by exchange of the 5 mm port for an 8 mm robotic port. This greatly minimizes the risk of injury during entry.

Instrumentation

The following instruments are used:

- Four 8 mm robotic ports if using the Xi robotic system
- A 5 mm assistant port
- 0 or 30 degree robotic camera
- DaVinci instruments: Curved monopolar scissors, Potts' scissors, fenestrated bipolar, two needle drivers, dual blade atrial retractor (which can be used for exposure if deemed necessary).
- Assistant instruments: 5 mm suction, needle driver, guide wire, flexible cystoscope and ureteroscope if stones are present.

Exposure

Adequate surgical exposure during laparoscopic or robotic pyeloplasty can be achieved via transperitoneal or retroperitoneal approach. During the transperitoneal approach, the white line of Toldt is reflected using the fenestrated bipolar forceps and the curved monopolar scissors, allowing access to the retroperitoneum. Then the colon is reflected medially, with care taken not to directly manipulate the bowel with the grasper. After observation of the psoas muscle, the ureter is identified just medial to the lower pole of the kidney and traced cephalad to the renal pelvis, which is dissected anteriorly and posteriorly up to the renal sinus [20]. On the other hand, transmesocolic exposure (Fig. 24.4) has been suggested as an alternative method in patients with left ureteropelvic obstruction and involves incising the mesocolon overlying the ureteropelvic junction and renal pelvis. A dilated renal pelvis is often easily recognizable posterior to the mesentery. The authors then first perform a retrograde pyelogram and place a balloon occlusion catheter into the renal pelvis at the outset of the procedure (Fig. 24.5). This is then gently brought down to the junction and is particularly useful in identifying the exact location of the ureteropelvic junction as movement of the catheter guides the surgeon to the precise point of interest. The advantage of the transmesocolic approach has been described extensively, as it has been shown to shorten operating time and leads to a faster recovery, even in obese patients [22, 23]. Overall, extensive ureterolysis should be avoided to preserve adequate blood supply and to avoid injury to the surrounding vasculature [18]. Ureteral peristalsis aids in differentiating the ureter from the gonadal vessels. Of note, normal planes of dissection are often obliterated in patients with prior surgical interventions and irradiated fields. While inspecting the ureteropelvic junction, the

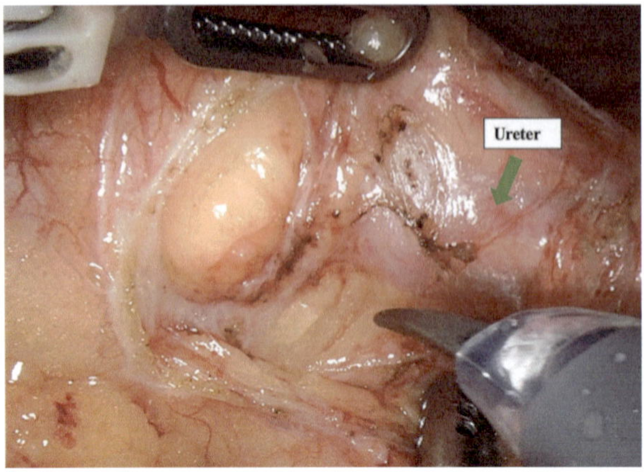

Fig. 24.4 Transmesocolic exposure in which the mesocolon is incised over the ureteropelvic junction which is accurately identified by gentle manipulation of the balloon occlusion catheter

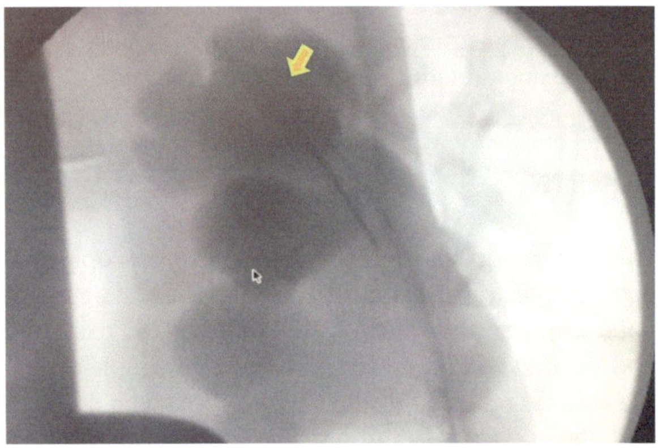

Fig. 24.5 Balloon occlusion catheter placed into the renal pelvis during surgical exposure. The balloon (yellow arrow) is then gently brought down to the ureteropelvic junction and is particularly useful in identifying the exact location of the ureteropelvic junction as movement of the catheter guides the surgeon to the precise point of interest

presence of crossing vessels should be evaluated, as they are present in almost 40% of cases of UPJO [19].

Pyeloplasty Techniques

Handling of Crossing Vessel

A crossing vessel (CV) is an ectopic or accessory renal artery, usually entering the kidney and accompanied by veins leading away from the renal hilum proper. Crossing vessels usually enter the lower pole of the kidney and pass ventral to the UPJ and may be implicated in causing mechanical compression and subsequent obstruction. Crossing vessels have been identified as a potential cause of extrinsic UPJ stenosis [19]. To date, there is still debate regarding what type of surgical technique should be employed and whether transposition of the vessels is always needed.

Ultimately, the decision is made by the surgeon intra-operatively. In the adult population, cephalad transposition is commonly performed as is reconstruction of the UPJ by anterior transposition. It is important to recognize that it is not necessary to skeletonize or separate anterior crossing vessels. One merely needs to identify the anterior surface of the renal pelvis superior to the vessels and the anterior surface of the ureter inferior to vessels and then join these two planes posterior to the vessels, leaving the perivascular tissues intact. This minimizes the risk of compromising the vasculature or causing vascular injury.

Anderson-Hynes

Initially introduced in 1949 by Anderson and Hynes (A-H) [24], this surgical technique is still considered the gold standard in the treatment of UPJ obstruction (Fig. 24.6), due to its reproducible and favorable outcomes, broad applicability including preservation of lower pole crossing vessels and long-term success rate, which ranges from 90% to 100% in multiple studies. Open pyeloplasty has been the preferred procedure over the years, as it allows treatment of all types of obstructions and removal of coexisting kidney stones [19, 20]. However with the introduction of laparoscopic pyeloplasty by Schuessler et al. [25] in 1993, and subsequently robotic pyeloplasty (Fig. 24.7) in 2002 [26], minimally invasive pyeloplasty has become a well-studied, commonly used technique, that results in minimal morbidity, decreased post-operative pain with similar functional success, and better cosmetic results. For this procedure, the renal pelvis is circumferentially transected above the UPJ. In patients with grade 3–4 hydronephrosis excess tissue may be excised but reduction is not mandatory. The proximal ureter is then spatulated laterally using the Potts' scissors. If needed, a concomitant pyelolithotomy is performed at this time before proceeding with the anastomosis, using a laparoscopic grasper or a flexible cystoscope with a stone basket through the assistant port. For the anastomosis an absorbable monofilament suture is preferred. The apex of the spatulated part of the ureter

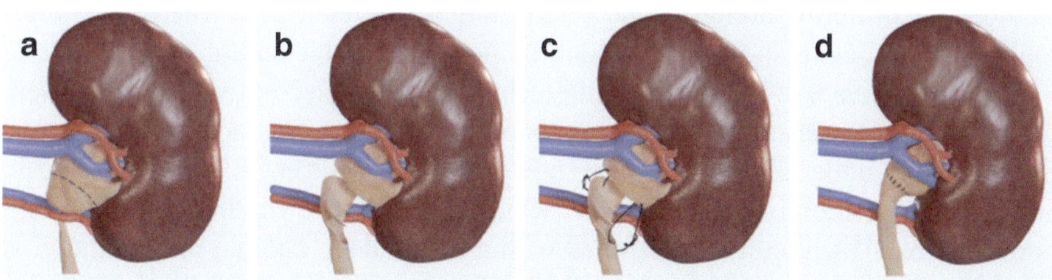

Fig. 24.6 Anderson-Hynes dismembered pyeloplasty surgical technique, in the setting of aberrant or accessory lower pole vessels, which allows transposition of the UPJ in relation to the vessels. (**a**) For this technique the renal pelvis is circumferentially transected above the UPJ. (**b**) The proximal ureter is spatulated laterally, (**c**) then the apex of the spatulated part of the ureter is brought to the most dependent and inferior part of the renal pelvis with the first suture. (**d**) The anastomosis is then performed with a running suture, and the most inferior part of the pelvis is joined to the upper part of the ureter

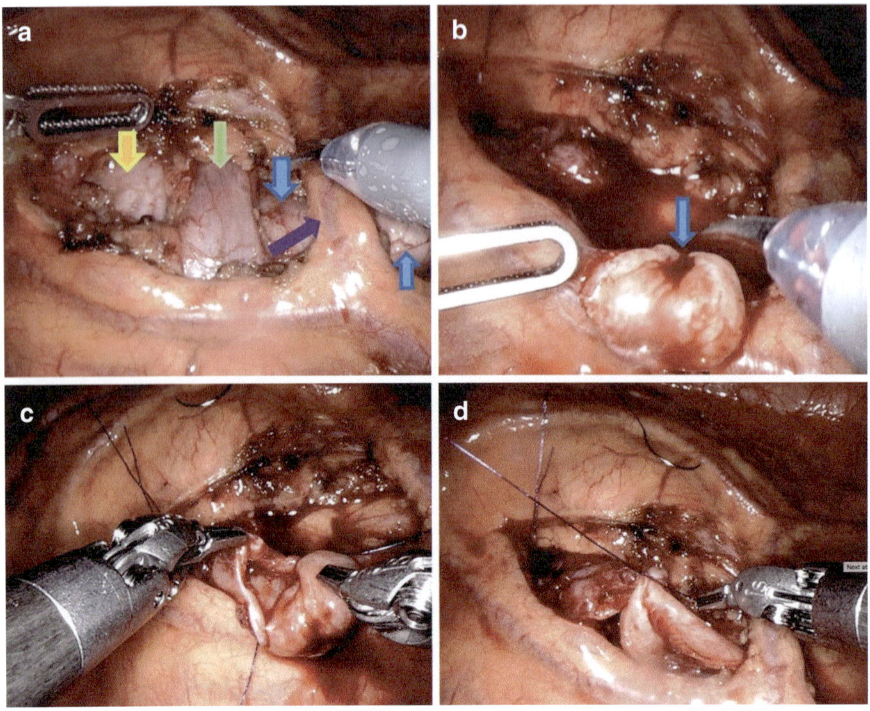

Fig. 24.7 32 year-old male who underwent uncomplicated robotic Anderson Hynes dismembered pyeloplasty due to a lower pole crossing vessel. (**a**) A transmesocolic exposure was achieved in which the renal pelvis (yellow arrow), the crossing vessel (green arrow), the ureter (blue arrow) and a crossing mesenteric vessel (purple arrow) were identified. (**b**) The proximal ureter was spatulated laterally (blue arrow) using Potts scissors. (**c**) Subsequently, the apex of the spatulated part of the ureter was brought to the most dependent and inferior part of the renal pelvis with the first suture. (**d**) The anastomosis was then performed in a running fashion

is brought to the most dependent, inferior part of the renal pelvis with the first suture. The posterior ureteropelvic re-anastomosis is then performed with interrupted or continuous 4–0 or 5–0 monofilament absorbable suture on a 1/2 circle 13 mm needle using a robotic suturing technique. If redundant tissue was excised, the remaining anterior pyelotomy incision is closed using additional sutures. Subsequently, under direct vision, an indwelling ureteral stent is usually placed in an antegrade fashion over a guidewire, which is introduced via the assistant 5 mm port. The distal stent coil is positioned within the bladder, and the proximal coil is carefully placed in the renal pelvis. With the ureteral stent in place, the anterior anastomosis is performed with a running suture and the most inferior part of the pelvis is joined to the upper part of the ureter. In recent years, a W type suture technique has been described with the aim of performing a more watertight anastomosis. For this technique, the first running suture is placed from the apex of the spatulated ureter to the upper part of the dorsal border of the ureter. The ventral border of the ureter is then brought to the dependent part of the renal pelvis with a running suture. With the same suture, the upper free part of the ureter is approximated to the renal pelvis using a W-shape stitch, which is created by going through the ureter from the outside to the inside, then from the inside to the outside and then performing the same type of stitch but including the renal pelvis. The remaining part of the renal pelvis is closed in a running fashion using the same suture. A recent study has shown that this novel approach may reduce the duration of post-operative abdominal drainage due to decrease urine leakage duration [27]. It is the author's preference to perform a continuous closure starting with the posterior suture line followed by positioning of the guide wire in the renal pelvis by passage through the existing balloon occlusion catheter, prior to closure of the anterior suture line. Then, the stent can be placed at the conclusion of the procedure using fluoroscopic guidance +/− a parallel flexible cystoscope alongside the guide wire in the bladder, to ensure the distal coil is correctly deployed. This eliminates any uncertainty as to whether the distal coil is correctly placed within the bladder.

Scardino-Prince

Developed in 1953 and also known as vertical flap pyeloplasty, this is a surgical technique recommended in patients with a dependent UPJ and a large extrarenal pelvis, associated with a long and narrow proximal ureter (Fig. 24.8). However, it has limited clinical application and, in most instances, has been replaced by the standard dismembered pyeloplasty. For this technique, the flap itself is created by creating a vertical incision from the base to the apex of the renal pelvis. The incision is then carried down the proximal ureter, completely traversing through the stenotic area and into normal-caliber ureter. The apex of the flap is then rotated down and approximated to the most inferior aspect of the ureterotomy. Finally, the flap is closed with interrupted or running fine absorbable sutures [19].

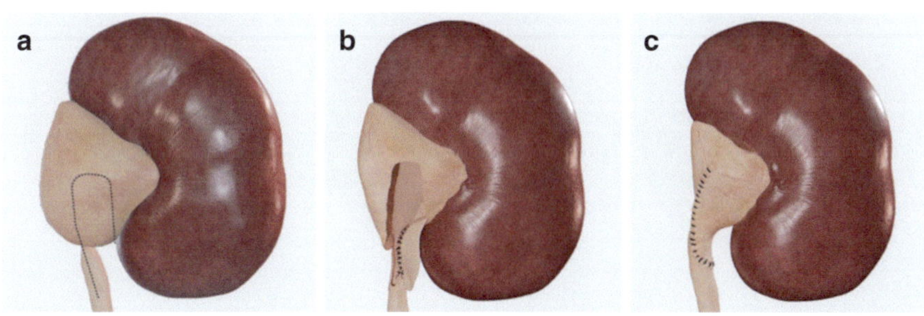

Fig. 24.8 Scardino-Prince or vertical flap technique is usually recommended in patients with a dependent UPJ and a large square-shaped extrarenal pelvis, associated with a long and narrow proximal ureter. (**a**) For this technique, the flap itself is created by doing a vertical incision from the base to the apex of the renal pelvis. The incision is then carried down the proximal ureter, completely traversing through the stenotic area and into normal-caliber ureter. (**b**) The apex of the flap is then rotated down and approximated to the most inferior aspect of the ureterotomy (C) the flap is then closed with interrupted or running fine absorbable sutures

Culp—DeWeerd

Also known as spiral flap pyeloplasty, is a surgical technique mostly used in patients with a large extrarenal pelvis with an oblique ureteral insertion, or in patients with both UPJ obstruction and a long segment of proximal ureteral stricture (Fig. 24.9). For this technique the proximal ureter is longitudinally incised, completely traversing through the obstructive segment. Subsequently, a spiral flap is obtained from the renal pelvis with a broad base positioned obliquely on the dependent aspect of the renal pelvis, which is then connected to the ureteral incision. For the flap, it's length depends on the length of proximal ureter to be bridged. To preserve vascular integrity of the flap, the ratio of flap length to width should not be greater than 3:1. In general, the outline of the flap should be made longer than what may initially be perceived as necessary, because the flap will shrink once the pelvis is incised. Once the flap has been created, the apex is rotated toward the most inferior aspect of the ureterotomy and the anastomosis is performed with absorbable sutures [19].

Foley Y-V Plasty

Originally described for the correction of UPJ obstruction in patients with a high ureteral insertion and an intrarenal pelvis (Fig. 24.10), it is usually performed whenever a tension free dismembered pyeloplasty is not possible. However, the Foley Y-V plasty is contraindicated when transposition of lower pole vessels is necessary and in patients that require concomitant reduction of redundant renal pelvis. For this

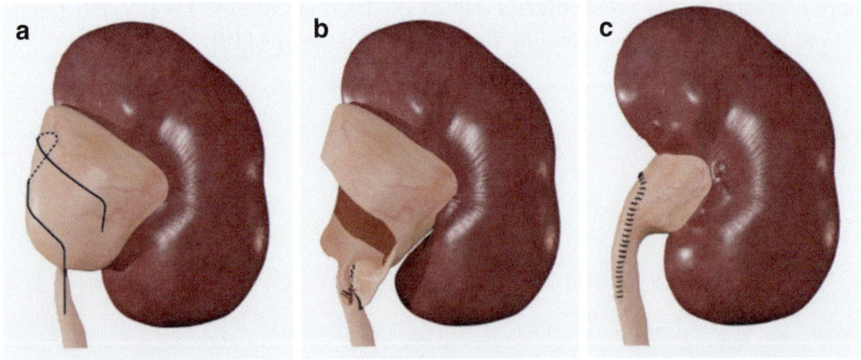

Fig. 24.9 Culp-De Weerd or spiral flap pyeloplasty is recommended in patients with large extrarenal pelvis with an oblique ureteral insertion, or in patients with both UPJ obstruction and a long segment of proximal ureteral stricture. (**a**) The proximal ureter is longitudinally incised, completely traversing through the obstructive segment. (**b**) A spiral flap is then obtained from the renal pelvis with a broad base positioned obliquely on the dependent aspect of the renal pelvis, which is then connected to the ureteral incision. (**c**) Once the flap has been created, the apex is rotated down to the most inferior aspect of the ureterotomy and the anastomosis is performed with absorbable sutures

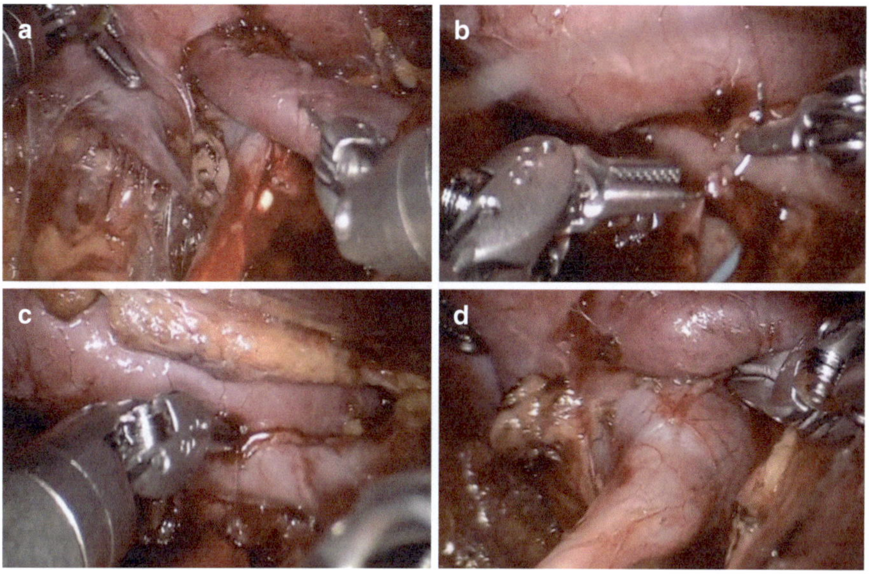

Fig. 24.10 (**a**–**d**) Robotic Foley Y-V plasty

technique Potts' scissors are most commonly used. The V flap is first delineated starting at the base on the lateral aspect of the renal pelvis, extending the apex of the flap to the level of the UPJ. Incision is then carried along the lateral aspect of the proximal ureter well into an area of normal caliber. Subsequently, the apex of the pelvic flap is brought to the most inferior aspect of the ureteral incision. The posterior walls are approximated using running or interrupted absorbable sutures, most preferably 4–0 or 5–0 monofilament absorbable suture. The senior author of this chapter has described the use of the 1/2 circle 13 mm needle in uretero-enteric anastomosis and this needle is preferred for all ureteral reconstructive work [28]. Lastly, the anterior wall of the pelvic flap is then approximated, completing the anastomosis [19, 29]. A stent can then be placed as previously described (Fig. 24.11).

Ureterocalicostomy

Initially described by Neuwirt [30] in 1948, Ureterocalicostomy is a salvage surgical intervention for recurrent UPJ obstruction, as well as upper ureteric injury and complete intrarenal pelvis. It typically includes complete amputation of the lower renal pole, preservation of periureteral blood supply and the creation of a widely spatulated, tension-free anastomosis of the ureter to the lower pole calyx [31]. The patient is positioned as previously described for pyeloplasty. A transperitoneal approach is used to gain access to the upper ureter and lower renal pole. The thin lower pole renal surface is identified and excised using cold scissors. A simple nephrotomy should be avoided, to prevent a secondary stricture, hence the

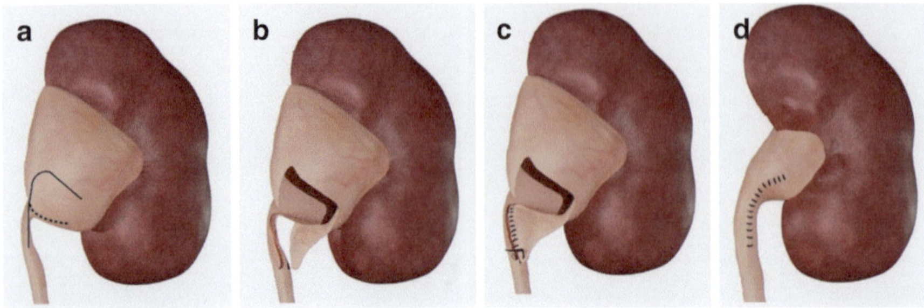

Fig. 24.11 Foley Y-V plasty was originally described for the correction of UPJ obstruction in patients with a high ureteral insertion, and is usually performed whenever a tension free dismembered pyeloplasty is not possible. However it is contraindicated in patients with transposition of lower pole vessels. (**a**) The V flap is first delineated starting at the base on the medial aspect of the renal pelvis, extending the apex of the flap to the level of the UPJ. (**b**) Incision is then carried along the lateral aspect of the proximal ureter well into an area of normal caliber. Subsequently, the apex of the pelvic flap is brought to the most inferior aspect of the ureteral incision. (**c**) The posterior walls are approximated using running or interrupted absorbable sutures. (**d**) Lastly, the anterior wall of the pelvic flap is then approximated, completing the anastomosis

parenchyma overlaying the lower pole calyx should be resected instead of simply incised. Subsequently, the UPJ is transected and then closed using 5–0 absorbable sutures at the level of the renal hilum. The ureter is spatulated laterally and a double-J ureteral stent is placed in an antegrade or retrograde fashion. End-to-end uretero-calyceal anastomosis with mucosa-to-mucosa apposition is performed in a running fashion using absorbable sutures. Overall, ureterocalicostomy has excellent long term outcomes, however a recent study by Srivastava et al. [32] in which 72 patients who underwent open or laparoscopic ureterocalicostomy, and who were followed for at least 2 years, showed that the rate of failed ureterocalicostomy was higher in patients with a low pre-operative glomerular filtration rate (less than 20 ml/min/1.73 m^2) and decrease cortical thickness (less than 5 mm).

Special Circumstances

Horseshoe Kidney

Horseshoe kidney (HSK) is the most common renal congenital abnormality, affecting 0.25% of the general population. Furthermore, it is more common in males, with a male to female ratio of 2:1. One-third of HSK cases are associated with UPJ obstruction due to a high incidence of aberrant crossing vessels, high-inserting ureter into the renal pelvis and its abnormal course over the isthmus. Because of inadequate rotation of the kidney, the renal pelvis and ureters are typically in an anterior position when compared to an orthotopic kidney. Additionally, HSK can also be associated with a duplicated collecting system and vesicoureteral reflux [33, 34]. In patients with HSK and UPJ obstruction, surgical technique varies because of anatomic complexities. However, in general, the patient is placed in a modified flank position and ports are placed in a similar fashion as for pyeloplasty in an orthotopic kidney as previously described. After incising white line of Toldt and reflecting the colon medially, the dilated renal pelvis is identified and isolated, as well as the UPJ and cranial portion of the ipsilateral ureter. On the left side a transmesocolic approach may also facilitate direct access to the left UPJ [35]. Careful attention should be paid during this step of the procedure, as commonly, aberrant crossing vessels are encountered. After the UPJ is carefully isolated, a dismembered Anderson-Hynes pyeloplasty (previously described in this chapter) is performed with ureteral transposition in the setting of an aberrant crossing vessel to avoid compression of the anastomosis. A double J ureteral stent is placed in an antegrade or retrograde fashion before completing the anastomosis. There is generally no need for isthmusectomy [36], however prior publications have shown that it can be a useful adjunctive measure to allow repositioning of the kidney and preservation of an unobstructed upper urinary tract in difficult surgical cases [37–39]. Overall, UPJ reconstruction in patients with HSK presents a challenging situation. However, there is enough evidence in the literature to support laparoscopic and robotic pyeloplasty, as a safe and feasible technique, with high success rates and good medium to long term outcomes [19, 40].

Simultaneous Stone Management

It has been shown that patients with UPJ obstruction have a 70 fold increased risk of developing renal stones, due to urinary stasis and the increased likelihood of upper urinary tract infections [41]. Furthermore, the coexistence of UPJ obstruction and stones may worsen symptoms and is therefore an absolute indication for pyeloplasty with pyelolithotomy. Each goal can be successfully achieved via laparoscopic or robotic approach [19]. In a retrospective study, Kadihasanoglu et al. [42]. reported 18 cases of laparoscopic pyeloplasty with concomitant pyelolithotomy. The results were compared to a similar cohort of patients undergoing laparoscopic pyeloplasty without concomitant stone extraction. For this study, the mean stone size was 13 + 5.24 mm, and the median number of stones was 1. Results showed that despite 30 min of stone extraction time, there was overall no significant impact on total operative time, estimated blood loss or complications. Additionally, all patients were stone free 3 months after the surgical intervention with no residual stones on imaging after surgery. In this study, once the upper ureter and renal pelvis were adequately exposed, an initial small pyelotomy incision was performed to remove all renal and calyceal stones. The incision was later incorporated into the final Anderson-Hynes pyeloplasty. A laparoscopic grasper was used to remove the stones, and irrigation was used to flush out the stones in the calyces. However, if stones could not be removed with the graspers, a flexible cystoscope was placed through a 12 mm port and stones were removed under direct vision using a nitinol basket. Intraoperative fluoroscopy was used to confirm stone clearance. After the pyelolithotomy, the initial pyelotomy incision was extended and an Anderson-Hynes pyeloplasty was performed, a ureteral double J stent was placed in an antegrade fashion before completing the anastomosis. As is more commonplace today, robotic assisted laparoscopic pyeloplasty with concomitant pyelolithotomy has also been extensively described. For this procedure, similar instruments such as laparoscopic grasper and flexible cystoscope are used. A recent study by Jensen et al. [43]. reported 18 cases of concomitant robotic pyeloplasty and pyelolithotomy, in which a flexible cystoscope was inserted via an assistant port and introduced into the renal pelvis through a minor incision. Stones were then grasped with a basket and removed through the assistant port or placed in a specimen retrieval bag. Next, pyeloplasty was performed using the standard robotic technique. In this cohort of patients, the overall stone free rate was 72%. The authors of this chapter recommend minimizing the use of irrigation during nephroscopy and careful suction so as the limit the contact of fluid with the intestine which may increase the risk of ileus, not to mention if stones are infected, the risk of contaminated fluid in the abdomen must be considered and avoided.

Post-Operative Management

Drains and Ureteral Stent Management

A closed suction drain (Jackson-Pratt/Blake) is placed in the retroperitoneum near the anastomosis before completing the procedure. On postoperative day 1, a drain fluid creatinine is ordered at 5 am, and if within normal limits the urethral catheter is removed. A repeat drain creatinine after two voids is sent and if it remains within normal limits the drain can be removed. If drain output remains elevated, or if drain creatinine is positive for a urinary leak, the closed suction drain should stay longer to prevent intra-abdominal collections and further post-operative complications. Ureteral stents are removed on an outpatient basis by cystoscopy 4–6 weeks after surgery. If a nephrostomy tube is placed, it can be removed at the end of the procedure, or at the surgeon's discretion based on the patient's history. In some instances, the nephrostomy can be left in situ and capped until one week after the stent removal at which time an antegrade nephrostogram is performed and once patent, the tube is removed. Patients are discharged home on post-operative 1 if no complications are encountered.

Pain Control

Although incisional pain associated with laparoscopic and robotic interventions is significantly lower compared with open interventions, pain is still present due to stretching of the intra-abdominal cavity, peritoneal irritation, creation of pneumoperitoneum and manipulation of abdominal viscera. In order to avoid postoperative narcotic use, and its attendant side effects including nausea, drowsiness and overall increased post-operative hospital stay, the use of local anesthetics is highly recommended. Infiltration of pre-peritoneal, transversalis abdominis muscle plane and each successive layer out to the skin with an intermediate to longer acting local anesthetic at each port site at the end of the procedure, has shown to significantly decrease post-operative narcotic use [44, 45]. Once patients are discharged home, a non-opioid treatment is prescribed with medications such as acetaminophen and ketorolac.

Follow-Up Imaging

A renal ultrasound and a diuretic renal scan are obtained 3 months post-operatively and an annual ultrasound thereafter.

Proximal and Mid Ureteral Reconstruction

Surgical Principles

Positioning and Port Placement

A similar position as for pyeloplasty is recommended (details described previously in this chapter), with patients in lateral decubitus or modified decubitus. The genitalia are prepped into the field to allow for access to bladder and urethra. For female patients, the leg is placed in a modified position to allow access to the urethra in case a ureteroscopy must be performed. Patients can also be initially placed in lithotomy position for stent placement, and then be transitioned to lateral decubitus or modified decubitus. Pneumoperitoneum is most frequently achieved using the Veress needle technique. If using the Xi DaVinci robotic system, 4 trocars are placed in a straight-line configuration between the pararectus line and the midclavicular line, starting 2 fingerbreadths below the costal margin and 2 fingerbreadths above the iliac crest. There should be approximately 8 cm between each trocar site, with the second port (from proximal to distal) been placed over the renal hilum. Additionally, a 5 mm or 12-mm assistant port is placed for the assistant surgeon (Fig. 24.3). Again, port placement may be modified as needed based on the presence of adhesions. The robot is then docked at a 90° angle to the patient.

Exposure

The line of Toldt is incised, allowing medialization of the colon. After localizing the psoas muscle, the ureter can then be easily identified just medial to the lower pole of the kidney and traced cephalad to the renal pelvis. Overall, extensive circumferential ureterolysis should be avoided to preserve adequate blood supply and to avoid injury to the surrounding vasculature [18]. Currently, there are several maneuvers that can aid in ureteral stricture identification, such as the near infrared feature of the daVinci system (Intuitive, Sunnyvale, CA). An ureteroscope is advanced up to the distal margin of the stricture, and transillumination of light from the ureteroscope is seen from the robotic camera, as it detects the near-infrared spectrum of the light emitted by the ureteroscope, allowing a better assessment of stricture length. The light from the ureteroscope whether digital or fiber optic is easily seen in the near infrared mode as an intense green fluorescence (Fig. 24.12). After the stricture has been satisfactorily identified, a stay suture marks the stricture and allows for retraction of the ureter. Intra-ureteral indocyanine green (ICG) (25 mg ICG in 10 mL water) is a real-time contrast agent (tricarbocyanide), which when activated by near-infrared fluorescence (NIRF), green light can be visualized using this specialized camera (Fig. 24.13). ICG is commonly used intraoperatively due to its ability to penetrate tissue and excellent safety profile. It can be injected into the ureter via nephrostomy tube or in a retrograde fashion using a 5 Fr ureteral catheter which is inserted into the distal ureter [46–48]. A retrograde pyelogram to localize the stricture, should be performed beforehand, as the ICG needs to be injected above and below the level of stenosis. In patients with a nephrostomy tube, antegrade and retrograde pyelogram are performed to guarantee that ICG is administered above and below the level of the stricture. After ICG is injected, the ureteral catheter and/or nephrostomy tube are clamped. The ureteral catheter is then secured to the Foley and left in the surgical field. A recent study by Lee et al. showed that intra-ureteral ICG injection facilitates rapid and accurate ureteral identification, as well as precise location of proximal and distal ureteral stricture margins [49]. A major disadvantage, however, is that once the incision has been made in the ureter, the ICG will stain the surgical field (Fig. 24.13). Intravascular ICG (10 mL × 1 mg/1 mL) is used to evaluate ureteral blood supply, as well-perfused tissue will show green fluorescence under NIRF. However, it is also important to

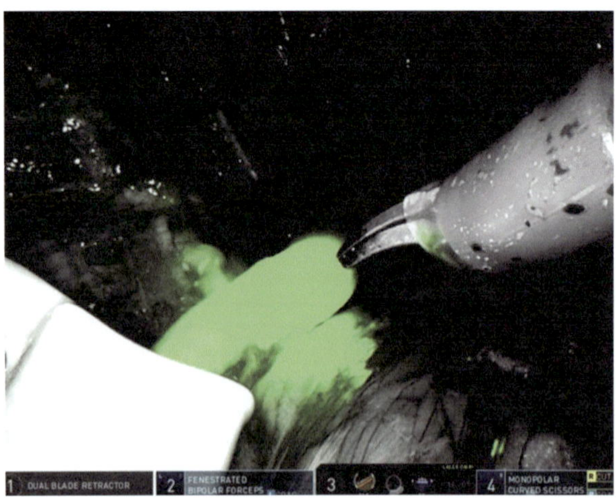

Fig. 24.12 Digital ureteroscope located in the ureter identifying a distal extent of an ureteral stricture

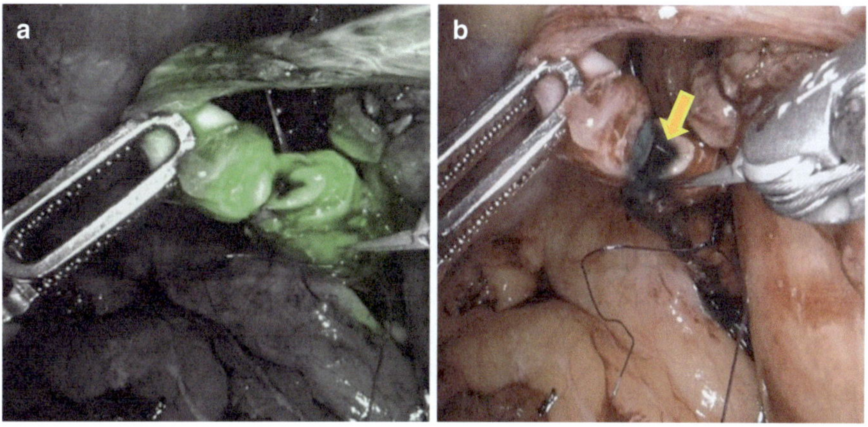

Fig. 24.13 (**a**) Intra-ureteral indocyanine green is a real-time contrast agent, commonly used intraoperative due to its ability to penetrate tissue and excellent safety profile. It can be injected into the ureter via nephrostomy tube or in retrograde fashion using a 5 Fr ureteral catheter which is inserted into the distal ureter. (**b**) A major disadvantage however, is that once the incision has been made in the ureter, the ICG will stain the surgical field (yellow arrow)

know that if intraureteral ICG is administered, and once in contact with the urothelium, intravascular ICG will not be useful for assessing ureteral vascularity [18]. As such if vascularity is deemed a concern, the stricture should be evaluated with the ureteroscopy and save the ICG for intravenous administration.

Reconstruction Techniques

Ureteroureterostomy

Robotic ureteroureterostomy is a safe and viable surgical technique, that has proven to have good outcomes for benign and malignant pathologies. It is traditionally used for short strictures (<3 cm) located proximal to the crossing of the iliac vessels [50]. For this surgical technique, once adequate ureteral exposure has been achieved, dissection of the ureter is performed in a circumferential fashion, allowing satisfactory ureteral mobilization. The exact margins of the stricture can be localized using NIRF as we have previously described. Once the stricture has been delineated, the diseased segment is excised. Subsequently, the remaining healthy ends of the ureter are widely spatulated. A watertight, end-to-end and tension free anastomosis is performed using 2 separate running absorbable sutures, like 4-0 or 5-0 monofilament absorbable suture in a tension free fashion. It is important to avoid excessive tissue manipulation or use of monopolar cautery to preserve the intricate peri-ureteral blood supply. After completion of the posterior anastomosis, a 0.035-inch hydrophilic tipped guidewire is then inserted through the previously placed ureteral catheter into the renal pelvis. Afterwards, the ureteral catheter is removed, and a double J ureteral stent is placed over the wire. Finally, the anterior part of the anastomosis is completed [19, 51].

Transureteroureterostomy

Initially described by Boari in 1894 [52], transureteroureterostomy has traditionally been used in patients with long mid-ureteral strictures and is contraindicated under the following circumstances: Insufficient length of the donor ureter to reach the contralateral ureter, patients with urothelial carcinoma; as it carries a high risk of tumor seeding into the recipient ureter, recurrent nephrolithiasis and retroperitoneal fibrosis. Given that the contralateral kidney and ureter will be used, the recipient ureter must be unobstructed and not affected by reflux. If reflux to the recipient ureter is present, it should be properly identified before surgery and corrected concurrently [19, 53]. For this surgical technique, once adequate ureteral exposure has been achieved, dissection of the ureter is performed in a circumferential fashion, allowing satisfactory ureteral mobilization. Once the stricture has been identified, the ureter is ligated proximally to the stricture, spatulated and then mobilized across the midline through a retroperitoneal tunnel, which is created with blunt dissection across the sigmoid colon mesentery, superior to the inferior mesenteric artery to avoid kinking. Subsequently, only the segment needed for the anastomosis in the recipient ureter is exposed, as optimal preservation of periureteral tissue and vasculature is essential. A longitudinal ureterotomy is performed at the medial aspect of the recipient ureter, which should be proportional to the lumen of the donor ureter. A watertight, end-to-end and tension free anastomosis is performed using 2 separate 4-0 or 5-0 monofilament absorbable sutures. After completion of the posterior anastomosis, a ureteral stent is placed across the anastomosis into the donor renal pelvis. In 2007, Piaggio and Gonzalez [54] initially described transperitoneal laparoscopic transureteroureterostomy; which was performed in three children successfully. Post-operative course was uneventful, except for urinary leak in one patient immediately after surgery. Mean operative time and estimated blood loss were 263 min and 47 ml respectively. At a mean follow up of 6 months, none of the patients developed recurrent stricture and had normal kidney function with no significant hydronephrosis. With the current breadth of techniques available to the urologist, this approach is rarely utilized today.

Ileal Ureter Replacement

Ileal ureteral replacement, is a surgical technique, initially introduced by Shoemaker [55] in 1906 and later popularized by Goodwin et al. in 1959 [56]. In 2008 the first extracorporeal robotic procedure was described by Wagner and colleagues, and later in 2014 the first laparoscopic and robotic fully intracorporeal cases were first published [57, 58]. Ileal ureter replacement has been traditionally used in long-segment ureteral strictures, in which the defect cannot be bridged, or the bladder is unfit for reconstruction. However, due to technical difficulties and major surgical complications such as bowel obstruction, enteric leak, fistula formation and long-term metabolic derangements, the use of this surgical technique is limited, and it is considered to be the last resort for strictures that are not amenable to reconstruction by other means [59]. Overall, ileal ureter replacement is contraindicated in patients with inflammatory bowel disease, short gut syndrome, neurogenic bladder and bladder outlet obstruction [18]. During this approach, once adequate ureteral exposure has been achieved, dissection of the ureter is performed in a circumferential fashion, allowing satisfactory ureteral mobilization. Once the stricture has been identified, the involved ureteral segment is dissected and the renal pelvis or the ureteral segment proximal to the resection site is widely spatulated to allow an adequate anastomosis to the end of the bowel. Afterwards, an appropriate ileal segment is divided 20 cm proximal from the ileocecal valve with a laparoscopic stapler. Bowel continuity is then restored with stapled side-to-side anastomosis. Proximally, the bowel can be anastomosed to the proximal ureter, renal pelvis or lower pole calyx, in an end-to-side, single layer technique using running or interrupted sutures in an isoperistaltic orientation between the renal pelvis and bladder. Distally, an ileocystostomy is performed in which a linear cystotomy is created at the bladder dome, to avoid angulation and obstruction of the ileum during bladder filling. The anastomosis is performed in a two-layered fashion using absorbable sutures, in a running mucosa-to-mucosa fashion and interrupted seromuscular-detrusor muscle sutures. After completion of the anastomosis, a ureteral stent is placed in a retrograde fashion over a guide wire, a 20 Fr indwelling Foley is placed and the bladder is filled to evaluate the anastomosis. If it is demonstrated that the anastomosis is water-tight, two suction drains are placed near the proximal and distal anastomoses. In 2018, Ubring and colleagues published a 7-patient series of completely intracorporeal ileal ureteric replacement, including a patient with a solitary kidney [60]. Of note, 5 patients underwent simultaneous psoas hitch. Mean operative time was 328 ± 66.3 min and median estimated blood loss was 100 cc, with a mean length of transposed ileum of 20.4 cm. Overall, no major complications were encountered, and all patients were stricture and symptom free 3 months after the procedure. Most recently, a 3-patient series was presented by Grosso et al. in which two patients underwent robotic intracorporeal ileal ureteric replacement of the entire ureter, while in one patient the lower ureteral stump was maintained and an ileal-ureter anastomosis was performed distally. Median operative time was 270 min, with no mayor complication in the post-operative period. However, at the 1-month follow up, stenosis was found at the level of the ileal-ureter anastomosis. The remaining two cases were successful. Overall, multiple studies have shown that intracorporeal robotic ileal ureter replacement can be performed with good results, within reasonable time and with low complication rates [61]. In 2015, Abhyankar and colleagues described the robotic reverse seven ileal ureter for bilateral strictures following extensive gynecologic surgery and retroperitoneal lymphadenectomy with subsequent radiation. These authors found it necessary to perform a side-to-side anastomosis for one of the ureters due to the inability to circumferentially mobilize the ureter as a result of very dense adherence to the retroperitoneum [62].

Appendiceal Onlay Flap

The appendiceal flap ureteroplasty technique was initially described by Melnikoff in 1912 [63]. However, it was an unpopular procedure, as an end-to-end anastomosis was required, carrying significant risk of stricture recurrence. However, in 2009, Reggio and colleagues reported the first successful laparoscopic appendiceal onlay flap ureteroplasty of a non-obliterated right ureteral stricture [64]. Unlike appendiceal interposition, in the onlay flap technique, the de-tubularized appendix is anastomosed to the posterior wall of the longitudinally opened ureter, therefore preserving posterior ureteral blood supply. Other advantages of the appendiceal onlay flap include: insignificant urine absorption, feasible appendiceal mobilization, lack of donor site morbidity, minimally disruption of the ureteral blood supply and the possibility of using a flap that carries its own blood supply [18]. Once adequate ureteral exposure has been achieved, the stricture is identified and the anterior wall of the strictured ureter is open longitudinally. Posterior ureteral dissection should be avoided to minimize the risk of ureteral devascularization. Subsequently, the appendix is identified and detached from the cecum, using a laparoscopic stapler to harvest the flap. Care must be taken to preserve the mesoappendix and appendices blood supply. Once the flap is harvested, the two ends of the appendix are transected and discarded. The appendiceal lumen is then cleared with suction and irrigation, and subsequently opened longitudinally along its antimesenteric border. Care must be taken to mobilize the appendix mesentery to aid in the creation of a tension free anastomosis. The appendiceal onlay flap is then sutured to the previously performed ventral ureterotomy using absorbable sutures. In a recent study by Duty and colleagues, 6 patients with a mean stricture length of 2.5 cm, underwent right laparoscopic appendiceal onlay flap ureteroplasty. Of note, three patients had failed pyeloplasty for congenital UPJ obstruction [65]. The mean operative time and estimated blood loss was 244 min and 175 ml respectively. Subjective and objective success was achieved in four patients at a mean follow up time of 16.3 months. However, two patients had recurrent abdominal pain without evidence of ureteral obstruction. Pain which was attributable to fibrosis near the gonadal vessels, resolved after laparoscopic ureterolysis and bladder advancement flap was performed. Overall, the authors concluded that laparoscopic appendiceal onlay ureteroplasty is a reasonable approach for complex mid and proximal ureteral strictures. Most recently Wang et al. published the first robotic experience performing robotic appendiceal onlay flap with a 100% objective success rate at 6 months [66].

Oral Mucosa Graft Onlay

Open ureteroplasty with buccal mucosa graft (BMG) was first described by Naude in 1999 as a less morbid and technically complicated surgical management in comparison to ileal ureter for management of complex ureteral strictures [67]. During the last 2 decades this procedure has gained increasing popularity due to its many advantages, such as well tolerated donor site morbidity, similar graft properties to the urinary tract mucosa, making it resistant to infections and compatible with a wet environment, as well as outstanding lamina propria vascularity, which makes it a worthy alternative for irradiated fields [18]. In 2015 Zhao and colleagues described their experienced with robotic BMG ureteroplasty (Fig. 24.14) on 4 patients with proximal ureteral strictures (median length 4 cm), showing no restenosis at 15.5 months and concluding that robotic BMG ureteroplasty is a viable and safe option for proximal or multifocal ureteral strictures [68]. Most recently Lee et al. retrospectively evaluated 43 patients who underwent an onlay BMG ureteroplasty and 11 patients who underwent an augmented anastomotic robotic ureteroplasty

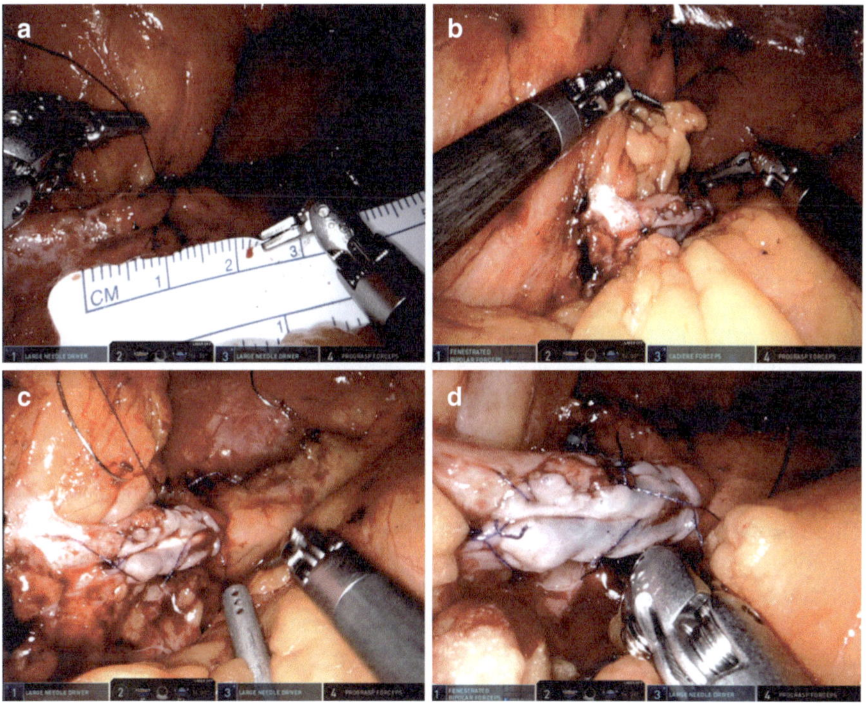

Fig. 24.14 (**a**) A 4 cm left ureteral stricture, which included a 2 cm segment of complete obliteration due to prior radiation. (**b**) An augmented ventral onlay buccal mucosal graft ureteroplasty was performed. (**c**) A ureteral stent (green arrow) was placed before completing the anastomosis (**d**) The anastomosis is performed using absorbable sutures in a running fashion suing 4-0 Vicryl on a RB 1 needle

with buccal mucosa graft with a median stricture length was of 3 cm [69]. Of note, 18 patients had previously failed ureteral reconstruction. Median operative time and estimated blood loss were 222 min and 75 cc respectively. Only one patient had an intra-operative complication consistent with a small serosal injury of the small bowel, which was repaired primarily during surgery. At a median follow up of 27.5 months, 87% of patients had no evidence of stricture recurrence. The authors then concluded that overall robotic ureteroplasty with buccal mucosa graft is associated with excellent intermediate-term outcomes and low morbidity.

For this procedure, after initial robotic access, adequate ureteral exposure is performed, as well as careful identification of the strictured ureteric segment. In patients with a narrowed lumen, an anterior ureterotomy is performed along the total stricture length and until pink, healthy ureteric mucosa is seen. This is done without circumferential mobilization. By incising only the anterior ureter, preservation of posterior ureteric blood supply is achieved and circumferential dissection is avoided. Afterwards, two sutures are placed at the midpoint on the ureterotomy opposite each other, exposing the ureteral plate. In patients with obliterative strictures, the obliterative section is excised and the ventral portion of the 2 ureteral ends is spatulated. Intravenous ICG can be used to assess blood supply to the remaining ureter (ICG use was previously described in this chapter). The required graft length is then measured intracorporeally with a ruler before the BMG is harvested. Buccal mucosa is prepped with iodine and the mouth is kept open using a Boyle-Davis retractor. A tongue blade can also be used for optimal exposure. Stenson's duct is identified and marked. A hydrodissection technique is used with lidocaine and epinephrine, and the graft is then sharply excised off the buccinator muscle. The submucosal tissue is then removed from the graft on the back table and tailored appropriately using a No. 11 blade or a fine, sharp tenotomy scissors. The buccal defect is then closed using absorbable sutures in an interrupted fashion or it can be left open to heal by secondary intention [70]. Subsequently, the BMG is delivered into the abdominal cavity through the 12-mm assistant port. It can be placed within a folded strip of Telfa to protect it during passage through the port. Additionally, a double armed fashioned suture can be passed through the apices to facilitate suturing of the graft. It is important to avoid using a suction device in close proximity to the graft once in the abdomen. The graft is then oriented over the ureterotomy with the mucosal surface facing the ureteral lumen. An anastomosis is performed using absorbable sutures in a running fashion using 4-0 or 5-0 monofilament absorbable suture. Next, the edges of the graft are trimmed. For patients with an obliterated ureteral lumen, the augmented anastomotic technique can be used in which after excising the strictured segment, an anastomotic posterior plate of healthy ureter is created using absorbable sutures in a running fashion. Subsequently, the BMG anastomosis is performed to the remaining ureteric defect using absorbable sutures in a running fashion. Of note, a double J ureteral stent is placed in all cases after completing half of the anastomosis. Lastly, omentum (supplied by the right or left gastroepiploic artery) or perinephric fat (which is generally only suitable for uretero-pelvic junction repair) is harvested and wrapped around the ureter, acting as a vascularized bed for the onlay BMG [18]. The tongue of omentum can be split and one half of it passed posterior to the ureter and the other anterior to ureter so as to avoid a bulky graft which may distort the site of repair.

Management of Retrocaval Ureter

Retrocaval or circumcaval ureter is a congenital abnormality secondary to the anomalous persistence of the right subcardinal vein, causing the right ureter to run posteriorly to the inferior vena cava (IVC) [19]. Symptoms such as recurrent urinary tract infections, lumbar pain and urolithiasis, usually present during the third or fourth decade of live. Traditionally, an Anderson-Hynes type dismembered pyeloplasty has been used for surgical correction of this condition if the proximal aspect is very dilated versus a more traditional uretero-ureterostomy if it is not very dilated, transecting and relocating the ureter anterior to the IVC [71]. In recent years, the use of robotic assisted surgery for management of retrocaval ureter has been increasingly reported, most commonly in the pediatric population [72, 73]. For this procedure, after initial robotic access, adequate ureteral exposure is obtained, as well as careful identification of the affected ureteric segment, taking care to minimize distal ureteral dissection to avoid stricture recurrence. Subsequently, the affected ureteral segment is carefully isolated and then transected. The normal ureter is then transferred anterior to the vena cava, and an end-to-end uretero-ureterostomy is performed using a monofilament 4-0 or 5-0 absorbable sutures in a running fashion. A double J ureteral stent is placed in all cases after completing half of the anastomosis. A recent multi-institutional study by Escolino and colleagues, which included 12 pediatric patients, compared outcomes of minimally invasive retrocaval ureter repair (laparoscopic and robotic assisted) vs open repair over a 5-year period [74]. The study outcomes suggests that minimally invasive surgical techniques should be the first choice compared to open surgery due to similar functional outcomes and decrease analgesia requirements with better cosmesis. Additionally, results showed that robotic assisted reconstruction was technically easier, safer and with less operative time compared to laparoscopic repair. Of note, all patients had complete resolution of symptoms and improvement of hydronephrosis.

Auto-transplantation

Renal auto-transplantation is a suitable option for patients with long upper ureteric or pan-ureteric strictures, however up to date it is still considered a salvage procedure. Initially described in 1963 as an open intervention (midline xiphopubic incision) by Hardy [75], it can offer good functional outcomes but is associated with high morbidity. Completely intra-corporeal robotic assisted kidney auto-transplantation was first reported in 2014 by Gordon and colleagues showing promising results and low morbidity compared to the traditional open approach [76]. For the first stage of the procedure, the patient is placed in lithotomy, steep Trendelenburg position. The bladder is then dissected off of the anterior abdominal wall and the ipsilateral external iliac vessels are exposed. Next, the external iliac artery and vein are dissected. For the second stage of the procedure, the patient is taken out of the Trendelenburg position and placed in a left lateral decubitus position. An irrigation tubing for intracorporeal cold perfusion is subsequently introduced through the 12 mm assistant port. The kidney is then harvested with maximal renal vessel length, and the collecting system is identified and transected at the level of the ureteral obstruction. After the donor nephrectomy is performed, the renal artery is intubated with the perfusion cannula, which is secured in placed using a Vicryl stitch, and 1 liter of histidine-tryptophan-ketoglutarate (HTK) at 4 °C is used for perfusion. Afterwards, the kidney is relocated in the ipsilateral iliac fossa and next to the previously dissected external iliac vessels. Lastly, the patient is repositioned in steep Trendelenburg position. The iliac vessels are then prepped, and the venous anastomosis is first performed. Subsequently the irrigation is stopped, and the arterial anastomosis is completed. Finally, the pyelovesicostomy is performed over a double J ureteral stent placed intracorporeally [20, 77].

Post-operative Management

Drains and Stent Management

Patients are admitted overnight for close monitoring and started on a regular diet immediately. If a closed suction drain was placed during the surgical intervention, a drain creatinine is ordered on post-operative day 1. If results are negative, drain can be removed, otherwise we preferred to keep the drain until the output is persistently low (less 100 cc/day) and the fluid sample can be re-analyzed for creatinine. If a nephrostomy tube was left in place, it is capped after completing the procedure. Patients are discharged home with the nephrostomy tube and are instructed to open it to gravity if they develop symptoms concerning for infection or obstruction. Nephrostomy tubes are removed in clinic 1 week after stent removal if the course was uneventful. Ureteral stents are removed in clinic via cystoscopy 4–6 weeks later. If no complications are encountered, patients can be discharged home on post-operative day 1.

Pain Control

Previously described in this chapter. Please refer to section “Pain control”.

Follow-Up Imaging

A renal ultrasound and a diuretic renal scan are obtained 3 months post-operatively followed by an annual renal ultrasound.

Distal Ureteral Reconstruction

Surgical Principles

Positioning and Port Placement

Positioning for patients undergoing distal ureteral reconstruction is similar as for robotic prostatectomy. Patients are therefore placed in a low lithotomy position with steep Trendelenburg (31 degrees). However, for patients with distal strictures extending up to the mid ureter, a lateral decubitus position can be adopted with the patient in modified low lithotomy position or supine with the legs only mildly abducted, allowing for cystoscopy or ureteroscopy to be simultaneously performed [78, 79]. All pressure points are adequately padded with an egg-create mattress and the patient is then safety secured to the bed using silk tape over the patient's arms and chest. Of note, genitalia and nephrostomy tubes should be adequately prepped and are included in the sterile field. Foley catheter is placed on the field. Pneumoperitoneum is most frequently achieved using the Veress needle technique, in which the needle is usually placed on the left side. Adequate placement of the needle in the peritoneum is confirmed either by the absence of blood during aspiration, and/or with maintenance of a low-pressure pneumoperitoneum (<10 mm Hg) with slow insufflation of carbon dioxide. Once an adequate pneumoperitoneum has been achieved, a 5 mm incision is made in the right upper quadrant to allow passage of a 5 mm visual port with a 5 mm 0-degree lens in place. After the peritoneal space is carefully examined, a transverse incision is made just above the umbilicus; approximately 21 cm from the pubic symphysis. An 8 mm robotic port is carefully placed through this incision under direct visualization. We then placed two additional 8 mm robotic ports; each approximately 17 cm form the pubic symphysis and approximately 8 cm from the midline. A fourth 8 mm robotic port is placed in the left lower quadrant. Lastly, a 5 mm or 12 mm is placed in the right lower quadrant for the assistant surgeon, allowing passage and retrieval of needles, as well as retraction and suctioning (Fig. 24.15). After port placement has been completed, the da Vinci Xi surgical system is docked.

Ureteric Exposure

For adequate distal ureteric exposure, the reflection of the peritoneum on the pelvic sidewall is incised longitudinally. In male patients the incision is made over the bifurcation of the common iliac vessels. The ureter is then isolated first proximal to the iliac vessels, and then traced both cranially and caudally as necessary and to the most proximal level of the stricture. Subsequently, the area of stricture is then identified, and the peritoneum along the anterior abdominal wall is incised in an inverted U-fashion to drop the bladder. The perivesical attachments can be released to allow better mobility [78].

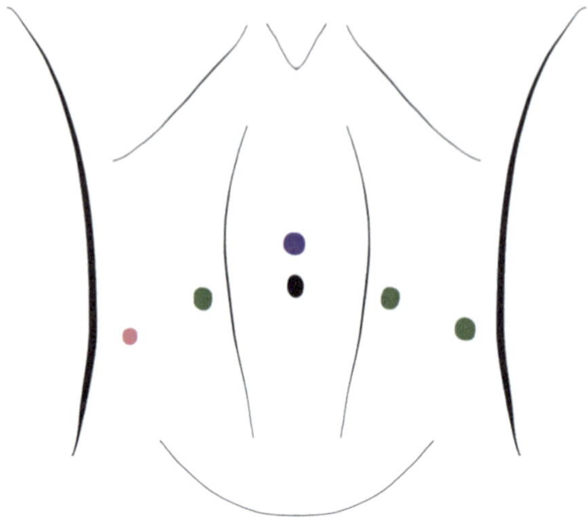

Fig. 24.15 Port placement for distal ureteral stricture
●8 mm Camera port
●8 mm Robotic port
●5 mm Assistant port

Reconstruction Techniques

Ureteral Reimplantation

Considered the gold standard surgical procedure for distal ureteral strictures located within 5 cm from the ureteral orifice, open ureteral re-implantation (ureteroneocystostomy) is associated with high success rates ranging from 70% to 100% and with a low rate of morbidity [80]. In 1994, the first laparoscopic ureteroneocystostomy was performed, and most recently robotic re-implantation (Fig. 24.16) has gained widespread acceptance [81, 82]. For this technique, the distal ureter is identified and carefully mobilized, avoiding extensive dissection of the peri-ureteral fat in order to preserve blood supply. Due to the magnification of the robotic system, it is easy to get very close to the ureteral wall and this should be avoided to preserve vascularity. In general, if the surgeon can see the micro-vasculature of the ureteral wall, the dissection is too close. Mobilization should be extended proximally as necessary to ensure tension-free anastomosis. Of note, in female patients who have undergone gynecological procedures, the dissection can be challenging given the formation of fibrotic tissue around the distal ureter. However, the bladder can usually be mobilized and brought over to the ureter rather than contrary. Subsequently, the ureter is transected just proximal to the stricture using the curved scissors and without the use of energy. Then the ureter is spatulated using Potts' scissors. The surgeon should be aware that the Potts' scissors' jaw length is 1.1 cm and use this as a guide to the adequacy of the spatulation. If necessary, a frozen section can be obtained to rule out malignancy. Next, the bladder is mobilized off the anterior abdominal wall by dividing the urachus and the medial umbilical ligaments at the umbilicus, and developing the retropubic space. The Heineke-Mikulicz technique can be also used to improve bladder mobilization, by incising the bladder horizontally and then closing

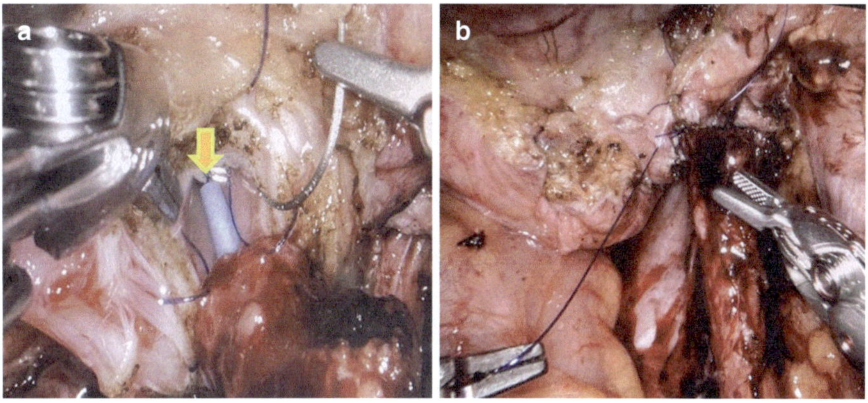

Fig. 24.16 Female patient who underwent hysterectomy with intra-operative right distal ureteral injury. Patient underwent robotic right ureteroneocystostomy. (**a**) 4–0 monofilament absorbable suture on a small half-circle needle was used to create a running watertight anastomosis along each side of the ureteral spatulation to the cystostomy incision. Upon completion of the posterior aspect of the anastomosis, a ureteral stent (yellow arrow) is placed. (**b**) The anastomosis is then completed

vertically towards the psoas muscle. After adequate bladder mobilization has been achieved, the bladder is filled with 200–300 cc of normal saline through the urethral catheter, and a cystotomy is performed at the dome using monopolar scissors. The bladder should be kept filled with normal saline for this step. At this point, the ureteroneocystostomy anastomosis is performed using two 4-0 or 5-0 monofilament absorbable sutures on a small half circle needle, placing sutures on each side of the apex of the bladder incision and the apex of the spatulated ureter. The anastomosis is performed in a running fashion, ensuring mucosal-to-mucosal apposition of the bladder and ureter. A ureteral stent is introduced through the assistant port and placed in an antegrade fashion over a guide wire. Yang et al. have described the "Modified Transurethral Stenting Technique" (Fig. 24.17), as an innovative and secure method for retrograde stent placement during robotic assisted laparoscopic ureteral re-implantation [83]. For this technique a Council catheter is inserted at the beginning of the case and advanced to the ureterovesical anastomotic site after completing one side of the anastomosis. A guide wire is then inserted through the catheter and into the ureteral lumen. Subsequently, a double J stent is then placed over a wire with a pusher catheter. This technique has been routinely utilized by the senior author for more than a decade, as it simplifies the retrograde ureteral stent placement during robotic ureteral re-implantation, and minimizes the risk of ureteral trauma and submucosal ureteral stent placement [84]. After the first layer of the anastomosis is completed, the bladder is filled with approximately 250 cc of normal saline to evaluate the integrity of the reimplant. Additional sutures are placed if necessary, and the anastomosis is completed with a second layer closure of the bladder serosa to the ureteral adventitia. Finally, a closed suction drain is placed near the anastomosis. Of note, the position of the ureteral stent should be confirmed in the recovery area with a plain x-ray film. Despite the fact that the traditional surgical

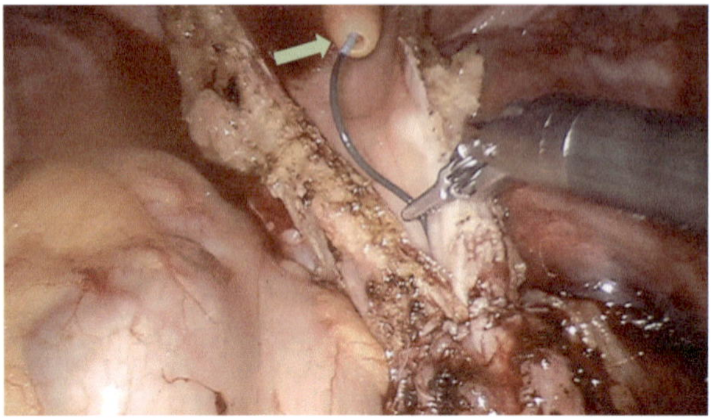

Fig. 24.17 The Modified Transurethral Stenting Technique: Is an innovative and secure method for retrograde stent placement during robotic assisted laparoscopic ureteral re-implantation. For this technique a Council catheter is inserted at the beginning of the case and pulled out from the ureterovesical stoma after completing the posterior anastomosis (green arrow). A guide wire is then inserted through the catheter and into the ureteral lumen. Subsequently, a double J stent is then placed over a wire with a pusher catheter

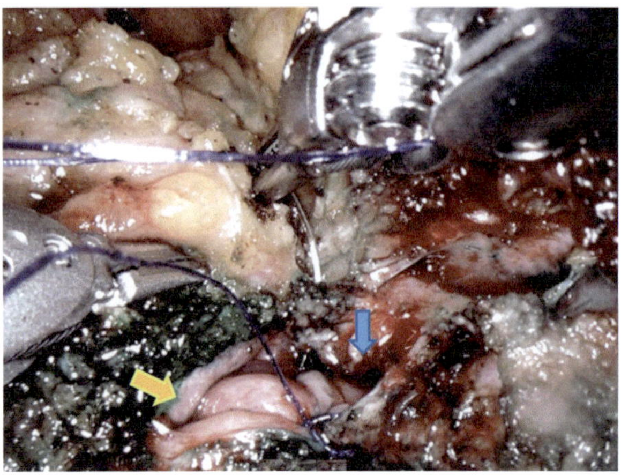

Fig. 24.18 For a distal ureteral stricture, a non-transecting side-to-side anastomosis was performed with the aim to maximally preserve distal ureteral blood flow. For this technique, a longitudinal ureterotomy (measuring approximately 2 cm) is performed proximal to the ureteral stricture (blue arrow), while leaving the distal strictured ureter in situ. An anastomosis is then performed between the ureterotomy and the cystotomy (yellow arrow) using absorbable sutures

technique for robotic ureteral re-implantation has high success rates [79], a modification of the technique has been described by Slawin and colleagues [85] in 16 patients, in which a non-transecting side-to-side anastomosis is performed with the aim to maximally preserve distal ureteral blood flow, reducing the risk of stricture recurrence. For this technique, a longitudinal ureterotomy (measuring approximately 2 cm) is performed proximal to the ureteral stricture, while leaving the distal strictured ureter in situ (Fig. 24.18). Operative time and estimated blood loss were

178 min and 50 ml respectively. At a median follow up of 12.5 months, all patients had radiographic improvement. Overall, multiple retrospective studies have supported the use of robotic ureteral re-implantation versus an open approach due to reduce estimated blood loss, length of stay and lower narcotic pain medication requirements, yet both approaches have durable outcomes and high success rates [86, 87]. Furthermore, conventional laparoscopic ureteral re-implantation has similar post-operative outcomes compared to the robotic approach, however the operative and anastomosis time were considerably longer [88].

Psoas Hitch

Psoas hitch vesicopexy is used in ureteroneocystostomy when the remaining ureter after appropriate resection is not long enough to reach the bladder and ensure a tension free anastomosis. Therefore it is considered a crucial maneuver in the management of distal ureteral strictures, allowing reconstruction of 6–10 cm gaps [78, 89]. Laparoscopic psoas hitch was first described two decades ago, and since then robotic assisted techniques have become more common place [83, 90, 91]. In 2008 Patil and colleagues [92] published the largest prospective series of robotic psoas hitch in 12 patients undergoing robotic assisted laparoscopic ureteral re-implantation. Mean operative time was 208 min, mean estimated blood loss was 48 ml and mean length of hospitalization was 4.3 days. After a mean follow up of 15.5 months, all patients were obstruction free on postoperative MAG-3 scan or intravenous urography. Most recently, Pugh and et al. reported an 8-patient series demonstrating that robotic ureteroneocystostomy with psoas hitch is an effective and safe alternative to other surgical techniques, due to precision of ureteral and bladder dissection, as well as efficiency and accuracy of intracorporeal suturing [93]. In this technique, the psoas tendon is identified immediately superior and lateral to the ipsilateral common iliac vessels. Subsequently, the bladder is mobilized in a cephalad direction towards the ipsilateral psoas muscle by incising lateral to the medial umbilical ligaments and transecting these and the median ligament to widely develop the space of Retzius. The psoas muscle and bladder's lateral wall are then sutured together using three to four 2-0 PDS stitches. Of note, it is recommended to pass the suture longitudinally and in a superficial manner along the psoas tendon to avoid injury to the femoral nerve within the psoas muscle belly and the genitofemoral nerve on the anterior surface of the muscle, which will cause femoral and/or genitofemoral neuropathy and severe post-operative pain [94]. Alternatively, the bladder can be attached to the side wall peritoneum for a similar effect. After the psoas hitch technique has been performed, the ureteral re-implantation technique is carried out similarly as explained in the above section [78]. Currently, due to the capability to widely dissect the space of Retzius and maximally mobilize the bladder, a psoas hitch is not always necessary. This is especially true in females with a more pliable bladder that will easily reach the ureter without tension.

Boari Flap

The Boari flap technique was initially described in dogs by Italian surgeon Achille Boari in 1896, however it was not until 1947 when the technique was described in humans by Ockerblad [95]. The Boari flap technique is indicated in patients with long distal ureteral strictures, when performing an isolated psoas hitch would be insufficient to reach the ureter and ensure a tension free anastomosis. The main principle is to bridge the gap with a tubularized tongue-shaped bladder flap, which can provide an additional 3–15 cm of length [19]. For this technique, after the bladder is fully mobilized and the space of Retzius is developed, the umbilical ligaments are transected. In the robotic era, it is rarely if ever necessary to have to address the contralateral vesical pedicle. The superior vesical artery can be used as a reference for the base of the flap, which extends towards the anterior bladder wall. It is then recommended to create a tongue shaped full thickness bladder flap with the pedicled base broader than the apex (approximately 7 cm in length with a 4 cm base and a 2.5 cm tip). The flap is then fixed to the psoas using a 2-0 absorbable suture in the direction of the muscle fibers. The senior author generally avoids performing a psoas hitch along with the Boari flap as this runs the risk of compromising flap vascularity. Subsequently, the ureter is spatulated posteriorly, and two 4-0 or 5-0 monofilament absorbable sutures on a small half circle needle are used to approximate the apex of the flap to the apex of the spatulated ureter. The posterior aspect of the Boari flap is anastomosed to the distal ureter using continuous suture technique. A guide wire is then advanced through the Council catheter (placed at the beginning of the case) and out through the cystotomy using the modified transurethral stenting technique previously described in detail in this chapter. A double J stent is then placed over a wire with a pusher catheter. The anterior aspect of the anastomosis is then closed using 4-0 or 5-0 monofilament absorbable suture, and the Boari flap is tubularized in two layers using 3-0 monofilament absorbable suture. We also preferentially use an 3-0 uni-directionally barbed suture to close the bladder. A closed suction drain is placed near the anastomosis [78, 83]. In 2016, Stolzenburg et al. reported the largest series to date of robotic ureteral re-implantation with Boari flap in 11 patients with distal ureteral strictures. The authors reported a 100% success rate at 15 months of follow up with minimal post-operative complications, therefore concluding that robotic ureteral re-implantation with Boari flap is a safe and effective method of ureteric re-implantation for long distal ureteral strictures [96]. Additionally, Sagalovich and colleagues [97] reported a case of robotic ureteroneocystostomy performed by bilateral Boari flap in a 82 year-old patient with bilateral mid ureteral strictures secondary to pelvis radiation therapy. Estimated blood loss was 50 ml and the patient was discharged home on post-operative day 4. Post-operatively, the patient did not report any de novo urinary symptoms. Given the significant degree of bladder reconstruction required for this intervention, the authors recommend assessing bladder capacity pre-operatively with gravity cystogram or video urodynamics.

Post-operative Management

Drains and Stent Management

Patients are admitted overnight for close monitoring and started on a regular diet immediately. If a closed suction drain was placed during the surgical intervention, a drain creatinine is ordered on post-operative day 1. If results are negative, the drain can be removed. Because there is a large cystotomy and repair, patients are discharged home with a Foley catheter. If a direct ureteral re-implant without flaps was performed, the Foley catheter usually remains in situ for 5–7 days, otherwise it is kept for 10–14 days and can be removed after a cystogram is performed and confirms healing without evidence of a leak. Ureteral stents are removed in clinic 4–6 weeks later. Barring any untoward circumstances, patients are discharged home on post-operative day 1.

Pain Control

Previously described in this chapter. Please refer to section "Pain control".

Follow-Up Imaging

A renal ultrasound and a diuretic renal scan are obtained 3 months post-operatively.

Summary

Over the last two decades, ureteral reconstruction techniques have significantly evolved with the advent of robotic surgery. Excellent visualization, improved dexterity and a less invasive approach, have greatly impacted morbidity, intra-operative blood loss, hospital stay and post-operative pain. This chapter describes in detail all the surgical techniques available for robotic ureteral reconstruction based on the location and length of the ureteral stricture. Overall, essential factors for achieving the best outcomes include selection of the most appropriate surgical technique, achieving a tension-free anastomosis and maintaining well vascularized ureteral tissue.

Tips and Tricks

- Meticulous ureteral dissection should always be performed; avoiding extensive circumferential dissection and preserving as much peri-ureteral tissue as possible, in order to maintain adequate ureteral vascular supply.
- One should strive for an atraumatic surgical technique, limiting ureteral handling, to maintain healthy tissue.
- Surgeons must be familiar with all types of reconstructive approaches and tissue substitutes.
- Surgeons should be prepared to use buccal mucosal grafts and intestinal segments for complex ureteral reconstruction, in which less invasive techniques are not feasible.
- Indocyanine green with Firefly technology, is a useful adjunct to accurately define the strictures ureteral segment limits and its vascular integrity.
- Concomitant ureteroscopy and other endourological techniques enhance the surgeon's ability to accurately define the pathology and select the most appropriate technique.
- Using a Council catheter may aid in retrograde trans-vesical guide wire access to the ureter prior to ureteral anastomosis.

Acknowledgement The authors would like to acknowledge Jacklyn Allen for renderings of Figs. 24.6, 24.8, 24.9 and 24.11.

References

1. Korobkin M. CT urography. Eur Radiol. 2005;15(Suppl 4):D82–4.
2. Potenta SE, D'Agostino R, Sternberg KM, Tatsumi K, Perusse K. CT urography for evaluation of the ureter. Radiographics. 2015;35(3):709–26.
3. Adams F, Qiu T, Mark A, Fritz B, Kramer L, Schlager D, et al. Soft 3D-printed phantom of the human kidney with collecting system. Ann Biomed Eng. 2017;45(4):963–72.
4. Taylor AT, Folks RD, Rahman A, Polsani A, Dubovsky EV, Halkar R, et al. (99m)Tc-MAG3: image wisely. Radiology. 2017;284(1):200–9.
5. Wood LN, Souders CE, Freedman AL. Is a reassuring MAG-3 diuretic renal scan really reassuring? Curr Urol. 2015;8(4):178–82.
6. O'Connor OJ, McLaughlin P, Maher MM. MR urography. AJR Am J Roentgenol. 2010;195(3):W201–6.
7. Paspulati A, Gupta A, Hill PA, Morgan MA. The utility of retrograde pyelography to follow up incompletely opacified ureters on CT urography. Abdom Radiol (NY). 2020;45(3):807–11.
8. Lightner DJ, Wymer K, Sanchez J, Kavoussi L. Best practice statement on urologic procedures and antimicrobial prophylaxis. J Urol. 2020;203(2):351–6.
9. Whitehurst LA, Somani BK. Semi-rigid ureteroscopy: indications, tips, and tricks. Urolithiasis. 2018;46(1):39–45.
10. Golan S, Nadu A, Lifshitz D. The role of diagnostic ureteroscopy in the era of computed tomography urography. BMC Urol. 2015;15:74.
11. De Coninck V, Keller EX, Somani B, Giusti G, Proietti S, Rodriguez-Socarras M, et al. Complications of ureteroscopy: a complete overview. World J Urol. 2020;38(9):2147–66.

12. Motola JA, Shahon RS, Smith AD. Anatomy of the ureter. Urol Clin North Am. 1988;15(3):295–9.
13. Frober R. Surgical anatomy of the ureter. BJU Int. 2007;100(4):949–65.
14. Lescay HA, Jiang J, Tuma F. Anatomy, abdomen and pelvis, ureter. Treasure Island (FL): StatPearls; 2021.
15. Stephens FD. Intramural ureter and ureterocele. Postgrad Med J. 1964;40:179–83.
16. Lee Z, Lee M, Lee R, Koster H, Cheng N, Siev M, et al. Ureteral rest is associated with improved outcomes in patients undergoing robotic ureteral reconstruction of proximal and middle ureteral strictures. Urology. 2021;152:160–6.
17. Dagli M, Ramchandani P. Percutaneous nephrostomy: technical aspects and indications. Semin Intervent Radiol. 2011;28(4):424–37.
18. Drain A, Jun MS, Zhao LC. Robotic ureteral reconstruction. Urol Clin North Am. 2021;48(1):91–101.
19. Nakada SY. Management of upper urinary tract obstruction. In: Wein AJKL, Partin AW, et al., editors. Campbell-Walsh urology. 11th ed. Philadelphia: Elsevier; 2016. p. 1104–47.
20. Bergersen A, Thomas R, Lee BR. Robotic pyeloplasty. J Endourol. 2018;32(S1):S68–72.
21. Cestari A, Buffi NM, Lista G, Sangalli M, Scapaticci E, Fabbri F, et al. Retroperitoneal and transperitoneal robot-assisted pyeloplasty in adults: techniques and results. Eur Urol. 2010;58(5):711–8.
22. Shadpour P, Nayyeri RK, Daneshvar R, Salimi H, Radfar H. Prospective clinical trial to compare standard colon-reflecting with transmesocolic laparoscopic pyeloplasty. BJU Int. 2012;110(11):1814–8.
23. Gupta NP, Mukherjee S, Nayyar R, Hemal AK, Kumar R. Transmesocolic robot-assisted pyeloplasty: single center experience. J Endourol. 2009;23(6):945–8.
24. Anderson JC, Hynes W. Retrocaval ureter; a case diagnosed pre-operatively and treated successfully by a plastic operation. Br J Urol. 1949;21(3):209–14.
25. Schuessler WW, Grune MT, Tecuanhuey LV, Preminger GM. Laparoscopic dismembered pyeloplasty. J Urol. 1993;150(6):1795–9.
26. Gettman MT, Neururer R, Bartsch G, Peschel R. Anderson-Hynes dismembered pyeloplasty performed using the da Vinci robotic system. Urology. 2002;60(3):509–13.
27. Janczak D, Szydelko U, Apoznanski W, Panek W, Szydelko T. W-type suture in Anderson-Hynes laparoscopic pyeloplasty: a novel approach to an old technique. Wideochir Inne Tech Maloinwazyjne. 2018;13(4):512–7.
28. Tan WP, Whelan P, Deane LA. Intentional omission of ureteral stents during robotic-assisted intracorporeal ureteroenteric anastomosis: is it safe and feasible? Urology. 2017;102:116–20.
29. Szydelko T, Kasprzak J, Apoznanski W, Zdrojowy R. Laparoscopic anterior y-v pyeloplasty: a valuable treatment option in patients with small or intrarenal pelvis. J Laparoendosc Adv Surg Tech A. 2010;20(7):627–30.
30. Neuwirt K. Implantation of the ureter into the lower calyx of the renal pelvis. Urol Cutan Rev. 1948;52(6):351.
31. Matlaga BR, Shah OD, Singh D, Streem SB, Assimos DG. Ureterocalicostomy: a contemporary experience. Urology. 2005;65(1):42–4.
32. Srivastava D, Sureka SK, Yadav P, Bansal A, Gupta S, Kapoor R, et al. Ureterocalicostomy for reconstruction of complicated Ureteropelvic junction obstruction in adults: long-term outcome and factors predicting failure in a contemporary cohort. J Urol. 2017;198(6):1374–8.
33. Esposito C, Masieri L, Blanc T, Manzoni G, Silay S, Escolino M. Robot-assisted laparoscopic pyeloplasty (RALP) in children with horseshoe kidneys: results of a multicentric study. World J Urol. 2019;37(10):2257–63.
34. Oderda M, Calleris G, Allasia M, Dalmasso E, Falcone M, Catti M, et al. Robot-assisted laparoscopic pyeloplasty in a pediatric patient with horseshoe kidney: surgical technique and review of the literature. Urologia. 2017;84(1):55–60.
35. Padilla W AD, Deane LA. Laparoscopic robotic-assisted transmesocolic left pyeloplasty in a Horshoe kidney. In: Endourology Jo, editor. 29th world congress of Endourology; Kyoto, Japan. 2011.

36. Kolln CP, Boatman DL, Schmidt JD, Flocks RH. Horseshoe kidney: a review of 105 patients. J Urol. 1972;107(2):203–4.
37. Lu L, Ma B, Zhong W, Yao B, Wang D, Qiu J. Laparoscopic transmesenteric pyeloplasty and isthmusectomy for adult horseshoe kidney with recurrent symptomatic hydronephrosis. IJU Case Rep. 2020;3(5):220–2.
38. Kawauchi A, Fujito A, Yoneda K, Soh J, Naitoh Y, Mizutani Y, et al. Laparoscopic pyeloplasty and isthmectomy for hydronephrosis of horseshoe kidney: a pediatric case. J Endourol. 2005;19(8):984–6.
39. Nadler RB, Thaxton CS, Kim SC. Hand-assisted laparoscopic pyeloplasty and isthmectomy in a patient with a horseshoe kidney. J Endourol. 2003;17(10):909–10.
40. Faddegon S, Granberg C, Tan YK, Gargollo PC, Cadeddu JA. Minimally invasive pyeloplasty in horseshoe kidneys with ureteropelvic junction obstruction: a case series. Int Braz J Urol. 2013;39(2):195–202.
41. Skolarikos A, Dellis A, Knoll T. Ureteropelvic obstruction and renal stones: etiology and treatment. Urolithiasis. 2015;43(1):5–12.
42. Kadihasanoglu M, Yucetas U, Karabay E, Sonmezay E. Comparison of the outcomes of laparoscopic pyeloplasty with and without concomitant pyelolithotomy. Int Braz J Urol. 2019;45(5):965–73.
43. Jensen PH, Berg KD, Azawi NH. Robot-assisted pyeloplasty and pyelolithotomy in patients with ureteropelvic junction stenosis. Scand J Urol. 2017;51(4):323–8.
44. Rivard C, Vogel RI, Teoh D. Effect of intraperitoneal bupivacaine on postoperative pain in the gynecologic oncology patient. J Minim Invasive Gynecol. 2015;22(7):1260–5.
45. Horodyski L, Ball B, Emile C, Rhodes A, Miao F, Reis IM, et al. Safe transition to opioid-free pathway after robotic-assisted laparoscopic prostatectomy. J Robot Surg. 2021;16:307–14.
46. Meershoek P, KleinJan GH, van Willigen DM, Bauwens KP, Spa SJ, van Beurden F, et al. Multi-wavelength fluorescence imaging with a da Vinci firefly-a technical look behind the scenes. J Robot Surg. 2020;15:751–60.
47. Bjurlin MA, Gan M, McClintock TR, Volpe A, Borofsky MS, Mottrie A, et al. Near-infrared fluorescence imaging: emerging applications in robotic upper urinary tract surgery. Eur Urol. 2014;65(4):793–801.
48. Lee Z, Simhan J, Parker DC, Reilly C, Llukani E, Lee DI, et al. Novel use of indocyanine green for intraoperative, real-time localization of ureteral stenosis during robot-assisted ureteroureterostomy. Urology. 2013;82(3):729–33.
49. Lee Z, Moore B, Giusto L, Eun DD. Use of indocyanine green during robot-assisted ureteral reconstructions. Eur Urol. 2015;67(2):291–8.
50. Andrade HS, Kaouk JH, Zargar H, Caputo PA, Akca O, Ramirez D, et al. Robotic ureteroureterostomy for treatment of a proximal ureteric stricture. Int Braz J Urol. 2016;42(5):1041–2.
51. Lee Z, Llukani E, Reilly CE, Mydlo JH, Lee DI, Eun DD. Single surgeon experience with robot-assisted ureteroureterostomy for pathologies at the proximal, middle, and distal ureter in adults. J Endourol. 2013;27(8):994–9.
52. Brown R, Barnes R, Wensell G, Asghar M. Ureteroureterostomy and cutaneous ureterostomy. J Urol. 1971;106(5):658–63.
53. Komninos C, Koo KC, Rha KH. Laparoendoscopic management of midureteral strictures. Korean J Urol. 2014;55(1):2–8.
54. Piaggio LA, Gonzalez R. Laparoscopic transureteroureterostomy: a novel approach. J Urol. 2007;177(6):2311–4.
55. Shoemaker GE. VIII. Removal of the ureter with a tuberculous kidney. Ann Surg. 1911;53(5):696–8.
56. Goodwin WE, Winter CC, Turner RD. Replacement of the ureter by small intestine: clinical application and results of the ileal ureter. J Urol. 1959;81(3):406–18.
57. Wagner JR, Schimpf MO, Cohen JL. Robot-assisted laparoscopic ileal ureter. JSLS. 2008;12(3):306–9.

58. Brandao LF, Autorino R, Zargar H, Laydner H, Krishnan J, Samarasekera D, et al. Robotic ileal ureter: a completely intracorporeal technique. Urology. 2014;83(4):951–4.
59. Zhong W, Hong P, Ding G, Yang K, Li X, Bao J, et al. Technical considerations and outcomes for ileal ureter replacement: a retrospective study in China. BMC Surg. 2019;19(1):9.
60. Ubrig B, Janusonis J, Paulics L, Boy A, Heiland M, Roosen A. Functional outcome of completely intracorporeal robotic ileal ureteric replacement. Urology. 2018;114:193–7.
61. Grosso AA, Di Maida F, Mari A, Campi R, Crisci A, Vignolini G, et al. Totally intracorporeal robotic ileal ureter replacement: focus on surgical technique and outcomes. Minerva Urol Nefrol. 2021;73:532–9.
62. Abhyankar N, Vendryes C, Deane LA. Totally intracorporeal robot-assisted laparoscopic reverse seven ileal ureteric reconstruction. Can J Urol. 2015;22(2):7748–51.
63. Melnikoff A. Sur le replacement de l'uretere par anse isolee de l'intestine grele. Rev Clin Urol. 1912;1:601.
64. Reggio ERL, Okeke Z, et al. Laparoscopic ureteroplasty using on-lay appendix graft. Urology. 2009;73(4):928–928.e10.
65. Duty BD, Kreshover JE, Richstone L, Kavoussi LR. Review of appendiceal onlay flap in the management of complex ureteric strictures in six patients. BJU Int. 2015;115(2):282–7.
66. Wang J, Xiong S, Fan S, Yang K, Huang B, Zhang D, et al. Appendiceal onlay flap ureteroplasty for the treatment of complex ureteral strictures: initial experience of nine patients. J Endourol. 2020;34(8):874–81.
67. Naude JH. Buccal mucosal grafts in the treatment of ureteric lesions. BJU Int. 1999;83(7):751–4.
68. Zhao LC, Yamaguchi Y, Bryk DJ, Adelstein SA, Stifelman MD. Robot-assisted ureteral reconstruction using buccal mucosa. Urology. 2015;86(3):634–8.
69. Lee Z, Lee M, Koster H, Lee R, Cheng N, Jun M, et al. A multi-institutional experience with robotic ureteroplasty with buccal mucosa graft: an updated analysis of intermediate-term outcomes. Urology. 2021;147:306–10.
70. Wood DN, Allen SE, Andrich DE, Greenwell TJ, Mundy AR. The morbidity of buccal mucosal graft harvest for urethroplasty and the effect of nonclosure of the graft harvest site on postoperative pain. J Urol. 2004;172(2):580–3.
71. Anderson JCHW. Retrocaval ureter: a case diagnosed preoperatively and treated successfully by a plastic operation. BJU Int. 1949;21:209–14.
72. Gundeti MS, Duffy PG, Mushtaq I. Robotic-assisted laparoscopic correction of pediatric retrocaval ureter. J Laparoendosc Adv Surg Tech A. 2006;16(4):422–4.
73. Smith KM, Shrivastava D, Ravish IR, Nerli RB, Shukla AR. Robot-assisted laparoscopic ureteroureterostomy for proximal ureteral obstructions in children. J Pediatr Urol. 2009;5(6):475–9.
74. Escolino M, Masieri L, Valla JS, Lopez PJ, Tokar B, Mushtaq I, et al. Laparoscopic and robotic-assisted repair of retrocaval ureter in children: a multi-institutional comparative study with open repair. World J Urol. 2019;37(9):1941–7.
75. Hardy JD. High ureteral injuries. Management by autotransplantation of the kidney. JAMA. 1963;184:97–101.
76. Gordon ZN, Angell J, Abaza R. Completely intracorporeal robotic renal autotransplantation. J Urol. 2014;192(5):1516–22.
77. Lee JY, Alzahrani T, Ordon M. Intra-corporeal robotic renal auto-transplantation. Can Urol Assoc J. 2015;9(9–10):E748–9.
78. White C, Stifelman M. Ureteral reimplantation, psoas hitch, and Boari flap. J Endourol. 2020;34(S1):S25–30.
79. Passoni N, Peters CA. Robotic ureteral reimplantation. J Endourol. 2020;34(S1):S31–S4.
80. Tyritzis SI, Wiklund NP. Ureteral strictures revisited...Trying to see the light at the end of the tunnel: a comprehensive review. J Endourol. 2015;29(2):124–36.
81. Reddy PK, Evans RM. Laparoscopic ureteroneocystostomy. J Urol. 1994;152(6 Pt 1):2057–9.
82. Babbar P, Yerram N, Sun A, Hemal S, Murthy P, Bryk D, et al. Robot-assisted ureteral reconstruction – current status and future directions. Urol Ann. 2018;10(1):7–14.

83. Yang C, Jones L, Rivera ME, Verlee GT, Deane LA. Robotic-assisted ureteral reimplantation with Boari flap and psoas hitch: a single-institution experience. J Laparoendosc Adv Surg Tech A. 2011;21(9):829–33.
84. Deane LA. Re: a modified transurethral stenting technique for (robot-assisted) laparoscopic ureteral reimplantation. Urol Int. 2021;105(3–4):336.
85. Slawin J, Patel NH, Lee Z, Dy GW, Kim D, Asghar A, et al. Ureteral reimplantation via robotic nontransecting side-to-side anastomosis for distal ureteral stricture. J Endourol. 2020;34(8):836–9.
86. Dirie NI, Wang S. Robot-assisted laparoscopic ureteroneocystostomy in adults: a single surgeon experience and literature review. Asian J Urol. 2020;7(1):37–44.
87. Kozinn SI, Canes D, Sorcini A, Moinzadeh A. Robotic versus open distal ureteral reconstruction and reimplantation for benign stricture disease. J Endourol. 2012;26(2):147–51.
88. Zhang Y, Ouyang W, Xu H, Luan Y, Yang J, Lu Y, et al. A comparison of robot-assisted laparoscopic ureteral reimplantation and conventional laparoscopic ureteral reimplantation for the management of benign distal ureteral stricture. Urol J. 2020;17(3):252–6.
89. Elbers JR, Rodriguez Socarras M, Rivas JG, Autran AM, Esperto F, Tortolero L, et al. Robotic repair of ureteral strictures: techniques and review. Curr Urol Rep. 2021;22(8):39.
90. Ahn M, Loughlin KR. Psoas hitch ureteral reimplantation in adults–analysis of a modified technique and timing of repair. Urology. 2001;58(2):184–7.
91. Fugita OE, Dinlenc C, Kavoussi L. The laparoscopic Boari flap. J Urol. 2001;166(1):51–3.
92. Patil NN, Mottrie A, Sundaram B, Patel VR. Robotic-assisted laparoscopic ureteral reimplantation with psoas hitch: a multi-institutional, multinational evaluation. Urology. 2008;72(1):47–50; discussion.
93. Pugh J, Farkas A, Su LM. Robotic distal ureterectomy with psoas hitch and ureteroneocystostomy: surgical technique and outcomes. Asian J Urol. 2015;2(2):123–7.
94. Muller C, van Houwelingen EE, Huygen F. Femoral neuropathy following a psoas hitch vesicopexy. BMJ Case Rep. 2018;2018
95. Ockerblad N. Reimplantation of the ureter into the bladder by a flap method. J Urol. 1947;57(5):845–7.
96. Stolzenburg JU, Rai BP, Do M, Dietel A, Liatsikos E, Ganzer R, et al. Robot-assisted technique for Boari flap ureteric reimplantation: replicating the techniques of open surgery in robotics. BJU Int. 2016;118(3):482–4.
97. Sagalovich D, Garisto J, Bertolo R, Yerram N, Dagenais J, Chavali JS, et al. Minimally invasive management of ureteral distal strictures: robotic ureteroneocystostomy with a bilateral Boari flap. Urology. 2018;120:268.

Chapter 25
Urinary Bladder Stones

Benjamin Van Parys, Thomas Tailly, and Senol Tonyali

Introduction

> *I will not use the knife, even upon those suffering from stones, but I will leave this affair entirely in favor of such men who are engaged in this craft.* (Hippocratic Oath, approx. 460 B.C. – 380 B.C.)

Bladder stones have been a torment to humankind since ages. Stone restings have been discovered in two ancient Egyptian mummies dating back to almost 5000 years B.C [1, 2]. Descriptions of its treatment belong to the first known medical procedures reported, and numerous examples survived time. Treatments for stones were recorded in ancient Egyptian medical writings from 1500 B.C., and in the texts of the Asutu in Mesopotamia between 3200 and 1200 B.C. An Indian surgeon, Sashruta, described the formation of bladder stones and, among other surgical procedures, a perineal lithotomy, around 60 B.C [3]. The famous Greek philosopher Hipprocrates mentioned bladder calculi in his eponymous oath in the fifth century B.C [4]. Several famous historical figures have been said to suffer from bladder lithiasis, most notably the Italian artist Michelangelo, the Italian anatomist Scarpa, the English scientist sir Isaac Newton, the philosopher Francis Bacon, the famous physicians Boerhaave and Harvey, the English nobleman Oliver Cromwell, tsar Peter the Great of Russia, king Louis XIV of France, king George IV of the United Kingdom, and king Leopold I of Belgium. The French emperors Napoleon Bonaparte and Napoleon III both were suffering from bladder stones on crucial

B. Van Parys
Department of Urology, General Hospital Alma, Eeklo, Belgium

T. Tailly
Department of Urology, University Hospital Ghent, Ghent, Belgium

S. Tonyali (✉)
Department of Urology, Istanbul University Istanbul School of Medicine, Istanbul, Turkiye

S. Tonyali et al. (eds.), *Current Endourology*,
https://doi.org/10.1007/978-3-032-00010-1_25

moments (the Russian campaign in 1812 of the first, and the Franco-Prussian war in 1870 of the latter), probably affecting their judgements, and historians nowadays discuss whether the whole European history might have been different if these two emperors had not had a bladder stone [2, 3].

Despite its ancient and well descripted history, bladder calculi nowadays are relatively rare and account for approximately 5% of all urinary calculi. However, their importance is not to be neglected, as bladder stones are responsible for 14% of hospital admissions and 8% of urolithiasis-related deaths in developed nations [5, 6]. They are rarely a diagnosis on their own; in children, they are prevalent in geographic areas where malnutrition, diarrheal disease, an/or chronic dehydration are endemic, and in adults, they are often diagnosed alongside other ailments resulting in urinary stasis (e.g. prostatic enlargement in elder males urinary dysfunction in neurologic patients) [7].

Aetiology

Primary Bladder Stones

Primary bladder stones occur in the absence of other urinary tract abnormalities. Typically, these are seen in children in areas with either a diet lacking animal protein and vitamins and/or excessive oxalate consumption, or poor hydration and recurrent diarrhea. Their exact pathogenesis is unclear, but involves most likely a combination of metabolic factors, such as decreased urine production, low urinary pH, low urine phosphate levels, and increased urinary uric acid or calcium oxalate excretion [7].

In the past, endemic bladder stones in children were common and predominant among childhood urinary stones. Epidemiological research in the 1930s both in the UK as in its colonies showed the link between a lack of vitamin A in the diet and the incidence of stones, proving malnutrition to be a risk factor of stone formation independent of the geographic region. Since the nineteenth century, the incidence of stones in childhood have been declining in the developed world. Nevertheless, in certain regions bladder stones in children remained common, especially in poor urbanized areas. The evolution from a rural towards an industrialized society, with more attention to the importance of healthy nutrition, for example pasteurization of milk and more equal distribution and availability of food, resulted in the disappearance of those "stone districts" in the Western world, which existed until the 1950s.

In contrast, endemic bladder stones remain prevalent in the developing world. Despite its incidence has been slowly declining in the last decades, a so-called Afro-Asian endemic bladder stone belt still exists, extending from Thailand and Indonesia, over India to the Middle east end further extending into Northern- and sub-Saharan Africa. The incidence of bladder stones in Central and South Africa, as well as in Latin-America is low.

Bladder stones are more common in boys (male: female ratio 10:1), probably due to the differences in the anatomy of the urethra. The most commonly affected age group is 1–5 years.

Secondary Bladder Stones

Bladder stone formation is mostly associated with other urinary tract abnormalities, which predispose for urinary stasis or other conditions facilitating stone formation. These stones are classified as secondary to these abnormalities.

- Bladder outlet obstruction
  - Benign prostatic enlargement (men)
  - Urethral stricture
  - Bladder neck contracture
  - Cystocele
  - Pelvic organ prolapse
  - Urethral kinking
- Underactive bladder
- Recurrent UTI
- Neurogenic bladder
- Bladder diverticula
- Foreign bodies
  - Prolonged bladder catheter
  - Bladder migration of intra-uterine devices, operative clips or tension-free vaginal tapes
- Bladder augmentation or urinary diversion.

Migratory Bladder Stones

Migratory bladder stones form in the upper urinary tract, and pass to the bladder. In the bladder, they may serve as a nidus for further bladder stone growth. In the absence of any anatomic conditions causing post void residual urine, these are usually spontaneously evacuated. If however, other underlying conditions such as benign prostatic obstruction or strictures, or hypocontractile detrusor, these stones may grow until spontaneous evacuation is no longer possible, and symptoms may present.

Clinical Presentation

Bladder stones present predominantly with lower urinary tract symptoms (LUTS), suprapubic pain and/or hematuria. Most commonly, patients mention perineal or suprapubic pain occurring at the end of the micturition, or sudden interruption of the urinary stream associated with radiating pain to the perineum or the urethra. Other symptoms include vague dull lower abdominal pain, terminal hematuria, and storage symptoms such as frequency and urgency. Detrusor overactivity is present in the majority of bladder stones, and more common in men and large stones. The symptoms are often provoked or aggravated by sudden movement or exercise. Bladder stones should be suspected in cases of recurring urinary tract infections, which may be the only symptom of the presence of these calculi.

Moreover, in children, symptoms may include pulling of the penis (caused by radiating pain due to irritation of the bladder trigonum, felt in the perineum, scrotum, and hip), nocturnal enuresis, straining (which may result in rectal prolapse caused by forced micturition), and urinary retention. Less specific signs may include anemia, signs of malnutrition or dehydration, conjunctival hemorrhage due to straining, and possibly fever due to an associated UTI.

According to the EAU guidelines, the clinical exam when suspecting bladder stones in adults, should include physical examination of external genitalia, digital rectal examination, and basic neuro-urologic evaluation (including peri-anal tone and sensation in men) In children, clinical examination may reveal a palpable bladder or a rectal prolapse.

Diagnostic Evaluation

Urinalysis

Urinary analysis usually shows presence of crystals and red blood cells. White blood cells may also be present, while urine culture demonstrates the absence of an infection.

Uroflowmetry and Post-void Residual Urine Assessment

Uroflowmetry is a necessary exam in the evaluation of bladder stone disease, since it is the main screening tool for bladder outlet obstruction.

Ultrasound

Bladder ultrasound, often available in the clinician's office, is mostly performed as the first consultation, and usually can diagnose the lithiasis. Typically, the stone moves with changing body position, and has a characteristic post-acoustic shadow. Stones in a diverticulum or a ureterocele do not move with body position. Ultrasound allows direct measurement of the stone size, and is able to identify all types of bladder stones. It has a sensitivity of 20–83% and an specificity of 98–100% for detection of bladder stones in adults [8].

Cystoscopy

A cystoscopy in the outpatient office is the most sensitive and specific diagnostic tool to detect bladder stones. Furthermore, it has the advantage of detecting the most frequent underlying causes of secondary bladder stone formation (e.g., bladder outlet obstruction due to prostate enlargement, strictures, foreign bodies). The macroscopic aspect of the stone can help in the decision which treatment options can be used.

Imaging

X-ray of kidney and/or bladder may show the presence of stones in the bladder. Calcium containing stones are usually well visible on x-ray, however, radiolucent stones (such as uric acid stones) can easily be missed. It has a sensitivity of 21–78% for detecting cystoscopically confirmed bladder stones [9]. However, it provides useful information of radio-opacity, which can help in the decision of the treatment options (combined with cystoscopic and/or ultrasound evaluation).

Need for Computed Tomography

In the western world, CT scan is widely used as an additional imaging technique. It provides great sensitivity, and the density of the stone can easily be calculated. This may help in the decision which technique to use in treatment. Furthermore, CT can also detect upper tract lithiasis [10].

Stone Composition

The composition of bladder stone is affected by several factors such as patient age, presence of infection, intravesical obstruction or anatomical abnormalities. There may also be a difference in composition between stones formed in the bladder and migratory stones [11]. Endemic bladder stones typically consist of ammonium acid urate and calcium oxalate. Ammonium acid urate is one of the important components in the nucleation of endemic bladder stones and requires high concentrations of both uric acid and ammonium to be precipitated [12]. In another study ammonium acid urate was found to be the main component of endemic bladders stones. Also, patients with sterile urine have shown to have significantly higher levels of ammonia compared to controls [13]. In a study by Douenias et al. [11] the urinary bladder stone composition was as follow: uric acid stone 50%, calcium oxalate stone 19%, mixed composition 31%. In their study including 273 patients having bladder stones, Takasaki et al. [14] reported that of those stones 50.0% consisted of magnesium ammonium phosphate, 39.9% calcium (oxalate and/or phosphate), 9.4% uric acid (urate), and 0.7% cystine. The most common disorders associated with bladder stones were prostatic hyperplasia and cancer (47.8%) in males, and neurogenic bladder (48.1%) in females.

Surgical Interventions

History [2, 3, 15]

Perineal Lithotomy

The first true lithotomist (stone cutter) was Ammonius "*Lithotomos*" of Alexandria, who lived around. 200 B.C. His technique, later described by the Roman philosopher and nobleman Celsus, and since known as the Celsian method, was commonly performed until into the renaissance. The patient was put on a special table, or sat in the lap of a strong person, with the legs spread to expose the perineum ("lithotomy position"). The operator inserted the forefinger of his left hand into the anus of the patient, pressing it upward and forwards the pubis, and used his right hand to push on the bladder in the suprapubic region, forcing the stone into the grip of his left forefinger, pushing it outwards to produce a perineal bulge. Then, a slightly curved transverse incision was made anterior of the anus, deep into the stone, the bladder cut into the trigonum, and the stone was pushed out by the left hand in the anus. For larger stones, Ammonius invented a tool, a hook-like instrument, to be slid into the bladder and hook the stone to withdraw it. If needed, the stone could be crushed using a second blunt tipped instrument. Nicknamed the "*apparatus minor*", since only few instruments were needed, this method was used only in young boys not older than fourteen years, as in older men the presence of an enlarged prostate would make the stone block. Many centuries later, around 1000 A.D., Albucasis of Cordoba (Ibn Abbas Alzahrawi), remarkably modified this technique, reducing its risks, and also invented a special lithotomy-scalpel with two sharp edges. However, the main principle remained the same for another 500 years.

Around 1520, based on the observation of easier stone evacuation through the short and relatively broad urethra in women, Franciscus de Romanis of Cremona invented a method to dilate the prostatic urethra. Incising the perineum, the membranous urethra was opened, using a metal urethral catheter as a guide; then, a "gorgeret" was put into the bladder to guide a series of dilatators, until the prostatic urethra was wide enough to extract the bladder stone. This method was known as the "*apparatus major*". Both methods commonly resulted in urethral stenosis, fistulas, incontinence and impotence, and mortality rates were as high as 30–50%.

In the seventeenth century, Jacques de Beaulieu invented a lateral perineal incision, hereby accessing the bladder wall directly avoiding the urethra. This "*sectio lateralis*" was later modified by the Dutch surgeon Johannes Rau, opening the bladder away from the sphincter, thus avoiding incontinence and impotence.

Sectio Alta

In the eighteenth century, the English surgeon William Chesselden and the French lithotomist Frère Côme independently described a technique to evacuate stones through a suprapubic incision, after realizing a distended bladder moved upward. The incision spot was indicated by inserting a hook-shaped instrument through the penis, which palpated the anterior bladder wall.

Lithotripsy

In 1824, French surgeon Jean Civiale, who later founded the first urology department in the world in the Necker hospital in Paris, was the first to treat bladder stones without incision. He invented a lithotrite, a trilabe, grasping and fragmenting instrument, to be inserted through the urethra into the bladder. After filling the bladder, the stones were crushed in situ so the patient could evacuate the fragments. This development, which can be considered as the beginning of the endo-urology, resulted in a dramatically drop in mortality rates, to 2.4%. It also lead to a series of discoveries, such as the "*percuteur courbe a Marteau*" by Heurteloup, and the curved lithotripter clamp by Charrière. The uprising of antisepsis and general anesthesia also helped to drop the morbidity of bladder stone treatment. In 1876, American surgeon Bigelow developed a powerful lithotripter to combine which a large evacuation catheter, an instrument still in use today, thus treating a bladder stone in a single procedure without any incisions.

Current Treatment Alternatives

Suprapubic Cystolithotomy

Patient is positioned in supine position, a foley catheter is placed to fill the bladder, and a 3–4 cm suprapubic midline incision is made. Muscles are split the bladder is exposed and a cystotomy is performed, without opening the peritoneum. Traditionally, an indwelling catheter and preperitoneal drain are left [16]. It is a very effective procedure, resulting in 100% stone free rates with a single surgical session in almost every study, and therefore remaining gold standard in regions where endoscopic treatments are not accessible. Although morbidity is not very high, open surgery has many disadvantages, such as visible scar, risk of wound infection, longer hospital stay (median 3.7 days, varying from 2 to 10 days), higher narcotic use, and duration of catheter (varying from 0 to 7 days) than percutaneous methods [17, 18]. Since the 1990s, the open cystolithotripsy has been progressively replaced by newer and less-invasive techniques. It is rarely performed on its own, but can be combined with another abdominal surgical treatment, such as an open Millin prostatectomy for very large prostate hyperplasia, or a bladder diverticulectomy. It may be the only option in cases with a difficult anatomy, or a contra-indication for transurethral or percutaneous access (e.g., after bladder augmentation with closed bladder neck and unsafe percutaneous access). Also, it can be considered a salvage option if minimally invasive approaches fail, especially in a very large stone burden (>4–5 cm) [7, 19, 20].

Transurethral Cystolihtotripsy

Transurethral cystolithotripsy is nowadays the most commonly used approach to treat bladder stones. Methods for stone disintegration include mechanical lithotripsy ("cystolitholapaxy", using a Mauermayer stone punch or a stone crushing forceps) or a range of modern energy sources, such as ultrasonic lithotripsy, electrohydraulic lithotripsy, pneumatic lithotripsy (e.g., Swiss LithoClast®(EMS)), laser lithotripsy, or a combination of techniques (e.g. Shockpulse-SE (Olympus) and Lithoclast Master® (EMS), combining ultrasound and pneumatic/ballistic energy).

Transurethral cystolithotripsy generally offers the same stone free rate as open suprapubic cystolithotripsy, with shorter length of hospital stay and fewer additional procedures.

Percutaneous Cystolithotripsy

Percutaneous cystolithotripsy is a minimally invasive, safe and effective treatment choice especially for large stone (>3 cm). Particularly it might be the choice of treatment in patients having anatomical disorders which prevent transurethral lithotripsy.

Percutaneous cystolithotripsy also might be preferred because it avoids urethral injury [21]. Laser lithotripsy, lithotripsy using ultrasound, pneumatic, electrohydraulic lithotripters as well as mechanical stone crusher might be utilized for stone fragmentation [20]. It has been shown that percutaneous pneumatic lithotripsy shortens operative time and decreases urethral and bladder trauma compared to transurethral pneumatic lithotripsy combined with transurethral resection of prostate [22]. Currently, using high power lasers might be useful in reducing stone fragmentation time which might encourage use of transurethral route.

Percutaneous cystolithotripsy can be performed with either general or local anesthesia. Patient positioning depends on patient characteristics. While dorsal lithotomy is the most commonly utilized position, the supine position may be preferred in patients having limb or spine deformities.

The procedure is initiated with cystoscopy using a rigid or flexible cystoscope to inspect the urethra and bladder and to distend the bladder with saline irrigation. Once the bladder is distended, an 18-gauge needle is utilized to puncture the bladder under direct vision approximately 2 cm above the symphysis pubis. Then a 0.036- or 0.038-inch hydrophilic guide is inserted into the bladder through the needle, and the needle is removed. A 1–2 cm skin incision is made at the puncture site. The percutaneous tract was formed using sequential Semirigid Amplatz dilators. The assistant monitors the dilation using the cystoscope to ensure that the dilator passes into the bladder and to prevent possible damage to the posterior bladder wall. The preferred size of the working sheath is advanced into the bladder, and the guide wire is secured as a safety wire.

Types of Lithotripsies

Mechanical Cystolithotripsy

Mechanical cystolithotripsy (stone crushing) is an age-old principle. Modern instruments allow direct endoscopic irrigation and visualization. It is a simple, fast and highly efficient method. However, mechanical lithotrites should always be used with caution to avoid bladder injury. It is essential to maintain a partially filled bladder and good endoscopic visualization of the bladder mucosa before closure of the jaws.

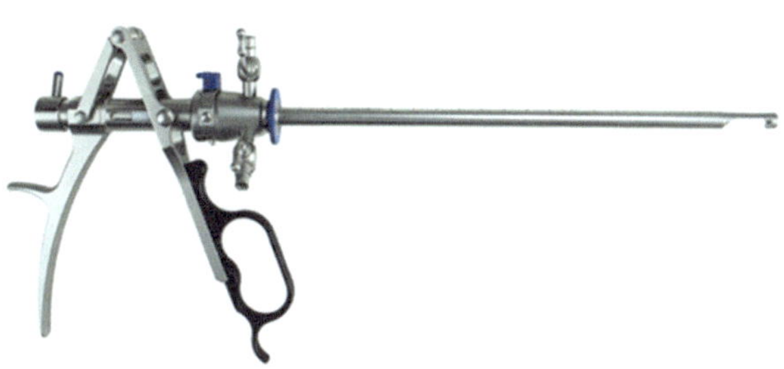

Mauermayer stone punch

Pneumatic Lithotripsy

Pneumatic or ballistic lithotripsy uses kinetic energy transferred by a rapid forward-moving rigid probe to produce a jackhammer effect on the stone. Several mechanisms are available on the market to generate the ballistic energy for this effect.

Until today, the cornerstone of pneumatic lithotripsy is the Swiss LithoClast® (EMS, Nyon, Switzerland), developed in 1991 by the Centre hospitalier universitaire vaulois in Lausanne, Switzerland. It includes a generator, a hand piece with metal probe, and a foot switch. It uses compressed air, available either via gas tanks or via the hospital air lines, to accelerate a projectile against the solid metal probe in the hand piece, with a pressure of approximately 3 atm. This way, ballistic energy is delivered at up to 12 cycles per second, with variable intensity. The probe exists in ranges from 2,4Fr to 9,6Fr [23].

A similar device is the LMA StoneBreaker (Cook Medical, Bloomington, IN, USA), which is no longer commercially available. It uses disposable cartridges of compressed carbon dioxide gas at high pressure as ballistic energy source, which are to be inserted in the handpiece. Since it is hand-activated and doesn't require an external energy source or electricity, portability and maneuverability of the device is improved. Each cartridge can deliver 80–100 shocks with a pressure of 31 atm [24]. According to a RCT by Chew in 2011 in 115 patients undergoing percutaneous nephrolithotripsy, LMA StoneBreaker offers similar stone free rates to the Swiss LithoClast (87% vs. 90% of patients are stone free or have residual fragments of <4 mm), and even faster stone fragmentation and total lithotripsy time [25], however, efficacy tends to decrease as the gas in the cartridge diminishes.

Pneumatic lithotripsy, generally using high kinetic energy and a low forward-backward movement frequency, results in fairly large stone fragments which can easily be removed. Since it transmits its energy like a jackhammer, contact with the stone is required to have effect. It has shown to be a safe and efficacious method for stone removal, with greater success for harder stones. The devices and generators are relatively low-cost and are easy and convenient in maintenance, compared to other methods. However, since all probes on the market are non-flexible, they can only be used through a rigid or semirigid scope (cystoscope, nephroscope), and applying some deflection may result in breakage of the probe. Moreover, as the probe is solid, pneumatic lithotripsy does not allow concurrent suction [24].

Ultrasonic Lithotripsy

Ultrasonic lithotripsy uses piezoceramic crystals, which convert electrical energy to mechanical energy, creating ultrasonic waves at 23–25 kHz. These are transmitted through a hollow metal probe that contacts the stone. As a result, ultrasonic lithotripsy produces heat, requiring continuous irrigation through the scope (and outflow through the lumen of the probe) to cool down the tip of the probe and avoid thermal effects on tissue. The rapid, low-energy vibrations result in small stone fragments, which can be aspirated continuously through the probe. As such, vibration against tissue results in minimal injury and is considered safe. Similar to pneumatic lithotripsy, contact between the probe and the stone is required to transfer its energy.

Laser Lithotripsy

Holmium-YAG and Thulium lasers (including Thulium fiber and pulsed Thulium YAG) are the most commonly utilized lasers in bladder stone lithotripsy. In has been shown that holmium laser could be utilized safely and effectively for transurethral urinary bladder stone lithotripsy even in stones larger than 2 cm [26–28]. In a systematic review Thulium Fiber laser lithotripsy of bladder stones was also found to be a safe and effective treatment choice [29].

Extracorporeal Shock Wave Lithotripsy

Extracorporeal shock wave lithotripsy (ESWL) has been used since the early 1990s for bladder stones, with good success rates, resulting in a full stone clearance between 72% and 99% in 1–5 sessions [20]. In a prospective study in 50 bladder stone patients with a stone size of <4cm^2, using ESWL monotherapy, elimination rate was 93%, with only a single session needed in 77% of cases, independent of the presence or absence of bladder outlet obstruction [21]. IPSS score dropped with 8 points. However, in approximately 10–25% of patients a second or third treatment is necessary, and up to 17% needed an adjunctive endoscopic procedure for evacuation of stone fragments [22].

Generally, the procedure is performed in an outpatient setting using no general anaesthesia or only mild analgosedation. Analgetic options include, amongst others, oral intake of non-steroidal anti-inflammatory drugs or mild opioids prior to the procedure, intravenous admission of a diclofenac infusion periprocedural, intravenous analgosedation using a midazolam infusion, or intravenous anesthesia using slow admission of propofol. The patient is generally positioned in supine position, with the lithotripter placed to the ventral side of the patient, in order to avoid the ileum and the sacrum. A foley catheter (16Fr in adults, 10–12Fr in children) is placed to first fill the bladder with 100–150 ml saline solution, in order to achieve good visualization. Then, the bladder is emptied to avoid stone displacement during the procedure, and intermittently irrigated to simplify fragment evacuation. Stone localization can be performed either fluoroscopy-guided or under direct ultrasound control. Direct ultrasound or postprocedural KUB can confirm fragmentation of the fragment before removing the foley catheter [23].

Antibiotic prophylaxis should be performed in accordance to a recent preprocedural urine culture. If sterile, no prophylaxis should be given.

The lack of publications about ESWL monotherapy for bladder stone results in failure to define the ideal stone volume for ESWL. Most authors report stone volumes up to 20–25 mm diameter. It is assumed efficacy of ESWL decreases with both higher volume sizes, as well as very small fragments.

Published results of studies using different types of lithotripters showed similar efficacy rates [20].

ESWL is generally well tolerated, but does not always result in immediate evacuation of stone fragments. Therefore, it is most commonly chosen in the setting of a high anesthetic risk, or to avoid urethral manipulation (e.g., in the presence of an artificial urinary sphincter) [24]. However, it's efficacy rate is still acceptably high and therefore it should be offered to those patients preferring no general anesthesia.

Chemolysis

There are also some chemodissolution strategies as the primary treatment of urinary bladder stones. As being time consuming and non-practical, those are rarely utilized in clinical practice. Hemiacidrin which is an irreversible inhibitor of urease Suby's G solution (Abbott Laboratories, Ltd., Saint-Laurent, Québec, Canada) can be used for dissolution of struvite stones. This compound acidifies urine and form calcium-citrate ion complexes thus might be useful in dissolving struvite and calcium phosphate stones. Oral administration of alkaline citrate may also be utilized for chemolysis of bladder stones consist of uric acid [20]. Oral intake of 1500–3000 mg L-methionine may also cause acidification of the urine and lead dissolution of struvite stones [30].

Concomitant Benign Prostate Hyperplasia and Bladder Stone Treatment

Conventionally co-existence of BPH and bladder stones constitutes the main indication for prostate surgery. However, the need for prostate surgery in presence of bladder calculi is debatable nowadays with the improved efficacy of medical treatments. In a recent study, it has been observed that only 41.9% of patients required prostate surgery whom bladder calculi was removed and medical treatment was initiated [31]. During endoscopic BPH surgery either percutaneous suprapubic or transurethral cystolithotripsy might be preferred depending on patient and stone characteristics.

Conclusion

Management of urinary bladder calculi is a multi-dimensional procedure including patient and stone characteristics and underlying pathology. There are several surgical treatment options which must be considered according to armamentarium and patient and stone characteristics.

References

1. Shah J, Whitfield H. Urolithiasis through the ages. BJU Int. 2002;89(8):801–10.
2. Ellis H. A history of bladder stone. J R Soc Med. 1979;72(4):248–51.
3. Tefekli A, Cezayirli F. The history of urinary stones: in parallel with civilization. Sci World J. 2013;2013
4. Dardioti V, Angelopoulos N, Hadjiconstantinou V. Renal diseases in the Hippocratic era. Am J Nephrol. 1997;17(3–4):214–6.
5. Allwright S. Hospital admissions for renal and bladder stone in Ireland. Ir Med J. 1978;71(4):112–6.
6. Kum F, Mahmalji W, Hale J, Thomas K, Bultitude M, Glass J. Do stones still kill? An analysis of death from stone disease 1999–2013 in England and Wales. BJU Int. 2016;118(1):140–4.
7. Soliman NA, Rizvi SAH. Endemic bladder calculi in children. Pediatr Nephrol. 2017;32:1489–99.
8. Ahmed FO, Hamdan HZ, Abdelgalil HB, Sharfi AA. A comparison between transabdominal ultrasonographic and cystourethroscopy findings in adult Sudanese patients presenting with haematuria. Int Urol Nephrol. 2015;47:223–8.
9. Linsenmeyer MA, Linsenmeyer TA. Accuracy of bladder stone detection using abdominal x-ray after spinal cord injury. J Spinal Cord Med. 2004;27(5):438–42.
10. Ather MH, Memon W, Aziz W, Sulaiman MN. Non-contrast CT in the evaluation of urinary tract stone obstruction and haematuria. In: Computed tomography-advanced applications. InTech; 2017.
11. Douenias R, Rich M, Badlani G, Mazor D, Smith A. Predisposing factors in bladder calculi: review of 100 cases. Urology. 1991;37(3):240–3.
12. Ashworth M. Endemic bladder stones. Br Med J. 1990;301(6756):826.
13. Thalut K, Rizal A, Brockis J, Bowyer R, Taylor T, Wisniewski Z. The endemic bladder stones of Indonesia—epidemiology and clinical features. Br J Urol. 1976;48(7):617–21.
14. Takasaki E, Suzuki T, Honda M, Imai T, Maeda S, Hosoya Y. Chemical compositions of 300 lower urinary tract calculi and associated disorders in the urinary tract. Urol Int. 1995;54(2):89–94.
15. Keeman J. Blaasstenen en lithotomie, een verdwenen kwaal als fundament van de urologie. Ned Tijdschr Geneeskd. 2006;150(51):2805–12.
16. Javanmard B, Karkan MF, Razzaghi MR, Ghiasy S, Ranjbar A, Rahavian A. Surgical management of vesical stones in children: a comparison between open cystolithotomy, percutaneous cystolithotomy and transurethral cystolithotripsy with holmium-YAG laser. J Laser Med Sci. 2018;9(3):183.
17. Ullah S, Chaudhary IA, Masood R. Comparison of open vesicolithotomy and cystolitholapaxy. Pak J Med Sci. 2007;23(1):47.
18. Deswanto IA, Basukarno A, Birowo P, Rasyid N. Management of bladder stones: the move towards non-invasive treatment. Med J Indones. 2017;26(2):128–33.
19. Miller DC, Park JM. Percutaneous cystolithotomy using a laparoscopic entrapment sac. Urology. 2003;62(2):333–6.
20. Philippou P, Moraitis K, Masood J, Junaid I, Buchholz N. The management of bladder lithiasis in the modern era of endourology. Urology. 2012;79(5):980–6.
21. Wollin T, Singal R, Whelan T, Dicecco R, Razvi H, Denstedt J. Percutaneous suprapubic cystolithotripsy for treatment of large bladder calculi. J Endourol. 1999;13(10):739–44.
22. Tugcu V, Polat H, Ozbay B, Gurbuz N, Eren GA, Tasci AI. Percutaneous versus transurethral cystolithotripsy. J Endourol. 2009;23(2):237–42.
23. Wisard M, Jichlinski P, Languetin J, Favre R, von Niederhäusern W. First clinical evaluation of the CHUV ballistic lithoclast. Helv Chir Acta. 1991;58(3):319–21.
24. Axelsson TA, Cracco C, Desai M, Hasan MN, Knoll T, Montanari E, et al. Consultation on kidney stones, Copenhagen 2019: lithotripsy in percutaneous nephrolithotomy. World J Urol. 2021;39:1663–70.

25. Chew BH, Arsovska O, Lange D, Wright JE, Beiko DT, Ghiculete D, et al. The Canadian StoneBreaker trial: a randomized, multicenter trial comparing the LMA StoneBreaker™ and the Swiss LithoClast® during percutaneous nephrolithotripsy. J Endourol. 2011;25(9):1415–9.
26. Garg M, Kumar M, Goel A, Sankhwar SN. Application of the holmium laser lithotripsy for bladder stones under local anaesthesia: a prospective analysis. Urologia J. 2015;82(4):219–22.
27. Karami H, Razaghi MR, Javanmard B, Yaghoob M, Hadad AH, Amani M, et al. Outpatient transurethral cystolithotripsy of large bladder stones by holmium laser. J Lasers Med Sci. 2016;7(1):12.
28. Nameirakpam S, Naorem S, Faridi M, Akoijam KS, Sinam RS. Transurethral cystolithotripsy of large bladder stones by Holmium laser as a day care procedure. J Clin Diagn Res. 2016;10(12):PC01.
29. Gao B, Bobrowski A, Lee J. A scoping review of the clinical efficacy and safety of the novel thulium fiber laser: the rising star of laser lithotripsy. Can Urol Assoc J. 2021;15(2):56.
30. Jacobs DH, Hesse AD. Chemolysis of struvite stones by acidification of artificial urine-an in vitro study. Scand J Urol Nephrol. 2001;35(5):345–9.
31. Anil H, Ünal U, Karamik K, Ortoglu F, Erçil H. Bladder calculi concomitant with benign prostatic enlargement: is prostate surgery mandatory in patients who have never received medical therapy? Asian J Androl. 2023;25(5):604–7.

Chapter 26
Lasers in Endourology

Hakan Bahadir Haberal and Senol Tonyali

The first laser was built and operated in 1960 and has since been used in medicine [1]. Ophthalmology was the first medical specialty to use lasers. The first use of lasers in urology occurred in the late 1960s, and the laser technology experienced a boom in the late 1990s [2–4], after Denstedt et al. reported the use of holmium:yttrium aluminum garnet in ureteroscopic laser lithotripsy [5]. Advances in laser systems that have made this technology suited for surgical procedures have played a major role in this increasing adoption. This section describes the features of the most common types of lasers used in urology. These include holmium: yttrium-aluminum-garnet (Ho:YAG), thulium: yttrium-aluminum-garnet (Tm:YAG), thulium fiber laser (TFL), potassium-titanyl-phosphate (KTP:YAG) / lithium triborate (LBO:YAG) (GreenLight), neodymium: yttrium-aluminum-garnet (Nd:YAG), erbium: yttrium-aluminum-garnet (Er: YAG) and diode lasers.

Holmium: Yttrium–Aluminum–Garnet (Ho:YAG) Laser

The Ho:YAG laser has been used in endoscopic urological procedures for over three decades [6]. The Ho:YAG laser beam originates from an optical cavity [7]. With each laser pulse, the light emitted by the flashlamp interacts with Holmium ions and causes the emission of new photons of a characteristic wavelength. These photons move freely in the optical cavity and are reflected by mirrors at both ends. Most of the emitted energy is lost and leads to heating of the optical cavity. Thus, Ho:YAG

H. B. Haberal (✉)
Department of Urology, Ankara Ataturk Sanatoryum Training and Research Hospital, Ministry of Health, University of Health Sciences, Ankara, Turkey

S. Tonyali
Department of Urology, Istanbul University Istanbul School of Medicine, Istanbul, Turkey

S. Tonyali et al. (eds.), *Current Endourology*,
https://doi.org/10.1007/978-3-032-00010-1_26

generators require a water-cooling system contributing to the large size of these generators. Ho:YAG lasers produce a pulsed laser energy at 2120-nm wavelength that is highly absorbed in water [7]. This absorption results in a penetration depth of 0.4 mm [8]. These characteristics make Ho:YAG lasers suitable for stone surgery for its lithotripsy effects and for endoscopic enucleation and endoscopic tumor procedures for its penetrating effects on soft tissue [7]. The major advantages of the Ho:YAG laser include its use of 200-μm fibers and efficacy in all types of kidney stones [9, 10]. These features have made it the gold standard lithotriptor in endoscopic stone surgery. Ho:YAG lasers have some disadvantages: they require multiple optical cavities to achieve high energy levels, the output beam is multimodal and it is a mirror-based generator, making it vulnerable to external shocks during manipulation or transportation [7].

The use of Ho:YAG lasers in lithotripsy has been shown to result in high stone-free rates and low complication rates, including in patients with comorbidities and those on anticoagulant therapy [11–13]. Results of its use in prostate enucleation have shown it to be effective and safe regardless of the prostate size [14]. It yields satisfactory functional results without increasing the risk of complications in elderly patients [15]. Another clinical use of the Ho:YAG laser is resection of bladder tumors. Studies comparing transurethral resection with Ho:YAG resection have found that the Ho:YAG laser results in better clinical outcomes in terms of length of hospital stay, bladder perforation and tumour recurrence and it may be a better option than transurethral resection in the treatment of non-muscle invasive bladder tumors [16].

One of the recent developments concerning the use of Ho:YAG lasers is the pulse modulation feature [17]. Recently, Lumenis® (Yokne'am Illit, Israel) has introduced the Moses technology, which enables the laser to produce two successive energy waves. The first wave splits the water in two allowing the second wave to be directed directly at the target [18]. Similarly, other manufacturers have introduced different pulse modulation technologies. Studies on lithotripsy have shown that although the Moses technology is associated with shorter laser delivery duration and faster stone ablation, it does not lead to a difference in stone-free and complication rates [19]. Also, some studies on laser prostate surgery showed that the Moses technology provided better intraoperative results in terms of enucleation time and hemostasis compared to the standard Ho:YAG laser [20]. However, further studies are needed to demonstrate the effect of the Moses technology on surgical outcomes in both lithotripsy and enucleation procedures [21]. Similarly, although there are promising results for other pulse modulation technologies, these data need to be further investigated.

Thulium: Yttrium–Aluminum–Garnet (Tm:YAG) Laser

The Tm:YAG laser works on a similar principle to the Ho:YAG laser. The laser beam is generated when thulium ions transition from a high-energy level to a low-energy level, releasing photons that move between the mirrors [22]. Tm:YAG generates laser energy at 2010-nm wavelength and in a continuous wave pattern [8]. It has been used for a range of soft tissue applications as part of urological procedures since 2005 [23]. It has a high surgical safety profile thanks to a tissue penetration thickness of 0.2 mm [8, 23]. It can be used for resection, enucleation, ablation and vaporization in transurethral procedures. Compared to the Ho:YAG laser, it has a lower tissue penetration depth, but a larger coagulation and total lasing area [24]. One of the developments concerning Tm:YAG lasers is the introduction of a Thulium laser using a pulsed mode.

Tm:YAG laser enucleation of the prostate has been reported to be safe and effective regardless of prostate size [25], with no reported negative effect on erectile function. Studies investigating the results of enucleation of the prostate with the Tm:YAG laser *vs.* the Ho:YAG laser have reported similar functional and perioperative results [26]. These results suggest that the Tm:YAG laser can be used effectively in endoscopic enucleation procedures.

A study in which the performance of the modified pulsed Tm:YAG laser in enucleation of the prostate was assessed by surgeons using it found this technique to be second only to the high-power Ho:YAG laser and better than the TFL [27]. Studies investigating its effectiveness in lithotripsy have found it to be effective both in dusting and fragmentation procedures [28, 29]. Moreover, a study investigating the use of this modified laser in stone surgery has shown it to produce a lower retropulsion force than the Ho:YAG laser [30].

Thulium Fiber Laser (TFL)

TFL is a type of laser developed in recent years as an alternative to the Ho:YAG laser. TFL uses long, thin thulium-doped silica fibers as the active laser medium [7]. TFL emits photons at 1940-nm wavelength and can be operated in both pulsed and continuous modes and with different energy and frequency settings [7, 31]. This wavelength is very close to the absorption peak of water and thus the water absorption coefficient of TFL is higher than both the Ho:YAG laser and the Tm:YAG laser [8]. This reduces the distance-dependent energy loss with the TFL. This means that the TFL only requires a simple fan system for cooling and, since it has no mirror system, it can also resist external shocks. Another advantage of the TFL over other lasers is related to the size of the laser fiber. Indeed, the smallest fiber thickness that can be used with the Ho:YAG laser is 200 μm, to be contrasted with extra small fibers (50 μm) that are available for the TFL [7, 32]. Smaller fiber sizes allow the TFL to generate more symmetrical, continuous and uniform energy waves compared to Ho:YAG lasers [7, 31]. This reduction in fiber size also enables a more miniaturized rigid and flexible ureteroscopy. The TFL has been shown to result in smaller bubble dimensions compared to the Ho:YAG laser [33]. This gives the TFL an advantage over the Ho:YAG laser in its lithotripsy performance in terms of stone retropulsion [32]. These features mean that the TFL may provide an advantage over the Ho:YAG in lithotripsy procedures.

The available body of literature shows that the TFL is superior to the Ho:YAG in terms of operation time, stone-free and complication rates [34, 35]. All in all, the TFL appears to be a safe and effective alternative for lithotripsy [36]. Studies investigating the performance of the TFL in laser enucleation surgery has shown it to provide satisfactory results with low complication rates and to yield comparable results to the Ho:YAG laser [37–39]. The TFL is believed to offer potential advantages in laser en bloc resection of bladder tumors thanks to its low penetration depth and lower likelihood of causing obturator reflex, but these results need to confirmed by further studies [40].

Potassium-Titanyl-Phosphate (KTP:YAG)/Lithium Triborate (LBO:YAG) Laser (GreenLight)

The KTP:YAG/LBO:YAG laser, also known as GreenLight, emits a beam at 532-nm wavelength that is absorbed by oxyhemoglobin [41, 42]. GreenLight lasers currently offer three different power settings: 80-W (KTP), 120-W High-Performance System (HPS) (LBO) and 180-W XPS (LBO) [42]. This type of lasers provide a very strong coagulative effect and, since they are absorbed only by hemoglobin, allow photoselective vaporization of the prostate. Studies have shown that the GreenLight laser can also be used in the enucleation of the prostate [43, 44].

GreenLight laser prostatectomy has been shown to provide satisfactory early and mid-term results in terms of complication rates and surgical outcomes [45]. Some studies have shown that the rate of patients requiring reoperation due to adenoma in the long term is higher compared to rates with transurethral resection [46]. Thanks to its hemostatic properties, it may be chosen particularly for patients at high risk of bleeding [47]. Although it has been shown to provide a potential advantage in terms of complications and intraoperative parameters compared to transurethral resection in the treatment of non-muscle invasive bladder tumors, long-term follow-up results are still needed to ascertain oncological outcomes [48].

Neodymium: Yttrium-Aluminum-Garnet (Nd:YAG) Laser

The Nd:YAG laser produces a laser beam at 1064-nm wavelength that penetrates deeply into tissue [8]. In 1994, Gillins et al. demonstrated its use in conjunction with the Ho:YAG laser in prostate ablation surgery [49]. Technological advances have allowed the addition of a KTP crystal to the Nd:YAG laser, resulting in the frequency-doubled double-pulse Nd:YAG (FREDDY) laser [50]. This allowed the new laser to be able to produce two laser beams, one at 532-nm and another at 1064-nm wavelength. In vitro studies have shown that this laser provides effective stone fragmentation with minimal effect on tissue [51]. While this feature makes it a safe laser option, it also means that this type of laser can only be used for stone fragmentation, precluding its use in tissue ablation procedures [9]. Also, it has been reported to have a significant disadvantage: it provides ineffective fragmentation of hard stones such as cystine [52].

Erbium: Yttrium-Aluminum-Garnet (Er:YAG) Laser

The Er:YAG laser produces a laser beam at 2940-nm wavelength [50]. In vitro studies have shown the Er:YAG laser to be more effective in lithotripsy than the Ho:YAG laser [53, 54]. This effectiveness was attributed to the Er:YAG laser's wavelength being compatible with the absorption peak of the stone, resulting in deeper craters on the stone. Although it has been reported to be effective by in vitro studies, the Er:YAG laser has been unable to get a foothold as a common laser technique in clinical practice due to problems with the development of suitable laser fibers.

Diode Lasers

Diode lasers refer to a heterogeneous group that produce laser beams at different wavelengths [55]. Various types of diode lasers at wavelengths of 940, 980, 1318 and 1470 nm are used in prostate ablation procedures [55–58]. They allow vaporization, resection and enucleation of the prostate. With its vaporization characteristics, diode lasers provide a high depth of tissue invasion and cause tissue necrosis [59]. Diode laser vaporization of the prostate has been reported to result in high rates of long-term complications as well as need for recatheterization and need for retreatment [55, 59, 60]. Diode lasers' use in enucleation procedures has been shown to provide similar results to the Ho:YAG [61, 62].

Tips and Tricks

- Every type of the laser currently used in clinical practice has its unique advantages for particular purposes. Thus, no type of laser can be qualified as the best. Selection of the appropriate type of laser should be guided by the surgical procedure to be performed, patient characteristics and technological suitability.
- Thulium fiber laser (TFL) has the potential to play a major role in both lithotripsy and enucleation procedures thanks to its advantages over other lasers in terms of power generation, transmission and practical use.
- Although pulse modulation technology appears to be promising for the future, further studies are needed to clarify its effects on surgical outcomes.
- In recent years, there have been significant technological advances in laser technology and the use of lasers in urological procedures. Science-industry cooperation is likely to result in further developments in this field.

References

1. Gibson KF, Kernohan WG. Lasers in medicine–a review. J Med Eng Technol. 1993;17:51–7.
2. Mulvaney WP, Beck CW. The laser beam in urology. J Urol. 1968;99:112–5.
3. Parsons RL, Campbell JL, Thomley MW. Carcinoma of the penis treated by the ruby laser. J Urol. 1968;100:38–9.
4. Kronenberg P, Traxer O. Update on lasers in urology 2014: current assessment on holmium:yttrium-aluminum-garnet (Ho:YAG) laser lithotripter settings and laser fibers. World J Urol. 2015;33:463–9.
5. Denstedt JD, Razvi HA, Sales JL, Eberwein PM. Preliminary experience with holmium: YAG laser lithotripsy. J Endourol. 1995;9:255–8.
6. Johnson DE, Cromeens DM, Price RE. Use of the holmium:YAG laser in urology. Lasers Surg Med. 1992;12:353–63.
7. Traxer O, Keller EX. Thulium fiber laser: the new player for kidney stone treatment? A comparison with Holmium:YAG laser. World J Urol. 2020;38:1883–94.
8. Enikeev D, Shariat SF, Taratkin M, Glybochko P. The changing role of lasers in urologic surgery. Curr Opin Urol. 2020;30:24–9.
9. Fried NM, Irby PB. Advances in laser technology and fibre-optic delivery systems in lithotripsy. Nat Rev Urol. 2018;15:563–73.
10. Kronenberg P, Traxer O. The truth about laser fiber diameters. Urology. 2014;84:1301–7.
11. Aboumarzouk OM, Somani BK, Monga M. Flexible ureteroscopy and holmium:YAG laser lithotripsy for stone disease in patients with bleeding diathesis: a systematic review of the literature. Int Braz J Urol. 2012;38:298–305; discussion 6.
12. Chen S, Zhou L, Wei T, Luo D, Jin T, Li H, Wang K. Comparison of holmium: YAG laser and pneumatic lithotripsy in the treatment of ureteral stones: an update meta-analysis. Urol Int. 2017;98:125–33.
13. Yang C, Li S, Cui Y. Comparison of YAG laser lithotripsy and extracorporeal shock wave lithotripsy in treatment of ureteral calculi: a meta-analysis. Urol Int. 2017;98:373–81.
14. Das AK, Han TM, Hardacker TJ. Holmium laser enucleation of the prostate (HoLEP): size-independent gold standard for surgical management of benign prostatic hyperplasia. Can J Urol. 2020;27:44–50.
15. Yilmaz M, Esser J, Suarez-Ibarrola R, Gratzke C, Miernik A. Safety and efficacy of laser enucleation of the prostate in elderly patients – a narrative review. Clin Interv Aging. 2022;17:15–33.
16. Li C, Gao L, Zhang J, Yang X, Liu C. The effect of holmium laser resection versus standard transurethral resection on non-muscle-invasive bladder cancer: a systematic review and meta-analysis. Lasers Med Sci. 2020;35:1025–34.
17. Sanchez-Puy A, Bravo-Balado A, Diana P, Baboudjian M, Piana A, Giron I, Kanashiro AK, Angerri O, Contreras P, Eisner BH, Balana J, Sanchez-Martin FM, Millan F, Palou J, Emiliani E. New generation pulse modulation in Holmium:YAG lasers: a systematic review of the literature and meta-analysis. J Clin Med. 2022;11
18. Ibrahim A, Badaan S, Elhilali MM, Andonian S. Moses technology in a stone simulator. Can Urol Assoc J. 2018;12:127–30.
19. Riveros CA, Chalfant V, Melchart T, Singh G, Forero AM, Ledesma B, Harnett S, Stec AA, Feloney M, Delto JC, Klett DE. Does Moses technology improve the efficiency and outcomes of standard holmium laser lithotripsy? A systematic review and meta-analysis. Cent Eur J Urol. 2022;75:409–17.
20. Gauhar V, Gilling P, Pirola GM, Chan VW, Lim EJ, Maggi M, Teoh JY, Krambeck A, Castellani D. Does MOSES technology enhance the efficiency and outcomes of standard holmium laser enucleation of the prostate? Results of a systematic review and meta-analysis of comparative studies. Eur Urol Focus. 2022;8:1362–9.

21. Corsini C, de Angelis M, Villa L, Somani BK, Pietropaolo A, Montorsi F, Goumas IK, Traxer O, Salonia A, Ventimiglia E. Holmium: yttrium-aluminum-garnet laser with Moses: does it make a difference? Curr Opin Urol. 2022;32:324–9.
22. Bozzini G, Berti L, Maltagliati M, Besana U, Micali S, Roche JB, Romero-Otero J, Pacchetti A, Perri D, Morini E, Saredi G, Mazzoleni F, Sighinolfi MC, Buizza C, Rocco B. Thulium: YAG vs continuous-wave thulium fiber laser enucleation of the prostate: do potential advantages of thulium fiber lasers translate into relevant clinical differences? World J Urol. 2023;41:143–50.
23. Kyriazis I, Swiniarski PP, Jutzi S, Wolters M, Netsch C, Burchardt M, Liatsikos E, Xia S, Bach T, Gross AJ, Herrmann TR. Transurethral anatomical enucleation of the prostate with Tm:YAG support (ThuLEP): review of the literature on a novel surgical approach in the management of benign prostatic enlargement. World J Urol. 2015;33:525–30.
24. Ortner G, Rice P, Nagele U, Herrmann TRW, Somani BK, Tokas T. Tissue thermal effect during lithotripsy and tissue ablation in endourology: a systematic review of experimental studies comparing holmium and thulium lasers. World J Urol. 2023;41:1–12.
25. Castellani D, Pirola GM, Pacchetti A, Saredi G, Dellabella M. State of the art of thulium laser enucleation and vapoenucleation of the prostate: a systematic review. Urology. 2020;136:19–34.
26. Hartung FO, Kowalewski KF, von Hardenberg J, Worst TS, Kriegmair MC, Nuhn P, Herrmann TRW, Michel MS, Herrmann J. Holmium versus thulium laser enucleation of the prostate: a systematic review and meta-analysis of randomized controlled trials. Eur Urol Focus. 2022;8:545–54.
27. Yilmaz M, Esser J, Kraft L, Petzold R, Sigle A, Gratzke C, Suarez-Ibarrola R, Miernik A. Experimental ex-vivo performance study comparing a novel, pulsed thulium solid-state laser, chopped thulium fibre laser, low and high-power holmium:YAG laser for endoscopic enucleation of the prostate. World J Urol. 2022;40:601–6.
28. Kraft L, Petzold R, Suarez-Ibarrola R, Miernik A. In vitro fragmentation performance of a novel, pulsed thulium solid-state laser compared to a thulium fibre laser and standard Ho:YAG laser. Lasers Med Sci. 2022;37:2071–8.
29. Kraft L, Yilmaz M, Petzold R, Gratzke C, Suarez-Ibarrola R, Miernik A. Dusting efficiency of a novel pulsed Thulium:Yttrium aluminum garnet laser vs a thulium fiber laser. J Endourol. 2022;36:259–65.
30. Petzold R, Miernik A, Suarez-Ibarrola R. Retropulsion force in laser lithotripsy-an in vitro study comparing a holmium device to a novel pulsed solid-state thulium laser. World J Urol. 2021;39:3651–6.
31. Kronenberg P, Traxer O. The laser of the future: reality and expectations about the new thulium fiber laser-a systematic review. Transl Androl Urol. 2019;8:S398–417.
32. Khusid JA, Khargi R, Seiden B, Sadiq AS, Atallah WM, Gupta M. Thulium fiber laser utilization in urological surgery: a narrative review. Investig Clin Urol. 2021;62:136–47.
33. Hardy LA, Kennedy JD, Wilson CR, Irby PB, Fried NM. Analysis of thulium fiber laser induced bubble dynamics for ablation of kidney stones. J Biophotonics. 2017;10:1240–9.
34. Ulvik O, Æsøy MS, Juliebo-Jones P, Gjengsto P, Beisland C. Thulium fibre laser versus Holmium:YAG for ureteroscopic lithotripsy: outcomes from a prospective randomised clinical trial. Eur Urol. 2022;82:73–9.
35. Corrales M, Traxer O. Retrograde intrarenal surgery: laser showdown (Ho:YAG vs thulium fiber laser). Curr Opin Urol. 2022;32:179–84.
36. Traxer O, Sierra A, Corrales M. Which is the best laser for lithotripsy? Thulium fiber laser. Eur Urol Open Sci. 2022;44:15–7.
37. Elmansy H, Hodhod A, Elshafei A, Noureldin YA, Mehrnoush V, Zakaria AS, Hadi RA, Fathy M, Abbas L, Kotb A, Shahrour W. Comparative analysis of MOSES(TM) technology versus novel thulium fiber laser (TFL) for transurethral enucleation of the prostate: a single-institutional study. Arch Ital Urol Androl. 2022;94:180–5.

38. Petov V, Babaevskaya D, Taratkin M, Chuvalov L, Lusuardi L, Misrai V, Sukhanov R, Scoffone CM, Enikeev D. Thulium fiber laser enucleation of the prostate: prospective study of mid- and long-term outcomes in 1328 patients. J Endourol. 2022;36:1231–6.
39. Doizi S. Lasers for benign prostatic hyperplasia (hybrid, blue diode, TFL, Moses). Which one to choose? Curr Opin Urol. 2022;32:438–42.
40. Enikeev D, Babjuk M, Shpikina A, Shariat S, Glybochko P. En bloc resection for nonmuscle-invasive bladder cancer: selecting a proper laser. Curr Opin Urol. 2022;32:173–8.
41. Dolowy L, Krajewski W, Dembowski J, Zdrojowy R, Kolodziej A. The role of lasers in modern urology. Cent Eur J Urol. 2015;68:175–82.
42. Mordasini L, Moschini M, Mattei A, Iselin C. GreenLight laser for benign prostatic hyperplasia. Curr Opin Urol. 2018;28:322–8.
43. Gomez Sancha F, Rivera VC, Georgiev G, Botsevski A, Kotsev J, Herrmann T. Common trend: move to enucleation-is there a case for GreenLight enucleation? Development and description of the technique. World J Urol. 2015;33:539–47.
44. Peyronnet B, Robert G, Comat V, Roupret M, Gomez-Sancha F, Cornu JN, Misrai V. Learning curves and perioperative outcomes after endoscopic enucleation of the prostate: a comparison between GreenLight 532-nm and holmium lasers. World J Urol. 2017;35:973–83.
45. Castellan P, Castellucci R, Schips L, Cindolo L. Safety, efficacy and reliability of 180-W GreenLight laser technology for prostate vaporization: review of the literature. World J Urol. 2015;33:599–607.
46. Castellani D, Pirola GM, Rubilotta E, Gubbiotti M, Scarcella S, Maggi M, Gauhar V, Teoh JY, Galosi AB. GreenLight laser photovaporization versus transurethral resection of the prostate: a systematic review and meta-analysis. Res Rep Urol. 2021;13:263–71.
47. Burtt G, Springate C, Martin A, Woodward E, Zantek P, Al Jaafari F, Muir G, Misrai V. The efficacy and safety of laser and electrosurgical transurethral procedures for the treatment of BPO in high-risk patients: a systematic review. Res Rep Urol. 2022;14:247–57.
48. Xu Z, Gan G, Chen G, Wu G. A systematic review and meta- analysis of green-light laser vaporization for superficial bladder. Urol J. 2020;17:578–86.
49. Gilling PJ, Cass CB, Malcolm AR, Fraundorfer MR. Combination holmium and Nd:YAG laser ablation of the prostate: initial clinical experience. J Endourol. 1995;9:151–3.
50. Marks AJ, Teichman JM. Lasers in clinical urology: state of the art and new horizons. World J Urol. 2007;25:227–33.
51. Zorcher T, Hochberger J, Schrott KM, Kuhn R, Schafhauser W. In vitro study concerning the efficiency of the frequency-doubled double-pulse Neodymium:YAG laser (FREDDY) for lithotripsy of calculi in the urinary tract. Lasers Surg Med. 1999;25:38–42.
52. Dubosq F, Pasqui F, Girard F, Beley S, Lesaux N, Gattegno B, Thibault P, Traxer O. Endoscopic lithotripsy and the FREDDY laser: initial experience. J Endourol. 2006;20:296–9.
53. Chan KF, Lee H, Teichman JM, Kamerer A, McGuff HS, Vargas G, Welch AJ. Erbium: YAG laser lithotripsy mechanism. J Urol. 2002;168:436–41.
54. Lee H, Kang HW, Teichman JM, Oh J, Welch AJ. Urinary calculus fragmentation during Ho: YAG and Er:YAG lithotripsy. Lasers Surg Med. 2006;38:39–51.
55. Lusuardi L, Mitterberger M, Hruby S, Kunit T, Kloss B, Engelhardt PF, Sieberer M, Janetschek G. Update on the use of diode laser in the management of benign prostate obstruction in 2014. World J Urol. 2015;33:555–62.
56. Kahokehr AA, Gilling PJ. Which laser works best for benign prostatic hyperplasia? Curr Urol Rep. 2013;14:614–9.
57. Tanaka EY, Barbosa FT, Murta CB, Claro JF, Manzano JP. Diode laser vaporization for benign prostate hyperplasia: outcome after 126 procedures. J Endourol. 2019;33:1025–31.
58. Rieken M, Bachmann A. Laser treatment of benign prostate enlargement–which laser for which prostate? Nat Rev Urol. 2014;11:142–52.
59. Rieken M, Ebinger Mundorff N, Bonkat G, Wyler S, Bachmann A. Complications of laser prostatectomy: a review of recent data. World J Urol. 2010;28:53–62.

60. Huang SW, Tsai CY, Tseng CS, Shih MC, Yeh YC, Chien KL, Pu YS, Tu YK. Comparative efficacy and safety of new surgical treatments for benign prostatic hyperplasia: systematic review and network meta-analysis. BMJ. 2019;367:l5919.
61. Das AK, Teplitsky S, Uhr A, Leong JY, Kucherov V, Shenot PJ. A retrospective comparison of diode to holmium for laser enucleation of the prostate. Can J Urol. 2019;26:9836–42.
62. He G, Shu Y, Wang B, Du C, Chen J, Wen J. Comparison of diode laser (980 nm) enucleation vs holmium laser enucleation of the prostate for the treatment of benign prostatic hyperplasia: a randomized controlled trial with 12-month follow-up. J Endourol. 2019;33:843–9.

Chapter 27
Ureteroscopy

Lazaros Tzelves, Alexandros Pinitas, Senol Tonyali, and Serdar Turan

Indications of Ureteroscopy

Ureteroscopy has both diagnostic and therapeutic goals.

Indications for performing diagnostic ureteroscopy are:

- Abnormal imaging findings for example a filling defect
- Obstruction and recognizing the cause
- Evaluation of hematuria originating from the upper urinary tract and/or lateralized "essential" hematuria
- Localizing source of positive urinary cytology results, culture results, or other test results
- Evaluation of ureteral injury
- Follow up of known history of urothelial malignancy

Indications for performing therapeutic ureteroscopy are:

- Endoscopic lithotripsy
- Retrograde endopyelotomy
- Incision of ureteral strictures
- Improvement of calyceal drainage

L. Tzelves (✉)
2nd Department of Urology, Sismanogleio General Hospital of Athens, National and Kapodistrian University of Athens, Athens, Greece

A. Pinitas
Department of Urology, Gennimatas General Hospital, Athens, Greece

S. Tonyali · S. Turan
Department of Urology, Istanbul University Istanbul School of Medicine, Istanbul, Turkey

S. Tonyali et al. (eds.), *Current Endourology*,
https://doi.org/10.1007/978-3-032-00010-1_27

- Treatment of calyceal diverticular lesions
- Treatment of malignant urothelial tumors
- Treatment of benign tumors and bleeding lesions

Ureteroscopy has no absolute contraindications. Active urinary tract infections should be treated before ureteroscopy [1]. If coagulopathy exists, then it should have been treated if possible. If blood coagulation cannot be improved and intervention is absolutely necessary then ureteroscopy is the most preferred option with lowest complication rates amongst the alternative option [1]. Pregnancy is a relative contraindication, because ureteroscopy have been shown to be safe during pregnancy [2].

Equipment

Not so long ago, upper urinary tract pathology was treated through large incisions. In the early 1980s the birth of Endourology reduced the morbidity of these patients. Rigid and flexible ureteroscopes brought revolution to diagnostic and therapeutic interventions. Constant breakthroughs in medicine and engineering led to a continuous improvement of instrumentation and technique of ureteroscopy.

Rigid Ureteroscopes

Rigid ureteroscopes are easy to use and to control, with wide working channels. The rod-lens system has provided excellent optical quality over the years, but scopes with this design require larger diameter and are susceptible to damage due to angulation of the ureteroscope. The angle of view originally was 0–70° degrees with interchangeable or integrated lens into the ureteroscope. Nowadays, the few remaining rod-lens ureteroscopes have a 0–5° degree integrated angle. This slight angulation has an advantage of reducing the possibility for damaging the urothelium and provide better visualization of the working instruments. Initially, ureteroscopes had standard eyepiece design in straight fashion. The introduction of rigid probes for ureteric lithotripsy led to an offset ocular configuration for easier entry and removal of the probe. Nowadays their optical system is fiberoptic, which enables their size to be smaller without compromising their durability, while preventing image distortion. Their size from 16 F with beaked tips has come down to 8.5–9F with the current tip designs to be beveled for easier and safer access into the ureter. Their working channel ranges between 3.5 to 5F. The working channel is triangular in cross-section to allow irrigation around the sides when a working instrument is being used.

Semi-rigid Ureteroscopes

Rod-lens provided image of adequate quality but only a minimal vertical variation was needed to impair intraoperative vision. Commonly scopes should be advanced through tortuous ureters, while preserving their image quality. This led to the introduction of fiberoptics into ureteroscope design. The semi-rigid ureteroscopes are comprised of fiber optic bundles with current pixel density to be >30.000, encased into a semi-rigid metal sheath. The size reduction of optical component freed up room for larger working channels. The offset eyepieces became necessary because many rigid instruments required a straight working channel through the ureteroscope. Offset eyepieces can be fixed or moveable and the angle of view is usually 0–10° degrees.

Size

The shaft of most semi-rigid ureteroscopes has tapered design with a distal tip ranging in size from 6 to 10F and a gradually increase in size toward the eyepiece, resulting in a proximal shaft size of 7.8–14.5F. The advantages of this design are the empowered strength and stability of the proximal ureteroscope and the gradually dilatation of the ureter as the ureteroscope is advanced proximally. Ureteroscopes have a length of 31-33 cm for accessing the mid-ureter in males and renal pelvis in females. In order to access the renal pelvis in males, a ureteroscope of 40 cm or more is needed. The tip of semi-rigid ureteroscopes is beveled with a round, oval tip or a smooth triangular tip.

Working Channel

Constant advances in construction of ureteroscope led to two options: either a larger single working channel for instrumentation and irrigation or two separate working channels. The single working channel permits the use of larger instrument, and its size is from 4 to 6F. Having two separate working channels can be advantageous on using on channel for the instrument passage and one for undisruptive irrigation, or on using two separate instruments simultaneously. The size of the dual working channels ranges from 2.1 to 5.4F, but they are usually 3.4F for introduction of rigid instrumentation and 2.4F for irrigation. In cross-section they are either triangular or oval, which allows irrigation through the sides of the instruments.

Camera and Image Transmission

Although the surgeon can view directly through the eyepiece, it is standard practice to use video camera and image transmission to large monitor. More commonly, analog images are used, because of the widely used fiberoptic bundles. The need to use digital distal sensor chip technology for digital imaging has not been the same in rigid ureteroscopes in comparison with flexible ureteroscopes, because of the high density of fiberoptic bundles that can be incorporated in semi-rigid ureteroscopes, which are more resistant to image degradation during excessive usage.

Irrigation

The simplest and most common irrigation method is gravity irrigation. There are other configurations that can achieve greater pressure and flow. One of them is the use of a pneumatic compressive device around the bag of fluid in a semi-automated setup. In addition, there is a foot-controlled device (Peditrol) which delivers bolus irrigation via foot pedal. There are devices that are assistant-based, and they can supply greater flow on demand either by using a pressure cuff or by attaching one or two 60 ml syringes for injecting fluid as needed. There is also an automated setup with the use of a continuous irrigation device that offers continuous saline irrigation in the preferred and chosen settings.

Flexible Ureteroscopes

Since Marshall's first report of flexible ureteroscopy in 1964, the flexible ureteroscope has undergone significant improvements in design and applications. Specifically, improvement of the optical system, increased secondary passive deflection, incorporation of active deflection and a working channel have established the flexible ureteroscope as a necessary tool to everyday practice. Moreover, advancements in energy sources and newer endoscopic instruments have led to miniaturization of the flexible ureteroscopes. The arrival of the digital sensor chip technology brought the era of state-of-the-art digital ureteroscopes.

Size

Flexible ureteroscopes have a working length from 60 to 70 cm and they can access the whole collecting system. They have tapered size from a thinner distal tip to an increased size proximal shaft. The tip diameter ranges from 4.9 to 9F and proximal shaft from 5.4 to 11F. Shaft's tapered size allows progressive dilation of the ureter as the shaft is passed further cephalad along the ureter. Nowadays, smaller diameter ureteroscopes (<9F) led to reduction of the need for active ureteral dilation to greater than 10F from 58% with 9.3F ureteroscopes to 25% with 7.5F ureteroscopes [3]. Use of the smaller diameter ureteroscopes has also been associated with a decrease in the ureteral complication rate.

Image Transmission

The use of 2 or 3 fiberoptic bundles is the standard. One to two bundles for light transmission and one bundle for image transmission. Two sets of bundles for light transmission increases illumination and decreases darkening. The light cord can either be plugged into the scope or incorporated in it. The most common angle of view is 0° degrees and active deflection can compensate for that. Some flexible ureteroscopes have an angle of view of 9° degrees and makes easier the visualization of the working instruments. The era of digital technology led to superior image quality of digital ureteroscopes in comparison with fiberoptic ones. Two different imaging chips are used for digital ureteroscopy: charge-coupled devices (CCD) and complementary metal oxide semiconductors (CMOS). CCD and CMOS image sensors both convert light into electronic signals. The biggest difference is that CCD sensors create high-quality images with low noise. CMOS imagers tend to be higher in noise, require less energy, process images faster, and are less expensive compared to CCD sensors. The digital signal for image processing and transmission is being done by a single wire who ends up on the "chip on the tip". There is no need of bulky camera head placed at the eyepiece of fiberoptic ureteroscopes. In addition, most digital ureteroscopes do not need an external light source, thanks to the LED (light-emitting diode) light source at their tip, minimizing shadowing and giving the sensation of depth of field. These two characteristics reduce the weight of the scope. This chip on the tip makes the distal tip of digital ureteroscopes bigger than fiberoptic counterparts. The same reason makes them less capable of accessing a sharp-angled calyx and have less deflection.

Working Channel

All flexible ureteroscopes have one working channel, 3.6 Fr in diameter, except the Cobra and the Cobra Vision by Wolf Company that have two working channels. Larger 4.5F do exist. The working channel ends up eccentrically at the tip. This eccentricity plays a key role because this design provokes less distortion of the working channel when deflected and allows easier passage of the instruments. The orientation of the working channel is different among the several flexible ureteroscopes and the option ranges among 3 o'clock, 9 o'clock, and 6 o'clock. Considering the anatomy of the right kidney, the calices are located at 9 o'clock, so it is better to use the flexible ureteroscopes with the working channel at 3 o'clock; and on the contrary the exact opposite it is the case for the left kidney. Stiffness and size of instruments passing through working channel plays an important role on reducing the endoscope's deflection and irrigation.

Deflection Mechanism

Currently flexible ureteroscopes have an active primary and passive secondary deflection mechanism. Active deflection of the tip is controlled by the deflection of the thumb lever located on the hand-held portion of the ureteroscope. The deflection can be intuitive (the tip moves the same direction as the lever) or counterintuitive (the tip moves the opposite direction of the lever's direction). The active deflection in flexible ureteroscopes ranges from 180 to 275° degrees. Secondary passive deflection is the flexibility of the proximal segment where the active deflection tip ends. Making this part more flexible than the rest of the shaft, lengthens the active deflection more proximally and permits to the surgeon to go deeper into the collecting system. Without passive deflection, Bagley et al. reported only a 71.4% success rate in accessing the entire intrarenal collecting system compared with a 90% to 95% success rate when using ureteroscopes equipped with active and passive deflection [4].

Disposable (Single – Use) Flexible Ureteroscopes

Durability and cost-effectiveness remain an issue despite the rapid advances in endourology. The durability of different instruments has been studied and shown that the number of procedures varies from 5 to 113, before there was a need for repair [5–7].

Ureteroscopes' durability depends on several factors such as the overall time of usage, location and size of the stone, use of other devices, surgeons' experience, and the sterilization method. Preferring single use ureteroscopes in difficult cases and for teaching purposes is cost-effective because it prevents damage to more costly reusable endoscopes. Any case with significant torque that will be applied to ureteroscope is perfect candidate for using single-use ureteroscope; cases such as those with a large stone burden requiring extended lasering times, hard to approach lower pole stones, cases needing antegrade ureteroscopic access and retrograde ureteroscopy through a urinary diversion are also eligible for single-use ureteroscopes.

Guidewires

Guidewires were first developed for vascular procedures, but they became an essential tool in endourology. In general, a guidewire ranges in diameter from 0.018″ to 0.038″ and in length from 145 to 260 cm, whereas the tips, which range from 3 to 15 cm, usually are flexible and soft to prevent tissue damage. Guidewires consist of two layers, one inner layer that determines the stiffness and flexibility of the wire and an outer layer that determines wire's lubricity. Most commonly wires are coated with polytetrafluorethylene (PTFE), which provides a higher rigidity to the wire, or a hydrophilic polymer, which offers a higher lubricity and lower friction characteristic. PTFE wires can kink permanently if handled roughly, whereas nitinol or super-elastic alloy (a nitinol alloy core with a polyurethane jacket and a hydrophilic polymer coating) do not kink. Also, hybrid guidewires, which come with a stiff shaft with proximal and distal hydrophilic tips, have the advantages of both PTFE and hydrophilic wires. Most commonly wires' diameter is 0.035″ or 0.038″, 150 cm in length with a 3 cm tip. Tips can be straight, angled or J-shaped. Each guidewire is developed for a specific task and the choice depends on the current goal. Overall, hydrophilic guide wires are preferable to get access to the urinary tract, particularly in tortuous or obstructed ureters, while PTFE coated guide wire are preferable for catheter or stent placement. If desired to work with only one guide wire, hybrid wires are an alternative.

Ureteral Catheters

Ureteral catheters, especially double J stents, have become an integral part of the urological armamentarium. Ureteral catheters are primarily being used for draining upper urinary tract, performing retrograde urography during surgery and maneuvering the direction of the guidewire. There are straight tip and torturable angled ureteral catheters. When it comes to double J stents, in the last decades, several synthetic polymeric materials have been used in their development, including latex rubber (polyisoprene), polyethylene, polyvinylchloride, polyurethane, and silicone. Moreover, various coatings have been introduced to improve lubricity and decrease biofilm formation and encrustation. Unfortunately, no currently available biomaterial is ideal. Stents should be inserted in patients who are at increased risk of complications (e.g., ureteral trauma, residual fragments, bleeding, perforation, UTIs, or pregnancy), and in all doubtful cases, to avoid stressful emergencies. Randomized prospective trials have shown after uncomplicated ureteroscopy stenting is not necessary. On the contrary, stenting might be associated with higher post-operative morbidity and costs [8–11]. A ureteral catheter with a shorter indwelling time (one day) can have similar results [12].

Ureteral Access Sheath

Ureteral access sheaths (UAS) have rapidly become an important accessory in flexible ureteroscopy. Their size ranges from 9 to 16F and allows to the surgeon multiple passages into the upper urinary tract with ease and without risk of damaging the ureter during ureteroscope's reinsertion. Ureteral wall ischemia, urothelial mucosal tears and subsequent strictures, as well as ureteral and renal pelvic perforations are some risks of UAS use, even though the possibility is low [13]. On the other hand, improved vision by establishing a continuous outflow, reduction of intrarenal pressure, and potentially reduction of operating time sums up the main advantages of ureteral sheaths [14, 15]. No data on long-term side effects are available [16]. Whilst larger cohort series showed no difference in stone-free rates (SFRs) and ureteral damage (stricture rates of about 1.8%), they did show lower post-operative infectious complications [17, 18]. For large and multiple renal stones or if long procedural time is expected, ureteral sheaths are safe and useful to use [19]. A 12/14F ureteral access sheath is the most common size utilized in adults. A 35 cm length sheath is preferred for women and 45 cm length sheath for men, as long as the goal is for the tip of the sheath to be at the level of ureteropelvic junction (UPJ). If the sheath cannot be promoted to the ureter, the inner dilator can be used alone first over a guide wire to dilate the ureter. Last but not least, suctioning ureteral access sheath is going to be a new trend which in its early steps shows reduced stone free rate from day 1 and reduced possibility for sepsis [20].

Intracorporeal Lithotripters

Despite there are a number of different types of lithotripters, such as pneumatic, ultrasonic, electrohydraulic (EHL), Holmium:YAG laser is established as the standard of care for intracorporeal lithotripsy. The ultrasound probe allows for continuous, simultaneous suction with stone ablation to reduce calculi retropulsion, but is considered the least effective option overall. Pneumatic probes may only be used through rigid and semi-rigid ureteroscopes and, while effective, they must be in direct contact with the stones to work. Pneumatic lithotripsy has a known disadvantage such as stone migration, which can be prevented by placement of special anti-migration tools proximal of the stone. In vitro, Holmium laser have demonstrated better efficacy in fragmenting all stone compositions and producing smaller stone fragments compared to pneumatic, EHL and pulsed-dye lithotripsy [21]. Thulium fibre laser (TFL) for stone disease offers at least not inferior clinical outcomes although more studies are needed [22].

Ureteral Balloon Dilators

Sometimes access to the ureter or advancing of the ureteral sheath are impossible due to ureteral stricture, spasm, or a tight ureteral orifice. In these cases, a ureteral balloon dilator is being utilized. The goal is to dilate 100% of the expected diameter regardless of any amount of radial constrictive force.

Stone Retrieval Devices

Stones can be extracted by endoscopic forceps or baskets. During flexible ureteroscopy only nitinol basket should be used, cause of their smaller size and their less negative impact on the scope's deflection [23]. A stone retrieval device is essential tool in endourology. Standard helical or flat wire baskets made of stainless steel can be difficult or even dangerous for grasping within a calyx. The widest opening between the wires is located significantly proximally from the tip. They are also stiffer and tend to perforate the mucosa. Nitinol-based baskets is the choice to go when using a flexible ureteroscope due to the unique pliability of the wires and the flexibility that allows full lower pole deflection in most cases. Alligator or rat tooth forceps characterized by their reversible grasp and reusability but their weak grasp limit their effectiveness. Because of their small diameter which ranges from 1.3–2.5F, they can be used simultaneously with a laser fiber when a captured large stone cannot be removed down the ureter, preventing stone migration.

Ureteral Occluding Devices

In order to prevent stone migration during lithotripsy, a variety of devices have been developed. These devices have to be adjusted in the ureter above the level of the stone. A biogel polymer, which is liquid in cold temperature and turns into a gel at body temperature, have been evaluated and shown some prospect. These devices and their manipulation add more maneuvers and manipulation before the ureteral lithotripsy and should be used wisely.

Innovations in Ureteroscopy

The increase of ureteroscopies performed each years mirrors the increasing incidence of urolithiasis, both due to adoption of a western lifestyle and due to utilization of more accurate imaging diagnostic techniques. Since its first introduction several technological innovations permitted excellent stone free rates (SFRs) with reduced complication rates.

The standard intracorporeal lithotripsy technique nowadays is with laser energy and specifically the use of Holmium: yttrium-aluminum-garnet (Ho:YAG) which has been a revolution in urolithiasis management. However even this paradigm has now shifted due to the discovery of more efficient laser platforms such as thulium fibre laser, (TFL) which demonstrate favourable physical characteristics. Ho:YAG has a low wall-plug efficiency due to a massive proportion of energy (98–99%) converted to heat, necessitating the coupling of these laser machines with powerful cooling systems [24]. TFL operates at a wavelength of 1940 nm, very close to the water energy absorption (1950 nm), which in comparison to Ho:YAG (2100 nm) leads to a fourfold lower threshold for laser disintegration [22]. TFL also enables the user to choose from a wider variety of settings, with energy ranging between 0.025–6 J and frequency up to 2000 Hz with a peak energy of nearly 500 Watts, compared to the peak Ho:YAG output of 120 W [24–26]. These energy settings may reduce the retropulsion met in Ho:YAG with the use of minimal energy coupled with higher frequency, while also permitting dusting, fragmentation and popcorn techniques [24]. Another important clinical implication is the ability to use smaller fibers up to 50 μm with TFL compared to 200 μm with Ho:YAG, which can lead to better scope maneuverability and increased irrigation flow, although the use of small fibers in very high frequency rates might obscure intraoperative view due to the "blizzard effect" from stone fragmentation [27]. Published randomized clinical trials (RCTs) detected less stone retropulsion with TFL (69% vs 4%), clearer endoscopic view, shorted operating times with similar long-term SFRs and complication rates [22, 28]. Newer Ho:YAG laser machines can also operate with newer technologies such as the Moses technology, during which energy is administered over two pulses with the first forming the bubble and second transferring the energy through the channel to the stone, thus reducing retropulsion and operative time in preclinical and clinical studies [29, 30]. VirtualBasker™ is another double-pulse setting, shown to lead to faster fragmentation with similar applied energy [31]. In order to draw safer conclusions regarding the effectiveness between TFL and newer Ho:YAG machines, clinical trials comparing TFL with high-energy lasers and those utilizing Moses or VirtualBasket™ technology should be designed [32].

Ureteroscopes' design has changed during the years with digital systems replacing fiberoptic, enabling improved visualization due to vanishing the "honeycomb" appearance and diminishing image flickering while applying laser energy [33–35]. Single-use flexible ureteroscopes have been well tested and proved to be non-inferior or even superior to reusable scopes for SFRs and complications, while improving ergonomics based on electromyographic data [36–38]. The risk of contamination is minimal due to single use nature of these scopes, while the cost-effectiveness is questionable. However, single use scopes seem to be ideal for training purposes and use for difficult-to-access stones, such as lower pole stones with steep infundibulopelvic access, due to high risk of damage [39].

Training-wise, several innovations have been achieved for educating novice endourologists, with 3D printed models based on CT images preoperatively and virtual-reality models depicting similar to real life conditions, showing adequate validity and ability to improve performance scores, without compromising patient safety [40–42]. Artificial-Intelligence based models demonstrated excellent prognostic accuracy regarding clinical outcomes for minimally-invasive stone treatment, as well as prediction of microorganism sensitivity based on clinical data before sensitivity results are released [32, 43, 44].

Irrigation fluid use is a necessary tool to improve visualization intraoperatively, but inevitably increased intrarenal pressure (IRP), especially with miniaturized ureteroscopes. The normal IRP ranging between 7.5–14.7 cmH20 can increase to more than 450 cmH20 if forceful irrigation is used, thus increasing pyelovenous, pyelolymphatic and pyelointerstitial backflow and leading to complications such as sepsis, collecting system rupture and kidney damage [45, 46]. Technological advancements led to incorporation of suction technology in ureteral access sheaths [45]. This technology seems to minimize operative time, length of stay post-URS, sepsis rates and immediate SFRs compared to traditional non-suctioning URS, according to clinical studies [47].

Implementing robotic systems in uro-oncology led to improved post-operative outcomes and reduced complications rates. The first robotic systems tested for URS, the Sensei robot, demonstrated improved ergonomics from a surgeon perspective regarding stability, reproducibility of access and auto-retraction [48]. Clinical studies shown no intraoperative complications, minor postoperative complications and excellent SFRs (89%), while comparative studies with standard URS showed lower re-treatment rates in favor of robotic systems (9.1% vs 15%) [48–50]. Although this technology is still in its infancy, accumulating evidence suggests excellent clinical outcomes and rapid incorporation into clinical practice.

Fluoroscopy use has been inextricably linked to minimally-invasive procedures for management of urolithiasis, aiding in guidance intraoperatively and detection of stones. However, exposure to ionizing radiation has detrimental effects on human tissues and research studies have shown that Urologists are not very compliant in use of protective equipment [51]. Although this does not represent a technological advancement per se, the development and testing of radiation-free protocols for performing URS can diminish these harmful effects of radiation. However, it should be highlighted that the majority of these studies was performed by expert surgeons and not-complicated cases such as those with anatomic abnormalities or impacted ureteral stones [51].

Technique

Irrespective of the reason for performing ureteroscopy, the initial stage involves obtaining access to the upper urinary tract. The patient is typically placed in the dorsal lithotomy position, although alternative positions such as prone or flank may be utilized, particularly when employing flexible endoscopes. The flank position is particularly advantageous in cases involving complex renal stones, as it promotes optimal gravitational drainage of the renal pelvis, thereby facilitating effective stone clearance [52].

Although local and spinal anesthesia, as well as intravenous sedation, are feasible alternatives, the use of general anesthesia is advocated due to its inherent benefits. General anesthesia mitigates potential renal movement induced by respiration during renal navigation and lithotripsy, as mechanical ventilation can temporarily suspend these concerns by inducing apnea [53–55]. Initially, cystoscopy is performed to examine the bladder, exclude gross malignancy, and identify the ureteral orifice. This initial step is crucial for accurate diagnosis and treatment planning. At this point, safety guidewire may be inserted through the ureteral orifice into the kidney to establish atraumatic access to the ureter and kidney, facilitating subsequent procedures. Accessing the ureteral orifice is generally uncomplicated, but caution must be exercised with the cystoscope at the bladder neck, especially in men whose prostates are both enlarged and vascularized [56]. In cases of challenging access, employing the ureteroscope to visually guide and insert the wire through direct visualization, positioning its tip precisely at the ureteral orifice (UO), can be advantageous.

Upon achieving successful guidewire access, the introduction of a ureteral catheter over the wire allows for the execution of retrograde ureteropyelography using fluoroscopic contrast dye by the endourologist. This catheter, commonly sized at 5–6 French with an open distal end, serves as a conduit for both dye injection and the retrieval of urine samples for cytology analysis [57]. In most cases, the initial step involves conducting a retrograde ureteropyelography to assess the upper tract anatomy. However, there are certain conditions where retrograde imaging is not feasible, and this determination should be made on a case-by-case basis. For patients with a distal ureteral stone detected on preoperative imaging, performing distal ureteroscopy before retrograde ureteropyelography may help prevent stone migration. If upper tract cytology specimens are to be collected, it is advisable to do so prior to administering contrast into the upper collecting tract. If purulent discharge is observed from the ureter at this juncture, the recommended course of action involves promptly inserting a stent to facilitate drainage of the infection, while deferring further intervention [58]. If the ureteroscope encounters resistance passing through the orifice, the next step may involve sequential dilation of the distal ureter, or alternatively, a balloon dilator may be utilized. Before usage, it is crucial to prepare the ureteric catheter to prevent the introduction of air into the renal system. Although fluoroscopy assists in delineating anatomy, in patients with distal stones confirmed by imaging, conducting distal ureteroscopy beforehand may be warranted to mitigate the risk of stone migration [59].

After visualizing a safe passage, the guidewire can be advanced into the renal pelvis under radiographic guidance. It is recommended to utilize brief “flash” of radiation, rather than continuous screening, to minimize radiation dose [58]. Following the successful insertion of the guidewire into the renal pelvis, if deemed appropriate, an assistant may anchor it to a secure sterile point to prevent kinking and inadvertent displacement during subsequent procedures [60]. At this point, the operating surgeon might consider replacing the initial guidewire, especially if it is hydrophilic coated, due to its propensity to unintentionally slip out of the urinary tract [57]. It is recommended to replace it using an open-ended catheter over the hydrophilic wire, as this ensures continued access to the renal pelvis. In certain scenarios, obstacles such as a J-hooked distal ureter or pathological conditions like impacted stones, tight strictures, or tumors can impede the advancement of the guidewire. Strategies to address this challenge include injecting dye at the obstruction site to delineate potential pathways for advancement or elongating the “floppy tip” of the guidewire to enhance flexibility at the obstruction site [57]. Difficulties in ureteroscope insertion can be addressed with techniques such as balloon or plastic dilators if necessary [56]. If accessing the ureter proves problematic, inserting a

JJ stent followed by delayed ureteroscopy after 7–14 days presents an alternative approach. This sequential method aids in gradual ureteral dilation, facilitating subsequent scope maneuverability.

Prior to introducing the scope, it is essential to ensure bladder voiding to prevent compression of the ureteric orifice and facilitate scope progression. The scope should be held by the endourologist's dominant hand, while the other hand stabilizes it at the urethral meatus. Maintaining the straight alignment of the ureteroscope and minimizing stress on its shaft is crucial. If accessing the ureteral orifice proves challenging, rotating the scope by 90°–180° can compensate for the curved beak at its tip. The initial safety guidewire maintains patency of the ureteral orifice, while adding a second "navigating" wire, typically made of PTFE, helps widen scope access. Following the path between the two wires facilitates navigation around any encountered obstacles. If the ureter is tightly constricted and scope advancement is difficult, it is imperative not to force the scope to avoid the risk of ureteric perforation. Upon encountering resistance, the endourologist should reassess the situation and cease all scope manipulation, with repeat fluoroscopic dye injection aiding in identifying obstructive causes. Hydrophilic wires are preferred for navigating obstructions, and if difficulties persist, attempting a wire with an angled tip may be considered. If contrast material extends beyond the obstruction, passing a hydrophilic wire through the ureteral catheter is warranted. For impacted stones hindering procedural advancement, displacement can be attempted cautiously using gentle maneuvers with the ureteric catheter or scope itself (Billiard Cue technique), or via scope manipulation post-stone fragmentation, with novices advised to abstain from these maneuvers. The detection of iatrogenic mucosal injury indicates the need to postpone endoscopic intervention, with stent insertion over the safety wire as a precautionary measure.

References

1. Skolarikos A NA, Petrik A, Somani B, Thomas K, Gambaro G, et al. EAU guidelines on urolithiasis. 2022.
2. Lifshitz DA, Lingeman JE. Ureteroscopy as a first-line intervention for ureteral calculi in pregnancy. J Endourol. 2002;16(1):19–22.
3. Elashry OM, Elbahnasy AM, Rao GS, Nakada SY, Clayman RV. Flexible ureteroscopy: Washington University experience with the 9.3F and 7.5F flexible ureteroscopes. J Urol. 1997;157(6):2074–80.
4. Bagley DH. Intrarenal access with the flexible ureteropyeloscope: effects of active and passive tip deflection. J Endourol. 1993;7(3):221–4.
5. Traxer O, Dubosq F, Jamali K, Gattegno B, Thibault P. New-generation flexible ureterorenoscopes are more durable than previous ones. Urology. 2006;68(2):276–9; discussion 80–1, 279.
6. Defidio L, De Dominicis M, Di Gianfrancesco L, Fuchs G, Patel A. Improving flexible ureterorenoscope durability up to 100 procedures. J Endourol. 2012;26(10):1329–34.
7. Knudsen B, Miyaoka R, Shah K, Holden T, Turk TM, Pedro RN, et al. Durability of the next-generation flexible fiberoptic ureteroscopes: a randomized prospective multi-institutional clinical trial. Urology. 2010;75(3):534–8.

8. Song T, Liao B, Zheng S, Wei Q. Meta-analysis of postoperatively stenting or not in patients underwent ureteroscopic lithotripsy. Urol Res. 2012;40(1):67–77.
9. Haleblian G, Kijvikai K, de la Rosette J, Preminger G. Ureteral stenting and urinary stone management: a systematic review. J Urol. 2008;179(2):424–30.
10. Nabi G, Cook J, N'Dow J, McClinton S. Outcomes of stenting after uncomplicated ureteroscopy: systematic review and meta-analysis. BMJ. 2007;334(7593):572.
11. Seklehner S, Sievert KD, Lee R, Engelhardt PF, Riedl C, Kunit T. A cost analysis of stenting in uncomplicated semirigid ureteroscopic stone removal. Int Urol Nephrol. 2017;49(5):753–61.
12. Moon TD. Editorial: Ureteral Stenting—An Obsolete Procedure? J Urol. 2002;167(5):1984.
13. Traxer O, Thomas A. Prospective evaluation and classification of ureteral wall injuries resulting from insertion of a ureteral access sheath during retrograde intrarenal surgery. J Urol. 2013;189(2):580–4.
14. L'Esperance JO, Ekeruo WO, Scales CD Jr, Marguet CG, Springhart WP, Maloney ME, et al. Effect of ureteral access sheath on stone-free rates in patients undergoing ureteroscopic management of renal calculi. Urology. 2005;66(2):252–5.
15. Stern JM, Yiee J, Park S. Safety and efficacy of ureteral access sheaths. J Endourol. 2007;21(2):119–23.
16. Aboumarzouk OM, Monga M, Kata SG, Traxer O, Somani BK. Flexible ureteroscopy and laser lithotripsy for stones >2 cm: a systematic review and meta-analysis. J Endourol. 2012;26(10):1257–63.
17. Traxer O, Wendt-Nordahl G, Sodha H, Rassweiler J, Meretyk S, Tefekli A, et al. Differences in renal stone treatment and outcomes for patients treated either with or without the support of a ureteral access sheath: the Clinical Research Office of the Endourological Society Ureteroscopy Global Study. World J Urol. 2015;33(12):2137–44.
18. Stern KL, Loftus CJ, Doizi S, Traxer O, Monga M. A prospective study analyzing the association between high-grade ureteral access sheath injuries and the formation of ureteral strictures. Urology. 2019;128:38–41.
19. Lima A, Reeves T, Geraghty R, Pietropaolo A, Whitehurst L, Somani BK. Impact of ureteral access sheath on renal stone treatment: prospective comparative non-randomised outcomes over a 7-year period. World J Urol. 2020;38(5):1329–33.
20. Qian X, Liu C, Hong S, Xu J, Qian C, Zhu J, et al. Application of suctioning ureteral access sheath during flexible Ureteroscopy for renal stones decreases the risk of postoperative systemic inflammatory response syndrome. Int J Clin Pract. 2022;2022:9354714–7.
21. Teichman JM, Vassar GJ, Bishoff JT, Bellman GC. Holmium:YAG lithotripsy yields smaller fragments than lithoclast, pulsed dye laser or electrohydraulic lithotripsy. J Urol. 1998;159(1):17–23.
22. Martov AG, Ergakov DV, Guseynov M, Andronov AS, Plekhanova OA. Clinical comparison of super pulse thulium fiber laser and high-power holmium laser for ureteral stone management. J Endourol. 2021;35(6):795–800.
23. Bach T, Geavlete B, Herrmann TR, Gross AJ. Working tools in flexible ureterorenoscopy--influence on flow and deflection: what does matter? J Endourol. 2008;22(8):1639–43.
24. Tzelves L, Somani B, Berdempes M, Markopoulos T, Skolarikos A. Basic and advanced technological evolution of laser lithotripsy over the past decade: an educational review by the European Society of Urotechnology Section of the European Association of Urology. Turk J Urol. 2021;47(3):183–92.
25. Traxer O, Keller EX. Thulium fiber laser: the new player for kidney stone treatment? A comparison with holmium:YAG laser. World J Urol. 2020;38(8):1883–94.
26. Kronenberg P, Hameed BZ, Somani B. Outcomes of thulium fibre laser for treatment of urinary tract stones: results of a systematic review. Curr Opin Urol. 2021;31(2):80–6.
27. Jones P, Beisland C, Ulvik Ø. Current status of thulium fibre laser lithotripsy: an up-to-date review. BJU Int. 2021;128(5):531–8.

28. Ulvik Ø, Æsøy MS, Juliebø-Jones P, Gjengstø P, Beisland C. Thulium fibre laser versus holmium: YAG for ureteroscopic lithotripsy: outcomes from a prospective randomised clinical trial. Eur Urol. 2022;82(1):73–9.
29. Elhilali MM, Badaan S, Ibrahim A, Andonian S. Use of the moses technology to improve holmium laser lithotripsy outcomes: a preclinical study. J Endourol. 2017;31(6):598–604.
30. Ibrahim A, Elhilali MM, Fahmy N, Carrier S, Andonian S. Double-blinded prospective randomized clinical trial comparing regular and moses modes of holmium laser lithotripsy. J Endourol. 2020;34(5):624–8.
31. Bozzini G, Maltagliati M, Berti L, Besana U, Calori A, Pastore AL, et al. "VirtualBasket" ureteroscopic holmium laser lithotripsy: intraoperative and early postoperative outcomes. Minerva Urol Nephrol. 2022;74(3):344–50.
32. Tzelves L, Geraghty RM, Hughes T, Juliebø-Jones P, Somani BK. Innovations in kidney stone removal. Res Rep Urol. 2023;15:131–9.
33. Juliebø-Jones P, Keller EX, Haugland JN, Æsøy MS, Beisland C, Somani BK, et al. Advances in Ureteroscopy: new technologies and current innovations in the era of Tailored Endourological Stone Treatment (TEST). J Clin Urol. 2022;16:20514158221115986–198.
34. Gridley CM, Knudsen BE. Digital ureteroscopes: technology update. Res Rep Urol. 2017;9:19–25.
35. Alexander B, Fishman AI, Grasso M. Ureteroscopy and laser lithotripsy: technologic advancements. World J Urol. 2015;33(2):247–56.
36. Mourmouris P, Tzelves L, Raptidis G, Berdempes M, Markopoulos T, Dellis G, et al. Comparison of a single-use, digital flexible ureteroscope with a reusable, fiberoptic ureteroscope for management of patients with urolithiasis. Arch Ital Urol Androl. 2021;93(3):326–9.
37. Ludwig WW, Lee G, Ziemba JB, Ko JS, Matlaga BR. Evaluating the ergonomics of flexible ureteroscopy. J Endourol. 2017;31(10):1062–6.
38. Dragos LB, Somani BK, Keller EX, De Coninck VMJ, Herrero MR, Kamphuis GM, et al. Characteristics of current digital single-use flexible ureteroscopes versus their reusable counterparts: an in-vitro comparative analysis. Transl Androl Urol. 2019;8(Suppl 4):S359–s70.
39. Bahaee J, Plott J, Ghani KR. Single-use flexible ureteroscopes: how to choose and what is around the corner? Curr Opin Urol. 2021;31(2):87–94.
40. Hameed BMZ, Somani S, Keller EX, Balamanigandan R, Mahapatra S, Pietropaolo A, et al. Application of virtual reality, augmented reality, and mixed reality in endourology and urolithiasis: an update by YAU Endourology and Urolithiasis Working Group. Front Surg. 2022;9:866946.
41. Matsumoto ED, Pace KT, D'A HONEY RJ. Virtual reality ureteroscopy simulator as a valid tool for assessing endourological skills. Int J Urol. 2006;13(7):896–901.
42. Cai JL, Zhang Y, Sun GF, Li NC, Yuan XL, Na YQ. Proficiency of virtual reality simulator training in flexible retrograde ureteroscopy renal stone management. Chin Med J. 2013;126(20):3940–3.
43. Tzelves L, Lazarou L, Feretzakis G, Kalles D, Mourmouris P, Loupelis E, et al. Using machine learning techniques to predict antimicrobial resistance in stone disease patients. World J Urol. 2022;40(7):1731–6.
44. Poulakis V, Dahm P, Witzsch U, de Vries R, Remplik J, Becht E. Prediction of lower pole stone clearance after shock wave lithotripsy using an artificial neural network. J Urol. 2003;169(4):1250–6.
45. Tzelves L, Skolarikos A. Suction use during endourological procedures. Curr Urol Rep. 2020;21(11):46.
46. Rattner WH, Fink S, Murphy JJ. Pressure studies in the human ureter and renal pelvis. J Urol. 1957;78(4):359–62.
47. Zhu Z, Cui Y, Zeng F, Li Y, Chen Z, Hequn C. Comparison of suctioning and traditional ureteral access sheath during flexible ureteroscopy in the treatment of renal stones. World J Urol. 2019;37(5):921–9.

48. Desai MM, Aron M, Gill IS, Pascal-Haber G, Ukimura O, Kaouk JH, et al. Flexible robotic retrograde renoscopy: description of novel robotic device and preliminary laboratory experience. Urology. 2008;72(1):42–6.
49. Desai MM, Grover R, Aron M, Ganpule A, Joshi SS, Desai MR, et al. Robotic flexible ureteroscopy for renal calculi: initial clinical experience. J Urol. 2011;186(2):563–8.
50. Geavlete P, Saglam R, Georgescu D, Mulţescu R, Iordache V, Kabakci AS, et al. Robotic flexible ureteroscopy versus classic flexible ureteroscopy in renal stones: the initial Romanian experience. Chirurgia (Bucur). 2016;111(4):326–9.
51. Tzelves L, Juliebø-Jones P, Manolitsis I, Bellos T, Mykoniatis I, Berdempes M, et al. Radiation protection measures during endourological therapies. Asian J Urol. 2022;10:215–25.
52. Herrell SD, Buchanan MG. Flank position ureterorenoscopy: new positional approach to aid in retrograde caliceal stone treatment. J Endourol. 2002;16(1):15–8.
53. Park HK, Paick SH, Oh SJ, Kim HH. Ureteroscopic lithotripsy under local anesthesia: analysis of the effectiveness and patient tolerability. Eur Urol. 2004;45(5):670–3.
54. Cybulski PA, Joo H, Honey RJ. Ureteroscopy: anesthetic considerations. Urol Clin N Am. 2004;31(1):43–7, viii:43–7.
55. Emiliani E, Talso M, Baghdadi M, Ghanem S, Golmard J, Pinheiro H, Gkentzis A, Butticè S, Traxer O. The use of apnea during ureteroscopy. Urology. 2016;97:266–8.
56. Tyritzis S, Wiklund N. Ureteral strictures revisited…trying to see the light at the end of the tunnel: a comprehensive review. J Endourol Endourol Soc. 2014;29:124–36.
57. Somani B, Aboumarzouk O, Srivastava A, Traxer O. Flexible ureterorenoscopy: tips and tricks. Urol Ann. 2013;5:1–6.
58. Rukin N, Somani B, Patterson J, et al. Tips and tricks of ureteroscopy: consensus statement Part I. Basic ureteroscopy. Cent Eur J Urol. 2015;68:439–46.
59. Basillote J, Lee D, Eichel L, Clayman R. Ureteroscopes: flexible, rigid, and semirigid. Urol Clin North Am. 2004;31:21–32.
60. Sprunger J, Herrell SD. Techniques of ureteroscopy. Urol Clin N Am. 2004;31:61–9.

Chapter 28
Extracorporeal Shock Wave Lithotripsy and Future Directions

Mustafa Karaaslan and Kemal Sarica

Urinary stone disease, the prevalence of which varies between 2% and 20%, according to the geographical and socioeconomic characteristics of different populations throughout the world, s an important health issue that increases the economic burden of countries' health systems of countries [15]. In the history of its treatment, open surgical treatments were the only option until the 1980s, but as technology has developed, extracorporeal shock wave lithotripsy (SWL), percutaneous nephrolithotomy (PNL), retrograde intrarenal surgery (RIRS) and laparoscopic surgical methods have taken their place [4, 19].

Shock wave lithotripsy is a non-invasive medical procedure used for the treatment of urinary tract stones, including kidney and ureteral stones. The procedure involves the use of high-energy shock waves to break up the stones into smaller fragments, which can then be passed through the urinary tract more easily. SWL has become a widely used and effective treatment option for urinary tract stones, and it is generally preferred over more invasive surgical procedures. It is also stated that SWL has several advantages over surgical procedures, including shorter hospital stays, lower healthcare costs, and a lower risk of complications [3, 26].

M. Karaaslan (✉)
Ankara Medipol University School of Medicine, Department of Urology, Ankara, Turkey
e-mail: mustafa.karaaslan@ankaramedipol.edu.tr

K. Sarica
University of Health Sciences, Prof I. Varank Research and Training Hospital, Department of Urology, Istanbul, Turkey
e-mail: kemalsarica@superonline.com

S. Tonyali et al. (eds.), *Current Endourology*,
https://doi.org/10.1007/978-3-032-00010-1_28

History and Development of Shock Wave Lithotripsy

The first SWL device was the Human Model 1 (HM1) device, developed by Dornier, an aircraft company, in the 1980s. This device began to be used in the treatment of urinary tract stones in 1982, after it was tested on humans by Chaussy et al. [5]. The first model to be used routinely for clinical purposes was the Dornier HM3 device (Dornier MedTech, Wessling, Germany), which received US Food and Drug Administration (FDA) approval in the United States in 1984. To perform SWL with this device, the patient had to be under general or spinal anaesthesia in a huge water tube [27]. However, research continued to provide a version that had painless application, was low cost, did not need the water pool and was electrodeless (time and cost advantageous) and multifunctional. After the introduction of second-generation lithotripters into clinical practice (Dornier: HM4, electrohydraulic, 1986; Siemens: Lithostar, electromagnetic, 1986; and Wolf: Piezolith 2300, piezoelectric, 1987), Dornier HM3 production stopped in 1990. Second-generation lithotripters were easier and more comfortable for both the patient and the practitioner. Without the need for a large water pool, the shock waves were transmitted through a water-filled reservoir in contact with the patient. Although devices using second-generation lithotripters, especially piezoelectric generators, provided painless application, insufficient energy required a greater shock wave rate and a longer session. Since the 1990s, these devices have been modified, and third-generation lithotripsy devices, in which fluoroscopy and ultrasonography can be combined as a focusing system, have been produced (Storz: Modulith SL20, electromagnetic, 1989; Siemens: Lithostar Plus, electromagnetic, 1989); Wolf: Piezolith 2500, piezoelectric, 1989; and Dornier: MFL5000-u (electrohydraulic, 1990) [7].

Shock Wave Lithotripsy Working Principles

SWL devices consists of an imaging unit (fluoroscopy and ultrasonography), a shock wave generator, a focusing system (ellipsoid reflector, lens system, piezoelectric crystals) and a contact membrane (water cushion and gel). Three different generator systems are used in shock wave generation: electrohydraulic, electromagnetic and piezoelectric (Fig. 28.1) [19].

A shock wave is a short acoustic vibration produced by an energy source. Each wave begins with a positive pressure wave (compressive phase), followed by a negative pressure wave(tensile phase). When the shock wave reaches the stone, it creates various forces, such as high-energy positive pressure (tear/shear forces), negative tensile force, spallation, semi-static compression (squeezing), dynamic compression and cavitation (explosion of the voids), and these forces fragment the targeted stone [22, 23].

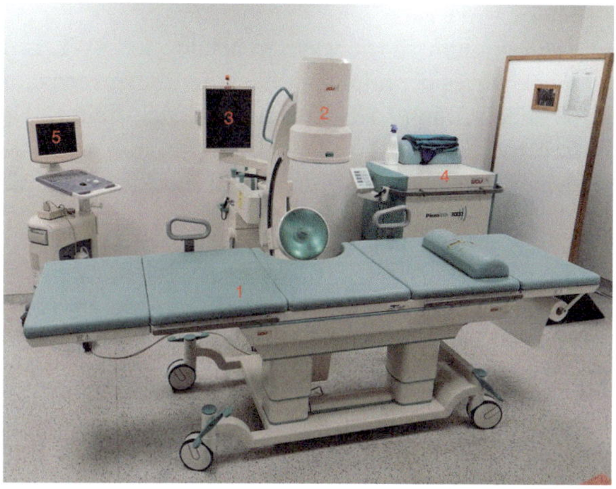

Fig. 28.1 SWL device with piezoelectric generator system. (1) Examination table, (2) X-Ray, (3) Operating unit, (4) Shock wave generator, (5) Ultrasonography

Principles for Device Use Affecting Outcomes in SWL Treatment

- **Coupling**
- It is important for the success of SWL to establish a bubble-free constant connection between the shock wave generator and the patient's body during the treatment. Even small air bubbles increase impedance and cause energy loss. Coupling can be achieved using oil or ultrasound gel. However, air bubbles may occur when using ultrasound gel, so be careful, otherwise the effectiveness of the treatment may decrease by 25% [21].
- **Focus size**
- Focus size is important for SWL success in focusable devices. Since the risk of ureteral stone migration is low, a shock wave will be applied with a smaller focus and thus treated with a higher energy level. However, kidney stones tend to have increased mobility due to many factors. Therefore, a greater focus is needed on kidney stones [18].
- **Ramping**
- To increase the safety and effectiveness of SWL, progressive energy increase(ramping) should be preferred instead of starting with high energy. Both in vivo and in vitro studies have shown that the ramping strategy increases the success of stone fragmentation and has a protective effect on the kidney. Lambert et al. achieved a stone-free rate (SFR) of 81% in the ramping group compared to 48% in the fixed energy group [13]. It is thought that starting with low energy causes vasoconstriction and that this has a protective effect on the kidney by increasing vessel stiffness and decreasing blood flow[8].

- **Shock wave rate**
- The optimum shock wave frequency for SWL is 1.0–1.5 Hz. The number of shock waves per minute in SWL varies between clinics. In meta-analyses, when 60 shocks/min (1 Hertz) and 120 shocks/min (2 Hertz) were compared, stone-free success was significantly higher in patients who received 60 shocks/min than in patients who received 120 shocks/min [11, 24].

Shock Wave Lithotripsy Indications in Kidney and Ureteral Stones

SWL, PNL and RIRS are current treatment modalities for kidney stones. While PNL efficiency is not much affected by stone size, SFR after SWL or ureterorenoscopy (URS) are inversely proportional to stone size. SWL is a simple, effective, non-invasive treatment modality with low complication rates and is the primary treatment option for kidney stones <2 cm. According to the EAU guideline, SWL is recommended as the first choice for stones with a size <2 cm located in the renal pelvis and the upper and middle calyx, while it is recommended to choose between endoscopic methods and SWL in lower calyx stones, considering unfavourable factors (lower calyx portion >1 cm, narrow calyx neck <5 mm and steep calyx angles) that may affect the treatment (Table 28.1) [25].

The success of SWL varies according to the lithotripter efficiency, the size, hardness and location of the stone, anatomical differences of the kidney, the patient's general physical characteristics and patient conformity [14].

Computed tomography (CT) is needed to evaluate the size, location and hardness of the stone and the anatomical features of the kidney when planning SWL treatment. Metabolic causes in the stone's aetiology determine its formation. Stone composition, which determines the hardness of a stone, is an important criterion in the treatment of SWL. Calcium oxalate monohydrate, brushite and cystine stones are seen as the main causes of ESWL failure. Imaging methods cannot accurately predict the composition of stones. However, the hardness of the stone is measured as

Table 28.1 Treatment recommendations for kidney stones (EAU 2022)

Stone localization	Stone size	Treatment modalities	
All but lower pole stone 10-20 mm	>20 mm	1. PNL	
		2. RIRS or SWL	
	10–20 mm	SWL or Endourology	
	<10 mm	1.SWL or RIRS	
		2. PNL	
Lower pole	> 20 mm and <10 mm	As above	
	10–20 mm Unfavourable factors for SWL	No	SWL or Endourology
		Yes	1. Endourology 2. SWL

Table 28.2 Treatment recommendations for ureteral stones (EAU 2022)

Stone localization	Stone size	Treatment modalities
Proximal ureteral stone	>10 mm	1. URS (ante- or retrograde)
		2. SWL
	<10 mm	1.SWL or RIRS
Distal ureteral stone	>10 mm	1. URS
		2. SWL
	<10 mm	1.SWL or RIRS

Hounsfield Units (HU) on CT, and studies have found a range of cut-off values (> 800–1000 HU) for SWL failure [16].

Patient compliance is an important factor in SWL success. The pain that may occur during the treatment will increase the patient's mobility, respiratory frequency and depth, leading to focusing problems and failure. Pain during SWL depends on many factors. Pain varies according to lithotripter type, shock wave frequency, applied voltage, age and gender of the patient. No routine analgesia protocol is used in the SWL procedure. Many agents are used, such as NSAIDs, opioids, topical agents, anaesthetic injections (local, epidural), intracutaneous sterile water injections, skin creams and non-traditional methods (i.e., music, acupuncture). Appropriate analgesic use before treatment increases the success of treatment by reducing the movement and respiratory irregularity caused by the patient's pain [2].

Currently, the most commonly used treatment modalities for the treatment of ureteral stones are SWL and URS (Table 28.2). When choosing the treatment method for ureteral stones, the ultimate goal is to make the patient completely stone-free with low morbidity. Stone (location and size) and patient-related factors, surgical experience and availability of certain technologies are important factors for targeted success. Shock wave lithotripsy is an effective treatment option for ureteral stones because it is non-invasive and practical. While the success of SWL is higher in proximal ureters, it tends to decrease for distal stones. With the development of endoscopic technology, a higher SFR and rapid decompression of obstruction in a single session are provided for ureteral stones compared to SWL. However, regarding complications, ureteroscopic techniques have been associated with higher complication rates than SWL (9–11% vs. 4%) [9].

Contraindications of Shock Wave Lithotripsy

There are several contraindications to the use of SWL, these are:

- Pregnancy due to potential effects on the fetus;
- Bleeding disorders that need to be compensated for at least 24 hours before and 48 hours after treatment;
- Uncontrolled UTIs;
- Severe skeletal malformations and severe obesity that prevent stone targeting;

- Arterial aneurysm around the stone;
- Anatomical obstruction distal to the stone [11].

In patients with bleeding disorders or taking antithrombolytic therapy, internal medicine and cardiology opinions should be sought for therapeutic measures before SWL is planned. In patients with uncorrected bleeding disorders, SWL is a high-risk procedure for perinephric hematomas. Shock wave lithotripsy is feasible and safe after the underlying coagulopathy has been corrected [11].

Complications of Shock Wave Lithotripsy

Shock wave lithotripsy has lower complication rates compared to PCNL and URS. After SWL, asymptomatic hematuria and cutaneous hemorrhage at the generator contact skin area are common but not clinically significant.

- Complications associated with stone fragmentation
  - Steinstrasse (4–7%)
  - Growth of residual stones (21–59%)
  - Renal colic (2–4%)
- Infection
  - Bacteriuria in non-infectious stones (7.7–23%)
  - Sepsis (1–2.7%)
- Acute extrarenal damage
  - Cardiovascular
    - Dysrhythmia (11–59%)
- Acute renal damage
  - Hematuria: This condition is seen in almost all patients, but it rarely reaches a serious proportion. Although hematuria is thought to be the result of damage to the urothelium as the stones break down, the most likely source is kidney damage. Shock waves have been shown to cause vascular rupture and damage to the surrounding renal tubule in dog and pig models.
  - Renal hematoma: It can be seen between 1% and 20%, depending on the type of lithotripter used. Some third-generation lithotripters have very high peak positive pressures; therefore, the reported rate of clinically significant renal hematomas is increasing. The appearance of renal hematomas can range from a mild contusion localised within the renal parenchyma to a large hematoma associated with severe bleeding, possibly requiring blood transfusion or, rarely, angiographic embolisation. Although some hematomas may persist for months or years, most have been reported to resolve within weeks and without long-term sequelae.

- Risk factors for acute renal injury
    - Age
    - Severe obesity
    - Coagulopathy
    - Thrombocytopenia
    - Diabetes mellitus, coronary artery disease and hypertension

- Chronic renal damage: Shock waves are known to cause vascular damage in human and animal models. In animal models, bleeding has been shown to initiate inflammation, leading to scarring. The relationship between SWL and hypertension, which is thought to be secondary to chronic renal damage, was investigated, but no clinically significant relationship was found.

In addition, morbid cardiac events, intestinal perforation and liver and spleen hematomas are rare complications secondary to SWL [11, 19].

Ureteral Stent Placement and Antibiotic Prophylaxis Before Shock Wave Lithotripsy

Shock wave lithotripsy successfully fragments stones as a safe and minimally invasive method. Most stone fragments successfully pass through the urinary tract after SWL. Particularly after SWL has been applied to large stones, steinstrasse can be seen and this may lead to kidney complications. However, there is still no consensus on whether ureteral stenting can be used to prevent Steinstrasse and other post-SWL complications. Studies have shown that ureteral stenting before SWL does not improve stone-free rates, and ureteral stenting is not routinely recommended. Standard antibiotic prophylaxis is not recommended prior to SWL. However, prophylaxis is recommended in patients with a stent before the procedure and in cases with bacterial load (such as permanent stent, nephrostomy tube and infection stones). Urine microscopy and urine cultures should be taken before SWL to minimise the risk of infection and sepsis [11, 20].

Specific Patient Groups and Shock Wave Lithotripsy

Shock wave lithotripsy can be applied to patients with pacemakers if appropriate precautions are taken. It would be appropriate to obtain a cardiology opinion before applying SWL to this patient group. Patients with implanted cardioverter defibrillators may need to temporarily adjust the firing mode during SWL, although it is emphasised that this is not necessary during the use of newer generation lithotripters [6].

Shock wave lithotripsy is a treatment option for transplanted kidney stones, in addition to flexible ureterorenoscopy (fURS) and PCNL. It is also an option for small calyx stones, with minimal risk of complications, but the stone is difficult to localise and the SFR is low [11].

Management and Follow-Up of Shock Wave Lithotripsy

For pain management following SWL, non-steroidal anti-inflammatory drugs (diclofenac, etc.) and opioids can be used if necessary. Randomized controlled trials(RCTs) and meta-analyses of the use of medical expulsive therapy (MET) support the idea that MET increases SFR by helping stone expulsion. In addition, MET can reduce the need for analgesia. Mechanical percussion and diuretic therapy can significantly improve stone-free rates and accelerate stone passage. Movement, plenty of fluid intake and if the stone is in the lower calyx, standing upside down at regular intervals can be recommended to the patients for easy removal of the broken stone particles [6, 11].

Since the removal of broken stones takes time, the most suitable time for the detection of residual stones is the fourth week. Kidney- ureter- bladder(KUB) radiography, ultrasonography and computed tomography can be used for follow-up imaging. CT has the highest sensitivity in the detection of residual stones. However, CT's showing clinically insignificant stones and radiation exposure should be kept in mind.

Shock Wave Lithotripsy Treatment in Children

Nephrolithiasis in children and adolescents is most common in non-Hispanic Caucasians, but its true incidence remains unclear due to the lack of extensive epidemiological studies. Since the first successful use of SWL in children in 1986, several studies have reported comparable success rates, complications, and safety to those observed in adult cohorts. SWL is the primary treatment option for most ureteral stones in children, with a success rate ranging from 68% to 84% when used as the first-line treatment for upper urinary tract stones. However, the success rate decreases in stones larger than 10 mm, impacted stones, calcium oxalate monohydrate or cystine stones, and children with unfavourable anatomy [11, 17, 19]. It is essential to note that the success rates may vary depending on specific patient and stone characteristics. As the size of the stone increases, the success of SWL decreases. Elsobky et al. [10]. reported a success rate of 91% for stones with a mean diameter of less than 10 mm, and 75% for larger stones with SWL treatment. It is more likely for SWL treatment under general anesthesia to be successful in children, but with advancements in modern lithotripters, successful treatment can be applied with intravenous sedation, analgesia, or no medication in select older, cooperative children. The location of a stone is a important factor in determining the success of SWL results. In retrospective studies, the SFR for lower pole stones ranged from 56% to 61%, with a retreatment rate of 40%. It's important to note that the success rates for SWL may vary depending on the location of the stone [11, 19].

Future Direction

In SWL treatment, imaging techniques are used to determine stone localisation and transmit the shock wave to the target. While fluoroscopy and ultrasonography are used as imaging methods, the most commonly used one is fluoroscopy. Improving the visual coupling of SWL can improve stone-free results by increasing the percentage of shock waves hitting the stone. However, fluoroscopy emits ionising radiation, and ultrasonography technologies are underway to reduce this radiation exposure. The new Visio-Track three-dimensional ultrasound stone locking system has the potential to increase stone fragmentation rates and reduce fluoroscopy time. This system is used together with the lithotripter to lock the lithotripter into the stone during the procedure. The Visio-Track locking system has been shown to achieve a higher SFR than standard ultrasound-guided SWL [1, 19].

Another new technology used in SWL is ultrasonic propulsion technology, which has emerged as a technology that can reposition kidney stones and expel small stones from the urinary tract. Other uses of this technology include moving the stone back into the kidney in the case of stone obstruction and colic pain. Ultrasonic propulsion technology became a clinical prototype device after 5 years of research and has been proven safe with minimal tissue destruction in the pig model. In the first human clinical trial in 2016, stones of 10 mm or less were successfully repositioned, with 93% success in 15 subjects. The potential use of this technology in the future will enable the movement of pre-SWL stones from an unfavourable location (lower pole of the kidney) to a favourable location (renal pelvis) [12, 19].

References

1. Abid N, Ravier E, Promeyrat X, Codas R, Fehri HF, Crouzet S, Martin X. Decreased radiation exposure and increased efficacy in extracorporeal lithotripsy using a new ultrasound stone locking system. J Endourol. 2015;29:1263–9.
2. Aboumarzouk OM, Hasan R, Tasleem A, Mariappan M, Hutton R, Fitzpatrick J, Beatty L, Jones GE, Amer T. Analgesia for patients undergoing shockwave lithotripsy for urinary stones–a systematic review and meta-analysis. Int Braz J Urol. 2017;43:394–406.
3. Bach C, Buchholz N. Shock wave lithotripsy for renal and ureteric stones. Eur Urol Suppl. 2011;10:423–32.
4. Chaussy C, Brendel W, Schmiedt E. Extracorporeally induced destruction of kidney stones by shock waves. Lancet. 1980;2:1265–8.

5. Chaussy C, Schmiedt E, Jocham B, Brendel W, Forssmann B, Walther V. First clinical experience with extracorporeally induced destruction of kidney stones by shock waves. J Urol. 1982;127:417–20.
6. Chaussy CG, Tiselius H-G. How can and should we optimize extracorporeal shockwave lithotripsy? Urolithiasis. 2018;46:3–17.
7. Cleveland RO, Mcateer JA. The physics of shock wave lithotripsy. In: Smith's textbook on endourology, vol. 1; 2007. pp. 529–558.
8. Connors BA, Evan AP, Blomgren PM, Handa RK, Willis LR, Gao S. Effect of initial shock wave voltage on shock wave lithotripsy-induced lesion size during step-wise voltage ramping. BJU Int. 2009;103:104–7.
9. Drake T, Grivas N, Dabestani S, Knoll T, Lam T, Maclennan S, Petrik A, Skolarikos A, Straub M, Tuerk C. What are the benefits and harms of ureteroscopy compared with shockwave lithotripsy in the treatment of upper ureteral stones? A systematic review. Eur Urol. 2017;72:772–86.
10. Elsobky E, Sheir K, Madbouly K, Mokhtar A. Extracorporeal shock wave lithotripsy in children: experience using two second-generation lithotripters. BJU Int. 2000;86:851–6.
11. Geraghty RM, Davis NF, Tzelves L, Lombardo R, Yuan C, Thomas K, Petrik A, Neisius A, Türk C, Gambaro G. Best practice in interventional management of urolithiasis: an update from the European Association of Urology guidelines panel for urolithiasis 2022. European Urology Focus; 2022.
12. Harper JD, Cunitz BW, Dunmire B, Lee FC, Sorensen MD, Hsi RS, Thiel J, Wessells H, Lingeman JE, Bailey MR. First in human clinical trial of ultrasonic propulsion of kidney stones. J Urol. 2016;195:956–64.
13. Lambert EH, Walsh R, Moreno MW, Gupta M. Effect of escalating versus fixed voltage treatment on stone comminution and renal injury during extracorporeal shock wave lithotripsy: a prospective randomized trial. J Urol. 2010;183:580–4.
14. Mi Y, Ren K, Pan H, Zhu L, Wu S, You X, Shao H, Dai F, Peng T, Qin F. Flexible ureterorenoscopy (F-URS) with holmium laser versus extracorporeal shock wave lithotripsy (ESWL) for treatment of renal stone< 2 cm: a meta-analysis. Urolithiasis. 2016;44:353–65.
15. Muslumanoglu AY, Binbay M, Yuruk E, Akman T, Tepeler A, Esen T, Tefekli AH. Updated epidemiologic study of urolithiasis in Turkey. I: Changing characteristics of urolithiasis. Urol Res. 2011;39:309–14.
16. Nakasato T, Morita J, Ogawa Y. Evaluation of Hounsfield Units as a predictive factor for the outcome of extracorporeal shock wave lithotripsy and stone composition. Urolithiasis. 2015;43:69–75.
17. Newman DM, Coury T, Lingeman JE, Mertz JH, Mosbaugh PG, Steele RE, Knapp PM. Extracorporeal shock wave lithotripsy experience in children. J Urol. 1986;136:238–40.
18. Paonessa JE, Lingeman JE. Extracorporeal shock wave lithotripsy: generators and treatment techniques. In: Urinary stones: medical and surgical management. Wiley; 2014. p. 216–26.
19. Partin AW, Peters CA, Kavoussi LR, Dmochowski RR, Wein AJ. Campbell-Walsh-Wein urology. 12th ed. Elsevier Health Sciences: Review E-Book; 2020.
20. Pengfei S, Min J, Jie Y, Xiong L, Yutao L, Wuran W, Yi D, Hao Z, Jia W. Use of ureteral stent in extracorporeal shock wave lithotripsy for upper urinary calculi: a systematic review and meta-analysis. J Urol. 2011;186:1328–35.
21. Pishchalnikov YA, Neucks JS, Vonderhaar RJ, Pishchalnikova IV, Williams JC, Mcateer JA. Air pockets trapped during routine coupling in dry head lithotripsy can significantly decrease the delivery of shock wave energy. J Urol. 2006;176:2706–10.
22. Rassweiler JJ, Knoll T, Köhrmann K-U, Mcateer JA, Lingeman JE, Cleveland RO, Bailey MR, Chaussy C. Shock wave technology and application: an update. Eur Urol. 2011;59:784–96.
23. Schmutz R, Birkhäuser F, Zehnder P, Schmutz R, Birkhäuser F, Zehnder P. Principles of SWL. Extracorporeal shock wave lithotripsy: In clinical practice; 2019. pp. 1–19.
24. Semins MJ, Trock BJ, Matlaga BR. The effect of shock wave rate on the outcome of shock wave lithotripsy: a meta-analysis. J Urol. 2008;179:194–7.

25. Tiselius H, Ackermann D, Alken P, Buck C, Conort P, Gallucci M. Guidelines on Urolithiasis1. Eur Urol. 2001;40:362–71.
26. Türk C, Petřík A, Sarica K, Seitz C, Skolarikos A, Straub M, Knoll T. EAU guidelines on interventional treatment for urolithiasis. Eur Urol. 2016;69:475–82.
27. Zhou Y, Cocks FH, Preminger GM, Zhong P. Innovations in shock wave lithotripsy technology: updates in experimental studies. J Urol. 2004;172:1892–8.

Chapter 29
Posterior Tibial Nerve Stimulations: Technical Methods and Outcomes

Mehmet Cetinkaya, Mesut Sengul, and Kadir Onem

Introduction

As of 2011, an estimated 29.8 million adults in the United States grappled with the challenges posed by overactive bladder (OAB) [1]. This condition, characterized by involuntary contractions of the detrusor muscle, manifests as frequent urination, urgency, and nocturia. Beyond the physical discomfort, OAB casts a shadow over quality of life, affecting sleep patterns, social interactions, and emotional well-being [2]. The American Urological Association (AUA) has created meticulous treatment guidelines similar to a stepwise algorithm. The initial step of OAB treatment involves behavioral modifications, emphasizing lifestyle adjustments such as fluid management, timed voiding, and pelvic floor exercises. Guidelines consider medical treatment such as anti-muscarinic agents and b3-adrenoceptor agonists as a second line treatment. These medications aim to decrease the hyperactivity of the detrusor muscle, allowing for greater bladder capacity and reduced urgency. Third-line therapies for OAB consist: chemical denervation, Sacral Neuromodulation (SNS), and the intriguing Peripheral Tibial Nerve Stimulation (PTNS). PTNS needle targets the tibial nerve just above of the medial malleolus. Through repeated electrical impulses, it stimulates the neural pathways, modulating bladder function.

M. Cetinkaya · K. Onem (✉)
Medicalpark Samsun Hospital, Department of Urology, Samsun, Turkey

M. Sengul
Gazi State Hospital, Department of Urology, Samsun, Turkey

S. Tonyali et al. (eds.), *Current Endourology*,
https://doi.org/10.1007/978-3-032-00010-1_29

The History of Percutaneous Tibial Nerve Stimulation (PTNS)

Acupuncture, a practice with roots in ancient Chinese medicine, has spanned thousands of years and left an indelible mark on the world of healing. Although its exact origins remain hidden in antiquity, the first recorded references to acupuncture appear in the Mawangdui Silk Texts [3]. These texts reference the art of sarcasm as a therapeutic method, like whispered secrets from the past.

But despite its consistent use in Asia, acupuncture remained a mystery to Western medicine for centuries [4]. Europeans' view of this ancient practice was not observed until 1683, when Dr. Willem ten Rhyne turned when he wrote his groundbreaking thesis. His observations stemmed from witnessing the needle dance of acupuncture in Japan. A century later, in the inaugural issue of The Lancet (November 1823), interest was intensified by an article titled "Acupuncturization" [5]. Dr. Philipp von Siebold recorded his observations with acupuncture during his travels in Japan between 1832 and 1850, solved its mysteries and brought them to the medical field [6] Remarkably, it was the essence of acupuncture that sparked Dr. Siebold's creativity: the hypodermic needle; a transformative breakthrough that is now in the annals of Western medicine.

But on the other side of the Atlantic, acupuncture remained a distant curiosity until the 1970s. In his touching article in The New York Times (July 26, 1971), James Reston describes how acupuncture applied in China after emergency appendectomy relieved his pain [7]. During their later journeys to the East, American physicians witnessed surgical achievements performed under the delicate influence of acupuncture anesthesia [4]. This developing fascination reached its peak in 1997, when a statement was issued by the National Institutes of Health (NIH) on the medical utility of acupuncture, particularly in the field of pain management [8].

Working Mechanism

It is not yet clear how activation of somatic afferents affects bladder function; The effect on the bladder generally depends on the frequency of the stimulus. In experimental studies in healthy cats, tibial nerve stimulation at 5–6 Hz (but not 15 or 30 Hz) resulted in a decrease in bladder activity by significantly increasing bladder capacity and reducing contraction amplitude [9–11]. Experimental studies using rat models also report the frequency specificity of tibial nerve stimulation, although this frequency has been reported differently in studies of different centers [12, 13]. Stimulation of both tibial and pudendal nerves at 5 Hz per second reduced the neuronal firing frequency caused by bladder dilation in spinal cord neurons, but the persistence of only tibial nerve-evoked effects after the end of stimulation suggests that the underlying mechanisms are not the same [13, 14]. In fact, tibial nerve stimulation is known to engage supraspinal brainstem pathways, in contrast to pudendal nerve-evoked effects, which are spinally mediated [15]. Interestingly, the effectiveness of tibial nerve stimulation may actually depend on the activation of fibers in the Saphenous nerve, possibly simultaneously, when the electrodes required for tibial nerve stimulation are placed [16, 17]. Additionally, Saphenous nerve stimulation produced frequency-dependent inhibition of bladder function in anesthetized cats [12, 18]. A recent clinical study shows that the procedure offers a promising new intervention for the treatment of OAB [19].

Although it is unclear how PTNS works, nowadays this treatment method has been widely preferred in the management of OAB associated symptoms, also non-obstructive urinary retention, neurogenic lower urinary tract dysfunction, pediatric patients with voiding disorders and bladder pain syndrome.

PTNS Application Technique

For PTNS, the patient is first placed in the supine position. In minors, pre-procedural application of a topical anesthetic (e.g., lidocaine) may reduce pain and anxiety associated with needle placement. A 34 G needle is inserted between the posterior edge of the tibia and the soleus muscle, ~3 fingers (4–5 cm) caudal to the medial malleolus. The goal here is to position the tip of the needle close to the PTN without actually touching the nerve. Considering that ankles are different for each person, the optimal depth and angle may differ from individual to individual. Additionally, a second electrode is attached near the arch of the foot on the same side (Urgent PC®; Cogentix Medical Inc., Minnetonka, MN, USA).

Stimulation of the fibers of posterior tibial nerve causes motor and sensory response . Flexion or fanning of the thumb is an efferent effect. The sensory afferent effect is the tickling sensation of the sole of the foot. During the initial stimulation, the amplitude is gradually elevated until the big toe is curled or the toes are ventrally flexed. Meanwhile, if the patient is uncomfortable with discomfort or “buzzing” around the area where the needle is inserted, the needle may not be deep enough. Conversely, if the stimulation is very uncomfortable, the needle may be placed close to the posterior tibial nerve. In this case, reinsertion of the needle into the ipsilateral or contralateral ankle may be recommended. Once the optimal position is achieved, stimulation is increased to level well tolerated and it can be changed during entire treatment period [20]. PTNS sessions can last up to 30 minutes and are reported in the majority of articles as once a week for 10–12 weeks. In an article by Finazzi Agrò et al., the treatment result achieved with a one weekly session was achieved in PTNS sessions performed more frequently, such as 3 times a week [21]. The advantage of more frequent sessions is that PTNS effects are achieved earlier, in 4 weeks instead of 12. The effectiveness of PTNS seems to correlate to the number of sessions performed and not on the entire duration of treatment [21]. Another study evaluated a treatment regimen consisting of weekly posterior tibial nerve stimulation sessions for six weeks in female patients with OAB. The writers reported that this short strategy achieved positive results in 69.7% of 43 patients [22].

The Effectiveness of PTNS

Those who defined PTNS evaluated techniques related acupuncture. One of publications reporting PTNS treatment for overactive bladder in humans, Edward J. McGuire et al. reported: "This traditional Chinese practice was the source of our idea to use transcutaneous stimulation at these points" [23]. In fact, the stimulation point which they chose is above the SP-6 point which is one of the acupuncture point is located 3 cun (about 4 finger widths) above the medial malleolus. The method they reported developed the points mentioned in ancient articles about acupuncture, while also using electrical stimulation. Surface electrodes on the tibial nerve have been shown to safely regulate bladder muscle reflex activity in T4-transfected primates [24]. In 1983, this research was reported in human subjects. One of the pivotal studies related to PTNS, posterior tibial nerve stimulation was applied with 5–8 volts, 2–10 cycles/second, width 5–20 msec to 22 patients with an "adhesive electrode". Of these, 17 (77%) reported full symptomatic benefit and 2 (9%) reported partial symptomatic benefit [23].

Additionally, PTNS studies was done on primates after a while. Most importantly, Marshall L. Stoller et al. performed these studies in monkeys in 1987 than at clinic in 1999 [25, 26]. The method, titled "Stoller Afferent Nerve Stimulation-(SANS)," consist puncture of a 34-G electrode "5 cm above the medial malleolus to the cephalad and posterior to the border of tibia". Later, Fred Govier et al. reported the first multicenter study on PTNS [20]. Fred Govier et al. used similar protocol as Stoller's; Differently, they extended the treatment period from 10 weeks to 12 weeks. 71% of the 53 pt. in the study reported a minimum 25% improvement in daytime incontinence. Enrico Finazzi-Agro and Kenneth M. Peterset al. both reported placebo-controlled studies in which similar results were obtained with 12 weeks of treatment [27]. As a result of these studies, PTNS was approved by the FDA for the treatment of OAB with its symptoms such as urgency, urinary frequency and urge urinary incontinence. After this approval, number of clinical studies on PTNS increased. In a meta-analysis conducted in recent years, the data of 28 studies were reviewed and as a result, it was emphasized that the cumulative success rate after PTNS treatment of 2461 patients was 0.68 (95% CI 0.59, 0.78) [28].

Another purpose of acupuncture is its analgesic effect. There was increasing interest in neuromodulation and acupuncture in the beginning of 1980s, using the PTNS in the management of chronic pelvic pain and painful bladder syndrome (CPS/PBS) came to the fore. Its effectiveness and safety in this context have been investigated in many studies and continue with more comprehensive studies. There is scientific evidence for the analgesic properties of PTNS and this evidence explains its analgesic effect. The cornerstone theory was the "gate control theory" of pain sensation [29]. In summary, it claims that nociceptive afferent impulses could be blocked by stronger, non nociceptive stimuli. As a result, electrical stimulation of peripheral nerve fibers can block painful sensation. Fumihiko et al. reported this interesting theory which stimulation tibial nerve to reduce pain in cats [30]. A literature review related to PTNS was made by Gabriele et al. They identified eight studies of IC/PBS therapy for the review. These eight studies reported success rates between 40% and 100% [31]. Maged M. Ragab et al. report that PTNS is not effective in the treatment of IC/BPS [32] This study reports that 75% of 20 patients treated with PTNS for 12 weeks experienced have still pain at week 6, and same score in pain at end of treatment. In light of the contradictory results, randomized controlled trials with a larger number of IC/BPS patients and more homogeneous groups are needed due to the limited number of IC/PBS patients and heterogeneity in the studies. According to these data, it is possible to say that PTNS may contribute to IC/PBS treatment, considering the minimal side effects of the treatment.

The treatment strategies for percutaneous tibial nerve stimulation has changed minimally since Dr. Stoller's description. The study of Peters and Finazzi-Agro still involves the prefer a 34G needle inserted 5 cm above to the medial malleolus (FA: 9 volts (S: 5–8 volts), FA: 5 cyc./sec. (S:2–10 cyc./sec.) and width FA: 20 msec (S:5–20 msec) [27, 33]. This strategy is very similar to acupuncture points in their approach. However, in recent years, many new products have found their place in the market and are used as current PTNS. BlueWind RENOVA iStim is a wireless, MRI-compatible implantable electro stimulator. In their clinical study, 71% of 34 patients were reported to achieve "more than a minimum significant difference of 10 points in health-related quality scores" [34]. One of the promising PTNS devices is eCoin. Ecoin is a PTNS device that can be placed under the skin. eCoin reported that 68% of 137 patients at 15 different centers showed at least a 50% improvement in UUI attacks 48 weeks after activation. The Bioness StimRouter is another new generation an implantable stimulator which approved for the treatment of IC/BPS and is used for neuromodulation for the management of overactive bladder.

In 1997, Sacral neuromodulation (SNM) was approved by The FDA for OAB treatment, for non-obstructive chronic urinary retention and also PTNS in 1999, and for non-neurogenic LUT dysfunction in 2005 [35, 36].

A review evaluating the effectiveness of posterior tibial nerve stimulation in patients with overactive bladder examined four randomized controlled trials involving 388 pt. (Table 29.1). One of these articles compared the effectiveness of posterior tibial nerve stimulation with tolterodine. The study organizers reported that, 79.5% of patients receiving PTNS therapy experienced improvement compared to 54.8% in the tolterodine arm at 3 months ($p = 0.01$) [37]. Another center compared the effectiveness of PTNS with placebo in 220 patients. They report treatment satisfaction for OAB symptoms at 3 months as 54.5% in the posterior tibial nerve stimulation and 20.9% in the placebo arm ($p < 0.01$) [33] Finazzi-Agrò et al. In a RCT designed by, 32 patients with urinary overactive bladder with urodynamically demonstrated detrusor overactivity reported superiority of PTNS to placebo over 4 months of treatment ($p < 0.001$) [27]. The conclusion of this clinical trial suggest that posterior tibial nerve stimulation may be an alternative treatment for patients with OAB with urinary incontinence. 71% of patients with incontinence have benefiting (>50% improvement in frequency of urge urinary incontinence) and the in placebo group treatment effect appearing negligible. Another randomized controlled study conducted by Güngör Uğurlucan et al., 52 patients were enrolled in this clinical trial. These patients had moderate lower urinary tract symptoms. In this

Table 29.1 Main characteristics of included studies assessing efficacy and safety in OAB patients treated with PTNS

Study	Design	Participants	Intervention (n)	Comparison	Follow-up	Assessment of improvement/ cure/success	Improvement rate/cure	p value	Pain rate/ complications
Peters et al. (2009) [7]	Prospective rando	84	PTNS = 41	Tolterodine = 43	3 mo	GRA VD	79.5% vs 54.8%	0.01	No major complications
Peters et al. (2010) [8]	Double blind, prospective rando, multi	220	PTNS = 110	Sham = 110	3 mo	GRA (primary endpoint: moderate or marked improvement in OAB symptoms)	54.5% vs 20.9%	<0.001	Six PTNS: ankle bruising, discomfort at the needle site, bleeding, tingling in the leg; no AE in the sham group
Finazzi-Agrò et al. (2010) [9]	Double blind, prospective rando, multi	32	PTNS (n = 17)	Placebo (N = 15)	After 12 treatments	VD (improvement of >50% in incontinence episodes)	71% vs 0%	<0.001	No major complications
Gungor Ugurlucan et al. (2013) [10]	RCT	52	PTNS = 17	ES = 35	12 wk	VD	Mean micturition/ d (7.4 + 2.6 vs 5.8 + 1.9)	0.03	–

study, the authors compared vaginal electrical stimulation versus PTNS [38]. If we look at the results of the trial, it was found that there was insignificant difference in both treatments compared to the initial level of stimulation and it was reported that no serious side effects of PTNS were detected. Side effects which were reported in the literature are generally mild, and the majority of side effects are associated with needle sticking, discomfort (1.8%), minor bleeding and bruising (0.9%), [20, 27, 33].

Available data support that transcutaneous tibial nerve stimulation (TTNS) is as effective as posterior tibial nerve stimulation in the treatment of OAB, and no adverse events have been reported In addition, prospective clinical trials with large numbers of patients are required to confirm this information [39].

PTNS improves lower urinary tract symptoms, as evidenced in two RCTs comparing PTNS with sham therapy in patients with overactive bladder. However, data from combination studies with PTNS and an anti-cholinergic prove that combination therapy results in greater improvement in symptoms. Non-comparative clinical studies reported that 70% of patients responded to treatment with 6 weeks of PTNS treatment. Long-term continuation of treatment is also a good alternative, especially in the group of patients who respond well to the first week of treatment to maintain symptom control [40]. There are clinical studies reporting that PTNS treatment in patients with multiple sclerosis and Parkinson's disease provides improvement in lower urinary tract symptoms both in a 12-week period and in patients receiving 3-month maintenance treatment. Various predictive factors of treatment success have been noted and patient utilization and stability have been shown to increase by incorporating PTNS into the treatment strategy as next-line therapy [41].

TTNS treatment achieved similar results to PTNS; There was no significant difference in cure rates compared to oxybutynin; However, the cure rate when used in combination with oxybutynin was much higher than when either was used alone. In general, the articles report that PTNS provides improvement in the lower urinary tract symptoms of overactive bladder patients in the short and long term. Adverse effects of PTNS appears to be more tolerable than those seen with anticholinergics, such as dry mouth and constipation. There are also concerns about cognitive impairment in elderly patients taking chronic anticholinergic medications. In parallel with advances in technology, personalized PTNS and implantable stimulators may increasingly replace OAB in the treatment of OAB. The potential exists to reduce transportation costs for patients coming to clinic visits for PTNS treatment and to provide a less invasive, one-step implant procedure compared to sacral neuromodulation therapy. However, it shows that more research is needed regarding long-term results and neuromodulation systems.

Overactive bladder is also common in children aged 6 to 16 years. PTNS may be a treatment alternative if standard treatment modalities (urotherapy, PMFT, and antimuscarinics) fail to cure the patient. Long-term outcomes of patients in the pediatric group treated with PTNS appear to be promising. In 44 children with lower urinary tract symptoms, the improvement rate after 1 year with PTNS was 41% for patients with overactive bladder and 71% for dysfunctional voiding [42]. Maintenance therapy was required in 29% of patients with dysfunctional voiding and in 50% of patients with overactive bladder [43]. Transcutaneous/percutaneous stimulation is promising in children with lower urinary tract symptoms unresponsive to drug therapy. However, studies with a larger number of patients are needed to determine more sensitive subjective and objective results. Data in recent publications report contradictory results.

Implantable Neurostimulator Devices

RENOVA iStim™ is a new implantable peripheral neuromodulation device developed by BlueWind Medical, Herzliya, Israel. Breda et al. conducted a study on 14 patients with OAB. In this study, an implantable device was placed in order to stimulate the posterior tibial nerve. The device was actively used for 30 minutes, six times a week [44]. A decrease in the frequency of daily urination was observed at third month. A significant increase in mean voided volume was achieved. Side effects included infectious pain and infection around the implantation site requiring oral antibiotics and analgesia. Heesakkers et al. evaluated the patients for six months in their prospective study with 36 patients with overactive bladder [45]. The device was used 6 sessions a week for 30 minutes for 3 months, or 3 times a week for 6 months. At the end of 6 months, 71% of the patients reported significant improvement in urination frequency, urgency, and urgency incontinence. Thirteen out of the 14 patients experienced a > 50% improvement in the number of severe urinary urgency episodes. When evaluated in terms of these two different regimens (3 months and 6 months), the 71% of patients who were clinically improved (>50% improvement) after 3 months. In 86.4 of them, this recovery lasted until the sixth month. Additionally, 41.7% of those who did not improve clinically at 3 months did so at 6 months. Clinical data is appearing to be promising. Wireless powered implantable tibial nerve technology remains an option for treating lower urinary tract symptoms without requiring any battery replacement of the implantable component. This device, which the patient can control himself, can also be personalized according to the patient's needs and different treatment strategies can be developed with longer or more frequent stimulation sessions.

Another newly launched device is eCoin®, developed by Valencia Technologies and approved by the FDA in 2022. eCoin® is a fully implanted, lead-free, nickel and small-sized device with a built-in battery to stimulate the tibial nerve. The implant can be easily performed in the office with local anesthesia. This device does not require an external power supply unit, as BlueWind implant. The stimulator, controlled by an external remote control, can provide stimulation amplitude between 0.5 and 15 mA, using the most appropriate and comfortable level for the patient. The implant can be programmed to automatically deliver 30-minute stimulation sessions every 2 days for 12 weeks and every 15 days thereafter. In a clinical study, 137 patients with urge urinary incontinence who did not benefit from drug treatment were included. Researchers reported that pretreatment UUI episodes were 4.3 ± 3.1 per day. It was reported that 68% of the patients (95% CI: 60–76%) had at least a

50% improvement in daily urge urinary incontinence after 48 weeks. 16% of patients reported device-related adverse effects after 52 weeks [46].

Cost Effectiveness of PTNS

Treatment may progress with difficulty in patients with overactive bladder that is unresponsive to medical treatment. In this case, the effectiveness and costs of second-line treatment options must be taken into account. Staskin and colleagues conducted cost analyzes of different treatment options for overactive bladder in the USA. PTNS has been reported as the least costly of these options ($4999 for 3 years of treatment), followed by intravesical Botulinumtoxin injection ($7651) and sacral neuromodulation ($26,269) for the same time period [47]. Martinson et al. also report that PTNS has significantly lower costs compared to Sacral Neuromodulation in the United States. Additionally, when SNS was used instead of PTNS, an additional 1% of patients would continue treatment for 2 years, but the average additional cost per patient would be >$500,000 [48, 49]. Considering the cost differences between countries, PTNS does not seem to be cost-effective as a first treatment option compared to antimuscarinics, but it is a good alternative in medical treatment non-responders patients. However, in the long term, due to the necessity of repeated clinic visits for PTNS, sacral neuromodulation may be more cost-effective.

Conclusion

PTNS delivers electrical stimulations to the sacral voiding center via the S2-S4 nerve roots. Stimulation is done percutaneously with a thin (34-G) needle (Percutaneous PTNS) placed just above the medial aspect of the ankle. There is also transcutaneous stimulation, which stimulates through surface electrodes that do not puncture the skin. Daily and weekly sessions are not considered standard strategy yet, and an optimal treatment plan has not been determined. Generally, 12 weekly treatment sessions are recommended. Tibial nerve stimulation is more accessible and less likely to cause side effects and complications than sacral neuromodulation [50, 51]. The most important undesirable effect of PTNS is pain at the needle entry point.

References

1. Coyne KS, Sexton CC, Vats V, Thompson C, Kopp ZS, Milsom I. National community prevalence of overactive bladder in the United States stratified by sex and age. Urology. 2011;77(5):1081–7.

2. Brown JS, McGhan WF, Chokroverty S. Comorbidities associated with overactive bladder. Am J Manag Care. 2000;6(11 Suppl):S574–9.
3. Lo V. Crossing the Neiguan 内關 "inner pass": a Nei/Wai 内外 "inner/outer" distinction in early Chinese medicine. East Asian Sci Technol Med. 2000(17):15–65.
4. Lu DP, Lu GP. An historical review and perspective on the impact of acupuncture on U.S. Medicine and Society. Med Acupunct. 2013;25(5):311–6.
5. Visca A, Lay R, Sessions AE, Rabinowitz R, Ajay D. History of peripheral tibial nerve stimulation in urology. Urology. 2023;174:3–6.
6. Omura Y. Some historical aspects of acupuncture and important problems to be considered in acupuncture and electro-therapeutic research. Acupunct Electrother Res. 1975;1(1–2):3–44.
7. Reston J. Now, let me tell you about my appendectomy in Peking. New York Times. 1971;1(6).
8. Health NIo, Health UDo, Services H. Acupuncture: NIH consensus statement. Consensus Development Conference Statement. 1997. pp. 1–34.
9. Ferroni MC, Slater RC, Shen B, Xiao Z, Wang J, Lee A, et al. Role of the brain stem in tibial inhibition of the micturition reflex in cats. Am J Physiol Renal Physiol. 2015;309(3):F242–50.
10. Theisen K, Browning J, Li X, Li S, Shen B, Wang J, et al. Frequency dependent tibial neuromodulation of bladder underactivity and overactivity in cats. Neuromodulation. 2018;21(7):700–6.
11. Wan X, Liang Y, Li X, Liao L. Inhibitory effects of a minimally invasive implanted tibial nerve stimulation device on non-nociceptive bladder reflexes in cats. Int Urol Nephrol. 2021;53(3):431–8.
12. Moazzam Z, Yoo PB. Frequency-dependent inhibition of bladder function by saphenous nerve stimulation in anesthetized rats. Neurourol Urodyn. 2018;37(2):592–9.
13. Park E, Lee JW, Kim T, Kang M, Cho BH, Lee J, et al. The long-lasting post-stimulation inhibitory effects of bladder activity induced by posterior tibial nerve stimulation in unanesthetized rats. Sci Rep. 2020;10(1):19897.
14. Yecies T, Li S, Zhang Y, Cai H, Shen B, Wang J, et al. Spinal interneuronal mechanisms underlying pudendal and tibial neuromodulation of bladder function in cats. Exp Neurol. 2018;308:100–10.
15. Xiao Z, Rogers MJ, Shen B, Wang J, Schwen Z, Roppolo JR, et al. Somatic modulation of spinal reflex bladder activity mediated by nociceptive bladder afferent nerve fibers in cats. Am J Physiol Renal Physiol. 2014;307(6):F673–9.
16. Mercer D, Morrell NT, Fitzpatrick J, Silva S, Child Z, Miller R, et al. The course of the distal saphenous nerve: a cadaveric investigation and clinical implications. Iowa Orthop J. 2011;31:231–5.
17. Elder CW, Yoo PB. Co-activation of saphenous nerve fibers: a potential therapeutic mechanism of percutaneous tibial nerve stimulation? Annu Int Conf IEEE Eng Med Biol Soc. 2016;2016:3129–32.
18. Li X, Wan X, Wang Z, Liang Y, Jia Z, Zhang X, et al. Frequency-dependent effects on bladder reflex by saphenous nerve stimulation and a possible action mechanism of tibial nerve stimulation in cats. Int Neurourol J. 2021;25(2):128–36.
19. MacDiarmid SA, John MS, Yoo PB. A pilot feasibility study of treating overactive bladder patients with percutaneous saphenous nerve stimulation. Neurourol Urodyn. 2018;37(5):1815–20.
20. Govier FE, Litwiller S, Nitti V, Kreder KJ, Rosenblatt P. Percutaneous afferent neuromodulation for the refractory overactive bladder: results of a multicenter study. J Urol. 2001;165(4):1193–8.
21. Campagna A, Sciobica F, Petta F, Germani S, Zuccalà A, Miano R. Posterior tibial nerve stimulation: is the once-a-week protocol the best option? Minerva urologica e nefrologica. 2005;57(2):119–23.
22. Yoong W, Ridout AE, Damodaram M, Dadswell R. Neuromodulative treatment with percutaneous tibial nerve stimulation for intractable detrusor instability: outcomes following a shortened 6-week protocol. BJU Int. 2010;106(11):1673–6.

23. McGuire EJ, Zhang SC, Horwinski ER, Lytton B. Treatment of motor and sensory detrusor instability by electrical stimulation. J Urol. 1983;129(1):78–9.
24. McGuire EJ, Morrissey SG. The development of neurogenic vesical dysfunction after experimental spinal cord injury or sacral rhizotomy in non-human primates. J Urol. 1982;128(6):1390–3.
25. Stoller M, Copeland S, Millard R, Murnaghan G. The efficacy of acupuncture in reversing the unstable bladder in pig-tailed monkeys. J Urol. 1987;137(6):104A.
26. Stoller M. Afferent nerve stimulation for pelvic floor dysfunction. Int Urogynecol J. 1999;10:P99.
27. Finazzi-Agrò E, Petta F, Sciobica F, Pasqualetti P, Musco S, Bove P. Percutaneous tibial nerve stimulation effects on detrusor overactivity incontinence are not due to a placebo effect: a randomized, double-blind, placebo controlled trial. J Urol. 2010;184(5):2001–6.
28. Wang M, Jian Z, Ma Y, Jin X, Li H, Wang K. Percutaneous tibial nerve stimulation for overactive bladder syndrome: a systematic review and meta-analysis. Int Urogynecol J. 2020;31(12):2457–71.
29. Melzack R, Wall PD. Pain mechanisms: a new theory. Science. 1965;150(3699):971–9.
30. Hanai F. Effect of electrical stimulation of peripheral nerves on neuropathic pain. Spine (Phila Pa 1976). 2000;25(15):1886–92.
31. Gaziev G, Topazio L, Iacovelli V, Asimakopoulos A, Di Santo A, De Nunzio C, et al. Percutaneous Tibial Nerve Stimulation (PTNS) efficacy in the treatment of lower urinary tract dysfunctions: a systematic review. BMC Urol. 2013;13:61.
32. Ragab MM, Tawfik AM, Abo El-enen M, Elnady M, El-Gamal OM, El-Kordy M, et al. Evaluation of percutaneous tibial nerve stimulation for treatment of refractory painful bladder syndrome. Urology. 2015;86(4):707–11.
33. Peters KM, Carrico DJ, Perez-Marrero RA, Khan AU, Wooldridge LS, Davis GL, et al. Randomized trial of percutaneous tibial nerve stimulation versus Sham efficacy in the treatment of overactive bladder syndrome: results from the SUmiT trial. J Urol. 2010;183(4):1438–43.
34. Dorsthorst MJT, Digesu GA, Tailor V, Gore M, van Kerrebroeck PE, van Breda HMK, et al. 3-year followup of a new implantable Tibial nerve stimulator for the treatment of overactive bladder syndrome. J Urol. 2020;204(3):545–50.
35. Siegel S, Noblett K, Mangel J, Griebling TL, Sutherland SE, Bird ET, et al. Results of a prospective, randomized, multicenter study evaluating sacral neuromodulation with InterStim therapy compared to standard medical therapy at 6-months in subjects with mild symptoms of overactive bladder. Neurourol Urodyn. 2015;34(3):224–30.
36. Levin PJ, Wu JM, Kawasaki A, Weidner AC, Amundsen CL. The efficacy of posterior tibial nerve stimulation for the treatment of overactive bladder in women: a systematic review. Int Urogynecol J. 2012;23(11):1591–7.
37. Peters KM, Macdiarmid SA, Wooldridge LS, Leong FC, Shobeiri SA, Rovner ES, et al. Randomized trial of percutaneous tibial nerve stimulation versus extended-release tolterodine: results from the overactive bladder innovative therapy trial. J Urol. 2009;182(3):1055–61.
38. Gungor Ugurlucan F, Onal M, Aslan E, Ayyildiz Erkan H, Kizilkaya Beji N, Yalcin O. Comparison of the effects of electrical stimulation and posterior tibial nerve stimulation in the treatment of overactive bladder syndrome. Gynecol Obstet Investig. 2013;75(1):46–52.
39. Yang D-Y, Zhao L-N, Qiu M-X. Treatment for overactive bladder: a meta-analysis of transcutaneous tibial nerve stimulation versus percutaneous tibial nerve stimulation. Medicine. 2021;100(20):e25941.
40. Bhide AA, Tailor V, Fernando R, Khullar V, Digesu GA. Posterior tibial nerve stimulation for overactive bladder-techniques and efficacy. Int Urogynecol J. 2020;31(5):865–70.
41. Rohloff M, Peifer G, Thompson JH. Patient navigation for overactive bladder improves access to care. Int Urogynecol J. 2020;31:1007–12.
42. Austin PF, Bauer SB, Bower W, Chase J, Franco I, Hoebeke P, et al. The standardization of terminology of lower urinary tract function in children and adolescents: Update report from

the standardization committee of the International Children's Continence Society. Neurourol Urodyn. 2016;35(4):471–81.
43. Capitanucci ML, Camanni D, Demelas F, Mosiello G, Zaccara A, De Gennaro M. Long-term efficacy of percutaneous tibial nerve stimulation for different types of lower urinary tract dysfunction in children. J Urol. 2009;182(4):2056–61.
44. van Breda HM, Martens FM, Tromp J, Heesakkers JP. A new implanted posterior tibial nerve stimulator for the treatment of overactive bladder syndrome: 3-month results of a novel therapy at a single center. J Urol. 2017;198(1):205–10.
45. Heesakkers JP, Digesu GA, van Breda J, Van Kerrebroeck P, Elneil S. A novel leadless, miniature implantable tibial nerve neuromodulation system for the management of overactive bladder complaints. Neurourol Urodyn. 2018;37(3):1060–7.
46. Rogers A, Bragg S, Ferrante K, Thenuwara C, Peterson DKL. Pivotal study of leadless tibial nerve stimulation with eCoin(R) for urgency urinary incontinence: an open-label, single arm trial. J Urol. 2021;206(2):399–408.
47. Staskin DR, Peters KM, MacDiarmid S, Shore N, de Groat WC. Percutaneous tibial nerve stimulation: a clinically and cost effective addition to the overactive bladder algorithm of care. Curr Urol Rep. 2012;13:327–34.
48. Barnett G, Ockrim J. Re: Cost of neuromodulation therapies for overactive bladder: percutaneous tibial nerve stimulation versus sacral nerve stimulation: M. Martinson, S. MacDiarmid and E. Black J Urol 2013; 189: 210-216. J Urol. 2013;190(4):1444–5.
49. Martinson M, MacDiarmid S, Black E. Cost of neuromodulation therapies for overactive bladder: percutaneous tibial nerve stimulation versus sacral nerve stimulation. J Urol. 2013;189(1):210–6.
50. Tutolo M, Ammirati E, Van der Aa F. What is new in neuromodulation for overactive bladder? Eur Urol Focus. 2018;4(1):49–53.
51. Ammirati E, Giammò A, Manassero A, Carone R. Neuromodulation in urology, state of the art. Urol J. 2019;86(4):177–82.

MIX
Papier aus verantwortungsvollen Quellen
Paper from responsible sources
FSC® C105338
FSC
www.fsc.org

If you have any concerns about our products,
you can contact us on
ProductSafety@springernature.com

In case Publisher is established outside the EU,
the EU authorized representative is:
Springer Nature Customer Service Center GmbH
Europaplatz 3, 69115 Heidelberg, Germany

Printed by Libri Plureos GmbH
in Hamburg, Germany